CW00456035

The I
Yoga Darśana

SUNY SERIES IN RELIGIOUS STUDIES
HAROLD COWARD, Editor

The Integrity of the Yoga Darśana

A Reconsideration of Classical Yoga

Ian Whicher

STATE UNIVERSITY OF NEW YORK PRESS

Cover photograph by Rose Montgomery-Whicher. View of the Beas River, Kullu Valley (Kullu, Himachal Pradesh, India).

Published by
State University of New York Press

1998 State University of New York

All right reserved

Printed in the United States of America

No part of this book may be used or reproduced in any manner whatsoever without written permission. No part of this book may be stored in a retrieval system or transmitted in any form or by any means including electronic, electrostatic, magnetic tape, mechanical, photocopying, recording, or otherwise without the prior permission in writing of the publisher.

For information, address the State University of New York Press, State University Plaza, Albany NY 12246

Marketing by Anne M. Valentine
Production by Bernadine Dawes

Library of Congress Cataloging-in-Publication Data

Whicher, Ian
The integrity of the yoga darśana : a reconsideration of classical yoga / Ian Whicher.
p. cm. — (SUNY series in religious studies)
ISBN 0-7914-3815-5 (alk. paper). — ISBN 0-7914-3816-3 (pbk. : alk. paper)
1. Patañjali. Yogasūtra. 2. Yoga. I. Title. II. Series.
B132.Y6W47 1998
181′.452—dc21 98-26388
CIP

2 3 4 5 6 7 8 9 10

In memory of my mother, Marjorie Whicher

CONTENTS

ACKNOWLEDGMENTS

This book is a much revised version of my Ph.D. thesis, "A Study of Patañjali's Definition of Yoga: Uniting Theory and Practice in the *Yoga-Sūtras*" (University of Cambridge, England, 1992). The project was brought to completion during my tenure as deputy director of the Dharam Hinduja Institute of Indic Research in the Faculty of Divinity at the University of Cambridge. As such, it can be regarded as a project of the Institute.

Many people, both directly and indirectly, have contributed to the production of this book. I am very grateful and indebted to Julius Lipner of the University of Cambridge for his many helpful comments and criticisms while he was my doctoral supervisor, and not least for his abiding friendship. More recently, in his capacity as director of the Dharam Hinduja Institute of Indic Research, Julius Lipner has offered me continued support and encouragement to publish this work. I express my gratitude to Christopher Key Chapple of Loyola Marymount University for his constructive comments and invaluable observations leading to a final draft of this book; I thank him as well for his friendship. I would like to thank Harold Coward of the University of Victoria, Klaus Klostermaier of the University of Manitoba, and Gerald Larson of Indiana University for their encouragement. To Georg Feuerstein, whose works on Yoga I have often drawn upon in this present study, and for his recent friendship, I express my thanks. I also thank Daniel Mariau of the University of Hull for being a continual source of intellectual stimulation on the subject of Yoga.

I am very appreciative of the many students who have studied with me while I was teaching at the University of Alberta and at the University of Cambridge. They never fail to challenge and inspire me along the way. I thank my parents, Ross and Jean Whicher, and my parents-in-law, Scott and Molly Montgomery, for their constant support and encouragement. I also express my gratitude to Denise and Philip Bilton for their painstaking efforts in typing the initial thesis manuscript. For the publication of the book, I wish to thank Nancy Ellegate, Bernadine Dawes, Anne Valentine, and others who were involved at the State University of New York Press.

I am very grateful to Swami Shyam of Kullu, Himachal Pradesh, India. Without his personal example and guidance I would not be personally engaged in an authentic living tradition of Yoga including the profound experiential and practical dimensions of Yoga, its philosophy and implications for daily life. Yet the ideas expressed in this book have not been formally discussed with Swami Shyam, nor has he read the manuscript itself. Thus, he cannot be held responsible for the conceptual proliferations that follow.

My deepest gratitude goes to my wife, Rose Montgomery-Whicher, whose love and support over many years has shown me the importance of integrating meditative practice and philosophical insight into the everyday world of embodied, lived experience. Our often-held discussions together have become an irreplaceable source of intellectual stimulation and inspiration.

Finally, I want to acknowledge the unique contribution of my newly born daughter, Sophia, whose delightful presence in my arms as I read through the final proofs of this book has rekindled, in such a tangible way, my original vision for a Yoga of embodied freedom.

I am grateful to various copyright holders for granting me permission to reproduce portions of previously published material. Chapter 3 is a revised version of material originally published as "The Mind *(Citta):* Its Nature, Structure and Functioning in Classical Yoga" in *Saṃbhāṣā (Nagoya Studies in Indian Culture and Buddhism)* 18 (March 1997): 35–62 and 19 (July 1998):1–50. Chapter 4 contains material much of which is a revised version of an article entitled "Nirodha, Yoga Praxis and the Transformation of the Mind" in *Journal of Indian Philosophy* 25.1 (February 1997): 1–67, and for which kind permission was granted from Kluwer Academic Publishers. Parts of chapters 4, 6, and the conclusion contain revised and expanded versions of material that appear as "Cessation and Integration in Classical Yoga" in *Asian Philosophy* 5.1 (March 1995): 47–58 (later published in Brian Carr, ed., *Morals and Society in Asian Philosophy* [Richmond, U.K.: Curzon Press, 1996]). Parts of chapters 2, 4, 6, and the conclusion contain revised versions of material that appear as "Yoga and Freedom: A Reconsideration of Patañjali's Classical Yoga" in *Philosophy East and West* 48.2 (April 1998): 272–322.

ABBREVIATIONS

TEXTS

BĀ Up	*Bṛhadāraṇyaka Upaniṣad*
BG	*Bhagavadgītā*
Chānd Up	*Chāndogya Upaniṣad*
Mait Up	*Maitrāyaṇīya Upaniṣad*
MBh	*Mahābhārata*
MD	*Mokṣadharma*
MP	*Maṇi-Prabhā* of Rāmānanda Yati
RM	*Rāja-Mārtaṇḍa* of Bhoja Rāja
ṚV	*Ṛg Veda*
ŚB	*Śatapatha Brāhmaṇa*
SK	*Sāṃkhya-Kārikā* of Īśvara Kṛṣṇa
SPB	*Sāṃkhya-Pravacana-Bhāṣya* of Vijñāna Bhikṣu
STK	*Sāṃkhya-Tattva-Kaumudī* of Vācaspati Miśra
Śvet Up	*Śvetāśvatara Upaniṣad*
Tait Up	*Taittirīya Upaniṣad*
TV	*Tattva-Vaiśāradī* of Vācaspati Miśra
YB	*Yoga-Bhāṣya* of Vyāsa
YS	*Yoga-Sūtra* of Patañjali
YSS	*Yoga-Sāra-Saṃgraha* of Vijñāna Bhikṣu
YV	*Yoga-Vārttika* of Vijñāna Bhikṣu
YYS	*Yoga-Yājñavalkya-Saṃhitā*

JOURNALS

ABORI	*Annals of the Bhandarkar Oriental Research Institute*
AJP	*American Journal of Philology*
ALB	*Adyar Library Bulletin*
AP	*Asian Philosophy*

BSOAS	*Bulletin of the School of Oriental and African Studies*
IIJ	*Indo-Iranian Journal*
IPQ	*International Philosophical Quarterly*
JAAR	*Journal of the American Academy of Religion*
JAOS	*Journal of the American Oriental Society*
JHR	*Journal of the History of Religions*
JIBS	*Journal of Indian and Buddhist Studies*
JICPR	*Journal of the Indian Council of Philosophical Research*
JIP	*Journal of Indian Philosophy*
JRAS	*Journal of the Royal Asiatic Society*
PEW	*Philosophy East and West*
WZKS	*Wiener Zeitschrift für die Kunde Süd- und Ostasiens (Südasiens) und Archiv für indische Philosophie*
YQR	*Yoga Quarterly Review*

Introduction

This book centers on the thought of Patañjali (ca. second–third century CE), the great exponent of the authoritative and classical Yoga school *(darśana)* of Hinduism and the reputed author of the *Yoga-Sūtra*. More specifically, the focus of this study is on Patañjali's central definition of Yoga (*YS* I.2), which states: "Yoga is the cessation of [the misidentification with] the modifications of the mind" *(yogaś cittavṛttinirodhaḥ)*. Our work is rooted in the conviction, implicitly expressed so it seems by Patañjali himself, that an in-depth examination of *Yoga-Sūtra* I.2 is helpful, indeed, we suggest crucial, for: (i) elucidating a clear response to the question, "What is the meaning of Yoga?" and (ii) exploring the integral relationship between *theoria* and *praxis* in the *Yoga-Sūtra*. Although *Yoga-Sūtra* I. 2 is acknowledged by Yoga experts and scholars to be of great importance for our understanding of Yoga, a thoroughgoing and systematic inquiry into its meaning and practical relevance is noticeably lacking.

What is classical Yoga philosophy and how can it enrich our understanding of human nature? What is the relationship between self-understanding, knowledge, morality, and spiritual emancipation in Patañjali's thought? As a response to these questions I will argue that Patañjali's philosophical perspective has, far too often, been looked upon as excessively "spiritual" or isolationistic to the point of being a world-denying philosophy, indifferent to moral endeavor, neglecting the world of nature and culture, and overlooking the highest potentials for human reality, vitality, and creativity. Contrary to the arguments presented by many scholars, which associate Patañjali's Yoga exclusively with asceticism, mortification, denial, and the renunciation and abandonment of "material existence" *(prakṛti)* in favor of an elevated and isolated "spiritual state" *(puruṣa)* or disembodied state of spiritual liberation, I suggest that Patañjali's Yoga can be seen as a responsible engagement, in various ways, of "spirit" (*puruṣa* = Self, pure consciousness) and "matter" (*prakṛti* = the source of psychophysical being, which includes mind, body, nature), resulting in a highly developed, transformed, and participatory human nature and identity, an integrated and embodied state of liberated selfhood *(jīvanmukti)*.

I have attempted a careful textual, historical, and interpretive study that, it is hoped, results in a plausible and innovative reading of the "intention" of the *Yoga-Sūtra,* namely, that it does not advocate the abandonment of the world for the successful yogin, but supports a stance that enables the yogin to live more fully in the world without being enslaved by worldly identification. In doing so I have tried to present a sustained argument for the above on the basis of a close (and cumulative) textual study within the tradition of classical Yoga itself. In this study I have endeavored to clarify the thought of Vyāsa (ca. fifth-sixth century CE), whose commentary on the *Yoga-Sūtra* entitled, the *Yoga-Bhāṣya,* illuminates our understanding of Patañjali's thought.

Thus I challenge and attempt to correct conclusions about classical Yoga philosophy drawn by traditional and modern interpretations of Patañjali's *Yoga-Sūtra.* From a critical perspective, it is necessary to make efforts to integrate theories of reality and knowledge per se with hermeneutical reflection and human motivation within which the theories were devised. There is a crust of preconceived ideas surrounding Patañjali's Yoga and to unfreeze the *Yoga-Sūtra* from the traditional reception that it has encountered in the Western world since the nineteenth century is no easy task. Millions of people today—both in the East (i.e., in India) and the West—practice some form or forms of Yoga influenced by or derived from Patañjali's *Yoga-Sūtra.* I have attempted to reinterpret a central feature of the *Yoga-Sūtra,* namely, the objective of *cittavṛttinirodha* or the cessation of the misidentification with the modifications of the mind, and provide a fresh vision of the spiritual potential present in this seminal text, thereby contributing to our understanding and reception of Yoga thought and spirituality. In order to do this I have felt it necessary to develop a comprehensive epistemological perspective in which the relation of identity and selfhood to the world is not severed due to a radical withdrawal from the world but is seen to be participatory in/with the world, allowing the yogin full access to the world through a mode of nonafflicted action. The interpretation of Patañjali's Yoga *darśana* presented in this study—which involves walking the line between an historical and a hermeneutic-praxis (or one might say here a theological or "systematic") orientation—counters the radically dualistic and ontologically oriented interpretations of Yoga presented by many scholars and suggests an open-ended, morally and epistemologically oriented hermeneutic that, I maintain, is more appropriate for arriving at a genuine assessment of Patañjali's system.

Chapter 1 presents a thematic portrayal of early forms of Hindu Yoga, showing how selected Hindu texts can be said to exemplify or emphasize different meanings of or approaches to the term "Yoga." No attempt has been made to analyze yogic disciplines within Jainism or Buddhism, although mention is made in chapters 1 and 2 (in the notes) of the parallels, association, or relationship between Buddhism, Jainism, and Hindu Yoga—in particular the *Yoga-Sūtra* of Patañjali. Admittedly, this is a very rich, diverse, and in many ways unexplored area of study, not least of which as it pertains to Jainism. However, it would require a necessary rigor and depth of analysis that, for want of space, lies outside the scope of this present study. While providing only a sketchbook account of Yoga that discloses a general view of Yoga within early Hinduism, the main purpose nevertheless of this background chapter is to act as a backdrop for the chapters that follow on Patañjali's Yoga. In fact, chapter 1 is perhaps most useful for those with little or no background in Yoga thought. It is not intended for scholarly experts in Yoga or for those who already have an adequate background in ancient and classical Hindu Yoga and its development.

The next two chapters deal with more theoretical issues in Patañjali's Yoga. Chapter 2 outlines Patañjali's basic philosophical stance and metaphysical schematic, while also referring to major similarities and differences between classical Yoga and classical Sāṃkhya. Chapter 3 elaborates on Patañjali's epistemology by examining the nature, structure, and functioning *(vṛtti)* of the mind *(citta)* through which the world and self-identity are experienced, perceived, and understood. The remaining chapters explore the notion of Yoga as a "theory-practice unification" by highlighting the transformative processes of the mind undergone by the yogin through the actual practice of Yoga. Chapter 4 presents a critical examination of the central term *nirodha* ("cessation") as used in *Yoga-Sūtra* I.2 and then proceeds with an analysis of the bipolar nature of the yogic path of practice *(abhyāsa)* and dispassion *(vairāgya),* including as well an overview of the "eight-limbed" *(aṣṭāṅga)* Yoga outlined by Patañjali. Chapters 5 and 6 discuss the meaning and practice of *samādhi* and show how the experiences and insight attained in the multileveled process of *samādhi* progressively lead to a disclosure of the soteriological goal of Yoga, that is, "aloneness" *(kaivalya)*.

Chapter 6 concludes with a section on "aloneness" and a consideration of the implications of Patañjali's Yoga for an embodied state of freedom. While I suggest that Patañjali adopts a practical and provisional dualistic metaphysics, there is no proof that his system stops at dualism or merely ends up in a radical dualistic closure in which *puruṣa* and *prakṛti* are incapable of "cooperating," establishing a "harmony," and achieving a "balance" together. Rather, as I argue, the *Yoga-Sūtra* seeks to "unite" these two principles by correcting a misalignment between them, thereby properly aligning them, bringing them "together" through a purification and illumination of consciousness leading to the permanent realization of intrinsic being, that is, authentic identity. Moreover, this study suggests that Patañjali's Yoga *darśana* can be seen to embrace a maturation and full flowering of human nature and identity, a state of embodied liberation—one that incorporates a clarity of awareness with the integrity of being and action.

chapter one

Selected Background Material on the Development of Yoga in Early Hindu Thought

This chapter will provide, within the context of early Hindu thought, an exposition of the term "Yoga," outlining some of the general and more specific meanings of "Yoga" as well as elaborating upon various Hindu spiritual disciplines that are intrinsic to, representative of, or related to yogic praxis. Thus we will review some of the earliest recorded scriptures within Hindu traditions of Yoga showing how selected primary, "revealed," canonical texts *(śruti)* as well as "remembered" texts *(smṛti)* exemplify different aspects of the development of ideas that lead into Patañjali's Yoga (ca. second-third century CE). The chapter will conclude with a look at Yoga in its pedagogical context, which functions as one of the foundations or crucial building blocks of Yoga philosophy and enriches our understanding of Yoga *theoria* and *praxis*. It is through the pedagogical dimension that ideas in Yoga are put into practice and authentically lived in daily life. While providing only a limited, sketchbook account revealing a panoramic view of Yoga within early Hindu thought, this background chapter, nevertheless, functions as an embedding matrix and contextual pointer for the study that follows on classical Yoga. In other words, this introductory chapter highlights and profiles certain key pointers that will come into their own over the full course of this study.

THE TERM "YOGA"

What is "Yoga"? As G. Feuerstein states, "the word *yoga* has a great many meanings which range from 'yoke' to 'mathematical calculus'."[1] If we accept a broad and very general definition of the term "Yoga," such as, according to M. Eliade, "any ascetic technique and any method of meditation,"[2] then there are as many kinds of Yoga as there are spiritual disciplines in India, for example: *bhakti-yoga, rāja-yoga, jñāna-yoga, haṭha-yoga, karma-yoga, mantra-yoga,* and so forth. Moreover, numerous traditions can be easily cited both in India and elsewhere in which the term "Yoga" in the above broad sense can be employed, for example: Buddhist Yoga, Vedānta Yoga, Jaina Yoga, Sāṃkhya Yoga, Integral Yoga, Taoist Yoga, Tibetan Yoga (Vajrayāna Buddhism), Chinese Yoga (Ch'an), Japanese Yoga (Zen), and even Christian Yoga. Yoga is thus the generic term for various paths of "unification," Hindu or otherwise. The term "Yoga" can thus become, according to G. Larson,

> indistinguishable from the general notion of spiritual *praxis* or *sādhana,* and in a secular environment *Yoga* may become any method of meditation for inhibiting heart disease, toning muscles, increasing concentration, fostering relaxation. . . . *Yoga,* then, becomes what Patañjali, Śaṃkara, Bhakti Vedānta, Agehananda Bharati, Maharṣi Mahesh Yogi, Baba Ram Das, Yogi Bhajan, Jack Lalane, the YMCA and the Roman Catholic Church all have in common. Admittedly the ecumenical possibilities are nearly endless.[3]

In its proper historical and philosophical context, however, Yoga refers to South Asian Indian paths of spiritual emancipation, or self-transcendence, that bring about a transmutation of consciousness culminating in liberation from the confines of egoic identity or worldly existence. Feuerstein calls Yoga, "the psychospiritual technology specific to the great civilization of India."[4] Within the Hindu tradition, six major forms of Yoga have gained prominence: classical Yoga or *rāja-yoga* (the "Royal Yoga" in later times often used to refer to Patañjali's school of Yoga in order to contrast it with *haṭha-yoga*), *jñāna-yoga* (the Yoga of "knowledge" or "wisdom"), *haṭha-yoga* (the "forceful Yoga" of the physical body), *bhakti-yoga* (the Yoga of "devotion") *karma-yoga* (the Yoga of "action"), and *mantra-yoga* (the Yoga of the "recitation of sound"). To this list can be added *laya-yoga* (the Yoga of "dissolution") and *kuṇḍalinī-yoga* (a discipline with Tantric associations that involves the intentional arousal of the "serpent energy" or *kuṇḍalinī-śakti*), which are closely associated with *haṭha-yoga* but are often presented as constituting independent approaches.[5] Historically speaking, the most significant of all the schools of Yoga is the system of classical Yoga as propounded by Patañjali. It is also known as *the* "perspective of Yoga" *(yoga-darśana)* and is classified among the so-called six *darśana*s or philosophical traditions of orthodox Brāhmaṇical Hinduism, the other five being: Nyāya, Vaiśeṣika, Sāṃkhya, Pūrva Mīmāṃsā, and Vedānta (Uttara Mīmāṃsā).

The word "Yoga" is etymologically derived from the verbal root *yuj* meaning "to yoke or join or fasten or harness"[6] and can have several connotations including: "union," "conjunction of stars," "grammatical rule," "endeavor," "occupation," "team," "equipment," "means," "trick," "magic," "aggregate," and "sum."[7] In fact, the English word "yoke" is acknowledged by the Oxford English Dictionary to be cognate to *yuj,* as is the word "join."[8] *Yuj* has other significant meanings for the purposes of this study, which include: "to connect," "to unite," "to restrain," "to keep under control," "to concentrate or fix the mind in order to obtain union with the Universal Spirit," "to make ready, prepare," and "to be absorbed or deeply engaged in meditation."[9]

Yoga has developed over a period of several millennia. Mircea Eliade has appropriately referred to Yoga as "a living fossil."[10] The *Bhagavadgītā*—written perhaps around the beginning of the Common Era—describes Yoga as being already ancient *(purātana).*[11] Studies by J. W. Hauer and Maryla Falk have provided convincing evidence that Yoga was not initially created by the adepts of the *Upaniṣad*s (i.e., in the sixth or seventh century BCE)—as had been assumed earlier by Indologists—but had already arisen in the form of rudimentary ideas and practices going back to the time of the *Ṛg Veda* (ca. 1200 BCE)[12] or, as some would argue, as far back as the Indus Valley Civilization between about 2500 and 1800 BCE.[13]

K. S. Joshi[14] informs us that one interpretation of Yoga (which we have traced to being that of S. Dasgupta)[15] specifically explains the word "Yoga" as a noun form derived from the root *yujir* meaning "to unite" or "connect." The noun "Yoga" was thus originally used to designate a union or connection between things. For example, in the *Ṛg Veda* a Vedic "seer" inquires about the "Yoga" (i.e., "connection") between the words of a verse.[16] According to Joshi, perhaps the most common example of "union" in the Vedic period was "the union of bullocks or horses, and the fact that these animals were kept together by means of the yoke seems to have made an impact on the meaning of the word *'Yoga'*. The word, in due course, began to denote the 'tool of the union'—the yoke"[17] or, it must be added, the animals even. For example, the term *ratha-yoga* was used to designate the "animals for yoking to chariots."[18]

There are numerous examples, however, where the word *"yuga"* has also been used instead to denote the "yoke,"[19] and we may understand the above usage of the term "Yoga" as only an intermediate step to a further shift of meaning that was more significant and lasting. This dramatic shift of meaning—from referring to the yoking of external objects or things like hymns, the 'gods,' and the Vedic sacrifice (*yajña,* see below), animals and carts, and so forth, to an internal "joining" or "harnessing" (e.g., the union between the senses and with the mind)—constitutes the most noteworthy change in the meaning of the term "Yoga" and is traceable to an apparent similarity between the human senses and horses: A well-controlled horse allows the rider to travel with ease; similarly, one can go through life more comfortably if one is not repeatedly and compulsively drawn to the objects of the senses, that is, if the senses are under "control," or are properly harnessed.

Hindu scripture often compares the human senses with horses.[20] It was thus that the term "Yoga" evolved to indicate the method by which the senses and, by implication, the mind could be controlled, mastered, and transcended. S. Dasgupta states: "The force of the flying passions was felt to be as uncontrollable as that of a spirited steed, and thus the word *'Yoga'* which was originally applied to the control of steeds began to be applied to the control of the senses."[21] The fact that the yoke was a tool used for bringing horses under control might have helped the meaning of the word "Yoga" to be shifted to the "tool," method of harnessing, or way of integration or union that can be utilized to bring the senses and the mind under control. It must be stressed, however, that the term "Yoga" as applied to the human senses and mind comes to refer to a philosophically sophisticated and highly technical meaning and presupposes the formation of a well-arranged program or system of practices capable of steadying the mind, bringing it under "control," and thereby transcending the trammels of worldly existence including the human (egoic) barriers to spiritual freedom *(mokṣa)*. Dasgupta explains that the techniques of controlling and steadying the mind were already developed and organized by the time of Pāṇini (ca. 400-500 BCE). To indicate these, Pāṇini thought it was necessary to derive the word "Yoga" from a root form different from *yuj-ir* (the original supposed root) and the root *yuj* was thus invented by him from the noun 'Yoga'.[22] Elsewhere, in his *History of Indian Philosophy,* Dasgupta writes: "In Pāṇini's time the word *Yoga* had attained its technical meaning and he distinguished the root *yuj samādhau* (*yuj* in the sense of concentration) from *yujir yoge* (root *yuj* in the sense of connecting). *Yuj* in the first sense is seldom used as a verb. It is more or less an imaginery root for the etymological derivation of the word *'Yoga'*."[23]

While the term "Yoga" was being used to denote simply a "union," the facts about controlling and steadying the mind were probably known. In the *Vedas* there are clear indications that the Vedic "seers" *(ṛṣis)* were familiar with various methods that, upon being followed faithfully, were known to bring about a state of self-transcendence, a transformation of consciousness and self-identity beyond the limitations of the ego-personality, resulting in an exalted and expanded sense of identity and being. These methods or techniques were spoken of variously as *dhyāna* (meditation), *dīkṣā* (spiritual initiation), *tapas* (asceticism), and so on.[24] Joshi notes that

> we find examples of Vedic seers aspiring to reach the heavens or even for attaining *Brahman,* through *dhyāna, tapas,* etc. But, in all probability, these practices were in the beginning in a more or less fluid form, lacking elaborate classification and differentiation. Later on, they were organized into a system, and it was possibly then that the name *"Yoga"* came to be associated with it. The word *"Yoga"* is thus older than the discipline or system of philosophy which goes by that name.[25]

YOGA IN THE VEDAS

The notion of sacrifice *(yajña)* is one of the foundational premises upon which Hinduism has developed. Sacrificial rituals played an integral and crucial role in the early Vedic age. Through the performance of sacrifice, the followers of the Vedas[26] attempted to attract and maintain the favor of the deities *(deva)*. Cosmic existence itself was seen to be molded on the principle of sacrifice. This is illustrated in *Ṛg Veda* X.90, where we are informed that the primordial Being *(puruṣa)* sacrificed "itself" in order to generate the cosmos. The transformative nature of cosmic existence, beginning with the creation and preservation of life in all its separate forms, inevitably leads to a dissolution of those forms. By analogy with the sacrifice of *puruṣa,* the dissolution of manifold existence is the way in which life continuously regenerates itself. In the celebrated hymn of the primeval sacrifice of the Cosmic Person, called the *Puruṣa Sūkta,*[27] the spiritual essence is as if sacrificed so that from out of the undivided "Oneness" the diversity or multiplicity of life-forms may come into being. The Vedic gods are shown as performing a sacrificial rite by immolating *puruṣa,* the Cosmic Person, as a result of which the world as we know it is generated. The *Puruṣa Sūkta* goes on to state that the various castes within society and the heavenly bodies such as the sun and the moon are all born from the various parts of *puruṣa*'s body. From the perspective of the seer or *ṛṣi,* cosmic order *(ṛta)*—with its regular movements and activities converging on the main purpose of upholding and sustaining life—was all laid in "heaven" *(svarga)* from the very beginning of its manifestation.[28]

Of this great oblation the human ritual is understood to be the microscopic reflection. The original idea, as implied in the *Puruṣa Sūkta,* simply expressed the offering, by the gods, of the divine life, the *puruṣa* as essence of all, the life-blood for the many (i.e., the spiritual essence that flows through all and animates all). It is split up into many forms but is one in essence. It both issues forth yet transcends its creation. The main word used for sacrifice—*yajña*—is derived from the root *yaj* meaning "to worship," "to pay honour to." It is an act of relatedness linking one level to another, making use of the concentration of mental power that "yokes" the mind to the object of worship. The wise, thus, are said to "integrate the mind, integrate spiritual insight."[29] In the sacrifice the mind is harnessed to a vision of the subtler realities, or to one god or other, or to the conception of the cosmic order *(ṛta);*[30] hence the interrelatedness of all, the rite being a framework or the means whereby the mind is directed toward, and can likewise attain insight into, the transcendent realm. As is expressed by R. Panikkar, "Worship does not consist solely in prayer . . . it is action, an action by which duality is transcended and dissimilarity banished. This act contains within itself, essentially, a sacrificial aspect, a death and a becoming, a doing, *karman.*"[31]

The prime function of the sacrifice is to generate heat within the body of the performer. This heat, called *tapas,* arises out of action[32] and is generated when the thoughts and intentions of the sacrificer are totally absorbed into that which is the object of the sacrifice. Through the performance of ritual action *(karman) tapas* is produced that allows the sacrificer to take on the qualities of the intended deity. For example, sacrifice performed to the god *Indra* may enable one to become a great warrior and achieve the desired goal. Through the application of *tapas,* creative intention *(kratu)* is cultivated that has the power to link the microscopic world of the sacrificer with the macrocosm, giving him or her the power to determine and alter circumstances, to bring forth new possibilities. This sacrifice has as its objective a "unification" of the sacrificer with the powers represented in what is sacrificed to. The performance of creative action generates a specific world symbolized by one of the various deities in the Vedic pantheon (e.g., *Indra, Agni, Varuṇa,* and so forth).[33] The deity to whom one sacrifices may change as one's needs and desires change. This sacrificial action, which is, according to Panikkar, "a death and a becoming," is the creative act par excellence. Ritualized in the sacrifice, it is sacred work performed according to certain well-attested rules, hence its identification with *rta*. The *Rg Veda* declares that cosmic order is maintained by sacrificial order: *rta* is upheld by *rta*.[34]

Based on her innovative study, which takes into account the role of spiritual practice and insight in Vedic times, J. Miller argues that meditative discipline as the core focus of Yoga praxis can be traced back to the period of the *Rg Veda:* "The Vedic bards were *seers* who *saw* the *Veda* and sang what they saw. With them vision and sound, seership and singing are intimately connected and this linking of the two sense functions forms the basis of the Vedic prayer."[35] By means of the performance of prescribed ritualistic sacrifices *(yajña),* the *rsis* directed their vision *(dhīh)* to the Divine.

In his work entitled *The Vision of the Vedic Poets,* Jan Gonda's examination of the Vedic word *dhīh* and its derivative *dhītih*[36] has provided ample evidence that *dhīh* is not just "thought" as it is usually translated, nor "hymn" or "devotion"; rather *dhīh* refers to "visionary insight," "thought-provoking vision," a spiritual power that enabled the seer-poets to see in depth what they duly expressed as songs, hymns, or prayers, so that the word has often the meaning of insight leading to song, hymn, or prayer. The term *dhyāna* (meditation), referring to a practice that is basic to Yoga, is derived from the root *dhyai* and is related to several Vedic terms derived from the root *dhī.*[37]

Miller understands meditative discipline in Vedic times as manifesting three distinct but overlapping aspects that she refers to as: mantric meditation, visual meditation, and absorption in heart and mind.[38] Mantric meditation corresponds with the absorption of the mind by means of sound or sacred utterance *(mantra)*. Visual meditation is exemplified in the concept of *dhīh* (which precedes the later related term *dhyāna*), in which a specific deity is envisaged. The subtlest meditative stage, called absorption in mind and heart, involves enheightened experiences in which the seer, on the basis of what Miller refers to as a "seed-thought," explores the mysterious psychic and cosmic forces that gave rise to the composition of the Vedic hymns, such as the *Purusa Sūkta* (mentioned above) and the *Nāsadīya Sūkta* ("hymn of creation," *Rg Veda* X.129). Successful meditation as disclosed in the Vedic hymns culminates in illumination wherein the seer perceives the "immortal light" *(jyotir amrtam)*.[39] Thus, in this highest form of meditative insight, the ancient sage Atri is said to have "found the sun concealed by darkness."[40] This occurs, according to Miller, in the course of the fourth degree of "prayer," which she equates with *samādhi*[41]—seen here as an ecstatic merging, as it were, with reality and the attainment of immortal knowledge. Miller points out that although the word *samādhi* does not appear in the *Ṛg Veda,* it is, however,

> almost certain that the *ṛṣis* experienced *samādhi* but they did not analyze this in terms used in later ages as Patañjali was to do; its culmination meant for them contemplation of and perhaps mergence with the sun.[42]

> There is no direct statement that the beholding of the "golden one" becomes a blending of the beholder and the object perceived but the knowledge of immortality which is part of the experience of *samādhi* is clearly stated.[43]

Scholarship does not easily acknowledge that yogic forms of contemplative discipline were known to the *ṛṣi*s of the early Vedic period thus failing to make a connection here with some of the core aspects of Yoga as expressed in its classical form, namely: concentration, meditation, and "unification." The integrating or harnessing of the mind (see n. 29 above) clearly points toward forms of yogic mental discipline insofar as it involves practices focusing on concentration, meditation, and the quest for a higher transcendent goal.

The very claim to seership entails the ability to see "within," which itself implies a contemplative perspective. That the overall aims of Yoga and of the Vedic seers may have been different is another question, the former purporting to lead to liberation from the limitations of worldly or cosmic existence, the latter emphasizing an expanded knowledge of the cosmos rather than freedom from its impediments. In view of the this-worldly, earthy nature of many of the Vedic hymns, it is easy to conclude that the Vedic prayers were only for material benefit[44] or selfish gain, and that forms of asceticism and contemplation that may have been intrinsic to the Vedic tradition were simply borrowed from the indigenous cultures. But to deny the Vedic Aryans any impetus for self-transcendence or capacity for metaphysical speculation could well prove to be an unwarranted position or oversight on the part of some scholars. As Miller's study indicates, the proto-Yoga of the Vedic *ṛṣi*s is an early form of sacrificial mysticism and contains many elements characteristic of later Yoga that include: concentration, meditative observation, ascetic forms of practice *(tapas)*,[45] breath-control practiced in conjunction with the recitation of sacred hymns during the ritual, the notion of self-sacrifice, impeccably accurate recitation of sacred words (prefiguring *mantra-yoga*), mystical experience, and the engagement with a reality far greater than our psychophysical identity or ego.

Although no form of Yoga is explicated in the Brāhmaṇas (1000–800 BCE)—exegetical works expounding and systematizing the Vedic sacrificial ritual and concerned with the significance of the *brahman,* the inner power of the sacrificial utterance—we can see contained in their sacrificial ritualism[46] one of the key contributing elements of the later Yoga tradition. Thus the treatment of the ceremony of the "fire sacrifice of the breaths" *(prāṇa-agni-hotra)*—consisting of the oblation of food to the different kinds of breath, reveals a form of practice and thinking that helped to lay a foundation for the full-blown yogic study and discipline of breath control *(prāṇāyāma)*. The *prāṇa-agni-hotra*[47] is a symbolic replacement for the earlier Vedic fire ritual *(agni-hotra),* one of the most frequently performed and therefore most popular of all the rites. In the *prāṇa-agni-hotra,* the more invisible, unobvious life-force or vital energy takes the place of the visible, obvious ritual fire. The *prāṇa* is associated with the transcendent essence—the *ātman* or spiritual Self. The more esoteric emphasis given here, however, does not as yet constitute the more fully developed form of self- or "mental" sacrifice as is the case in yogic forms of meditation. It was enacted through one's body. Nevertheless, this important sacrifice was a major stepping-stone toward a most interesting phenomenon that has been referred to as the interiorization of sacrifice: the transformation or conversion or redirection of attention from externally oriented rites to internally oriented or mentally enacted rites.

YOGA IN THE UPANIṢADS

The sages of the early Upaniṣads (800–500 BCE) presented a real challenge to the normal, formalized sacrificial cult of Vedic society by instigating what was to become an ideological—one might even say a spiritual—"revolution" by "internalizing" the ritualistic norms of the Vedas and Brāhmaṇas and establishing the path of intense thought, reflection, and meditation as the "inner sacrifice." Once it is understood that life perpetuates itself through its transformative or changing nature, that is, the creation, maintenance, and dissolution of separate life-forms, the only appropriate and spiritually mature response is to relate to existence as a continual sacrifice of the sense of separate selfhood or individuality. While the external rituals of orthodox Brāhmaṇism were acknowledged as having a proper place in the social order, the Upaniṣadic adepts denied outright their soteriological efficacy. If the externalized forms of sacrifice involving a variety of rituals were the means to attain "heaven" for the Vedic people, then the sacrifice of the self, or egoic identity, is the means par excellence to liberation for the Upaniṣadic sage and, as we will see, the authentic Yoga practitioner. What is interesting to note is that the means of achieving both heaven *(svarga)*[48] and liberation *(mokṣa)* can be seen as converging on basic yogic-oriented practices such as concentration, meditation, absorption, and unification. The internalization of the Vedic ritual in the form of meditational praxis is well illustrated, for example, in the *Kauṣītaki Upaniṣad* (II.5) (ca. 800 BCE) which refers to the "inner fire sacrifice" *(āntaram agni-hotram)*.[49]

Like the Vedas, the Upaniṣads are looked upon as sacred revelation *(śruti)*. Yet in contrast to the Vedas, the Upaniṣads are regarded as belonging to the "wisdom part" *(jñāna-kāṇḍa)* as opposed to the "ritual part" *(karma-kāṇḍa)* of the Vedic heritage. The knowledge that "behind" our ever-changing universe—the reality of multiple forms and phenomena—there abides an eternally unchanging and unfractured (single) Being was communicated already in Vedic times. For example, the *Ṛg Veda* (I.164.46) clearly discerns a unitary principle in which the personal gods to whom people sacrifice are seen as merely names for, or manifestations of, this unitary principle ("To that existence which is one *[ekam sat]* the sages give many a name."). However, the Upaniṣadic seekers disclosed, so it appears, a new or fresh insight: that the single transcendent Being is nothing more and nothing less than the essential core of one's own existence or Self. This finds clear expression, for example, in the *Bṛhadāraṇyaka Upaniṣad,* by one of the most profound thinkers of ancient India, Yājñavalkya (ca. 800 BCE).[50] Yājñavalkya was asked how that Self is to be conceived, to which he responded:

> You cannot see the seer of seeing. You cannot hear the hearer of hearing. You cannot think the thinker of thinking. You cannot understand the understander of understanding. He is your Self, which is in everything. Everything else is irrelevant.[51]

This passage epitomizes one of the essential teachings from the Upaniṣads that was transmitted orally from an enlightened preceptor *(guru)* to disciple *(śiṣya)*: the transcendent Source of the world is identical with the transcendent core of the human being; *brahman* and *ātman* are one in identity.[52] There is no possible way to exhaustively describe or define that supreme Reality. One must simply realize it, and in this state of the fully awakened consciousness of Self *(ātman)* or *brahman* one could doubtlessly declare, as did Yājñavalkya, "I am the Absolute (the Whole)." This ultimate essence of life is described as being pure Selfhood, that is, the knower who is unknowable, the seer who cannot be seen, and so forth, as being the One—

transcendent of all multiplicity—as being pure consciousness, that is, consciousness that is free from any enslavement or limitation within the subject-object duality of ordinary experience.

How can the infinite, eternal, utterly free and real, and immeasurably blissful Self be realized? The Upaniṣadic sages emphasized the need for renunciation *(saṃnyāsa)* and intensive meditation *(dhyāna),* but the earliest Upaniṣads reveal very few practical instructions about the actual practice of meditation. It appears this was a matter to be settled between teacher and disciple. But the purpose of meditational praxis, as Patañjali was later to explain,[53] is to transcend saṃsāric existence and its afflicted modes of mistaken identity and spiritual ignorance *(avidyā)* that ensconce one in the repeated drama of birth, life-span, and death and that merely result in pain, distress, and dissatisfaction, that is, suffering *(duḥkha).* There being no real relief in this cycle *(saṃsāra),* the Upaniṣadic sages taught the necessary means by which saṃsāric existence, that is, the world of change, unending rounds of rebirth and ignorance of one's true identity, could be transcended. Yājñavalkya urges one to see that the true Self *(ātman)* is beyond all action *(karma)* and not to be deceived by ideas of what is ritually right and wrong, so that what one has done and what one has not done do not bind or affect one[54] as in the saṃsāric condition of selfhood. Through this attainment, having seen that the Self is "not this, not this" *(neti neti),* the Self is then seen in all things, in fact everywhere, making one free from evil, impurity, doubt, fear, and confusion.

Elsewhere in the same scripture, Yājñavalkya proclaims:

> He who has found and awakened to the Self that has entered this perilous and inaccessible place [psychophysical being or body-mind], is the creator of the world, for he is the maker of the universe and of all. The world belongs to him. He is indeed the world.[55]
>
> It should be seen as only one [i.e., as single], immeasurable, perpetual. The Self is taintless, unborn, great, perpetual, and beyond [the subtle element of] space.[56]

The realization of the unchanging, ever-pure Self *(ātman)*—an immortal state of existence—is itself emancipation *(mokṣa).* This awakening coincides with the transcendence of the identifications with the limited sense of self or ego-personality and thus of conditional existence *(saṃsāra)* itself. Moreover, Self-realization is the *telos* of human existence and the universe.[57] Being in truth all that there is, the Self, or *brahman,* cannot be an object of knowledge. Therefore, Yājñavalkya argues that, ultimately, all descriptions of of the Absolute amount to being mere words, ideas, or concepts of reality. Repeatedly he responds to all positive characterizations of the Self by exclaiming "not this, not this" *(neti neti)*.[58] This famous method of approaching the undivided nature of Reality is an attempt to liberate the disciple from clinging to any erroneous predications about Reality and open the way to an unbound, unmodified state of existence and identity beyond all description. It is later adopted even in the nondualist schools of Yoga and Vedānta, where it is known as *apavāda* ("refutation").[59] Yogins who embark on this more Vedāntic approach to spirituality are asked to remind themselves constantly of the fact that all the states, functions or modes of our psychophysical existence are, in themselves, not the transcendent Reality. Neither the body, as it is ordinarily experienced, nor our thoughts and feelings as they normally present themselves are our true identity. The Self is no-thing or object that could be located in the external or experiential (empirical) finite world. This form of alert discrimination is called *viveka*. Through vigilant cultivation of *viveka* the yogin develops an inner watchfulness or attentiveness to what is of a changing nature, that is, what is within the realm of experience, as well as to the eternal Being or Source of all experiences, the unchanging identity or experiencer. By this form of practice the yogin cultivates a steadfast will to renounce all attachment to the changing, phenomenal world. Discrimination and renunciation *(saṃnyāsa)* ultimately are said to lead to the discovery of the formless dimension of Self, the *ātman,* beyond all conceptual understanding and imagery. Moreover, the true purpose of life and highest knowledge to be attained is not of the manifest sphere of existence, but rather is of the imperishable *(akṣara),* the unknown, unreflective Self or knower *(avijñātaṃ vijñātṛ),* which itself gives rise to the outer world of manifestations.[60] The seeker of truth and lasting fulfillment must be free of all attachment to the knowable (or seeable), must learn to sacrifice all egoic identification with what is experienced in order for authentic identity and, thus, liberation to arise.

The *Chāndogya Upaniṣad* (ca. seventh or eighth century BCE) also gives us valuable insights into the early development of metaphysical ideas within Hinduism and the transformed nature of sacrifice *(yajña)* as articulated in the Upaniṣads. As we have seen, the external sacrificial ritual so prominent in early Vedic times was largely shunned by the Upaniṣadic sages who emphasized disciplines that brought about an interiorization of attention resulting in the internalization of the sacrificial ritual. This in turn opened the door for the development of Yoga within orthodox Brāhmaṇism. In the *Chāndogya,* Ghora Āṅgirasa explains to Kṛṣṇa that austerity *(tapas)*, charity *(dāna)*, rectitude *(ārjava)*, nonviolence *(ahiṃsā)* and truthfulness *(satya)* are themselves the sacrificial gift *(dakṣiṇa)*,[61] thus implying that the inner attitudinal dimension as well as the way in which one lives one's life are the best recompense for what one has imbibed from one's teachers. The above idea clearly links up with an earlier notion presented in the same scripture: insofar as one is spiritually motivated, that person *is* a sacrifice.[62] This recognition led to the full-fledged perspective of the internalized or spiritualized sacrifice, which entails the dedication of one's life to an intrinsic, higher, transcendent purpose in contrast to the more extrinsically motivated ritual offerings of libations to the deities.

In an illuminating section in the *Chāndogya Upaniṣad,* Prajāpati instructs Indra as follows:

> When the eye is directed toward space, that is the seeing witness *(cākṣuṣa puruṣa);* the eye is but the instrument for sight. . . .
>
> The one who knows "Let me think this"—that is the true self; the mind *(manas)* is the divine eye *(daiva cakṣu)*. That one, with the divine eye, the mind, sees desires here, and experiences enjoyment.
>
> Those gods who are in the Brahmā world reverence the Self. Therefore all worlds and all desires have been appropriated by them. He obtains all worlds and all desires who has found out and who understands that Self *(ātman)*.[63]

While the *Bṛhadāraṇyaka Upaniṣad* articulates the unspeakable or indescribable aspect of the Self *(ātman, puruṣa)*, the *Chāndogya Upaniṣad* reveres the Self as the context for the unlimited obtainment of worlds, and the fulfillment of desires. In both instances, the Self is not found in what is seen, but in the one who sees—the seer: detachment from the objects of the senses is a prerequisite to the realization of the Self. These important insights, which point to a practice *(abhyāsa)* involving a high-level form of discernment capable of distinguishing between the seer/knower and the seeable/knowable coupled with the need for dispassion *(vairāgya)* toward worldly existence *(saṃsāra)*, are crucial in the context of Yoga philosophy as will be seen in our examination of Patañjali's Yoga.

In the *Taittirīya Upaniṣad,*[64] another of the older Upaniṣads (but not as old as the *Bṛhadāraṇyaka Upaniṣad* or the *Chāndogya Upaniṣad*), one of the earliest technical references of the term Yoga is found, probably standing for the sage's mastery of the body and senses. However, the tradition of Yoga in its classical sense would not emerge and assume its place alongside other Hindu soteriological perspectives until several centuries later.[65] The *Kaṭha Upaniṣad* (fifth century BCE) can perhaps be acknowledged as the oldest *Upaniṣad* that deals explicitly with Yoga. In the *Kaṭha Upaniṣad* one of the key doctrines relating to Yoga is called *adhyātma-yoga,* the "Yoga of the inner self." The goal of this form of Yoga is the realization of the supreme Being, which is concealed within the "cave" of the heart. As this *Upaniṣad* states:

> The wise one relinquishes joy and sorrow, realizing, by means of the Yoga of the inner self that primal God who is difficult to be seen, immanent, seated in the cave [of the heart] residing in the body.[66]

> This Self cannot be attained by instruction, or by thought, or by much hearing. It is attained only by the one whom it chooses. To such a one the Self reveals its own nature.[67]

In the above, the author (anonymous) explains that the Self *(ātman)* is not an object like other objects we can experience, speculate on, or analyze. As the transcendent essence—in effect, the authentic nature, being and identity of everything—there is nothing anyone can do to "acquire" or "obtain" the Self. For how can one "acquire" *that* which one already *is?* Thus the realization of the Self must be a matter of the *ātman* disclosing itself to itself. In religious terminology, this means that spiritual emancipation is dependent upon the element of "grace." The *ātman,* as the *Kaṭha* surmises in the above passage, is attained by "one whom it chooses." This should not be misconstrued to imply that the spiritual practitioner should therefore relinquish all efforts for attaining salvation. On the contrary, the practitioner must undergo the necessary preparation for the reception of grace. Practice is valid as a means for someone who is progressing on the path to enlightenment. Until the "goal" of liberation is reached, efforts toward its attainment, including purification of mind and body, are not rendered invalid.

In chapter three of the *Kaṭha Upaniṣad,* the *ātman* is said to be at the summit of a hierarchy of levels of existence. By way of a metaphor, the instruction is given to: "Know the Self as lord of the chariot, and the body as the chariot. Know further that the intellect *(buddhi)* is the driver, whereas the mind-organ *(manas)* is the rein. The senses, they say, are the horses, and the sense-objects their arena."[68] By understanding spiritual practice as a return to the transcendent origin of being or retracing in consciousness, in reverse order, of the various stages of the evolutionary unfoldment of manifest existence only to "arrive" at the origin of all, the *Kaṭha* distinguishes seven levels that comprise the hierarchy of existence: the senses *(indriya);*

the sense-objects *(viṣaya);* the mind-organ *(manas); the intellect (buddhi);* the "great self" *(mahān ātmā)* or "great one" *(mahat)*—the initial level of manifest existence; the unmanifest *(avyakta)*—the transcendent source or unmanifest ground *(prakṛti)* of all manifest existence (including nature/the cosmos and psychophysical being); and the Self *(puruṣa)*—our intrinsic identity which is an immortal state of consciousness.[69] *Puruṣa* is eternally beyond the dynamics of *prakṛti* in her manifest and unmanifest aspects. In the *Kaṭha* one finds both the old Upaniṣadic notion of the Self *(ātman)* together with the beginning of the Sāṃkhya notion of *puruṣa.* The above ontological scheme is characteristic of the Sāṃkhya tradition. In the context of the *Kaṭha* it was probably never intended as mere metaphysical speculation, rather it served to provide contemplative directives, a "map" as it were, for the yogic processes of "interiorization" (i.e., the sacrifice of saṃsāric identity) involving the expansion or ascent of consciousness to subtler levels of identity, terminating with the ubiquitous/omnipresent Being, *puruṣa* itself. The disclosure of authentic identity as *puruṣa,* the transcendent Self, is the purpose of all efforts to transcend saṃsāric identity and the finite realm.

A clear definition of Yoga is given in *Kaṭha Upaniṣad* II.3.11, which states: "This they consider to be Yoga: the steady holding of the senses. Then one becomes attentive *(apramatta),* for Yoga can come and go."[70] Here Yoga means the condition of inner steadfastness or equilibrium that depends on one's one-pointedness of attention. When the mind is undistracted and stabilized, then one can discover the "inner" or subtler dimensions of existence and consciousness that are revealed to the diligent aspirant. Ultimately, however, as we have seen, even this subtle exploration and disclosure of inner awareness and space does not result in liberation. It is merely a precondition for the reception of grace (see n. 67 above). Sheer determination (will power) and successful effort must be tempered with considerable patience and humility. The pedagogy of the *Kaṭha Upaniṣad* represents an important breakthrough in the tradition of Hindu Yoga. Some of the fundamental ideas underlying Yoga *theoria* and *praxis* are found. The *Kaṭha* marks a definite transition between the esoteric, monistic trends of proto-Yoga as expressed in the early Upaniṣads and preclassical forms of Yoga as illustrated in later Upaniṣadic works such as the *Śvetāśvatara* and *Maitrāyaṇīya* as well as the famous epic, the *Mahābhārata*—especially as revealed in the *Bhagavadgītā* (see below for a discussion on these scriptures). Notwithstanding the obvious lack of any formal structure or systemization of Yoga, the recordings in the *Kaṭha Upaniṣad* helped to mold together some of the crucial building blocks and central philosophical ideas so basic to the enterprise of Yoga. The consequence of this clear development of Yoga was nothing less than Yoga becoming a recognizable tradition that could stand more or less on its own.

In the *Śvetāśvatara Upanisad* (ca. third century BCE), a form of Yoga is proclaimed that is indicative of the panentheistic teachings of the epic age. The Lord *(īśa, īśvara)* is portrayed as dwelling eternally beyond "His" own creation. This *Upanisad* states:

> Following the Yoga of meditation, they perceived the inner power of God concealed by "its" own qualities. God is the one who presides over all the causes associated with time and the self.[71]
>
> By knowing God there is a dwindling of all fetters. When the afflictions are destroyed, there is cessation of birth and death [i.e., changing identity]. By meditating on "Him," there is a third state, universal lordship, upon separation from the body. Being alone, [the yogin's] desire is fulfilled.[72]

The process of meditation recommended in this scripture involves the recitation of the sacred syllable *Om* (called the *pranava*). Meditation generates a necessary churning process by which the inner fire, likened to the Self, is rekindled. This in turn leads to the revelation of the intrinsic glory of the Self or God.[73] The disciplined practice of meditation *(dhyāna)* can lead to a variety of inner experiences that, as the text cautions, must not be confused with liberation itself. The culminating realization is described as follows: "I know that supreme Self *(purusa)* effulgent like the sun beyond the darkness. Only by knowing 'Him' does one pass beyond death. There is no other way for passing [beyond *samsāra*]."[74] Here, like the *Katha Upanisad,* the highest goal is the realization of the supreme, transcendent Self. Far from being portrayed as a colorless or dry ascetic, the yogin is placed in the role of a devotee *(bhakta),* that is, where devotion (*bhakti:* VI.23) to God and to one's spiritual teacher *(guru)* is an integral component of yogic practice. Spiritual growth and emancipation are seen not as a calculated or mechanistic enterprise stemming from self-effort alone, but rather the fruit of one's spiritual discipline is perceived to be enveloped in a mysterious process that is clearly dependent on some measure of "divine grace" as the sage—Śvetāśvatara himself—comes to experience and speak about to others.[75]

The later *Maitrāyanīya Upanisad* (ca. second century BCE)[76] presents a more concrete, formalized, and systematic portrayal of Yoga than had previously been developed. In the *Maitrāyanīya* we can read about many intriguing ideas pertaining to Yoga which easily suggest a further breakthrough in the development of Yoga. Included here are a series of practices that laid much groundwork for the classical formulations contained within the *Yoga-*

Sūtra of Patañjali (see below). As this scripture discloses, the "elemental self" or *bhūtātman* (referring to our psychophysical being or empirical self) is ineluctably entrenched within the saṃsāric world implying afflicted states of identity leading to struggle and conflict due to the "pairs of opposites" *(dvandva)* such as loss and gain, or pleasure and pain. As a result, our sense of self, irrevocably confined to the forces—constituents or qualities *(guṇas)*—of nature and existence *(prakṛti)* as we normally know it to be, is constantly undergoing change[77] and sets itself up for inevitable pain and dissatisfaction *(duḥkha),* which follows until it appears to disintegrate at death. The transcendent Self, however, always remains unaffected by these ongoing changes.[78] Moreover, the Self can be realized through knowledge *(vidyā),* austerity *(tapas),* and deep contemplation *(cintā).*[79] The revered Śākāyanya explains this realization in terms of a union *(sāyujya)*[80] of the elemental (individual) self with the intrinsic Self, the "ruler" *(īśāna),* and later proclaims the "sixfold" Yoga *(ṣaḍaṅga-yoga):*

> This is the rule for effecting this [oneness or union with the Self]: breath control *(prāṇāyāma),* withdrawal of the senses *(pratyāhāra),* meditation *(dhyāna),* concentration *(dhāraṇā),* reflection *(tarka)* and unification *(samādhi);* [this is] said to be the sixfold Yoga. When the seer sees the brilliant Maker, the Lord, the Person, the Source of the Creator-God *(Brahmā),* then, being a knower, shaking off good and evil, collapses everything into unity in the supreme Imperishable.[81]

The above list (excluding *tarka*) mentions five of the eight limbs *(aṅgas)* of the later classical Yoga—the philosophical system that has developed around Patañjali's *Yoga-Sūtra*[82] and its commentarial literature. Also some of the physiological theories of later Yoga begin to appear in the *Maitrāyaṇīya Upaniṣad* (chapter VI) along with meditations on the mystical syllable *Om.*[83] S. Dasgupta writes, "The science of breath had attracted notice in many of the earlier *Upaniṣads,* though there had not probably developed any systematic form of *prāṇāyāma* . . . of the *Yoga* system." He goes on to state that it is not until the *Maitrāyaṇīya* "that we find the *Yoga* method had attained a systematic development."[84]

YOGIC THEMES IN THE *BHAGAVADGĪTĀ* AND THE *MOKṢADHARMA*

The *Bhagavadgītā* (lit., "Song of the Lord") is the most popular and famous of all Yoga scriptures and forms part of the great Hindu epic, the *Mahābhārata* (VI.13-40). The *Bhagavadgītā* (like the *Mahābhārata* as a whole) is not formally a part of primary, revealed scripture (*śruti*, the canonical *Veda*) but belongs to the noncanonical sacred literature called "tradition" or *smṛti* (lit. "remembering" past wisdom). Yet in its own context, in Sanskrit or in translation, the *Bhagavadgītā* has for centuries functioned as revealed or primary scripture for a large number of Hindus. It was composed probably between 150 BCE and 250 CE. This widely acclaimed scripture has often been regarded as a self-contained text by a long line of Hindu thinkers and spiritual preceptors *(gurus)*. The *Bhagavadgītā* is a seminal text for much of Vaiṣṇavism, the tradition centering on the worship of the Lord in the form of Viṣṇu, specifically the descent by Viṣṇu in the embodied form (i.e., *avatāra*) of Kṛṣṇa. Placing before us a rich and challenging body of moral, mystical and metaphysical teachings in the form of a dialogue between Kṛṣṇa and his close friend, Arjuna, the *Bhagavadgītā* on the whole recommends an approach to spiritual liberation that incorporates *karma-yoga, jñāna-yoga* and *bhakti-yoga*. Though not disposing of the kind of world-renouncing asceticism that characterizes much of the earlier Upaniṣadic literature, the *Bhagavadgītā* nevertheless advocates the ideal of "actionless-action" (i.e., non-self-centered or ego-transcending action = *naiṣkarmya-karma*)[85] as being superior to the renunciation of all action. A central aspect of Kṛṣṇa's teaching to Arjuna on *karma-yoga* is encapsulated in the following verse: "Steadfast in Yoga be active, relinquishing attachment and having attained equilibrium in success and failure, O winner of wealth. Yoga is called 'evenness' (*samatva*) [of mind]."[86] As Kṛṣṇa affirms, in order to attain enlightenment and supreme peace it is unnecessary to abandon the world or one's responsibilities even when they summon one into battle, as in the case of Arjuna. To be sure, renunciation *(saṃnyāsa) of* action is, in itself, a legitimate means. Kṛṣṇa, however, declares a superior approach, that being the path of renunciation *while engaged in action* or "actionless-action," which results in freedom from the bondage of action *(naiṣkarmya)*. In other words *naiṣkarmya-karma* refers to a special "kind" or "quality" of action that comes into being through a particular inner attitude toward action, a mental form of activity that can be classified as a kind of action itself. Life in the world can be spiritualized; one's commitment to spiritual discipline and engagement in the world can be, indeed should be, cultivated simultaneously thereby establishing a basis for an integrated life through Yoga:

> Not by abstention from actions does a person enjoy freedom from the bondage of action, nor by mere renunciation does one attain perfection.[87]
>
> He who restrains his organs of action but continues to remember in his mind the objects of the senses is deluded and is called a hypocrite. But

> he excels, O Arjuna, who controlling the senses with the mind engages the organs of action in *karma-yoga.*[88]

Kṛṣṇa points to his own activity as an enlightened example of *karma-yoga:* "For Me, O Pārtha [Arjuna], there is nothing whatever to be done in the three worlds, nothing unobtained which is to be obtained—and yet without fail I engage in action."[89] The secret to *karma-yoga* lies not in the action itself but rather in the state or quality of the human mind which gives rise to the action. If the mind is pure, that is, the yogin having sacri-sacrificed all selfish or inordinate desire *(tṛṣṇā)* and attachment *(rāga)* to the self-centered fruit of deeds, it cannot be defiled by actions even as they are engaged in daily life. What sets in motion the dynamic of *karma* through which a person is bound in *saṃsāra* is not action itself, but, rather, attachment. The mind that remains "even" yet alert, lucid and free of the stain of attachment[90] born of ignorance *(avidyā),* allows for a mode of selfless or non-covetous action *(niṣkāma karma)* through which salvation is attained. *Niṣkāma karma* integrates *samatva* (evenness, serenity of mind) with the resolution to act with detachment. The perfected yogin enjoys a vision of the everywhereness *(sarvatra samadarśana)* of Self: all things are revealed as they truly are, that being of the Self *(ātman):* "One whose self is disciplined by Yoga and who sees everywhere the same, sees the Self abiding in every being and every being in the Self."[91]

Acts must not only be carried out in the spirit of detachment or selflessness, they must also be ethically sound and reasonable, that is, have a high degree of moral content and value. For, as G. Feuerstein incisively states, "If action depended solely on one's frame of mind, it would be the best excuse for immoral behaviour. The *[Bhagavadgītā]* does not propound such a crude subjectivism. For action to be wholesome *[kṛtsna]* it must have two essential ingredients: subjective purity (i.e., nonattachment) and objective morality (i.e., moral rightness)."[92] Kṛṣṇa elaborates on the true nature of action as follows:

> Indeed, one must understand not only action, but improper action *(vikarman)* and inaction *(akarman)*. The way of action is impenetrable. He who sees action in inaction and inaction in action is a wise person performing whole actions in a disciplined way.[93]

Having relinquished the attachment to the fruit of action *(karmaphalāsaṅgaṃ),* the yogin is freed from compulsive desire and abides in a state of constant satisfaction and without dependence on any object. Such a person is said to do nothing whatever (as a separate agent) even though engaged in action.[94] Sacrifice is cited as the model for proper action; the sacrifice of knowledge *(jñāna-yajña)*—superior to the sacrifice of material things—brings about the completion of action (i.e., all action culminates in knowledge).[95] The doctrine of *karma-yoga* states that one is no longer effected by the enslaving power of *karma* if action is done in the spirit of sacrifice. One is free to live as the Self *(ātman)* rather than be bound to an egoic identity. Thus, *naiṣkarmya-karma* liberates the yogin from a misidentified, separate sense of self and is a special form of action in which the ego is transcended. As such it must not be confused with mere action *(karman)* or inaction *(akarman)*.

The final vision or liberated state of Being that the *Bhagavadgītā* acknowledges is union with the Lord. For Kṛṣṇa, Yoga consists essentially in the complete alignment of one's practical, daily life to the divine Being, Kṛṣṇa. In short, every aspect of the yogin's life must become engaged or "yoked" in Yoga.[96] By discarding all attachments in the form of personal volitions, intentions and expectations, and by seeing everywhere and in everything the Divine, the yogin's life is purified and illuminated. Kṛṣṇa is revealed as the ultimate source of all including the unmanifest and the manifest existence in all its diversity. The ethical teachings of the *Bhagavadgītā* basically stem from a panentheistic metaphysical understanding of reality: All is in God, while God transcends everything. Kṛṣṇa embraces the indestructible nature of Being as well as "becoming"—the ever-changing, destructible realm of existence. As Kṛṣṇa professes:

> This whole universe is pervaded by Me in my unmanifested form. Though all beings abide in Me, I do not subsist in them.
>
> Yet beings do not abide in Me. Behold my lordly Yoga: Generating all beings, yet not being generated by them, My Self is the source of beings.[97]

Since the Lord is everywhere and in everything, the idea of renouncing or extricating the world in order to seek salvation or enlightenment ultimately becomes superfluous. What one needs to do is to cultivate a higher intelligence *(buddhi)*,[98] the "eye of wisdom" *(jñāna-cakṣus)*[99] in order to discern the purity of Being, the knower, and thereby attain liberation.

Complementary to, and as some would argue, integral with, while yet even surpassing the insights and realizations attained through *karma-yoga* and *jñāna-yoga*, is the highly recommended "path" in the *Bhagavadgītā* of the Yoga of "devotion" or *bhakti-yoga*. Interestingly, in chapter II Kṛṣṇa discusses a type of emancipation called *brahma-nirvāṇa* ("extinction in the

Absolute") where the yogin transcends the realm of time and space and abides in "his" true nature as peace *(śānti)*.[100] In chapter VI we are told: "Thus continually disciplining himself, the yogin of restrained mind attains peace, the supreme extinction [of deluded identity], that which exists in Me."[101] Moreover, in chapter XVIII Kṛṣṇa appears to distinguish between two degrees of liberation: one in which devotion is absent, the other in which devotion is central. As Kṛṣṇa states, "Having become one with *Brahman,* and being tranquil in oneself, one neither grieves nor desires. Beholding the same [essence] in all beings, one attains supreme devotion to Me. Through this devotion, one comes to know Me in essence. Then having known Me, one forthwith enters into Me."[102]

Yet the high-level state of *brahma-nirvāṇa* of which Kṛṣṇa speaks appears to lack the full-blown devotional element of *bhakti.* A vital and personal connection with the divine personality of Kṛṣṇa, the all-encompassing suprapersonal (in contrast to impersonal) reality, does not appear to come into play or at least is not an essential component of this level of awakening. The supreme Person *(puruṣa-uttama),* who is said to surpass both the perishable *(kṣara)* and the imperishable *(akṣara),*[103] is realized only in what is perhaps a higher form of emancipation, a higher devotion *(para-bhakti),* when the yogin fully awakens in the Lord. For, as Kṛṣṇa says: "One who standing in oneness and worships Me, abiding in all beings, dwells in Me in whatever state one exists."[104] Devotion *(bhakti)* is a major aspect of Kṛṣṇa's teaching, being the surest path by which the devotee-yogin approaches the supreme Person and thereby attains grace *(prasāda).* Thus Kṛṣṇa declares: "Of all yogins, one who worships Me full of faith and whose inner self abides in Me—that one I consider to be nearest to my vision."[105] Thus the "path" of *bhakti-yoga* attained great status as one of the central teachings on Yoga in the *Bhagavadgītā,* and indeed, in much of the Brāhmaṇic devotional literature that followed.[106]

Other significant material that illuminates our understanding of the development of Yoga can be found in the *Mokṣadharma (MD)* section in the *Mahābhārata,* which comprises chapters 168-353 of the twelfth book *(Śāntiparvan).* Important clues are given especially about Yoga and Sāṃkhya in their "epic" forms prior to their classical systematizations by Patañjali and Īśvara Kṛṣṇa respectively. Notwithstanding obvious similarities between Sāṃkhya and Yoga, a careful examination of the the *Mokṣadharma* reveals that both of these traditions were already developing into distinct, independent "views" around the time of the final composition of the *Mahābhārata.* Later in our study it will be noted where the contrast between these two perspectives is apparent.

One important yogic approach that is utilized in the *Mokṣadharma,* termed *nirodha-yoga* (the "Yoga of cessation"), is the progressive transcendence or de-identification with the contents of empirical consciousness—from sensations, to thought, to even subtler experiences—until the culminating realization of authentic identity *(puruṣa)* takes place. Here, sense-withdrawal, concentration, and meditative disciplines are considered the "inner core" or primary methods of Yoga. One can read, for example, that

> the ascetic should fix the thought-organ (mind), closely united with study, on a single point, rolling together the group of the senses (in the thought-organ), sitting like a stick of wood (XII.188.5).
>
> When he rolls together the senses and the thought-organ, this is described by me (Bhīṣma) as the first course of meditation (XII.188.10).[107]

After describing a period wherein the thoughts of the yogin may become unsteady, the speaker, Bhīṣma—a wise teacher and heroic warrior—instructs the practitioner not to be discouraged and to persist in meditation: "Undespondent and undistressed, free from weariness and selfishness, the one who knows the discipline (Yoga) of meditation *(dhyāna)* shall again concentrate his thought by meditation" (XII.188.14).[108] In the next verse several levels of meditation are distinguished that are close to Patañjali's classical terminology. Thus, Bhīṣma briefly mentions the meditative stages of *vitarka* ("cogitation," "discursive thought"), *vicāra* ("subtle reflection"), and *viveka* ("discrimination") without explaining them further.[109] The yogin who is successful at meditation enters the state of complete inner peace and bliss: "Endowed with that bliss he will abide happily in the process of meditation. For thus possessors of Yoga go to that *nirvāṇa* which is free from disease."[110]

It is not unreasonable to assume that the didactic passages of the *Mahābhārata* epic, notably the *Mokṣadharma,* were probably composed between the third century BCE and the third century CE. The fact that teachings such as the above-mentioned "Yoga of meditation" *(dhyāna)* as well as "breath control" *(prāṇāyāma),* concentration *(dhāraṇā),* and not least the cultivation of moral virtues (e.g., truthfulness, nonviolence, compassion) were incorporated in the *Mahābhārata* clearly alludes to their importance and indeed popularity during this time. As can be seen from our brief look at Upaniṣadic and epic literature, Yoga developed into a strong and challenging presence within the Hindu fold thereby laying a solid foundation for what was to manifest as a coherent, successful and enduring formulation of

Yoga philosophy and practice, namely as contained in the *Yoga-Sūtra* of Patañjali.

YOGA AND *SAMĀDHI*

Yoga can refer to both the method that "joins" and the "harnessed" state—sometimes referred to as "union." Viewed from another angle, Yoga can denote the process of becoming liberated as well as the final "goal" of liberation *(mokṣa, mukti, apavarga)* or Being itself. However, what are thus "joined together" in Yoga must be understood according to the specific context. G. Feuerstein writes:

> In the *Ṛg-veda* the root *yuj* and its derivative *Yoga* are still predominately used in the sense of "yoking, harnessing." *Yoga* is the restraining of the senses for the purpose of magically attracting the numinous forces in the universe. However, the mythic form of *Yoga,* as we have known it since the time of the early *Upaniṣads* intends to be a path of return to the primordial source *(yoni)* by way of "re-linking" *(saṃyoga)* with the Origin.[111]

"Yoga" is frequently interpreted as the "union" of the individual self *(jīvātman)* with the transcendent Self *(paramātman),* as can be seen in the nondualist tradition of Vedānta, a tradition which has influenced a large number of Yoga schools. Yājñavalkya[112]—a Yoga adept who is often mentioned or quoted in the later Upaniṣads (and who may have been the author of the *Yoga-Yājñavalkya-Saṃhitā*)—tells us that Yoga is "the union of the *jīvātman* with the *paramātman.*"[113] In the *Mahānirvāṇa Tantra* ("Treatise on the Great Extinction"), dating from the eleventh century CE, Yoga has been defined as "the unity of the *jīva* with the transcendent Self *(ātman).*"[114] Abhinavagupta's (tenth to eleventh century CE) *Tantrasāra* (702) states: "Yoga is undoubtedly the union of *Śiva* (the transcendent pole representing the "possessor" of power) and *Śakti* (the dynamic pole of creative power and energy)."[115] The idea of "union" is also highlighted in the *Viṣṇu Purāṇa* (VI.7.31), where Yoga has been defined as the union of the purified mind with *brahman.*[116]

Not only the "joining" or "union" but also the methods and practices leading to the "joining" or "union" are called Yoga. If the methods are divided into the main and the subsidiary, then even the subsidiary methods are part of Yoga. In addition to the six main forms of Yoga previously mentioned (see p. 6 above), there are in the Sanskritic tradition of Hinduism various compound words that end in *-yoga.* On the whole these do not represent autonomous schools of Yoga. In the above context, the term "yoga" refers to a specific form or method of "practice." For example, the compound *buddhi-yoga*[117] means the practice of discernment, and *saṃnyāsa-yoga*[118] denotes the practice of renunciation. Other examples include: *dhyāna-yoga*[119] (the practice of meditation), *kriyā-yoga*[120] (the Yoga of ritual action), and *nāda-yoga*[121] (the Yoga of the inner sound).

Within the fold of Hinduism, all authentic forms of Yoga can be conceived as ways to an unchanging "center" of Being, the transcendent Reality of spirit or authentic identity *(ātman, puruṣa),* which may be defined variously depending on the particular school of Yoga one is examining. The genuine practitioner (yogin) of Yoga is thus motivated by a recognition of the necessity for self-transcendence (i.e., the transcendence of ordinary human consciousness), also understood as the desire to realize one's true nature or intrinsic identity as an immortal state of being (i.e., the realization of the Self or "God"). Yoga cannot be reduced to any one *system* of thought and practice. There can be no totalization of Yoga for in all its rich diversity Yoga proper is not a uniform whole. Even just a cursory look at Yoga in its historical context reveals that methods/techniques/practices and philosophies of Yoga can vary from school to school and from preceptor to preceptor.

Yet despite the complex nature and diverse range of ideas in Yoga, it must be emphasized that the various branches and schools of Yoga do share an essential concern, that being with a state of consciousness and immeasurable identity that clearly transcends our normal boundaries of empirical identity or selfhood. This crucial orientation is evident in the definition of Yoga given by the great Yoga authority Vyāsa (ca. fifth–sixth century CE) where, in his commentary on the *Yoga-Sūtra,* the *Yoga-Bhāṣya,* he states: "Yoga is *samādhi.*"[122] The word *samādhi*[123] literally means "placing, putting together." What is "put together" or "unified" is the sense of self or subject along with the object of contemplation. *Samādhi* is both the practice or "technique" of the unification of consciousness and the resulting state of "union" with the perceived object. Mircea Eliade suggested[124] that *samādhi* be appropriately rendered as *"enstasy"* rather than *"ecstasy."* Derived from Greek origin, the term "ecstasy" means to stand *(stasis)* outside *(ex)* the ordinary self or ego, whereas the term "enstasy" ultimately denotes one's standing in *(en)* the Self—the transcendent essence or source of contingent identity, that is, the ego-personality. Both interpretations, however, are entirely valid according to the degree or depth of *samādhi* being experienced. As we will see later in this study (chapters 4–6), there are forms of *samādhi* in Yoga that resemble more ecstasy than enstasy. We can permanently abide in and as spirit or Self only when we transcend the barriers of empirical selfhood, the egoic claim to authentic being. Exactly how this unconditional identity is interpreted and what means are recommended for its realization again vary from school to school.

The definition of Yoga as "union" is popular among Vedānta and neo-Vedānta followers and, as we have seen, generally implies a union between the individual self and the supreme Self, an identity that can be equated with *brahman* (the underlying, transcendent Reality). According to some scholars, the notion of "union," while making sense within the context of Vedānta, is not representative of all forms of Yoga. It is valid in regard to earlier schools of Yoga, that is, as seen, for example, in the *Kaṭha, Śvetāśvatara,* or *Maitrāyaṇīya Upaniṣad*s, and the *Bhagavadgītā* and *Mokṣadharma* section of the *Mahābhārata,* and it also generally applies to the later, postclassical schools of Yoga as given expression in the *Yoga Upaniṣad*s, tantric forms of Yoga and *haṭha-yoga,* all which basically subscribe to a form of Vedāntic, nondualist, or panentheistic philosophy. G. Feuerstein argues that the metaphor of "union" does not have any real place in the system of classical Yoga: "it is definitely inapplicable to Patañjali's [Yoga] . . . whose essence consists rather in a 'disunion,' namely the disjunction of the Self *(puruṣa)* and the world *(prakṛti).* There is no question of any union with the Divine."[125] Max Müller also observes that the aim and culmination of Patañjali's Yoga in not to unite, as is generally understood, but to disunite, to separate, to isolate the spirit or Self *(puruṣa)* from "matter" *(prakṛti),* thereby "returning" to the Self its essential and original purity.[126] This understanding of Yoga was expressed by Bhoja Rāja (eleventh century CE), a Śaivaite yogin and commentator on the *Yoga-Sūtra,* who states that Yoga means "separation" *(viyoga).*[127] Bhoja Rāja argued that the foundational technique or method utilized in Patañjali's classical Yoga is the "discrimination" *(viveka)* between the transcendent, spiritual Self *(puruṣa)* and the "nonself" *(anātman)*—the realm of "matter" *(prakṛti)* that includes our psychophysical being.

Etymologically, the word *samādhi* can mean the "settling down" or one-pointedness of the intellect *(buddhi)* or mind *(citta)* on some object,[128] which in turn gives rise to a steady, peaceful state of mind. In this regard *samādhi* has very clear affinities with the meaning of Yoga. In the *Kaṭha Upaniṣad* (II.3.11; see n. 70 above) Yoga has been described as "steadiness" or "attentiveness" *(apramatta)* of mind. The *Bhagavadgītā* (II.48; see n. 86 above) defines Yoga as "equanimity" or "evenness" *(samatva).* This special state of mind allows the yogin to function in the world through a mode of activity described by Kṛṣṇa as "skill in action";[129] that is to say, the yogin performs alloted actions without any attachment to the results, without being obsessively concerned with the fruits of the activity (*BG* IV.20). Thus it is not difficult to see how and why Yoga could be equated (as Vyāsa has done) with *samādhi, samādhi* signifying a state of steadiness or evenness allowing for an alertness and lucidity of mind that culminates in the "unification" or identity of the subject or "seer" with the object or "seeable." This view is again reinforced in the *Bhagavadgītā* where Yoga is said to be attained when the intellect is no longer distracted by what is heard and stands immovable and steady in a state of *samādhi*.[130]

According to Vyāsa's definition ("Yoga is *samādhi*"), the word Yoga—as Patañjali uses it in *Yoga-Sūtra* I.1—is derived not from *yuj* meaning "yoking" or "joining," but from the verb whose meaning is similar to *samādhi.* The learned commentator Vācaspati Miśra (ninth century CE) notes that the term Yoga should be derived from the root *yuja* (in the sense of "concentration") and not from *yujir* (in the sense of "conjunction").[131] Vācaspati may have been compelled to make this remark because in the nondualist tradition of Vedānta with which he was familiar the term *yoga* is frequently explained as the union *(saṃyoga)* between the individual self and the transcendent Self. This understanding of Yoga does not formally apply to Patañjali's classical school, which emphasizes the distinction between unchanging identity and the changing identity of empirical selfhood and, it is often argued, culminates in an absolute separation between pure consciousness or Self *(puruṣa)* and the realm of nature, psychophysical being and its source *(prakṛti).* One may ask, however, why it is generally acknowledged that the word *yoga* may be derived from the verb meaning "joining" or "yoking." This may be explained by the fact that the sages of the Upaniṣads experienced *samādhi* as a union of the individual and the universal Self, thereby lending a secondary meaning to the same verb. The primary meaning was probably "concentration," as seen, for example, in the *Ṛg Veda* (V.81.1);[132] but elsewhere the Vedic and Upaniṣadic literature is replete with usage of the verbs meaning "concentration" (i.e., *samādhi*) in the sense of "uniting," and "joining," as well as "restraining" and "yoking."[133] A study of the ancient texts shows therefore that the forms are used interchangeably. Why the outstanding grammarian, Pāṇini, chose to differentiate them so substantially can only be answered by hazarding the guess that perhaps by his time (ca. fourth-fifth century BCE) the conjugational forms of the verbs had settled into fixed meanings as recorded by him.

The oral tradition does not indulge in the artificial rules of grammar, but in his major work on grammar, the *Mahābhāṣya,* Patañjali[134] (ca. second century BCE) admits that grammarians only acknowledge the usage of words as found in the Vedas and voiced among the people. Therefore, it would appear that any conflicts between grammarians and philosophers need not arouse undue concern. Furthermore, since philosophy is central to this present study, it will be necessary to inquire into the meaning of Vyāsa's statement that the word "Yoga" in the *Yoga-Sūtra* means *samādhi.*[135]

Mādhavācārya (fourteenth century CE) advocates in the "Patañjali-Darśanam" chapter of his *Sarva-Darśana Saṃgraha,* that Yoga is to be equated with *samādhi.*[136] It is generally the case, Mādhavācārya explains, that the process leading to awakening in *samādhi* begins with restraining the senses and yoking the mind to the inner self; and that the experience of *samādhi* itself is joining the individual self and the supreme Self.[137] All of these various stages or levels of the endeavor and experience are, according to Mādhavācārya, meant to be included in the process of Yoga. Since "restraining," "yoking," or "joining" used separately would have been incomplete, one could hypothesize that Vyāsa chose to derive the word from the verb whose meaning is similar to *samādhi.* As U. Arya informs us, the above approach "falls within the convention of Indian logic known as *aṅgāṅgi-bhāva:* that is to say, when a statement is made concerning a complete entity (*aṅgin* 'one who owns *aṅga*s, or parts'), each one of its parts *(aṅga*s*)* is already included."[138] Mādhavācārya asserts that the practice and experience of *samādhi* is inclusive of "restraining," "yoking," or "joining" since these are all contained within the eight *aṅga*s (*YS* II.29) or "limbs" of Yoga as outlined by Patañjali.[139] If, in the above context, Bhoja Rāja's definition of Yoga is also taken into consideration (see n. 127 above), then not only the dynamic of "joining," "harnessing" or a "union," but even a "separation" *(viyoga)* may be included among the "parts" that constitute the complete process of *samādhi.* But a further in-depth exploration into the meaning of *samādhi* will be reserved for the later chapters (4–6) on the classical Yoga of Patañjali.

THE PEDAGOGICAL DIMENSION OF YOGA: (i) THE PRACTITIONER (YOGIN) AND THE COMMITMENT TO PRACTICE

The practitioner of Yoga is designated by the term *yogin* (in the nominative: *yogī*), which, like the word *yoga,* is derived from the verbal root *yuj* (see n. 6 above). A yogin may be broadly classified as: (1) a novice or beginning student, (2) an advanced or mature student, or (3) an enlightened adept *(guru),* implying one who has arrived at the highest level of spiritual awakening. A female practitioner is called a *yoginī.* The masculine noun *yogin,* however, can be generically applied to all spiritual practitioners of Yoga. Throughout our study the term *yogin* has been adopted as there is nothing inherent in the context of Yoga which asserts that *yogin* cannot refer to a male or a female practitioner.

The spiritual development of the yogin is often portrayed hierarchically in an attempt to distinguish between levels of commitment, growth (i.e., self-transcendence) and awareness. Vijñāna Bhikṣu (sixteenth century CE), a yogin and Vedāntic philosopher, differentiates between the following levels in his *Yoga-Sāra-Saṃgraha* ("Summary of the Essence of Yoga"): (1) *Ārurukṣu*—referring to one who is desirous of a life based on Yoga; (2) *Yuñjāna*—referring to one who is actually practicing; and (3) *Yogārūḍha*—referring to one who is advanced or "ascended" in Yoga, also called *yukta* ("yoked one") or *sthita-prajñā* ("one of firmly established wisdom").[140] The *Bhagavadgītā* characterizes the latter two—the aspirant-practitioner and the more accomplished adept—in these words:

> Action is stated to be the medium for the sage who desires to ascend to Yoga. For one who has already ascended to such Yoga, serenity is said to be the medium.[141]
>
> When one does not cling to actions or to the sense-objects and has renounced all compulsive intention and expectation, then one is said to have ascended in Yoga.[142]
>
> When one whose mind controlled abides in the Self alone and is freed from yearning, then one is said to be "yoked" (disciplined).[143]

In the second chapter of the *Bhagavadgītā,* the yogin who is of firmly established wisdom (*sthita-prajñā, BG* II.54), is described as follows: "One whose mind is not affected in the midst of sorrow and is free from desire in the midst of pleasure, and who is without attachment, fear and anger, is said to be a sage of steadied vision."[144]

An interesting fourfold division is presented in the *Yoga-Bhāṣya* of Vyāsa, which describes the yogin at four different levels of accomplishment: (1) *Prāthama-kalpika*—the beginner or neophyte in the first stages of Yoga; (2) *Madhu-bhūmika*—one who has arrived at the "honeyed" or delightful stage; (3) *Prajñā-jyotis*—one who has attained the "light" of knowledge or illuminative insight; and (4) *Atikrānta-bhāvanīya*—one who has gone beyond all that was to be cultivated.[145] Vyāsa elaborates on these four stages of yogic attainment as follows:

> The first is the practitioner for whom the light of knowledge has just begun to dawn. The second is one who has attained to "truth-bearing" insight. The third is one who has subjugated the elements and the sense-organs and has developed means for securing all that has been and is yet to be cultivated [by that one]. . . . While the fourth who has passed beyond that which may be cultivated has as one's sole aim the "resolution" of the mind [into its source—the unmanifest *prakṛti*]. One's insight then attains to the seven final stages [*YS* II.27][146] [whereupon the Self abides in its intrinsic purity or own form/identity].[147]

The last stage of transcendence leads to the culminating goal of classical Yoga—the liberated state of "aloneness" *(kaivalya)*. This is the realization of the Self *(puruṣa)*, the eternal, spiritual essence of our human identity that transcends the ever-changing manifest or the unmanifest dimension of the cosmos *(prakṛti)*. *Kaivalya*—which will be examined in detail in chapter 6—is the state of spiritual liberation and the highest "attainment" in the life of the yogin who follows Patañjali's teachings on Yoga.

Once more, in his *Bhāṣya,* Vyāsa explains that there is a ninefold classification of yogins, according to the intensity of their quest, which may be mild *(mṛdu)*, moderate *(madhya)*, or ardent *(adhimātra)*.[148] Vācaspati Miśra (ninth century CE) explains that the degree of intensity and momentum of progress depends on the yogin's accumulated impressions *(saṃskāra*s*)* from past experiences, even lifetimes, as well as hidden karmic influences *(adṛṣṭa)*.[149] The depth of one's attraction to the realization of authentic identity *(puruṣa)* is preconditioned by one's karmic past in that one's actions, volitions and intentions not only in the present lifetime but also in past lives determine one's future embodiments or states of being (i.e., one's genetic composition and psychophysical as well as social identity).[150] One's commitment to Yoga discipline or practice *(sādhana)* is not entirely under one's control, and especially in the beginning stages of practice the yogin must persist in self-discipline in the face of any adversities. One's rate of progress is dependent upon the intensity of one's method *(upāya)* and the degree of one's momentum, energy or intensity *(saṃvega)*. For one whose rate of progress is fast—whose practice is strongly intense with ardent energy—Patañjali tells us that *samādhi* is very near.[151] Yogins at this level of practice soon attain *samādhi* and the fruit of *samādhi,*[152] which is "aloneness" *(kaivalya)*.[153] This intense level of commitment, however, refers to those yogins who practice at the highest level of intensity, for as *Yoga-Sūtra* I.22 informs us, "Hence, even [among the ardent] there is a distinction of the mild, moderate and ardent."[154] The highest level of intensity spoken of does not refer to "excessive asceticism or pathological mortification." Rather, it involves genuine "enthusiasm"[155] and a commitment that, as I later argue, is properly grounded in an integral approach to life.

THE PEDAGOGICAL DIMENSION OF YOGA: (ii) THE SPIRITUAL GUIDE OR PRECEPTOR *(GURU)*

In his well-known study of Yoga, M. Eliade rightly declares, "What characterizes Yoga is not only its practical side, but also its initiatory structure."[156] Yoga presupposes the guidance of a spiritual preceptor or adept who has direct experience of the insights and realizations as well as the distractions or obstacles that may arise on the path of Yoga. Ideally, the teacher or *guru* should be a "true teacher" *(sad-guru),* having attained the ultimate realization informing all yogic endeavor, which, in the language of different yogic schools, can be referred to as enlightenment *(bodha),* liberation *(mokṣa),* or "aloneness" *(kaivalya).* The *sad-guru* is looked upon as an invaluable agent of grace *(anugraha, prasāda)* and compassion *(karuṇā).* However, as the author of the *Śiva Purāṇa*[157] observes, if a preceptor is only nominal, so is the enlightenment thus bestowed on the disciple *(śiṣya).* Yoga does not conceal its criticisms of false teachers or *gurus* (see n. 172 below). Moreover, contrary to popular conceptions of Yoga adopted by many Westerners, authentic forms of Yoga are *never* a self-appropriating endeavor or "do-it-yourself" undertaking. As Eliade wisely remarked, "One does not learn *Yoga* by oneself."[158] Yoga entails a profound pedagogical commitment involving periods of study during which preceptors can communicate and transmit their wisdom to worthy disciples or devotees. This crucial pedagogical context is exemplified in the *Bhagavad-gītā* where Kṛṣṇa instructs Arjuna: "Know this [knowledge] by obeisance, by inquiry and by service to them. Those of wisdom, who themselves have seen the truth, will instruct you in this knowledge."[159] Mere conceptual knowledge, words or metaphysical speculation cannot contain or exhaust the knowledge *(jñāna)* spoken of by Kṛṣṇa. In a succinct description of the central role of the Hindu *guru,* J. D. Mlecko writes:

> Primarily . . . the guru is the personal teacher of spirituality, that is, of the basic, ultimate values perceived within the Hindu tradition. Further, the guru possesses experiential knowledge, not only intellectual knowledge, of these values. In a word, the guru is indispensable for spiritual development. In early Hinduism he was a vital factor in imparting *Vedic* knowledge; in

> later thought the guru became the visible embodiment of truth and in some cases he was worshipped as an incarnate deity.[160]

The "heavy" authority given to the *guru* or "weighty one" places the preceptor at the hub of the entire initiatory and pedagogical structure of Yoga. The Upaniṣads have preserved examples of some of the more profound teacher/disciple relationships, in which the pinnacle of spiritual wisdom, not merely intellectual knowledge, was pursued. Having experienced directly the scriptural revelation, the enlightened adept is thus deemed fit to prepare others for the same realization. Hence the *Śiva-Saṃhitā* declares: "[Only] knowledge imparted by way of the teacher's mouth is productive; otherwise it is fruitless, weak and leads to much suffering."[161]

Spiritual initiation *(dīkṣā)*[162] is a crucially important notion in Yoga for it involves an essential transference of knowledge *(jñāna)* or spiritualized power *(śakti)* from the *guru* to the disciple *(śiṣya)* enabling the transforming processes of Yoga to come into their own. Through initiation, the disciple gains access to the *guru*'s state of consciousness and even mysteriously becomes a part of the *guru*'s line of transmission *(paraṃparā)*. The transmission of spiritual energy and awareness to the aspirant through the *guru*'s "proximity" or "nearness" has been noted from ancient to modern times:

> Education has been aptly defined as the transmission of life from life to life. This ideal seems to have been literally realized under . . . [the] ancient pedagogic system.[163]

> Merely to be in this man's presence [his *guru*'s] seemed to be enough to dissolve all problems, to make them non-existent, like darkness in the presence of light.[164]

> When one enters into right relationship with a Spiritual Master, changes happen in the literal physics of one's existence. . . . The transforming process is . . . through that Living Company.[165]

The synonym for *dīkṣā, abhiṣeka,* refers to the ritualistic "sprinkling" of consecrated water on the devotee—a form of baptism. By means of initiation the spiritual process is either activated or intensified in the practitioner. It is a direct empowerment in which the adept effects in the disciple a transformation or turnabout of consciousness, a metanoia.[166]

The initiatory teacher/disciple system dates back to the early Vedic period (ca. 1200–900 BCE) where a young boy would spend his youth and adolescence in the home of a teacher of the sacred canonical scriptures, a teacher whose authority represented the wisdom of the holy texts. Vedic knowledge was transmitted orally to the student by the teacher and had to be properly memorized. The interpersonal dimension of education was highly regarded. It was the teacher's responsibility to guide and counsel the disciple through study and understanding of the Vedas, and to attend to the disciple's welfare. In the *Ṛg Veda*[167] the *guru* is described as the source and inspirer of spiritual knowledge, or the essence of reality, for the seeker. In the *Yajur-Veda*[168] the *guru* is described as the one who blesses and enhances the seeker's spiritual life. The formalized relationship between teacher and disciple is referred to as the *guru-kula* ("teacher's household") system. The following statement by R. K. Mookerji describes this original model of education:

> The school . . . is the home of the teacher. It is a hermitage, amid sylvan surroundings, beyond the distractions of urban life, functioning in solitude and silence. The constant and intimate association between teacher and taught is vital to education as conceived in this system. The pupil is to imbibe the inward method of the teacher, the secrets of his efficiency, the spirit of his life, and these things are too subtle to be taught.[169]

Its rationale is given in the *Taittirīya Upaniṣad* as follows: "The teacher is the first form. The student is the latter form. Knowledge is their junction. Instruction is the connection."[170] The key role and necessity of a *guru* became more and more explicit throughout the Upaniṣads. As the *Chāndogya Upaniṣad* puts it, only by knowledge received directly from the *guru* can one attain the purest, most beneficent and subtle truth.[171] In the *Kaṭha Upaniṣad*, the guru is represented as being indispensible to the attainment of knowledge.[172] Study by oneself, perceived as an end in itself, is repeatedly disapproved of in the Upaniṣads for even exclusive self-study cannot give one liberating knowledge.

Composed of the verbal root *sad* ("to sit") prefixed with *upa* and *ni* (together meaning "near"),[173] the term *upaniṣad* thus conveys the idea of "sitting down near" the teacher, who instructs the disciple. The Upaniṣadic dialogues involving the teacher or *guru* figure are clearly didactic (such as the dialogue in the *Kaṭha Upaniṣad* between the *śiṣya,* Naciketas, and the *guru,* Yama). They reveal little about the actual character of the *gurus*. However, the methods espoused by the *gurus* are clear and varied and they all have a soteriological goal. For example, in the *Bṛhadāraṇyaka Upaniṣad,* the teacher Yājñavalkya, instructing his wife Maitreyī, used the *neti neti* ("not this, not this") method through which it is revealed that all positive descriptions of the Self *(ātman)* can only act as pointers to that Reality which transcends all thought. All affirmations about Reality are not ultimately true. When all attachment to ideas is eliminated, the unmodified and ineffable Self alone remains.[174] In the *Taittirīya Upaniṣad,*[175] Varuṇa—the guardian of cosmic order and overseer of moral action—urges his disciple *(śiṣya)* (and son), Bhṛgu, to perform asceticism *(tapas),* to strive for, discover, and directly experience the truth of *brahman.* On the other hand, in the *Chāndogya Upaniṣad* the *guru,* Uddālaka, made use of analogies to enable his students to gain insight into the nature of *ātman* as the invisible essence of life, and then concluded with the famous expression to his son Śvetaketu, *"tat tvam asi"* or "That thou art."[176]

The formal method of teaching included a dialectical approach whereby the student asked questions and the teacher discoursed upon them. There was, however, more to the method than simply asking and listening. There was the insistence, as the *śiṣya* advanced, on contemplating ultimate reality and realizing or actualizing it in one's own life. The responsibility of spiritual growth ultimately devolved on the *śiṣya* and not on the *guru.* R. K. Mookerji relates the following:

> The *[Bṛhadāraṇyaka Upaniṣad]* clearly states that education in the highest knowledge depends upon three processes following one another. . . . *[Śravaṇa]* is listening to what is taught by the teacher. . . . *Manana* is defined as constant contemplation of the One Reality in accordance with the ways of reasoning aiding in its apprehension. *Nididhyāsana* is concentrated contemplation of the truth so as to realize it.[177]

The *śiṣya* must be seriously engaged in the above three disciplines, all of which demand a great deal of focus and commitment.

Many of the yogic practices within Tantrism (ca. fifth century CE) necessitate the guidance of an accomplished preceptor. Shashibhusan Dasgupta observes, "Because of their stringent nature these practices have repeatedly been declared in all the *Tantras* as the secret of all secrets . . . and, therefore there is no other way of being initiated into this method of yoga save the practical help of the *guru.*"[178] There are many functional types of *guru*s, and the Yoga scholar M. P. Pandit, in his translation of the *Kulārṇava Tantra* (a medieval text), mentions no fewer than twelve.[179] Eventually, the *guru*'s presence, energy and personality affect the whole spiritual life of the yogin as the passage cited below seems to imply: "The form of the guru is the root of *dhyāna,* the lotus feet of the guru is the root of *pūjā,* the word of the guru is the root of *mantra,* and the grace of the guru is the root of *siddhi* [supernatural power]."[180] The tantric *guru* is not just a learned person but in the eyes of the disciples has attained, embodies and *is* the highest Reality.[181]

Moreover, within the Hindu fold in general, it is the perfected *guru,* the fully liberated preceptor, the true "dispeller of darkness [i.e., ignorance],"[182] who is extolled in the yogic scriptures above all others; and it is the qualified disciple *(adhikārin* or *sādhaka)*—competent and worthy of instruction—who is eligible for formal spiritual initiation. By empowering the initiation process, the *guru* undertakes his/her responsibility to function as a catalyst in order to undermine the disciple's ignorance *(avidyā)* of authentic identity *(ātman, puruṣa)* and awaken the disciple to spiritual freedom. Thus the pedagogical dynamic embodied in the *guru*-disciple relation constitutes one of the essential building blocks of the Yoga tradition and is itself an integral component of Yoga theory and practice. The soteriological and practical orientation in Yoga is inseparable from the pedagogical context in which it has arisen.

CONCLUDING REMARKS

As can be seen from the above preliminary, background, albeit sketchbook look at Yoga, it is important to acknowledge that the classical formulation of Yoga within Hinduism as given shape in the *Yoga-Sūtra* did not appear in a vacuum but rather was preceded by many centuries of ingenuity and profound investigation into the possibilities for self-transcendence and ultimate freedom *(mokṣa).* The early development of Yoga within Hinduism as, for example, given expression in the Upaniṣads, pointed to the necessity for direct experience of Reality or rather permanent abiding as the Self *(ātman, puruṣa),* an all-pervading, omniscient identity in which the normal, conventional, and empirical boundaries confining our sense of self to the conditional, saṃsāric realm were transcended. Thus, through the transformation and illumination of consciousness involving a sacrifice of mistaken identity or egoity, a radical identity shift or change in perspective—from that of the mortal ego-personality to that of the immortal Self—could take place.

Notwithstanding the above overall emphasis given to Yoga, that is, of self-transcendence, a study of Yoga's richly textured history, its traditional goals and purposes, reveals that Yoga cannot be properly conceived as a monolithic system but rather as a tradition that has been burgeoning since its incipience in ancient times. In its long complex evolution Yoga can be seen as a vast tradition (or, rather, as several traditions within a tradition) that has incorporated a diverse and rich body of teachings within Hinduism and indeed other religious traditions[183] over a period of many centuries. What does become clear is that Yoga achieved a philosophical maturity in the classical period (ca. 150–800 CE) when the appearance of the *Yoga-Sūtra* of Patañjali (ca. second–third century CE) provided a foundational text on the formal philosophical system of Yoga *(yoga-darśana).*

The purpose of our broadly based exposition has not been to provide a detailed exploration into the complexity of Yoga as a multifaceted phenomenon that embraces a number of spiritual paths and orientations "with contrasting theoretical frameworks and occasionally incompatible goals."[184] Nor has it been the concern of this brief introduction on Yoga to conduct an exhaustive review of the history, literature, and branches of even the early (pre-classical) Hindu tradition of Yoga: its metaphysical ideas, related practices, and soteriological perspectives. Rather, this chapter has focused and elaborated on a select range of ideas, texts, and disciplines that can enhance our understanding and appreciation of early forms of Yoga as they have evolved mostly within a Hindu context. The material presented profiles some of the simple, basic contributing ideas on Yoga and is meant to act as a backdrop and an embedding matrix by highlighting certain relevant pointers that will come into their own over the course of the study on Patañjali's Yoga, to which we will now turn.

chapter two

The Yoga-Sūtra:
Introduction and Metaphysical Perspective

INTRODUCTION TO PATAÑJALI AND THE *YOGA-SŪTRA*

Few scholars, if any, would disagree that a precise analysis of the human condition from the perspective of the sophisticated *darśana* known as *Pātañjala Yoga* remains a desideratum in Indological studies. In the Western world few things are more confused about Indian thought than the understanding of the term "Yoga," which as one scholar succinctly states, "is a Sanskrit word which everybody knows, but in spite of *haṭha-yoga* classes and widespread curiosity about oriental mysticism, there is little sound information available about the main authority on *Yoga*—the *Yoga-Sūtra* of Patañjali."[1] What can generally be acknowledged as a Western misconstrual of Yoga is also true for India, the motherland of Yoga. K. S. Joshi writes: "It is an amazing fact that even in the land of *Yoga,* superstitious and fanciful notions of the subject seem to have wide currency. The philosophy of *Yoga* is perhaps one of the least known of its aspects."[2] After giving a brief introduction to Patañjali and the *Yoga-Sūtra,* our discussion will focus on the basic philosophical stance of Patañjali's Yoga, highlighting some of the major differences as well as similarities between classical Yoga and classical Sāṃkhya, and outlining Patañjali's metaphysical schematic.

The classical formulation of the Yoga *darśana* by Patañjali (ca. second-third century CE)—the reputed author of the *Yoga-Sūtra*—is truly a climactic event in the long development of yogic practice and philosophy (see previous chapter). Out of all the various yogic schools in existence around the time of the composition of the *Yoga-Sūtra,* it was Patañjali's that was to become recognized as *the* authoritative perspective *(darśana)* of the Brāhmaṇic Yoga tradition. The *Yoga-Sūtra* represents an attempt to provide succinct and soteriologically effective definitions, explanations and descriptions of key concepts and terms relating to *theoria* and *praxis* in Yoga, thereby providing Yoga with a systematic, comprehensive, and foundational grounding and formulation that led to its legitimization as one of the six *darśana*s or philosophical schools within Brāhmaṇical Hinduism. As can be gathered from numerous sources including the extensive commentarial literature on the *Yoga-Sūtra* and references—of both a praiseworthy and critical nature—to the *Yoga-Sūtra* in the literature of orthodox and nonorthodox Hindu schools, this text had early on gained considerable influence and was recognized as the source text *(prasthāna-vākya)* that established Yoga as an independent perspective within the arena of Hindu soteriological thought.[3]

Historically, little if anything of certainty is known about Patañjali, and scholars have been unable to ascertain whether he is the same or different from the Patañjali who is the celebrated author of the *Mahābhāṣya* (ca. second century BCE), the great commentary on Pāṇini's grammar. Scholars such as R. Garbe[4] and S. N. Dasgupta[5] maintain that the grammarian and the Yoga writer are identical. The traditional identification of Patañjali with his namesake the grammarian was first made by Bhoja Rāja (eleventh century CE) in his *Rāja-Mārtaṇḍa.*[6] Following along the lines of S. N. Dasgupta, T. S. Rukmani states that the date "can be accepted as between the second century BC and the first century AD,"[7] thereby allowing for the possibility of the composer of the *Yoga-Sūtra* and the grammarian of the same name being identical. Scholarly opinion, however, seems to have arrived at a consensus that renders the above possible identification unlikely. The historicality, contents and the terminology of the *Yoga-Sūtra* suggest the period between 150-500 CE as a probable time-frame for Patañjali, although the traditions from which its author draws are undoubtedly older[8] (see introductory chapter and below). Dates within this time period have been argued for by scholars such as: Jacobi,[9] Keith,[10] Woods,[11] Hauer,[12] Frauwallner,[13] von Glassenapp,[14] Winternitz,[15] Larson,[16] and Feuerstein.[17] Based on the evidence at hand, it would appear that the *Yoga-Sūtra* is a product of the second[18] or third century CE.

Again, according to Hindu tradition, Patañjali was an incarnation of Ananta or Śeṣa, the "thousand-headed" leader of the serpent race. Ananta, desiring to teach Yoga on earth, is said to have fallen *(pat)* from "heaven" onto the palm *(añjali)* of a noble woman called Goṇikā. Ananta is often depicted in iconography as the couch on which Lord Viṣṇu takes repose. The numerous heads of the Lord of Serpents are said to symbolize infinity *(ananta)* or omnipresence.[19] The name, Śeṣa ("Remainder"), is explained by the fact that Śeṣa remains after the destruction of the cosmos. Feuerstein informs us that: "Legend . . . knows of him [Patañjali] as the incarnation of the serpent-king Ananta, a manifestation of god Viṣṇu, who is believed to encircle the earth. This identification is at least of symbolic interest. For the serpent race over which Ananta or Śeṣa presides is associated, in mythology, with the guarding of the esoteric lore and Yoga is . . . the secret tradition *par excellence*."[20] To this day, many yogins bow to an image of Ananta before they begin their daily round of yogic exercises.

It is reasonable to assume that Patañjali, as head of a school of Yoga, was an active preceptor or *guru* and, judging from the *Yoga-Sūtra,* a great authority on Yoga whose approach was sympathetic toward philosophical inquiry and exposition. It would not seem unlikely that Patañjali taught a community of disciples *(śiṣya*s*)* devoted to the study and practice of Yoga. Thus, it would follow that there must have been adherents to Patañjali's school who carried on the tradition in the formal context of a particular teaching lineage *(paraṃparā)*.[21] Adopting basically a classical format written in *sūtra* style, Patañjali composed the *Yoga-Sūtra* at a time of intense debate and ongoing philosophical speculation in India. As such, "he supplied Yoga with a reasonably homogenous framework that could stand up against the many rival traditions," including Nyāya, Vedānta, and Buddhism.[22]

The *sūtra* style of writing is employed in the source books *(prasthāna-vākya*s*)* of the so-called six orthodox systems *(ṣaḍ-darśana*s*)* of philosophy within Hinduism. The word *sūtra* has the literal meaning of "thread" (from the root *siv,* to sew). In the above context a *sūtra* means a more or less short thread of sounds (consisting of as little as one word) conveying meaning in a condensed form. A *sūtra* composition is a work comprised of mostly simple, pithy aphoristic statements that taken altogether provide one with a "thread" linking together all the noteworthy ideas representative of that traditional perspective. It attests to the fact that Hindu wisdom schools have traditionally been transmitted by word of mouth thus facilitating such transmission. Moreover, the *sūtra* style within Brāhmaṇic traditions points to an important pedagogical concern: that wisdom was on the whole safeguarded and was not, therefore, to be indiscriminately transmitted. Within the tradition of classical Yoga, a *sūtra* contained within the *Yoga-Sūtra* functions as a mnemonic device for the purpose of recalling and investigating into specific and sometimes complex yogic doctrine and practices, the detailed explanation and instruction being supplied orally by the teacher.[23] Often unintelligible by itself, a *sūtra* requires elucidation by means of an exposition or commentary (see below). However, it should be noted that a *sūtra* functions not only as a mnemonic device because it is taught in an oral tradition. It is both an inspired utterance and a mnemonic formula in need of much background information. Such crucial information was imparted to mature disciples within the tradition in daily study and often in the company of the *guru*—a special gathering referred to as *sat-saṅga* ("contact/company with the Real/Truth"). In order to shed light on the meaning and perhaps relevance of the theory and practice contained in the *Yoga-Sūtra,* later adepts, practitioners and/or scholars of Yoga, from Vyāsa (fifth century CE) onward, wrote extensive commentaries, some of which—such as those by Vācaspati Miśra (ninth century CE) and Vijñāna Bhikṣu (sixteenth century CE)—were commentaries on Vyāsa's own composition.[24]

Turning to Patañjali's work itself, the text of the *Yoga-Sūtra* consists of 195 *sūtra*s distributed over four chapters:

1. *Samādhi-Pāda,* the chapter on ecstasy/enstasy comprised of 51 *sūtra*s;
2. *Sādhana-Pāda,* the chapter on the "path" or "practice" of Yoga made up of 55 *sūtra*s;
3. *Vibhūti-Pāda,* the chapter on the "powers" in Yoga also totaling 55 *sūtra*s;
4. *Kaivalya-Pāda,* the chapter on the liberated state of "aloneness" and consisting of 34 *sūtra*s.

Scholars have, for some time now, questioned the unity of the work, viewing the above division of chapters as somewhat arbitrary and as appearing to be the result of an inadequate reediting of the text. The conclusion reached by some is that in its present form the *Yoga-Sūtra* cannot possibly be considered as unitary.[25] Thus there have been scholarly attempts to reconstruct the original by dissecting the available text into subtexts of presumably independent sources.[26] These efforts, as Feuerstein argues, "have not been very successful, because they leave us with inconclusive fragments."[27] Their approach is justifiably criticized by C. Pensa, who writes:

> In contrast to the approach adopted by many Orientalists who *a priori* tend to deny the unity of the text under examination, fragmenting it into so many parts or heterogeneous strata until nothing remains, Feuerstein

> rightly asks in his methodological study whether this compulsive search for incongruencies and textual corruptions is not the expression of an ethnocentric rationalising mentality which inclines to project everywhere its own need for abstract and absolute logic, and hence is particularly prone to misinterpret paradoxical expressions so common in eastern thought which has a *penchant* for transcending dualism and therefore in part also rational language as such.[28]

The present study takes the overall position that the *Yoga-Sūtra* is a coherent text and that it need not warrant the supposition of multiple authorship or composition over several segments of time. Therefore, the approach that I have adopted accepts the text on its own authority as a complete whole.[29] Many scholars fail to comprehend the inner connections or "threading links" among the *sūtra*s, as well as their relationship with the steps of a guided practice.[30] There is, I submit, an internal coherence or continuity running throughout the text where the meanings of key yogic terms are seen to be interdependent and interrelate with each other. It is preferable, therefore, to take a more sympathetic view of Patañjali's work and acknowledge the possibility that it is far more self-contained and integrated than some scholars have tended to assume.[31] There are different understandings of what constitutes the unity of a text, and without going further into the question I shall treat the *Yoga-Sūtra* as a "unity" for purposes of analysis, suggesting further reasons for an appreciation of its "unity." Even just a cursory reading of the *Yoga-Sūtra* reveals that Patañjali outlines and summarizes a plurality of practices—more than twenty different techniques are specified[32]—and, some would argue, a concatenation of philosophical perspectives or distinct schools of Yoga (e.g., *nirodha-yoga, samādhi-yoga, kriyā-yoga, aṣṭāṅga-yoga*) that provide us with seemingly contrasting descriptions and characteristics of Yoga.[33] Frauwallner has stated that the *Yoga-Sūtra* "is composed of different constituents or elements which, in no way, give a homogeneous picture."[34]

Yet, throughout its long history Patañjali's *Yoga-Sūtra* has proved to be a successful work, and to this day the text remains a highly influential and authoritative spiritual guide in schools of Yoga and Hinduism in general. As C. Chapple rightly argues, the various and extensive methods of practice, perspectives, and attainments explained by Patañjali—although all endeavoring to bring about yogic experience—are meant to "stand in juxtaposition and in complementarity"[35] rather than to compete with each other. It should also be emphasized—even at the risk of disabusing some—that the practice-orientation so prominent in Yoga does not warrant the reduction of Yoga to a purely technical (and somewhat mechanical) enterprise, and we must guard against the tendency, so prevalent today, in which Yoga is perceived merely as a series of "practices." This more modern and popular misconception of Yoga can often result in an overemphasis on "technique" at the expense of developing a sound philosophical understanding of Yoga. In order for it to be properly engaged, Yoga demands our available energy and attention, which includes a high level of study. Patañjali's Yoga is not about the glorification of "technique," which by virtue of bypassing the processes of reflection enables the yogin to supersede or override philosophical investigation. Nor does Yoga attempt to demarcate or separate out theory from practice, taking one and discarding the other. Rather, Patañjali's whole approach unites theory and practice, bridging and healing any rifts between thinking and acting, metaphysics and ethics, transcendence and immanence. This study intends to show that the text of the *Yoga-Sūtra* strives for and achieves a basic unity of conception, including a theory-practice unification, founded in direct yogic experience and given expression in Patañjali's central definition of Yoga (*YS* I.2).

The conciseness and condensed nature of the *sūtra* style of writing used by Patañjali is illustrated in the opening aphorisms of the *Yoga-Sūtra*. In the first four *sūtra*s of the first chapter *(Samādhi-Pāda)* the subject matter of the *Yoga-Sūtra* is mentioned, defined, and characterized. The *sūtra*s run as follows:

Yoga-Sūtra I.1: "Now [begins] the discipline of Yoga."
Yoga-Sūtra I.2: "Yoga is the cessation of [the misidentification with] the modifications of the mind."
Yoga-Sūtra I.3: "Then [when that cessation has taken place] there is abiding in the Seer's own form (i.e., *puruṣa* or intrinsic identity)."
Yoga-Sūtra I.4: "Otherwise [there is] conformity to (i.e., misidentification with) the modifications [of the mind]."[36]

The first four *sūtra*s lay the foundation for the entire system. Having introduced and defined the subject matter, Yoga, the *sūtra*s continue to explain a number of technical terms. The third *sūtra* states what is philosophically most important in the system: One who succeeds in "bringing about" the cessation *(nirodha)* of the misidentification with the modifications *(vṛtti*s*)* of the mind *(citta)* is liberated from any mistaken identity of self and abides as the real Seer or spiritual Self, that is, is established in the true nature and identity of pure, immortal consciousness *(puruṣa)*. The fourth *sūtra* supplements this by declaring that one who is not established in the true form or nature of authentic selfhood *(puruṣa)* "fails to see" or "forgets" intrinsic being by misidentifying with the modifications of the mind, thereby, in effect, conforming to an extrinsic, deluded, and confused self-identity—a changing , empirical, and mortal (perishable, material) sense of selfhood.

The opening *sūtra,* "Now [begins] the discipline of Yoga," states the subject matter and nature of Patañjali's treatise. The two great commentators on Vyāsa's *Bhāṣya,* Vācaspati Miśra and Vijñāna Bhikṣu, consider Patañjali to be not the founder of the Yoga tradition but, according to S. Dasgupta, "an editor."[37] Dasgupta goes on to state that the *Yoga-Sūtra* does "not show any original attempt, but a masterly and systematic compilation which was also supplemented by fitting contributions."[38] Although Patañjali presents his compilation of Yoga as an "exposition" of existing materials[39] that, in effect, constitutes a discipline *(anuśāsana)* of Yoga, his work nevertheless does not lack originality. To be sure, much of the philosophical and praxis-orientation presented in the *Yoga-Sūtra* has its roots in the Upaniṣadic-Brāhmaṇic tradition of early Hinduism, reflecting ideas and practices from, for example, the *Kaṭha, Maitrāyaṇīya,* and *Śvetāśvatara Upaniṣad*s and the *Mahābhārata*. In addition, as some scholars have been keen to point out, the *Yoga-Sūtra* does incorporate techniques/practices that around the time of Patañjali were undoubtedly an integral part of Buddhist and Jain discipline.[40] In his effort to clarify and formalize the yogic tradition, Patañjali compiled and systematized existing knowledge within the Yoga tradition elaborating upon Yoga theory and practice. In his own voice, Patañjali presented major yogic themes, concepts, and terms—largely consistent throughout the text—in a clear and convincing manner, whereby Yoga became recognized as one of the leading schools or classical philosophical systems of India. However, it is not correct to regard Patañjali as the "father of Yoga." There must have been both prior to and during Patañjali's time more nonsystematic Yogas and other yogic compositions that disappeared over time and are now lost. What is clear, however, is that Patañjali's *Yoga-Sūtra* has superseded all earlier *sūtra* works within the Yoga tradition and that this is probably due to the overall comprehensive and systematic nature of Patañjali's presentation of Yoga. In a clear response to those who suggest that Patañjali has made no specific philosophical contribution in his presentation of Yoga, C. Chapple, likening Patañjali's method to the multiplicity of liberating perspectives and practices employed in the *Bhagavadgītā,* writes, "[Patañjali's] is a masterful contribution communicated through nonjudgmentally presenting diverse practices, a methodology deeply rooted in the culture and traditions of

India."[41] Further discussion on the issue of Patañjali's philosophical contribution will be reserved for a later chapter.

Considering that Hiraṇyagarbha[42] is acknowledged as the original teacher of Yoga, why is so much importance given to Patañjali? Why does Patañjali present himself as such a figure of authority? The questions may be responded to in two ways:

1. At the beginning of some manuscripts of Vyāsa's commentary (*YB* I.1), the text says that Patañjali is the same who incarnates again and again to teach the knowledge of Yoga, even though he may bear different names from one lifetime to another. The authenticity of the opening verse of Vyāsa's commentary is controversial because some manuscripts include it[43] and others do not. Most begin with a prayer verse to Āhīśa who is the Lord of Serpents.[44]
2. The other way lies in examining the meaning of the word *anuśāsana,* which has been translated as "discipline."[45]

The word *anuśāsana* (*YS* I.1) is derived from the prefix *anu* and the verb root *śās*. The prefix *anu* denotes that something is subsequent, a follow-up to something else that has formerly occurred or existed.[46] The verb *śās* means "to teach, instruct, inform"[47] and the noun *śāsana* denotes "teaching, instruction, discipline, doctrine."[48] A teaching without an attendant discipline would not be properly expressed by the word *anuśāsana*. From the verb *śās* is derived the word for a disciple *(śiṣya),* one who is instructed with and within a discipline. The prefix *anu* can be understood as having two main connotations in the context of *anuśāsana:* (1) The discipline of Yoga is being imparted only after the student has demonstated a necessary degree of "fitness," that is, through observances of self-discipline, and is fit or prepared for advancing along the "path" of Yoga; and (2) *anuśāsana* means to teach that which has been taught before within an existing tradition, not claiming that anything new has been created by the author.

Vyāsa (*YS* I.1) states that *atha,* meaning "now," has the purpose of indicating *adhikāra*.[49] *Adhikāra* means "authority," "qualification," "entitlement." Since *atha* has other meanings such as "afterwards," "questioning," and "auspiciousness," Vyāsa specifically mentions that in the context of *Yoga-Sūtra* I.1 *atha* is used in the sense of *adhikāra*. Considering Vyāsa's statement, *atha* can be understood as an implicit recognition of Patañjali's authority and a declaration of Patañjali's teaching. By using the prefix *anu,* Patañjali issues a disclaimer to his own authorship of the teaching even though by the word *atha* he has stated his authority to teach it. Implied here, however, are the two essential factors that contribute to the authentic *guru-śiṣya* relationship as applied to Yoga: (i) there is a desire to know *(jijñāsā)*,[50] through critical inquiry and meditative discipline, on the part of the student, and (ii) Patañjali possesses the authoritative "knowledge" of Yoga and wishes to convey it. The "knowledge" is open to one who has the necessary desire *(mumukṣu)* for spiritual liberation and, who being sufficiently qualified to progress on the "path" of Yoga, can therefore be referred to as an *adhikārin*. Such a text taught within a tradition and with a discipline is called a *śāstra;* hence the entire "science" or body of knowledge is known as *yoga-śāstra*.

It may be argued that, unlike the schools of Vedānta (Uttara Mīmāṃsā), Pūrva Mīmāṃsā, and Nyāya, the Sāṃkhya and Yoga systems have no continuing traditional schools where the in-school knowledge may be imparted. Whatever may be the case with Sāṃkhya, Yoga is a living tradition and *guru*s to this day continue to teach the *Yoga-Sūtra* in the *āśrama*s, homes, and monasteries in an unbroken lineage and primarily as an experiential discipline because Yoga philosophy exists on the basis of its practices. As many of the categories of Sāṃkhya philosophy are so closely allied to the Yoga system, the Sāṃkhya tradition has survived as a supportive school in association with Yoga. The Yoga school of philosophy is often referred to as *Sāṃkhya-Yoga*,[51] but a note of caution must be maintained in doing so. Not all the categories of Sāṃkhya are used in Yoga, as even a cursory look at the *Sāṃkhya-Kārikā (SK)* and the *Yoga-Sūtra* will show. The categories of Sāṃkhya are employed practically by all the schools of orthodox Hindu philosophy. Patañjali may well have prefigured or integrated ideas appropriated by the Sāṃkhya tradition as he understood it, Sāṃkhya later being refined and systematized into its classical form in the *Sāṃkhya-Kārikā* of Īśvara Kṛṣṇa (ca. fourth century CE). Sāṃkhya philosophy proper (i.e., in its classical form outlined in the *Sāṃkhya-Kārikā*) does not refer to much of the practical systems of Yoga and cannot return the compliment by calling itself *Sāṃkhya-Yoga*. Classical Yoga philosophy, as formulated by Patañjali in the *Yoga-Sūtra* and later expounded on by Vyāsa, does depend on parts of the Sāṃkhyan system and, it must be emphasized, even gives it a new interpretation. Yoga does not thereby lose its independent status as an autonomous philosophical school *(darśana)*. Thus, in the above context, Vyāsa's commentary can be understood as *Sāṃkhya-pravacana-bhāṣya:* "An Exposition that Enunciates Sāṃkhya." *Sāṃkhya-pravacana*[52] ("Enunciation of Sāṃkhya") is an alternative title of the *Yoga-Sūtra*.

It is not, therefore, that "Vyasa . . . often foist[s] on *Yoga* the philosophy of *Sāṃkhya,*"[53] or that one needs to "combat the overpowering influence exercised by Vyāsa's scholium,"[54] but rather that Vyāsa, having studied and mastered both the Yoga and Sāṃkhya systems, clarifies Patañjali's work within its proper context of Yoga. It must be remembered that both Patañjali and Vyāsa are regarded by Hindu tradition as "seers" *(ṛṣi*s*),* their words equally authentic. In the lineage of Yoga philosophy the two names have been inseparably linked together so that in spite of the existence of later independent commentaries the word *"Yoga-Sūtra"* evokes the name of Vyāsa. Yet, perhaps two or even three centuries separate the two Yoga authorities, and as such it would be inappropriate to accept the *Yoga-Bhāṣya* at face value and without some degree of caution. Vyāsa is often more reflective and systematic than Patañjali and elaborates sometimes at great length.[55] Suffice it to say, however, that like much of the Yoga tradition in India this study regards the *Yoga-Sūtra* and the *Yoga-Bhāṣya* as a single composite whole, the two parts of which complement each other and on which alone rests the authority of all other *vṛtti*s and *ṭīkā*s because it is thus that the Yoga tradition would have it. Moreover, it is not in any way apparent that scholars have fathomed the depth of Vyāsa'a commentary.[56] The purpose of our examination of Vyāsa's work is not to offer a critical analysis of the *Yoga-Bhāṣya* that would try to determine the extent to which Vyāsa correctly explains the *Yoga-Sūtra.* Rather, our study is an attempt to draw upon and clarify the wealth of philosophical knowledge and experiential authenticity that the *Yoga-Bhāṣya* offers in order to aid and deepen our understanding of Patañjali's thought.

DISTINGUISHING SĀṂKHYA AND YOGA, AND THE TRANSITION TO THE *YOGA-SŪTRA*

Preclassical[57] developments of Sāṃkhya[58] (e.g., in the *Mahābhārata,* and Upaniṣadic texts such as the *Kaṭha, Śvetāśvatara,* and *Maitrāyaṇīya,* ca. 500–200 BCE) show a close association with the tradition of Yoga, to the extent that both are mentioned together—as *Sāṃkhya-Yoga* (see below). Sāṃkhyan cosmological speculations are often combined with elaborate descriptions of yogic experience.[59] In contrast to methods of spiritual discipline that emphasize yogic-oriented practices as in the *Śvetāśvatara Upaniṣad* (II.8–10)[60] (i.e., posture, breath control, a favorable place for practice, asceticism *[tapas]*), Sämkhya tends to adopt an intellectual or reasoning method: "The follower of Sāṃkhya is one who reasons or discriminates properly, one whose spiritual discipline is reasoning."[61] This is probably the sense of the term *sāṃkhya* in, for example, *Śvetāśvatara Upaniṣad* VI.13, where the compound *sāṃkhya-yoga-adhigamya*[62] ("to be understood by proper reasoning and spiritual discipline") is used. The enumeration of basic principles *(tattva)* of existence in a hierarchical order[63] is a fundamental aspect of the Sāṃkhyan methodology of salvation by reasoning. On occasion the highest principle is the old Upaniṣadic *brahman* or *ātman,* or it may be "God" *(īśvara).* In varying contexts the Sāṃkhyan methodology implies a monistic, theistic, or dualistic perspective. Early references to Sāṃkhya seem to indicate that pre-*Kārikā* Sāṃkhya (prior to the *Sāṃkhya-Kārikā*) acknowledged *brahman* as the universal Self and regarded it to be the goal of life. In *Mahābhārata* XII.211, the teacher Āsuri, while addressing an assemblage of his followers, is said to have explained *brahman* as one immutable being assuming diverse forms. Aśvaghoṣa and Caraka mention *brahman* as the ultimate goal in their brief expositions of the Sāṃkhya (*Buddhacarita* XV.65 and Caraka on *Śarīra* I.99). In the list of sixty different topics of the *Ṣaṣṭitantra* (attributed to either Kapila or Pañcaśikha, ca. 100 BCE–200 CE) given by the *Ahirbudhnya Saṃhitā* (XII.20), the first topic is stated to be *brahman.* It is mentioned in the *Mahābhārata* (XII.212) that Pañcaśikha held the view that liberation is the union of the individual being with *brahman.*[64] Some Sāṃkhyan passages such as *Mahābhārata* XII.290 (3) and elsewhere throughout the *Bhagavadgītā* are clearly theistic.

In the formative period of the *Bhagavadgītā,* and later epic literature such as the *Mokṣadharma,* Yoga was very closely allied with Sāṃkhya. This fact is reflected in the *Mahābhārata,* which utilizes the compound *sāṃkhya-yoga* (chapter II of the *Bhagavadgītā* is entitled *"Sāṃkhya-Yoga"*) and also asserts that Sāṃkhya and Yoga can be looked upon as being identical (*Mahābhārata* XII.293.30 and *Bhagavadgītā* V.5)[65] or as being "one" because they have the same practical result (*MBh* XII.304.24–26)[66]—liberation *(mokṣa).* The epic schools of Sāṃkhya and Yoga gave rise in part to the Sāṃkhya-Yoga syncretism. However, both traditions were likewise asserted as being already distinct and independent developments at the time of the final composition of the *Mahābhārata.* This is epitomized in the following statement: "The method of the yogins is immediate [mystic] perception, [whereas] of the Sāṃkhyas it is scriptural [accepted] tradition" (XII.189.7). "These [two approaches] are not the same,"[67] as we are informed two stanzas later. The important distinction made at this point in the *Mahābhārata* epic is between the experiential and pragmatic approach of the yogins, and the reliance on traditional doctrine in conjunction with a rational form of inquiry into the nature of reality and human existence that characterizes the adherents of Sāṃkhya. Elsewhere, in the *Mahābhārata* (XII.289.3), Sāṃkhya is rejected by the followers of Yoga because the former does not believe in a saving Lord *(īśvara)*.[68]

In several key passages from the *Mokṣadharma* (XII.189) Sāṃkhya is presented thus: as being nontheistic and as relying on accepted teaching as a means of knowledge, and rational knowledge *(vijñāna)*[69] is given as the means of salvation. Yoga, however, is presented as being theistic, as relying primarily on immediate perception as a means of knowledge, and as emphasizing strength[70] (or power, *Mahābhārata* XII.304.2)—resulting from practical psychophysical disciplines (i.e., meditation, breathing exercises, posture). In the *Bhagavadgītā* (V.4), Yoga is equated with *karma-yoga* (the Yoga of action) and Sāṃkhya with the path of renunciation *(saṃnyāsa)*,[71] though in the next stanza (V.5) their essential unity is stressed. However, we are then informed (*Bhagavadgītā* V.6) that renunciation is difficult to attain without Yoga and that one who is earnest in Yoga (i.e., the path of action) soon attains the supreme spiritual being *(brahman)*.[72]

In subsequent times, Yoga and Sāṃkhya[73] developed into their separate philosophical and classical schools founded by Patañjali and Īśvara Kṛṣṇa respectively. In their metaphysical ideas Sāṃkhya and Yoga are closely akin. Dasgupta asserts that it was Patañjali who collected the different forms of Yoga practices, gleaned the diverse ideas that were or could be associated with Yoga, and "grafted them all on the Sāṃkhya metaphysics."[74] In the above sense, Sāṃkhya is often characterized as the theoretical aspect of Yoga praxis, but this is inaccurate.[75] Nor is Yoga simply a borrowed form of Sāṃkhya. G. Feuerstein[76] has convincingly shown that "there can be no justification whatever for deriving Classical Yoga from Classical *Sāṃkhya*."[77] Despite the seemingly radical nature of Feuerstein's arguments to challenge the idea that Sāṃkhya and Yoga are two sides of the same coin, his overall claim is not as strong as it sounds. When we examine his arguments closely, he is not asserting that the two systems have virtually nothing in common, but merely that some scholars have gone too far in their claims that Yoga is a subschool of Sāṃkhya. In this he is correct and Hindu tradition obviously agrees with him since it classes Sāṃkhya and Yoga as two philosophical schools *(darśana)*, not one. As we have seen in connection with the *Mahābhārata* (notably the *Mokṣadharma* section), it was in this earlier period (200 BCE–200 CE) that Yoga and Sāṃkhya assumed separate identities from their more or less common Vedāntic (Upaniṣadic) base. Moreover, the *Yoga-Sūtra* (ca. second–third century CE) is probably older than the *Sāṃkhya-Kārikā* (ca. 400 CE), and if any borrowing has occurred it is more likely to be on the part of Īśvara Kṛṣṇa.[78]

In spite of the similarity between these schools in their approach to the basic structure of reality, they in fact present different systems of thought, holding divergent views on important areas of doctrinal structure such as theology, ontology, psychology, and ethics, as well as differences pertaining to terminology. The numerous philosophical differences between classical Yoga and classical Sāṃkhya derive, however, from the different methodologies adopted by the two schools of thought. Sāṃkhya relies primarily on the exercise of the discernment *(viveka)* of *puruṣa* (spirit, pure consciousness) from *prakṛti* (matter, nature, psychophysical being and its source) on the basis of prefabricated categories of differentiation, stressing a theoretical/intellectual analysis in order to bring out the nature of final emancipation. This emancipation is often understood as an "isolation" *(kaivalya)* of *puruṣa* from *prakṛti, puruṣa* conceived as the uninvolved *(mādhyasthya),* inactive *(akartṛbhāva)* witness *(sākṣin)* of the evolutions of *prakṛti.*[79] However, Sāṃkhya's overt conceptual means of discrimination *(vijñāna)* is not sufficient enough for the aspiring yogin. The ontological categorization of what represents the "nonself" *(prakṛti)* must become the object of direct experience and perception. Without praxis and its experiential and perceptual dimension, philosophy would have no meaning in Yoga. Yoga is a practical spiritual discipline for mastering the modifications of the mind (*YS* I.2) and abiding as the changeless identity of the Self *(puruṣa).* In Yoga, immortality is realized through consistent practice and self-discipline, and is not something to be demonstrated through inference, analysis, and reasoning. Classical Yoga emphasizes the necessity of personal experimentation and practical meditational techniques for the cultivation of *samādhi* (*YS* I.17–18) in which insight *(prajñā),* disclosed within the deeper levels of the mind, progressively leads to a clearer understanding and realization of one's intrinsic identity as *puruṣa.*

Even just a cursory look at the *Yoga-Sūtra* reveals that Patañjali makes no attempt, as does Īśvara Kṛṣṇa, to speculate upon a metaphysical explanation of the nature of reality. In the first chapter of the *Yoga-Sūtra (Samādhi-Pāda),* no formal ontological schematic is given by Patañjali. It is not until the second chapter on the "means" or "path" of Yoga *(Sādhana-Pāda)* that a more formalized ontological scheme is explicitly outlined.[80] Assuming the text to be unitary, we can, however, conceive of an implicit metaphysics in chapter I, which can be explained by the fact that Patañjali falls back on a world view that he does not need to make explicit. Patañjali's overriding concern, however, is to show *how* to bring about the realization, freedom, and glory of an immortal state of consciousness and being as one's own identity or Self *(puruṣa),* a state that can be described in terms of freedom from suffering *(duḥkha)*.[81] This "showing how" culminates in "clear seeing," which in turn reveals our true identity as *puruṣa.* Patañjali begins the discipline of Yoga by addressing his listeners where they "are" from a yogic perspective, that is, as human beings desirous of freedom, yet who are subject to a mistaken identity, ensconced within the subject-object duality of empirical existence *(prakṛti),* and who conceive of themselves and the world from the limited perspective of ego-consciousness.

For Yoga, as well as other soteriological traditions of India, the ultimate concern of a human being is not understood to be separate from humanity itself. That is to say, the highest goal to which a human being can and ought to aspire does not lie in some separate realm or "outer," extrinsic world, but is, rather, "within" oneself, as one's "core" intrinsic being. Yoga tries to express this concern in a truly human way beginning with the psychophysical nature and experience of our humanness with its weaknesses, vulnerabilities, and virtues, and describes the human condition by incorporating our multileveled understandings and concepts of self-identity *(cittavṛtti).* Through a process of transformation of the mind, or *metanoia,* termed *nirodha* (*YS* I.2), Yoga expands, purifies, and illuminates our understanding of self and world. By grasping the nature of our personal experiences: *how* we think, feel, act, understand, and *why* we have assumed ourselves to be finite, temporal beings when, according to Yoga our authentic nature is infinite and unchanging, we can more easily discern how Yoga philosophy applies to our own perception and to our day-to-day existence.

Classical Yoga informs us of the fundamental defining characteristic of empirical selfhood as essentially being a misidentification with or conformity to *(sārūpya, YS* I.4) the mental processes or modifications *(vṛttis)* of the mind *(citta).* Yet, the process of identification (and misidentification—which is a form of identification) with thought and personality takes place for the purpose *(artha)* of experience *(bhoga)* and spiritual emancipation *(apavarga),* that is, for the purpose of realizing the *puruṣa* (*YS* II.21). As a cross-reference to assess the aspirant's standard of awareness, and to enable one to grow and develop, classical Yoga also offers the ideal of the *jīvanmukta,* one established in the true nature of *puruṣa* (*YS* I.3) and who embodies that enlightened perspective. Vyāsa's reference[82] to the enlightened being, the yogin free while yet living, places before us the ultimate "human" potentiality for the transformation of consciousness and identity of all aspirants of Patañjali's Yoga.

One of the problems confronting any study of the *Yoga-Sūtra* is that there is no obvious reference (excluding the *Yoga-Bhāṣya*) from which to base an analysis of Patañjali's thought. Some of the fundamental philosophical concepts of the Sāṃkhyan system of Īśvara Kṛṣṇa can provide a useful backdrop or cross-reference point from which to facilitate understanding and a greater appreciation of Patañjali's metaphysical and soteriological perspective. Vyāsa's *Bhāṣya,* which was probably written after the *Sāṃkhya-Kārikā* (and other major Sāṃkhyan works) has unhesitatingly drawn upon Sāṃkhyan doctrine for the purpose of expounding yogic principles taught by Patañjali.

Following from our previous discussion on Sāṃkhya and Yoga, we will now highlight some of the basic similarities and differences between classical Sāṃkhya and the Yoga of Patañjali. It is often said that, like classical Sāṃkhya, Patañjali's Yoga is a dualistic system, understood in terms of *puruṣa* and *prakṛti.* Yet, I submit, Yoga scholarship has not clarified what "dualistic" means or why Yoga had to be "dualistic." Even in avowedly nondualistic systems of thought such as Advaita Vedānta we can find numerous examples of basically dualistic modes of description and explanation.[83] It does not seem inappropriate to suggest the possibility of Patañjali having asserted a provisional, descriptive, and "practical" metaphysics, that is, in the *Yoga-Sūtra* the metaphysical schematic is abstracted from yogic experience, whereas in classical Sāṃkhya "experiences" are fitted into a metaphysical structure. This approach would allow the *Yoga-Sūtra* to be interpreted along more open-ended, epistemologically oriented lines without being held captive by the radical, dualistic metaphysics of Sāṃkhya. Despite intentions to render the experiential dimension of Yoga, purged as far as possible from abstract metaphysical knowledge, many scholars have fallen prey to reading the *Yoga-Sūtra* from the most abstract level of the dualism of *puruṣa* and *prakṛti* down to an understanding of the practices advocated. Then they proceed to impute an experiential foundation to the whole scheme informed not from mystical insight or yogic experience, but from the effort to form a consistent (dualistic) worldview, a view that culminates in a radical dualistic finality[84] or closure due to its hierarchically structured tendency toward abstractive reduction.

It should be noted that the contrast, suggested above, between the philosophical perspectives of Īśvara Kṛṣṇa and Patañjali is of crucial importance. Nevertheless, the theoretical connections and parallels between the *Yoga-Sūtra* and Sāṃkhya remain significant. Patañjali's philosophy, however, is not based upon mere theoretical or speculative knowledge. It elicits a practical, pragmatic, experiential/perceptual (not merely inferential/theoretical) approach that Patañjali deems essential in order to deal effectively with our total human situation and provide real freedom, not just a theory of liberation or a metaphysical explanation of life. To this end Patañjali outlined, among other practices, an "eight-limbed" path of Yoga (*aṣṭāṅga-yoga, Yoga-Sūtra* II.29) dealing with the physical, moral, psychological, and spiritual dimensions of the yogin. Yoga is not content with knowledge *(jñāna)* perceived as a state that abstracts away from the world removing us from our human embodiment and activity in the world. Rather, Yoga emphasizes knowledge in the integrity of being and action and as serving the integration of the "person" as a "whole." Edgerton concluded in a study dedicated to the meaning of Yoga that: "Yoga is not a 'system' of belief or of metaphysics. It is always a way, a method of getting something, usually salvation."[85] But this does not say enough, does not fully take into account what might be called the *integrity* of Patañjali's Yoga. As a major philosophical *darśana* within Hinduism, Yoga derives its real strength and value through an integration of theory and practice, implying a philosophy of "life"—incorporating both *puruṣa* and *prakṛti*—grounded in the direct experience of "life."

Patañjali's Yoga derives its insights from a process of introspection into the nature of *prakṛti* not unlike that of Sāṃkhya. According to Sāṃkhya and Yoga our "inner" world of thought, feeling, imagination, and so forth, parallels the structure of the cosmos itself. It is made up of the same fundamental layers of existence (i.e., *prakṛti, traiguṇa*) that compose the hierarchy of the external world. Therefore the so-called "maps"[86] utilized by Patañjali and Ïśvara Krsna are guides to both the "inner" and the "outer" dimensions of existence, and also function—certainly in the case of Yoga—as heuristic devices in the form of contemplative directives for facilitating understanding and meditative insight. Their principle purpose, thus, is to point beyond the levels and limitations of psyche and cosmos reminding us that the true nature and identity of human being—the spiritual component of our person—is a transcendent yet immanent reality, pure consciousness *(puruṣa)*, sometimes referred to as the witness *(sākṣin)* behind all content of consciousness. Patañjali's Yoga philosophy incorporates the Sāṃkhyan idea of a multilayered or hierarchical cosmos where *prakṛti* is seen to encompass: (1) on the one hand, the grosser levels of manifestation and actualization resulting in the material forms of manifest reality *(vyakta)*, and (2) on the other hand, the transcendent ground of *prakṛti* herself. Beyond *prakṛti*'s realm of existence is the unmodified dimension of pure identity/consciousness, the formless *puruṣa*-principle. As we will soon discover, the ontological categories outlined in the *Yoga-Sūtra* provide one with a provisional "map" consisting of contemplative directives that enable the yogin to pass through different levels of experience *(bhoga)* culminating in emancipation *(apavarga)* whereupon one transcends the binding influence or effects of *prakṛti* altogether.

The psychocosmological "map" structure put forward by Patañjali is, in the true sense of yogic experimentation that results in first-hand evidence *(pratyakṣa)* or experiential verification, no doubt profoundly informed by the territory he discovered in the course of his own explorations of human consciousness or mind *(citta)*—levels of consciousness, self-understanding, and identity that can be correlated to the dimensions of *prakṛti*. Īśvara Kṛṣṇa's sketched account or "map" of reality appears to be shaped by more formalistic, rationalistic, and theoretical considerations interwoven no doubt with Sāṃkhya's long history (i.e., several centuries) of metaphysical speculation. I shall be alluding to this and other philosophical differences or points of divergence between the two systems throughout our study (see, for example, n. 87 below). Both "maps," of course, are intended to guide the practitioner to the realization of *puruṣa* and are thus ultimately derived for *soteriological* purposes. The above intention notwithstanding, scholars have often questioned the efficacy of the classical Sāṃkhyan "means" for attaining freedom *(mokṣa, kaivalya)* especially in comparison to yogic methods.[87]

Within the context of Yoga, hierarchical "maps" of reality served a very practical, psychological, pedagogical, and soteriological purpose.[88] G. Feuerstein states: "The ontogenetic models were originally and primarily maps for meditative introspection intended to guide the yogin in his exploration of the *terra incognita* of the mind . . . [and] are records of internal experiences rather than purely theoretical constructions. They are descriptive rather than explanatory."[89] C. Pensa rightly describes the approach of Yoga as an "homologisation between cosmological and psychological structures."[90] To be sure, the categories used in Yoga are both descriptions and contemplative directives for the ways in which the mind, identity, and world are actually experienced through meditative awareness and insight.

If one is to grasp how Yoga philosophy can be lived on a practical level, one must understand how *puruṣa* and *prakṛti* relate to one in practical, experiential, and personal terms. To this end Patañjali translated a "universal," macrocosmic perspective into subjective, microcosmic terms. Yoga philosophy, being historically rooted in a pedagogical context, functions in part as a teaching method skillfully aimed at transforming, purifying, and illuminating human consciousness (i.e., the mind or *citta,* which can be described as a grasping, intentional, and volitional consciousness) and thus our perception and experience of reality. The metaphysics is united to the teaching tradition of spiritual preceptor *(guru)* and disciple *(śiṣya)* and is soteriological as well as practical in nature and purpose. The distinction between the two major categories in Yoga: *puruṣa* or *draṣṭṛ* (the "seer"), and *prakṛti* or *dṛśya* (the "seeable"), may not have been intended by Patañjali as a metaphysical theory of truth. Moreover, despite the fact that Patañjali initially adopts a Sāṃkhyan metaphysical orientation, there is no proof in the *Yoga-Sūtra* that his system stops at dualism (i.e., the dualism may be said to be open to the criterion of falsifiability playing only a provisional role in his system), or merely ends up, as many scholars have concluded, with a radical dualism in which *puruṣa* and *prakṛti,* absolutely disjoined, are unable to "cooperate," establish a "harmony" and achieve a "balance" together. In this sense the *Yoga-Sūtra* can be understood not so much as contradicting Sāṃkhya but more so as accommodating and subsuming the philosophical stance in the *Sāṃkhya-Kārikā* by extending the meaning of purification and illumination of human identity to incorporate an enlightened mode of action as well as being. As such, Yoga philosophy helps to resolve some of the tensions inherent in a radically dualistic perspective—as is exemplified in interpretations of classical Sāṃkhya—wherein *puruṣa* and *prakṛti* are utterly separate and incapable of "uniting" through an integration of being and activity, that is, as an embodied state of freedom, consciousness and being.

PRAKṚTI AS VIEWED IN THE *YOGA-SŪTRA*

In Patañjali's Yoga, as in classical Sāṃkhya, *prakṛti* refers to both the primordial ground *(mūlaprakṛti)* of the innumerable manifest forms and those forms themselves. Also termed *pradhāna* (or *avyakta*), which denotes the transcendent matrix of *prakṛti* as apart from the consciousness principle *(purusa), prakṛti* is defined by Vācaspati Miśra as that by which the mutiplicity of evolutes *(vikāra)* is brought forth *(pradhīyate)*.[91] It is the primordial, undifferentiated continuum that contains in potential the entire cosmos in all its levels and categories of being.

Prakṛti is frequently defined in Sāṃkhya as the state of balance or equilibrium of the three *guṇas (tri-guṇa-sāmya-avasthā)*.[92] When this state of balance is disturbed or disrupted by the presence of pure consciousness *(puruṣa),* the process of the "creation" or manifestation of the ordinary world takes place. The theory of homogeneous equilibrium *(sāmyāvasthā)* formulated by later Sāṃkhyan thinkers proceeded more from speculation concerning the drive for liberation; it flowed only indirectly from an analysis of the phenomenon of observation. The perfectly balanced substrata of *prakṛti* ("matter") was an unevolved and unmanifest state wherein the three *guṇa*s—the basic strands or qualities of *prakṛti* ("matter," see below)—were thought to revolve in "palpitating"[93] balanced movement within unmanifest *prakṛti* while yet being completely separated from the light of *puruṣa*. This theory, which does not appear to be upheld in the *Yoga-Sūtra* or the *Yoga-Bhāṣya,* is not without its difficulties. Can the *guṇa*s in the undifferentiated state of *prakṛti* really be described as "moving"? Do the *guṇa*s of unmanifest potentiality possess the reality of the actual, manifest observable world of experience that the Sāṃkhyan claims to analyze? If the *guṇa*s are only unevolved potentiality, then what can claim the attribute of movement or dynamism and manifestation? The above questions hint at only a few of the unresolved issues that arise for those who wish to hypothesize a theoretical state of perfect, unmanifest equilibrium in contrast to the imbalanced and disharmonius state of manifest existence, that is, the world we normally perceive and experience. An even more serious problem for such speculators would be to explain how such a hypothetical state of equilibrium actually becomes unbalanced.[94] Is imbalance or disequilibrium an intrinsic characteristic of the reality of manifestation, actualization, and the "evolution" of the universe in all its diversity? Is the suffering (*duḥkha, YS* II.16), misidentification, and confusion that should be overcome or discarded in order for authentic identity to arise an intrinsic aspect of any "movement" within *prakṛti* herself? If suffering is an inherent aspect of manifest existence, would spiritual liberation necessitate a return to the original unmanifest ground dissolving away or withdrawing from our human, manifest nature and identity? Or, is the state of human conflict and sorrow (*YS* II.15; see n. 121 below) that Yoga seeks to remove the result of a malfunctioning factor within *prakṛti* including the various phenomena of mind *(citta)* or consciousness through which we perceive and experience reality? If the latter be the case, it would then follow that the cause of this malfunction or distortion operating within *prakṛti* and leading to sorrow would need to be uprooted and discarded. Is *prakṛti*'s two-tiered existence consisting of: (1) an unmanifest potentiality that is in itself a state of homogeneous equilibrium, and (2) manifest existence implying disharmony and imbalance, meant to be understood with an ontological emphasis, that is, as an ontological description of reality? Can the homogeneous equilibrium, referred to as *sāmyāvasthā,* as well as the processes of "disequilibrium" resulting from its actualization and manifestation be more appropriately rendered with an epistemological emphasis? Much of the remainder of our study will be addressing these as well as other related questions not from a purely Sāṃkhyan orientation but rather from within the context of Patañjali's Yoga philosophy.

Patañjali subscribes to the Sāṃkhyan theory of "evolution" or manifestation, called *satkāryavāda,* according to which an effect *(kārya)* is preexistent *(sat)* in its cause *(kāraṇa);* and also *prakṛti-pariṇāma-vāda,* which signifies that the effect is a real transformation *(pariṇāma)* of *prakṛti,* not merely an appearance or illusory change as is thought in the idealist schools of Vedānta[95] and, some would argue, Mahāyāna Buddhism. The *satkārya* doctrine maintains that whatever comes into manifestation is not a completely new reality or production[96] thereby rejecting the notion of creation *ex nihilo.* Yoga holds that what is nonexistent can never be produced; what is existent can never perish.[97] The causes must be of the same fundamental substance as the effects.[98] The effects are thus already latent in the material causes and manifest as transformations resulting from, as Patañjali states, the outflow or implementation of their material causes *(prakṛtyāpūra).*[99] The disappearance of a previous transformation and the rise of a subsequent one takes place as a result of the integrating pervasion of the constituent parts of the material cause.[100]

In Yoga, differentiation and actualization (or what may be referred to as "creation") is always only the manifestation *(āvirbhāva)* of latent possibilities. The ultimate material cause is thought to be *prakṛti.* All unmanifest and manifest forms are simply developments, transformations, or actualizations *(pariṇāma, vikāra, vikṛti)* of that primal "substance" or *prakṛti.* Moreover, the disappearance of an existing object does not mean its total annihilation, but merely its becoming latent again *(tirobhāva).* "Destruction" is nothing but "dissolution" into the unmanifest, a withdrawal from manifestness or return to the "origin." This theory may well have been derived from the kind of metaphysical speculation found, for example, in the *Bhagavadgītā* (II.16–17), where Kṛṣṇa instructs Arjuna as follows:

> Of the nonexistent there is no coming to be. Of the existent there is no ceasing to be. Also, the final truth of these is known by the seers of Truth. Yet, know as indestructible that by which all this is pervaded. Nothing is able to accomplish the destruction of that which is imperishable.[101]

Like *puruṣa,* the transcendent core of *prakṛti—pradhāna, avyakta,* or what Patañjali calls *aliṅga*[102]—is also indestructible. Yet it has the capacity to undergo modification and it does so in the process of actualization or manifestation during which it gives birth to the multidimensional universe. In Sāṃkhya (*SK* 20–21) the ubiquitous presence of *puruṣa* as unchanging, contentless, and pure (that is, unaffected by the changes within *prakṛti*) consciousness, "solicits" this process. According to Patañjali (*YS* III.13),[103] the transformation and development *(pariṇāma)* of *prakṛti,* denoting serial change, is of three basic types: (1) *dharma-pariṇāma,* the change or development in the form of a substance; (2) *lakṣaṇa-pariṇāma,* or the change of characteristic implicit in the fact that time *(kala)* consists of past, present and future; and (3) *avasthā-pariṇāma,* the state or stage of development or the qualitative change or condition due to the effects of time (i.e., aging), as when an earthen vessel breaks and turns to dust. Patañjali seeks to apply these insights to the mind *(citta)*—the locus of empirical consciousness and personality—and its transmutation through the practice of Yoga. The above three types of change are universally applicable to the phenomena of consciousness as well as to material objects, the elements, and the senses. While recognizing the changelessness of pure spirit or awareness *(puruṣa),* Yoga (unlike Sāṃkhya) explicitly allows for fluctuation between potentiality or pure power *(śakti)* and actuality *(abhivyakti)* within the mind, such modification or transition within the phenomena or content of consciousness referring to the transformation from an unconscious "nonviewed" *(aparidṛṣṭa)* state to a conscious "viewed" *(paridṛṣṭa)* one.[104]

In *Yoga-Sūtra* (III.13) Patañjali employs the term *dharma* in the technical sense of "form," which is of changing nature. This he contrasts (*YS* III.14) with the concept of "*dharma*-holder" *(dharmin),* the underlying essential nature or unchanging "substance" (as opposed to the changeable form).[105] *Prakṛti* is the permanent "substance" *(dharmin)* and its series of manifestations are the forms *(dharma).* Applying the *satkāryavāda* doctrine, which states that change affects only the form of an object, not its underlying substance, Patañjali distinguishes between three forms or states of an object: its "subsided" *(śānta)* or past aspect, its "arisen" *(udita)* or present aspect, and its "undetermined" *(avyapadeśya)* or future aspect.[106] All three are related to the same "substance" or "*dharma*-holder," which is permanently present in, yet cannot be contained by (and therefore is different from) its forms or modifications, that is, it assumes many changes but is not wholly defined or consumed by these changes. Vyāsa explicitly contrasts this view with the Buddhist doctrine of *anātman,* no-self or inessentiality, according to which there is a multiplicity of changing forms but no underlying being or substance.[107] In contrast to the Yogācāra school of Buddhism, for example, classical Yoga does not attempt to reduce "being" to "being experienced." Yet classical Yoga "tends to ascribe a more constitutive role to awareness or experience than the Sāṃkhya and to interpret it as an efficient factor of manifestation and actualization."[108] The above three kinds of transformation can be understood as different ways of looking at the change affecting a single substance.

To illustrate the concept of *pariṇāma* (as used in *YS* III.13), Vyāsa describes the three modalities *(dharma, lakṣaṇa, avasthā)* in the following manner: a lump of clay is made into a water jar, thus undergoing a change in external property or form *(dharma);* in its present condition as water jar it is thus able to hold water *(lakṣaṇa);* finally, the jar gradually becomes "old," thus undergoing "stages of development" *(avasthā).*[109] Vyāsa, furthermore, associates the notions of actuality and potentiality, manifest *(vyakta)* and subtle *(sūkṣma),* with time and temporality: Present phenomena are manifest or actual; past and future phenomena are considered subtle or in potential form.[110] Thus, there is an attempt in Yoga to clarify the nature of time in the light of the concepts of actuality and potentiality and as it applies to the structure and functioning of the mind. The reality of time and its three "paths" *(adhvan)*—past, present, and future—is the reality of the ever-changing nature and forms arising from the unmanifest ground of *prakṛti.*[111]

Patañjali's philosophy of the change and development of *prakṛti* as applied to empirical consciousness *(citta)* disallows intrinsic stability or permanency to the phenomena of the mind and the empirical sense of self. Only *puruṣa* is able to enjoy the status of immutability *(apariṇāmitva),*[112] meaning that its authentic, immortal identity is never really "lost" throughout all the changes and identifications that take place in the mind and the perceived world. Yoga reminds us that even though our psychophysical being is an apparent composite of the forces of *prakṛti* and is merely a temporary modification, it is also associated with an eternal, transcendent, yet immanent and essentially unaffected aspect, the *puruṣa* or spiritual Self.

Patañjali makes use of the *guṇa* theory, one of the most original contributions of the Sāṃkhya tradition. The three *guṇa*s—the basic "constituents" of *prakṛti*—compose all cosmological as well as physical and psychological principles. Without the manifestation of the *guṇa*s there would be nothing to be experienced. The most common denotation for the tripartite process *(traiguṇa)* of *prakṛti* given in the *Yoga-Sūtra* is the term *dṛśya,* the "seeable" (*YS* II.17, 18, 21, and IV.23), which includes the unmanifest, nondifferentiated potentiality as well as the manifest, differentiated universe or diverse aspects of *prakṛti.* This concept has a strong epistemological resonance to it and signifies anything that is capable of becoming an object of the *puruṣa,* meaning here anything that pertains to *prakṛti* in her diverse modes including the causal source *(pradhāna, aliṅga)* itself. Descriptions of the *guṇa*s (cf. Sāṃkhya) point to an interpretation that would stress that their psychological and even moral components are both indispensible for the definition and existence of individual entities or persons within the world. The *guṇa*s encompass the entire personality structure including the affective and cognitive dimensions involving various qualities and states such as pleasure, pain, intelligence, passion, dullness, and so on.[113] The *guṇa*s also function like cosmological proto-elements (cf. *MBh* XII.187[114] and *SK* 15–16), as generative/creative factors involved in and responsible for the evolution of life-forms. Patañjali employs the term *dṛśya* in the above possible ways where he delineates its main characteristics in *Yoga-Sūtra* (II.18).[115] Here, he mentions the three characters or dispositions of the "seeable" in a clear reference to the interdependent nature of the three *guṇa*s: namely, *prakāśa* or "luminosity"/"brilliance" (pertaining to *sattva*), *kriyā* or "activity" (belonging to *rajas*), and *sthiti* or "fixity"/"inertia" (connected with *tamas*). The "seeable" has the nature of the elements *(bhūta)* and the senses *(indriya)* and serves the dual purpose of experience *(bhoga)* and emancipation *(apavarga)*.[116]

Patañjali appears to conceive of the *guṇa*s as three types of psychophysical force, "matter," or energy whose existence can be deduced from the "behavior" patterns of *prakṛti*. Vyāsa provides us with a lucid commentary on the tripartite process where he describes the *guṇa*s in the following manner:

> *Sattva* tends towards luminosity; *rajas* towards action; *tamas* towards fixity. Though distinct, these *guṇa*s mutually affect each other. They change, they have the properties of conjunction and disjunction, they assume forms created by their mutual co-operation. Distinct from each other, they are identifiable even when their powers are conjoined. They deploy their respective powers, whether of similar or dissimilar kind. When one is predominant, the presence (of the others) is inferred as existing within the predominant one from the very fact of its operation as a *guṇa*. They are effective as engaged in carrying out the purpose of the *puruṣa*.[117]

G. Koelman notes: "The *guṇa*'s nature is throughout expressed in terms of functional qualities, kinetic dispositions and causal urges."[118] To summarize the above, we can say that the *guṇa*s underlie all physical, material, cosmological, psychological, and moral realities.[119] From the *Yoga-Bhāṣya* (II.18 above) we are informed that: (1) although the *guṇa*s are to be distinguished according to their qualities, (2) they are nevertheless interdependent and (3) in combination generate cosmic existence/the phenomenal universe, whereupon (4) everything must be regarded as a "synergization"[120] of these three factors. Constituting the realm of the "seeable" *(dṛśya),* the *guṇa*s exist for the purpose of *puruṣa* (i.e., for experience *[bhoga]* and emancipation *[apavarga]*), which suggests that from a yogic perspective the guṇic processes do not ultimately result in delusive forms of self-identity, worldly identification, conflict, destruction, and dissatisfaction *(duḥkha).* Rather, they can function as a vehicle for liberating self-identity from the bondage of worldly existence.

In *Yoga-Sūtra* II.15 Patañjali portrays these three types of fundamental prakṛtic forces as being in continual conflict with each other: "Because of the dissatisfaction and sufferings due to change and anxieties and the latent impressions, and from the conflict of the modifications of the *guṇa*s, for the discerning one, all is sorrow alone."[121] As a result of this inherent tension between them, and due to their dynamic, energetic nature associated with "transformation" *(pariṇāma),* the *guṇa*s are said to form the different ontological levels *(parvan)* of prakṛtic reality.[122] From the perspective of the discerning yogin *(vivekin)* human identity contained within the phenomenal world of the three *guṇa*s amounts to nothing more than sorrow and dissatisfaction *(duḥkha).*[123] The declared goal of classical Yoga is to overcome all suffering (*duḥkha, YS* II.16) by bringing about an inverse movement or counterflow *(pratiprasava)*[124] understood as a "return to the origin"[125] or "process-of-involution"[126] of the *guṇa*s, a kind of reabsorption into the transcendent purity of being itself. What does this "process-of-involution"—variously referred to as "return to the origin," "dissolution into the source,"[127] or "withdrawal from manifestation"—actually mean? Is it a definitive ending to the perceived world of the yogin comprised of change and transformation, forms and phenomena? Ontologically conceived, *prasava* signifies the "flowing forth" of the primary constituents or qualities of *prakṛti* into the multiple forms of the universe in all its dimensions, that is, all the evolutionary process or "creation" *(sarga, prasarga). Pratiprasava,* on the other hand, denotes the process of "dissolution into the source" or "withdrawal from manifestation" of those forms relative to the personal, microcosmic level of the yogin who is about to attain freedom *(apavarga).*

Does a "return to the origin" culminate in a state of freedom in which one is stripped of all human identity and void of any association with the world including one's practical livelihood? The ontological emphasis usually given to the meaning of *pratiprasava*—implying for the yogin a literal dissolution of *prakṛti*'s manifestation—would seem to support a view, one that is prominent in Yoga scholarship, of spiritual liberation denoting an existence wholly transcendent (and therefore stripped or deprived) of all manifestation including the human relational sphere. Is this the kind of spiritually emancipated state that Patañjali had in mind? At this rather early stage in our study it suffices to say that in *Yoga-Sūtra* II.3-17—which sets the stage for the remainder of the chapter on yogic practice *(sādhana)*—Patañjali describes *prakṛti,* the "seeable" (including our personhood), in the context of the various afflictions *(kleśa*s*)* that give rise to an afflicted and mistaken identity of self. Afflicted identity, as we shall see later on (see chapters 3 and 4), is constructed out of and held captive by the root affliction of ignorance *(avidyā)* and its various forms of karmic bondage. Yet, despite the clear association of *prakṛti* with the bondage of ignorance *(avidyā),* there are no real grounds for purporting that *prakṛti* herself is to be *equated* with or subsumed under affliction itself. To equate *prakṛti* with affliction itself implies that as a product of spiritual ignorance, *prakṛti,* along with the afflictions, is conceived as a reality which the yogin should ultimately avoid or discard completely. Patañjali leaves much room for understanding "dissolution" or "return to the source," with an epistemological emphasis thereby allowing the whole system of Yoga *darśana* to be interpreted along more open-ended lines. In other words, what actually "dissolves" or is ended in Yoga is the yogin's *misidentification* with *prakṛti,* a mistaken identity of self that—contrary to our true identity as *puruṣa*—can be nothing more than a product of the three *guṇa*s under the influence of spiritual ignorance. Understood as such, *pratiprasava* need not denote the definitive ontological dissolution of manifest *prakṛti* for the yogin, but rather means the eradication of misidentification—the incorrect world view born of *avidyā*—or incapacity of the yogin to "see" from the yogic perspective of the seer *(draṣṭṛ),* our true identity as *puruṣa.* However, in order to appreciate this line of argument, which gives an epistemological emphasis to the meaning of key yogic terms, it is necessary to outline in greater detail Patañjali's metaphysical schematic.

Within *prakṛti*'s domain, Patañjali recognizes four hierarchic yet interrelated levels of existence whose characteristics and qualities are determined by the relative predominance of any of the three *guṇa*s. The levels are, according to *Yoga-Sūtra* II.19:[128]

1. The "Unmanifest" *(aliṅga)*
2. The "Designator" *(liṅga-mātra)*
3. The "Unparticularized" *(aviśeṣa)*
4. The "Particularized" *(viśeṣa)*

The following excerpt from the *Yoga-Bhaṣya* (II.19) shows Vyasa's correlations of Patañjali's four-level model with the more familiar (Sāṃkhyan) series of principles of existence *(tattvas):*

> Of these [four divisions], space, air, fire, water and earth are the gross elements which are the particularizations of the unparticularized subtle elements *(tanmātras):* sound, touch, form-precept, taste and smell. Ears, skin, eyes, tongue and nose are the sense-organs, and mouth, hands, feet, organs of evacuation and generation are the five action organs. The eleventh organ, the mind-organ *(manas),* is multi-objective. These are the particularizations of the unparticularized I-am-ness. This is the sixteen-fold transformation of the *guṇas* into particulars *(viśeṣa).* The unparticularized *(aviśeṣa)* are six. They are the subtle elements of hearing, touching, seeing, tasting and smelling, distinguished (respectively) by one, two, three, four and all five, beginning with hearing. The sixth unparticularized is mere I-am-ness *(asmitā-mātra).* These are the six unparticularized transformations of the great principle *(mahat-tattva),* whose nature is mere being *(sattā-mātra)* which is bare form *(liṅga-mātra).* Beyond the unparticularized is that great (self) which is mere being; supported in it these fulfil their development to the limit. And in the reverse process they are supported in that great (self) which is mere being and go back to that *pradhāna,* the formless *(aliṅga)* which is neither being-non-being, nor yet existent-non-existent.[129]

In classical Yoga, *aliṅga* (the "signless," "formless") is the most subtle level—because of its utter unmanifest nature—of the hierarchical levels of *prakṛti.* It is the state of undifferentiated existence and corresponds with the Sāṃkhya concept of *avyakta* or the "unmanifest" (also termed *mūlaprakṛti*). Vācaspati Miśra defines it *(aliṅga)* as the equilibrium *(sāmyāvasthā)* of the three primary constituents *(guṇas)* of *prakṛti.*[130] Being the transcendent core of *prakṛti,* which is pure potentiality, it is without any "mark" or "sign." Only a small part of *prakṛti* is at any time undergoing manifestation and actualization. The rest remains in unmanifest existence.

From out of the "unmanifest" emerges the "(mere) designator," or *liṅga-mātra,* as the first cosmic principle or level of manifest existence. This is the level of cosmic manifestation prior to the mergence of specific objects. Vyāsa identifies it as the "great principle" *(mahat-tattva),* whose nature is "mere being" *(sattā-mātra).*[131] Vācaspati Miśra also refers to *liṅga-mātra* as the "great principle" *(mahat-tattva).*[132] *Mahat* is the most sattvic, finest, and purest production of *prakṛti.* On the one hand, it is that first manifestation of *guṇas* in which no other form or shape yet emerges. As the "designator" *mahat* is also the *buddhi,* the faculty of discernment that serves as a vehicle of *puruṣa*'s (reflected) consciousness.[133] Because it is the most subtle and sattvic modification, it is fit to serve as a medium between *puruṣa* and the phenomena of *prakṛti.* In Sāṃkhya (*SK* 22, 23) a "spark" of the universal *mahat* is also the individual or personal aspect of *buddhi,* the faculty of intelligence and discernment in a sentient entity, and the highest power in the process of sensation.

Following from *liṅga-mātra* is the "unparticularized" *(aviśeṣa)* composed of six categories, namely, the five subtle elements or potentials (*tanmātra*s, lit., "that only") and the principle of individuation *(asmitā-mātra)* or mere I-am-ness.[134] The last level of guṇic manifestation is the "particularized," which, according to Vyāsa, is composed of the five elements *(bhūta*s*),* the ten senses *(indriya*s*),* and the mind-organ *(manas),* and is a product of the unparticularized I-am-ness.[135]

Whereas, in a cosmological context, *liṅga-mātra* is a category of which nothing can be predicated except that it exists—the first sign that *prakṛti* gives of her presence—*asmitā-mātra,* in the words of G. Koelman, "differentiates and pluralizes the indetermined and universal principle of being *(sattā-mātra)* into so many different centres of reference, so many sources of initiative."[136] Koelman continues: "These centres of reference constitute, so to say, distinct nucleations within the one *Prakṛti,* in such a way that there arise different suppositions or subjectivations or numerically distinct units of centralisation adapted to the needs of each particularised Self. This supposition is sufficiently stable to be called a substantial entity, a *tattva* or a *dravya.*"[137] *Asmitā-mātra* is the principle and agency that splits the primary substratum into subjects vis-à-vis objects in the form of a bifurcate line of development and transformation. It corresponds with Īśvara Kṛṣṇa's notion of *ahaṃkāra* ("I-maker" or sense of self; see below). The author of the *Yuktidīpikā* (on *SK* 4) wrongly maintains that Patañjali does not know *ahaṃkāra* as a separate principle but includes it in *mahat.*[138] As is the case with the Sāṃkhyan principle of *ahaṃkāra, asmitā-mātra* brings forth the subjective sensorial world and the objective sensed world. It is the generic pool of all individualized empirical selves that according to the Sāṃkhyan system is the cosmic differentiator of subject and object; *ahaṃkāra* is a self-awareness *(abhimāna)* giving rise to the human sense "I am."[139]

We must guard against generalized statements such as that made by S. Radhakrishnan who asserts that Yoga "does not recognize *ahaṃkāra* and *manas* as separate from *buddhi.*"[140] Prior to his commentary on *Yoga-Sūtra* II.19 (see above), Vyāsa already refers to the sixth unparticularized principle as *ahaṃkāra,* which strongly suggests that *ahaṃkāra* is the equivalent of *asmitā-mātra:* "Subtler than these [the *tanmātra*s] is the *ahaṃkāra,* and subtler than that is the great principle *(liṅga-mātra).*"[141]

Patañjali's vocabulary, while not being a mere replica of Sāṃkhyan terminology, can be seen as accommodating the Sāṃkhyan metaphysical schematic. Much of this hinges on how we understand Patañjali's important concept of *asmitā* ("I-am-ness") which, being one of the five afflictions *(kleśas)* in Yoga, is defined in *Yoga-Sūtra* II.6 as follows: "I-am-ness is when the two powers of seer and view [i.e., what is viewed] as if (appear) as one self."[142] Vyāsa's commentary states:

> *Puruṣa* is the power of the seer; mind *(buddhi)*[143] is [understood here to be] the power of seeing. The taking on of a single nature, as it were, by these two, is called the affliction of I-am-ness. When there comes about a failure, as it were, to distinguish between the experiencer and what is experienced, which are utterly distinct and have nothing to do with each other, that is the condition for experience. But when the true nature of the two is recognized, that is aloneness. Then how could there be experience? So it has been said: 'Not seeing *puruṣa* beyond the mind and distinct from it in such things as form, disposition and knowledge, one will make there a mental self out of delusion.'[144]

In *Yoga-Sūtra* III.35 Patañjali defines experience *(bhoga)* as "an idea (i.e., intention or cognition) that does not distinguish between *sattva* and *puruṣa,* though they are absolutely unmixed."[145] Vyāsa has clearly understood *asmitā* as taking place, or finding its primal locus of identification in the *buddhi* (i.e., *liṅga-mātra*), which in Sāṃkhya is also called *mahat*. To facilitate an understanding of the practical processes leading to meditational praxis, Patañjali employs terminology a little differently from that of Sāṃkhya. For example, the *Sāṃkhya-Kārikā* discusses *mahat* but not *asmitā.* In the *Yoga-Sūtra* it is in *asmitā* that the impression of a "union" (*saṃyoga, YS* II.17) between *puruṣa* and *prakṛti,* between consciousness and insentience, first occurs. *Asmitā* is that process in which *mahat* or *buddhi,* being the purest and most sattvic evolute of *prakṛti,* becomes a recipient of a "reflection" of pure consciousness. This reflected state of consciousness (which will be explained in chapter 3), masquerading in the garb of *asmitā,* assumes itself to be Self/*puruṣa*. It is, by analogy, like the union of a crystal mirror with a reflection of the sun. *Puruṣa,* like the distant sun in the sky, remains unaffected by the union of its "reflection" in the mirror, but at the interface between *puruṣa* and *prakṛti* all the processes of the composite personality begin. Consciousness and life flow through this *asmitā,* which lends to the ego-principle *(asmitā-mātra, ahaṃkāra)* and to the mind *(citta)* a semblance of awareness. This reflected awareness generates a deluded sense of selfhood and must be understood as arising from a mistaken identity, that is the misidentification of *prakṛti* with *puruṣa* (authentic identity), beginning with *mahat*. The *puruṣa*-principle in Sāṃkhya and Yoga is not a supreme creator and does not reappear in the cosmos as a personal world-soul. Our empirical sense of self misidentifies with the prakṛtic, "created" world thereby veiling *puruṣa,* resulting in a failure "to distinguish between the experiencer and what is experienced" (*YB* II.6; see n. 144 above). Thus, what is seen as real cosmogony in the Upaniṣads (for example, *Kaṭha Up* III.2), is described in the *Yoga-Sūtra* (II.3-5) as a process taking place under the influence of spiritual ignorance *(avidyā).* This does not mean to imply that the cosmogony of Yoga is itself an illusory process. *Prakṛti* does, in full reality, transform herself into the created essences, headed by *mahat/buddhi.* The *seeming* aspect of this "flowing forth" *(prasava)* or "creation" *(sarga)* refers to *puruṣa*'s *seeming* bondage within *prakṛti.* The cosmos itself is experienced as if pervaded by consciousness. Patañjali describes *prakṛti* in terms of how the world is experienced by one who is ensconced in the condition of ignorance. When one falsely identifies or misidentifies with the principles of "matter" or any of *prakṛti*'s modifications, those *tattva*s and mental processes *(vṛtti*s*)* are experienced as pervaded by an "I-am" consciousness (i.e., "I am *buddhi,*" "I am *ahaṃkāra*") that is wholly identified within *prakṛti* thereby masking or excluding *puruṣa. Puruṣa* does not *do* anything in this process. *Asmitā* thus is an afflicted state of consciousness and identity that permeates and sustains our notions or sense of authentic identity *(puruṣa)* as a bound "entity" under the sway of prakṛtic existence.

Asmitā-mātra, the sixth category of the level of the "unparticularized" *(aviśeṣa),* is a product of the "designator" *(liṅga-mātra)* and can have no "direct contact" (as does *mahat* or *buddhi*) with *puruṣa*'s reflection of consciousness that produces the "I-am-ness" located in *buddhi* (*YB* II.6). H. Āraṇya correctly addresses the meaning of *asmitā-mātra* as used in Vyāsa's commentary (II.19) as follows: "Here it means ego *[ahaṃkāra].* It has been said before (*YS* II.6) that identity of the instrument of reception with . . . consciousness is *asmitā.* From that point of view *buddhi* is pure *asmitā* or final form of egoism. In every case, however, *asmitā-mātra* is not *mahat [buddhi]*."[146]

Patañjali uses the term *asmitā-mātra* once (in *YS* IV.4), where it is described as that principle from which the multiple individualized or fabricated minds *(nirmāṇa-citta*s*)*[147] are projected. Patañjali merely asserts that the individualized minds arise from the unparticularized I-am-ness.[148] *Asmitā-mātra* is an ontological concept, and is ontologically real. In contrast, *asmitā* is an afflicted state of self-identity—of our having mistaken *prakṛti* (or prakṛtic identity) for *puruṣa*—and is a psychological concept (as given in *YS* II.3, 6 and III.47) whose meaning can be rendered with an epistemological emphasis.

In disagreement with S. Dasgupta,[149] our study maintains that *mahat* or *buddhi* is a synonym of *sattā-mātra* (*YB* II.19), not *asmitā-mātra*. Both Koelman[150] and Feuerstein[151] understand I-am-ness *(asmitā)* as a psychological experience of "I-am" rooted in *asmitā-mātra*. However, in doing so it appears that both of the above scholars have restricted the meaning of *asmitā* to the notion of an individualized subject with a particular *buddhi.*[152] This study understands *asmitā* as taking root in *mahat,* the cosmic, pre-individual (or, from another perspective, trans-individual) aspect of *buddhi*. As in Sāṃkhya, the intellect *(buddhi)* has a dual role to play, individual and pre-individual or cosmic (which can also be designated as trans-individual). While *asmitā-mātra* is the cosmic (ontological) principle of individuation that produces both the psychomental and physical realities of the individual self, *asmitā* (egoity, I-am-ness)—as an afflicted psychological functioning of the mind *(citta)*—is also responsible for the root or pre-individual identification of self-identity with *mahat* (cosmic knowing). When *puruṣa* seemingly "comes into" relationship with insentient *prakṛti* in the form of *prakṛti*'s first created essence, *buddhi (mahat),* that essence becomes "as it were" (*iva, YS* II.6), conscious as cosmic "I-am-ness."[153] The "insentient" cosmic knowing (transcending individual cognition)—a reflected consciousness or semblance of *puruṣa*'s awareness—is experienced as the location of self: "I am *mahat/buddhi.*" This misidentification results in a transformation *(pariṇāma)* of cosmic knowing into personal volitional knowing; it makes cosmic *buddhi (mahat)* into "my intellect" (which is the usual definition of the term). Cosmic knowing is experienced as my intellect when I identify with it as myself.

From *asmitā-mātra* ("individuation"), which follows from *mahat,* issues forth the subjective and objective world (cf. *SK* 24). *Asmitā-mātra* is that principle which differentiates unified cosmic knowing (*mahat* or *buddhi,* where the affliction of *asmitā* originates) into ascertaining subject and the ascertained object. *Mahat* is the cosmic principle of unification, of pure cosmic being *(sattā-mātra)*. S. Chennakesavan observes: "The *mahat* [great one or *buddhi*] is the last limit, in an ascending order, up to which the subjective and objective are differentiated. Or, in other words, at this stage of evolution [creation] the subject and object aspects of experience had not yet emerged."[154] However, by misidentifying with *asmitā-mātra* we wrongly consider the subjective to be *puruṣa* or true identity itself: "I am this 'myself' of which I am aware." "This myself is me." Mistaken identity of *puruṣa* transforms cosmic subjectivity/objectivity into individual self-awareness. *Asmitā-mātra (ahaṃkāra)* is experienced as my ego, personal individualized fabricated consciousness *(nirmāṇa-citta),* when I am identified with it as myself. This modified yet contracted and egoistic sense of self can be dissolved or purified through Yoga into its cosmic source, *mahat,* whereby one's understanding of selfhood is transformed and expanded into cosmic "I-am-ness"[155] which is still first personal but not egoistic as is *ahaṃkāra.* Based on our analysis above it would appear that Feuerstein's assertion[156]—that the Sāṃkhyan term *ahaṃkāra* is probably replaced in the *Yoga-Sūtra* by *asmitā*—is inaccurate. We must bear in mind that *asmitā* is an affliction *(kleśa)* that arising out of spiritual ignorance permeates the entire realm of our seeing or prakṛtic consciousness, individual and cosmic. As such, it along with its root cause (ignorance) must be discarded in order for the *puruṣa* or pure seer to shine in its true light.

The notion of mistaken identity or misidentification with *buddhi* and *ahaṃkāra* makes it easy to understand how these *tattva*s can be depicted as both cosmic and psychological, for it is the very false identification that turns the cosmic into the psychological. It would be a grave mistake to assert, as does S. Dasgupta,[157] that the cosmic and individual *buddhi* for example, have the same ontological status. *Mahat* or cosmic knowing is the first created essence of *prakṛti,* as real as *prakṛti* herself. *Mahat* brings forth the rest of *prakṛti*'s essences—not personal intellects. Personal intellects are not generated from *prakṛti* in the real causal process but are "created" when the prakṛtic sense of self "imagines" or conceives *mahat* to be the locus of authentic identity. The identification with "I am *mahat*" (uttered by the sattvic component of *prakṛti*), not the ontological causal process in itself, creates a personal or self-appropriated intellect. Personal intellect, egoity, and so forth, have no ontological reality, only psychological. Thus, the psychological terminology used in Yoga results from an apparent ("as if") identification of *puruṣa* with *buddhi, ahaṃkāra,* and so on. *Puruṣa* and *prakṛti seemingly* "come together" in the prakṛtic "condition" of misconception or ignorance *(avidyā).* Through discerning knowledge *(viveka-khyāti)* Yoga brings about a retrieval of our true identity as *puruṣa.*

Although Vyāsa does not state in *Yoga-Bhāṣya* II.19 that the subtle elements arise out of *asmitā-mātra,* it can be inferred from *Yoga-Bhāṣya* I.45 that this is the case; that is, Vyāsa states that *ahaṃkāra* is subtler than the *tanmātra*s, implying that the subtle elements arise out of the I-principle.[158] It seems reasonable to assume then that *asmitā-mātra* (as is the case for *ahaṃkāra* in the *SK*) also acts as the source of the *tanmātra*s (assuming that they are a part of Patañjali's ontology), and the elements *(bhūta*s*)* and the senses (*indriyas*). Koelman, taking his cue from Vācaspati Miśra, asserts that "Yoga . . . maintains that the objective universals [*tan-mātras*] are derived directly from the 'function-of-consciousness' *[buddhi].*"[159] Vācaspati Miśra places *asmitā-mātra* and the *tanmātras* on the same ontological level in as much as he regards both as evolutes of *buddhi (liṅga-mātra)*.[160] However, there is no reason not to follow the basic Sāṃkhyan scheme[161] in this regard. Thus, H. Āraṇya writes:

> The commentator (Vyāsa) says that Mahat undergoes six undiversified modifications in the shape of Tanmātra and ego. Sāṃkhya says that from Mahat arises ego and from ego come the Tanmātras. Some say that this is a point of difference between Sāṃkhya and Yoga philosophies. There is, however, no real difference. . . . In the commentaries on Sūtra I.45 the author of the Bhāṣya has said that the ego is the cause of the Tanmātras, and the cause of the ego is the Mahat principle. . . . Therefore it is not quite right to say that the six Aviśeṣas have arisen straight out of Mahat. The commentator also does not mean it. From Mahān Ātmā (the great self) or Mahat to ego, from ego to the five Tanmātras and from Tanmātras to the five Bhūtas, this is the correct order of succession.[162]

It is important to note that, like Sāṃkhya, Yoga distinguishes between the material *(upādāna)* and the efficient or instrumental *(nimitta)* cause. New categories of existence and other species or forms of life must all necessarily be developments, transformations *(pariṇāma),* or differentiations *(vikāra, vikṛti)* of the same fundamental substance *(prakṛti)*. Moreover, as Vyāsa informs us: "The change of body and senses into another life, when they are transformed into the other life, is implemented by their *prakṛti*-natures. With the disappearance of the earlier transformation, the corresponding rise of the later transformation comes about by an integrating pervasion of the new parts."[163] The material or substrative cause does not produce its effects without the aid of motivating causes known as efficient causes *(nimitta)*.[164] Every effect requires for its actualization an appropriate combination of the material cause along with efficient causes such as place, time, and form (i.e., virtue).[165] Thus a particular place aids in the production of a particular effect. For instance, Kashmir produces (Kashmiri) saffron, which will not be produced at other places in the world even though other causes of its growth may be present at those other places. Likewise, in certain regions of the world, rain may not fall at appropriate times thereby impeding the growth of certain crops later on. Similarly, an elephant cannot give birth to a human being, as the form of an elephant cannot give birth to a form different from its own. In the same way, a nonvirtuous person does not experience any kind of pleasure in the absence of the motivating cause of virtue. Owing to the operation of place, time, and form and motivating causes, the essential nature of things do not become manifest all at once.[166]

According to the tradition, *Yoga-Sūtra* IV.2–3 concerns the way in which the virtues or merits *(dharma)* of the yogin cause that yogin to enter another body, that is, by rebirth or even yogic powers.[167] In *Yoga-Sūtra* IV.3 the term *prakṛti* is used in the plural (in its two other occurrences in the *Yoga-Sūtra*—I.19 and IV.2—its number is unmarked since it is the first member of a compound). This plural use is common in earlier texts such as the *Bhagavadgītā* (VII.4–5) and the *Buddhacarita* (XII.18). The *Sāṃkhya-Kārikā* uses the term *prakṛti* in both the singular and plural, speaking of *mūlaprakṛti* (in the sense of an ultimate first principle) and of the various *prakṛti*s and *vikṛti*s, that is, the various primary and secondary evolutes and differentiations of primordial *prakṛti* (*SK* 3). The plural use in the *Sāṃkhya-Kārikā* refers to the first eight "creative" *tattva*s, namely, *avyakta, buddhi, ahaṃkāra,* and the five *tanmātra*s, while *prakṛti* in the single *(mūlaprakṛti)* refers to the eight collectively.[168] Patañjali seems to apply the use of the term *prakṛti* in a similar twofold way. According to Vācaspati Miśra[169] the term *prakṛti* as used in *Yoga-Sūtra* IV.2 refers to the five elements that are the *prakṛti* of the body, and the "I-am-ness" that is the *prakṛti* of the senses. These are thought to continue from one embodiment to the next, thus corresponding to what the *Sāṃkhya-Kārikā* calls the *liṅga-śarīra* (*SK* 39). The compound *prakṛtyāpūra* in *Yoga-Sūtra* IV.2 (see n. 99 above): "implemented by [the] *prakṛti*[s]," refers to the process whereby the *prakṛti*s of the yogin's previous body "fill" a new body. Vācaspati explains[170] that the *prakṛti*s of the first body "fill" the parts of the new body, while the *prakṛti* of the first set of faculties *(asmitā)* fills the new faculties. The *prakṛti*s in the form of mental impressions *(saṃskāra*s*)* that remain cause future experiences to take place. *Prakṛti* as material cause is not, however, the sole cause; it operates according to certain efficient causes *(nimitta)* such as the yogin's merit *(dharma).* Vācaspati tells us that the process is analogous to the passage of a body through childhood, growth, and old age (where the body follows a predetermined pattern of change, but only at certain times), or the growth of a banyan seed into a banyan tree (which can only happen if it is in the earth and suitably watered), or the way a spark dropped on a heap of grass suddenly rises to the sky.[171] In each case the tendency inherent in the material cause is only manifested when an efficient cause arises.

In *Yoga-Sūtra* IV.3 Patañjali tells us how the implementation of *prakṛti* takes place: "The efficient cause does not actuate the *prakṛti*s, but removes obstacles from them like a farmer [for irrigation]."[172] The various pathways of manifestation are determined by impressions *(saṃskāras)* already in motion. From the implementation of *prakṛti* comes transformation into other births. According to Yoga, an efficient cause does not set the material cause into action nor, as in *Nyāya-Vaiśeṣika,* does it make the effect a different existence from the cause *(anyathākaraṇa).* It is not that the cause produces something new as it is held by the Vaiśeṣikas.[173] In Sāṃkhya and Yoga the efficient cause removes the barriers or obstacles *(varaṇa)* to the manifestation of the effect latent in its material cause. The analogy of the farmer in *Yoga-Sūtra* IV.3 refers to the practice of irrigation, as Vyāsa explains:

> The farmer, in order to irrigate a terraced field by flooding it with water from another (higher) field, does not take the water in his hands, but makes a breach in its retaining barrier, after which the water pours into the lower field of itself. Similarly, virtue breaches nonvirtue, the retaining barrier of the *prakṛtis.* When it is breached the *prakṛtis* flow out into the respective effects or differentiations.[174]

As an alternative explanation of the analogy one could say that the farmer cannot himself force the nourishment from the water or earth into the roots of his crop, but permits it to penetrate the roots by removing the weeds.[175] Efficient causes can obstruct or aid the manifestations of the material causes.[176] The fact that for instance a potter, the efficient cause, turns the potter's wheel does not detract from the inherent capacity of the wheel to help shape the pot. In the psychological context of the mind and its functioning (see chapter 3), it will be seen that the *prakṛtis* in the form of *saṃskāras*—the deep-rooted impressions that mysteriously shape our lives—are canalized by our good or evil actions.

While admitting the subtlety of both the unmanifest *(aliṅga)* or undifferentiated *prakṛti* and pure consciousness *(puruṣa),* Vyāsa points out the considerable difference between these two in that *puruṣa* is not a subtle cause of the great principle *(mahat, liṅga-mātra)* in the same way that *aliṅga (pradhāna)* is. Not being the material cause of *liṅga-mātra, puruṣa* is however considered to be a final cause of prakṛtic reality.[177] Moreover, in his commentary on *Yoga-Sūtra* II.19, Vyāsa informs us that "the unmanifest *(aliṅga)* is not caused by any purposefulness of *puruṣa;* no purpose of *puruṣa* brings it about, nor is there any purpose of *puruṣa* in it. Hence it is classed as eternal. But purposefulness of *puruṣa* is a cause of the three differentiated states. This purpose being their final (and efficient) cause, they are classed as non-eternal."[178]

The *guṇas* are the material cause of everything prakṛtic and they also act as efficient causes to actualize or manifest their latent determinations.

On this issue, Koelman writes: "*Prakṛti* is the universal cause of all genetic realities, a root-cause both substrative in nature and efficient. . . . All other causes have only an assisting causality."[179] The purposefulness of *puruṣa* is evidently a cause. Vācaspati's comments are worth noting here. He argues that

> it cannot be supposed that it is the purpose of *puruṣa* that sets all in motion. It is only the Lord *(īśvara)* who does this with this purpose in view. For the purpose of *puruṣa* is described as setting all in motion in the sense that it is the final end. While this purpose of the *puruṣa* is yet to be realized, it is correct that the unmanifest *prakṛti* should be the cause of stability (of things). . . . In the case of the Lord, we must understand that his functional activity is limited to the removal of obstacles with a view to securing a basis for the manifestation of forms.[180]

While virtue is an efficient cause for removing unvirtue (see n. 174 above), it is not, however, the cause which sets the material cause in motion. In the same sense, there is a view in Yoga that the Lord *(īśvara)* favors the yogin through the yogin's special devotion (*YS* I.23). All barriers themselves are causes in the sense that they block the manifestation of another form. Thus place, time, form, and other factors are required for the manifestation of some change of modality.[181]

In the condition of misidentification (*YS* I.4), human identity is ensconced in the ever-changing saṃsāric world of the three *guṇa*s. Vyāsa tells us that virtue and nonvirtue, pleasure and pain, attachment and aversion are the causes of the six-spoked "wheel" *(cakra)* of *saṃsāra*. Ignorance, the root cause of all affliction, is said to be the driver of this "wheel."[182] Everything within the purview of saṃsāric experience is thus reduced to different functional dispositions of the three *guṇa*s.

According to the commentaries (see, for example, Vācaspati Miśra on *YS* IV.3) the *Yoga-Sūtra* reconciles the idea of *karman*[183] ("action" in a moral context as determiner of future embodiments) with that of a self-operating *prakṛti* (or set of *prakṛti*s). The topic is discussed in the context of the yogin's power to change or multiply his body, but there is no reason for not assuming that the same principles apply elsewhere, as Vācaspati has shown by the examples of the maturing and aging of the body, and so forth. The *sūtra*s (IV.2–3) are not primarily concerned with cosmology; the term *prakṛti* refers here to the makeup of the empirical self rather than to the primary "stuff" of the cosmos. This is a clear indication of Yoga's practical, psychological, and integrative approach, or what J. W. Hauer appropriately termed "experienced metaphysics."[184] In the chapters that follow we will see how this integrative or wholistic approach displayed by Yoga finds congenial expression in Patañjali's conception of mind *(citta).*

The above metaphor of a "wheel" (used by Vyāsa) seems an apt description of saṃsāric self-identity and existence. The term *duḥkha* (i.e., suffering, dissatisfaction, pain, sorrow) is comprised of *duṣ* meaning: difficult, bad, doing wrong,[185] plus *kha* meaning: axle hole, cavity, cave, space[186] and can literally mean "having a bad axle-hole." Such a wheel is unable to function properly or smoothly leading to an unsteady ride or journey in life, perhaps even disabling completely the vehicle (the body-mind) it is helping to propel. With spiritual ignorance *(avidyā)* "driving" the wheel of self-identity, consisting of the mind and its perceptions, concepts, memories, and so on, human consciousness (the mind) is molded into, shaped by a mistaken identity of self that has become this wheel of *saṃsāra* and its future sorrow/dissatisfaction. This "wheel of saṃsāric life" or "bad/ afflicted space" manifesting as self-identity in the form of the mental makeup of the mind (i.e., of impressions *[saṃskāra*s*],* habit patterns *[vāsanā*s*]* and mental modifications *[vṛtti*s*]*) including egoity *(asmitā)* with its self-appropriated virtues and nonvirtues, attachments and aversions, pleasures and pain, is the product of a malfunctioning of consciousness in the mind. Can this malfunctioning of the "wheel" of the mind and its mental processes be corrected? Or is it necessary for this wheel of life—in the form of the mind, personal identity, morality, likes and dislikes—to be utterly removed, dissolved, negated, or snuffed out of the yogin's life? Are our embodied, sensorial, thinking apparatus and empirical existence as well as relationships and participation in society an inherently or ultimately dissatisfying, sorrowful state of affairs? Are the *guṇa*s, by definition, a reality of dis-ease, disharmony? Is the "wheel of *saṃsāra*" a limitation, distortion, or contracted *form* of human life in the world?

The discerning yogin sees (*YS* II.15) that this world or cycle of saṃsāric identity is itself dissatisfaction *(duḥkha).* But we must ask, what exactly is the problem being addressed in Yoga? What is at issue in Yoga philosophy? Is our ontological status as a human being involved in day-to-day existence forever in doubt, in fact in need of being negated, dissolved in order for authentic identity *(puruṣa),* an immortal consciousness, finally to dawn? Having overcome all ignorance (*avidyā,* the "driver" of the wheel and cause of all afflicted identity), is it possible for a human being to live in the world and no longer be in conflict with oneself and the world? Can the *guṇa*s cease to function in a state of ignorance and conflict in the mind? Must the guṇic constitution of the human mind and the whole of prakṛtic existence disappear, dissolve for the yogin? Can the ways of spiritual ignorance be replaced by an aware, conscious, nonafflicted identity and activity that transcends the conflict and confusion of ordinary, saṃsāric life? Can we live, according to Patañjali's Yoga, an embodied state of freedom?

The following chart (see below) constitutes a summary of the different ontological levels comprising *prakṛti.* On the left-hand side is the general scheme outlined in the system of classical Sāṃkhya (i.e., the *SK*), and on the right-hand side are the alternative explanatory titles given in the *Yoga-Sūtra* (II.19) and as explained by Vyāsa (*YB* II.19):

Classical Sāṃkhya		Classical Yoga
1	*prakṛti (avyakta)*	*aliṅga,* the unmanifest
2	*mahat (buddhi)*	*liṅga-mātra,* the designator: *sattā-mātra* or *mahat/buddhi*
3-8	*ahaṃkāra* ("I-maker") 5 *tanmātra*s (subtle senses)	6 *aviśeṣa*s, the unparticularized: *asmitā-mātra* and 5 *tanmātra*s
9-24	*manas* and: 5 cognitive senses and 5 conative senses (=10 *indriya*s) 5 *bhūta*s (gross elements)	*viśeṣa*s, the particularized: the final 16 products as in Sāṃkhya

We note that in classical Yoga *asmitā-mātra* can be understood as fulfilling a similar function as *ahaṃkāra* in classical Sāṃkhya, that is, its sattvic illuminative nature giving rise to *manas* (the mind-organ), the five cognitive senses *(buddhīndriya*s*)*, and the five senses of action *(karmendriya*s*)*; and its tamasic "inert" nature as generating the five subtle elements *(tanmātra*s*)* and the five gross elements *(bhūta*s*)*.[187]

The twenty-three evolutes or manifestations of which the cosmos is constituted and which also form our psychophysical being/personality are all *prakṛti,* matter-energy or "nonself" (i.e., extrinsic identity or *anātman*), as is *aliṅga,* the unmanifest. The whole of the guṇic realm (including all the evolutes) does not constitute intrinsic identity *(puruṣa)* and is therefore classified as "nonself." In order of subtlety, intelligence or the faculty of discernment *(buddhi)*, sense of self *(ahaṃkāra)* and the mind-organ *(manas)*, including all the things or content of the mind such as cognitions, volitions, inclinations, emotions, and so forth, all the senses *(indriya*s*)* as well as their objects, the components as well as the states of the physical body—they are all "nonself" (i.e., are not to be mistaken for *puruṣa*). This realization or discriminative discernment is the key to the eradication of ignorance, misidentification, and dissatisfaction *(duḥkha)* and it ushers one into a state of freedom termed *kaivalya:* the "aloneness of seeing"[188] or *puruṣa* established in its true nature or form *(svarūpa)*.

THE *PURUṢA*-PRINCIPLE IN THE *YOGA-SŪTRA*

As in Sāṃkhya, Patañjali's Yoga regards *puruṣa* as the witness *(sākṣin)* of *prakṛti,* that is, the three *guṇas*. More specifically, *puruṣa* is affirmed as being the "seer" *(draṣṭṛ)* of all mental content or psychomental experiences,[189] and the "knower" of all the mental processes or modifications *(vṛtti)* of the mind *(citta).*[190] The most common term used by Patañjali to designate *puruṣa*—authentic Selfhood—is the "seer," as can be observed in *Yoga-Sūtra* I.3 and II.17 as well as II.20 and IV.23. In the *Yoga-Sūtra* the gender of *puruṣa* must be seen merely as a linguistic or grammatical convenience. This masculine word meaning the "seer" or Self (i.e., pure consciousness) is used interchangeably with the feminine words: *śakti*[191] (power, energy, force), *citi*[192] (consciousness), *citiśakti*[193] (power of consciousness), and *dṛśi*[194] (sight, seeing). Also termed the "power of seer" *(dṛś-śakti),*[195] *puruṣa* is described as being absolutely unmixed with[196] or distinct from[197] even the finest, most subtle aspect of *prakṛti*—the *sattva* of consciousness or mind—which can still allow the yogin to misidentify with prakṛtic existence, the "seeable" *(dṛśya).* The "seeable" is, in itself, insentient and lacks all consciousness or self-luminosity.[198]

Yet what we call worldly existence including our ordinary human identity is due to the conjunction *(saṃyoga)* between the "seer" *(puruṣa)* and the "seeable" *(dṛśya, prakṛti).*[199] That conjunction, which is the cause of suffering and dissatisfaction (*YS* II.16–17), is to be undermined through yogic praxis until the *puruṣa* shines forth in its original and untainted glory. It is the *puruṣa* that the yogin seeks to realize and thereby liberate identity from any "entanglement" or "concealment" within "matter." *Puruṣa* is often described as being totally opposite to manifest or unmanifest *prakṛti (vyaktāvyakta)* and as such is unaffected by *prakṛti*'s intricate web or network of traces or strands of materiality. Due to its "otherness," *puruṣa*—the principle of consciousness—is not to be confused with the transactions of human awareness (intellect, memory, and so on) as it transcends all object (worldly) orientation; and unlike *prakṛti, puruṣa* is said to be uncharacterizable, conscious, and nonproductive.[200] As witness, and possessing freedom and the quality of clear vision or "seeing," *puruṣa* can be conceived (i.e., from *prakṛti*'s perspective) as being indifferent and inactive,[201] thus laying emphasis on an existence whose nature appears wholly transcendent, uninvolved, and invariably aloof from *prakṛti*'s realm. Whereas change characterizes all "matter" including our psychophysical being, changelessness is the very essence of *puruṣa.* Dasgupta writes:

> Puruṣa is the constant seer of the mind when it has an object, as in ordinary forms of phenomenal knowledge, or when it has no object as in the state of nirodha or cessation. Puruṣa is unchanging. It is the light which remains unchanged amidst all the changing modifications of the mind. . . . Its knowing is manifested in our consciousness as the ever-persistent notion of the self, which is always a constant factor in all the phenomena of consciousness. Thus puruṣa always appears in our consciousness as the knowing agent.[202]

Since such a *puruṣa,* as contentless consciousness, could not be fully at home within the world of evolved matter, its ideal state is conceived of as being separate and apart from its apparent entanglement by the bonds of *prakṛti.*

In the Sāṃkhyan ontological duality of *puruṣa* and *prakṛti,* which Patañjali—at least on a provisional basis—utilizes, it appears to be the case that the former category comprises countless *puruṣa*s (cf. *SK* 18) that are omnipotent, omniscient, and passive spectators of the cosmos. The *Mahābhārata* (XII.338.2)[203] states that both Yoga and Sāṃkhya proclaim the existence of multiple *puruṣa*s in the world but that these many *puruṣa*s all have their origin in the one Self *(ātman),* which is eternal, immutable, and incommensurable. That Self is described in the same section as being *both* the "seer" *(draṣṭṛ)* and the "seeable" *(draṣṭavya).* While this view is generally characteristic of the schools of preclassical Yoga it is not on the whole the acknowledged scholarly understanding of classical Yoga. According to Vyāsa, Yoga does admit many liberated beings *(kevalin*s*)*[204] although it is not stated in the *Yoga-Bhāṣya* whether a plurality of *puruṣa*s is ontologically intended or is not derived from a single *ātman* or the *puruṣa*-principle as spiritual essence.

What is the metaphysical status of *puruṣa?* Being eternal and omnipresent (*YS* III.54) a *puruṣa* has no particular locus but is ubiquitous, pervading everywhere. However, that a *puruṣa* is all-pervading leads to problems for both Sāṃkhya and Yoga (unlike, for example, Vedānta) since there is supposedly an infinity (or at least a very large number) of completely distinct, unrelated *puruṣa*s. How can they all occupy the same infinite space without affecting each other in some way? Transcending all objectification, how can *puruṣa* be conceived as an entitative being? Given that, as pure consciousness, *puruṣa*s are devoid of any attributes, how are they to be distinguished from each other? Furthermore, each liberated *puruṣa,* being ubiquitous, must coexist with all of *prakṛti* yet remain unaffected by her realm. Vācaspati Miśra (*TV* I.41) emphasizes that there is no distinction between these many Selves.[205] But is the doctrine of a plurality of *puruṣa*s really a part of Patañjali's system of thought?

Following the cues provided in Vyāsa's *Yoga-Bhāṣya* and especially Vācaspati Miśra's *Tattva-Vaiśāradī,* S. Dasgupta[206] argues on the basis of *Yoga-Sūtra* II.22 that Patañjali recognized a plurality of *puruṣa*s. The text of *Yoga-Sūtra* II.22 runs as follows: *kṛtārthaṃ prati naṣṭamapyanaṣṭaṃ tadanyasādhāraṇatvāt,* "For one whose purpose is accomplished, it [the nature of the seeable/extrinsic identity] has ceased, but not for others [i.e., the deluded, empirical selves], due to it being common."[207] In agreement with Feuerstein,[208] I submit that it cannot be conclusively demonstrated based on the above *sūtra* that Patañjali subscribed to the doctrine of plurality as, for example, is more explicitly set out in classical Sāṃkhya (*SK* 18). In fact, I cannot locate any clear reference to the effect that there is a multiplicity of *puruṣa*s. There is no reason why *Yoga-Sūtra* II.22 could not be read in the same light of the preclassical tradition, where the term *kṛta-artha* also signifies the enlightened person who has attained *puruṣa*-realization thereby recovering authentic identity of Self beyond all plurality.[209]

The Sanskrit commentaries on the *Yoga-Sūtra* do imply that *puruṣa*s are somehow countable entities and, if such is the case, then it must be admitted that the ancient Yoga masters or *guru*s allowed themselves to fall into ineluctable difficulty. According to G. Larson's reading of classical Sāṃkhya, there may be as many disclosures of pure consciousness *(puruṣa)* as there are intellects *(buddhi)* capable of reflective discernment *(adhyavasāya),* that is, the intellects are following various life "paths" and are functioning at various times and under varying circumstances in accordance with the various manifestations of the *guṇa*s.[210] In classical Sāṃkhya pure contentless consciousness in its immanence accompanies every intellect (unlike the cosmic *ātman* of the Upaniṣads), and thus it is stressed that

> the awareness of consciousness is an achievement of the intellect and is a negative discernment of what the intellect is not. The Sāṃkhya arguments for a plurality of pure consciousness . . . appear to be directed at epistemological concerns rather than ontological matters. Because contentless consciousness can never be a content and cannot be characterized as are materiality or the tripartite process, it is hardly likely that the Sāṃkhya teachers were thinking of the plurality of consciousness as a set of knowable entities to be counted. They were thinking, rather, of the plurality of intellects through which the disclosure of contentless consciousness occurs.[211]

The only Sāṃkhya textual support for the above view is given by Vijñāna Bhikṣu in his commentary (entitled the *Sāṃkhya-Pravacana-*

Bhāṣya) on *Sāṃkhyasūtra* I.154. Vijñāna Bhikṣu raises a similar issue in his *Yoga-Vārttika* (II.22), which seems to suggest that for him the intention in Yoga with its so-called plurality of *puruṣa*s is also largely epistemological. Bhikṣu understands the meaning of the expression *"kṛtārtha"* in *Yoga-Sūtra* II.22 as referring to "one whose object or purpose is supplied by the intellect,"[212] which can imply a plurality of intellects leading to the existential sense of there being multiple individualized selves or persons (because each individual self has a particular mind) through which pure consciousness discloses itself. Bhikṣu suggests that the Sāṃkhya notion of a plurality of *puruṣa*s does not contradict the evidence of the Veda that there is only one Self *(paramātman)* or essential identity. Bhikṣu makes the arguable claim that in the Veda oneness or uniformity refers to the essential nature *(svarūpa)* of selfhood in terms of genus *(jāti)* and therefore Vedic references to oneness or selfhood need not be construed as implying singularity.[213] Bhikṣu further maintains that many passages in the Veda (i.e., *śruti*) show that selfhood presents itself under limiting adjuncts *(upādhi)* and as such there is no contradiction between Vedic testimony and the Sāṃkhyan notion of the plurality of *puruṣa*s.[214]

One way, therefore, to approach the notion of the "plurality" of *puruṣa*s is to adopt a somewhat suspicious attitude toward Yoga interpreters (in both the extant native textual tradition and in modern scholarship) and approach the issue (as mentioned above by Larson) by laying emphasis on the epistemology of the intellect *(buddhi)* or mind *(citta)* rather than the ontology of the *puruṣa*s. *Puruṣa,* by definition being ever-free, ever-wise, unchanging, and so on, could never be in actual bondage, and its intrinsic nature is therefore quite unaffected by any apparent loss of true identity or by any form of limitation. Vyāsa (*YB* II.18) reveals that: "These two, experience and emancipation, are created by the mind (i.e., *buddhi*) and function only in the mind. . . . In the mind alone are bondage, which is the failure to fulfill the purpose of *puruṣa,* and emancipation, which is completion of that purpose."[215] Metaphysically speaking, the universe has meaning only insofar as it serves the purpose of *puruṣa,* that is, for experience and liberation.[216] According to Vyāsa's statement (n. 215 above), it would make more sense to understand spiritual emancipation as referring to a liberated state of mind (i.e., the mind—including the individual consciousness and personality—is liberated from its former condition of spiritual ignorance) and not literally as referring to a *puruṣa,* which is by definition already free and therefore has no intrinsic need to be liberated from the fetters of worldly existence. One of the implications of multiple *puruṣa*s for Patañjali's system would be to underscore the uniqueness of each individual's perspective or consciousness. Whether or not Patañjali actually adhered to the notion of a plurality of *puruṣa*s appears to be an open question.

Any consideration of Patañjali's "metaphysics" would be incomplete without reference to the third major "principle" of his ontology, the concept of *īśvara* or "Lord" (God). The term *īśvara* is found as early as the *Bṛhadāraṇyaka Upaniṣad* (e.g. I.4.8).[217] In some Vedānta-inspired schools of Yoga, *īśvara* refers to the Supreme Being as it rules over the cosmos and individuated beings. This idea is illustrated in the *Bhagavadgītā* (XVIII.61): "The Lord abides in the heart of all beings, Arjuna, by his power *(māyā)* causing all beings to revolve [as if they were] mounted on a wheel."[218]

In the Hiraṇyagarbha "school" of Yoga outlined in XII.296 of the *Mahābhārata* epic,[219] the noteworthy distinction is made between the Self that is recovering or awakening to its innate enlightenment, that is, the *budhyamāna,* and the ever-enlightened *buddha* ("awakened one") or *prabuddha.*[220] The later principle, *buddha,* is considered the twenty-sixth principle *(tattva)* and is also referred to as "Lord," *īśvara.*[221] The *budhyamāna* is the twenty-fifth principle *(tattva)*—the principle of conscious existence. When it fully "awakens" and realizes its intrinsic nature as being already enlightened, it becomes the Absolute.[222] There does not appear to be, however, any clear and simple identification of the twenty-fifth principle *(budhyamāna)* with the twenty-sixth principle—the supremely enlightened state *(buddha* or *īśvara)*. The *budhyamāna* partakes, as it were, in the realm of the twenty-sixth principle without necessarily attaining an identity *as* it. Maintaining a constant state of transcendence, *īśvara* "never becomes involved with the lower *tattva*s. Thus emancipation can be said to be a condition of the *[budhyamāna] qua* the *[budhyamāna]* in the 'company' *(samiti)* of the lord."[223]

In the above we have seen that the epic yogins allowed twenty-six fundamental categories of existence *(tattvas*), *prakṛti* and its modes comprising the first twenty-four principles. Many passages in the *Mokṣadharma* section of the *Mahābhārata* that assert a twenty-sixth principle do not necessarily imply the classical Yoga notion of a "Lord" *(īśvara).* Such passages could simply refer to the *puruṣa* (or *kṣetrajña*) in its intrinsically enlightened state.[224] However, it is obvious from examining sections of the *Mahābhārata,* especially the twelfth *parvan,* that the conceptualization of *īśvara* in Patañjali's Yoga has its epic antecedents. In his pioneering study, P. M. Modi rightly points out, "The idea of God in the Yoga System was not arrived at by superimposing it on an atheistic Sāṃkhya System with twenty-five principles but by distinguishing the Jīva [individuated self] from God on practical grounds."[225]

While classical Sāṃkhya is said to be *nir-īśvara* or "nontheistic," classical Yoga appears to incorporate a *sa-īśvara* or theistic stance. However, it is simply not appropriate to label the *Sāṃkhya-Kārikā* as being nontheistic. Īśvara Kṛṣṇa, rather like the Buddha, chooses not to mention or make any statement about God at all. According to the *Sāṃkhya-Kārikā,* if there be a God (there being no positive denial of God's existence in the *Sāṃkhya-Kārikā*), then such a Being has little or nothing to do with the actual path of salvation as propounded by Īśvara Kṛṣṇa.[226]

According to several scholars, the theistic stance of Yoga is clearly acknowledged by Patañjali.[227] The "Lord" *(īśvara)* is not a creator (i.e., an anthropomorphic deity) like the Judeo-Christian God. Neither Patañjali nor Vyāsa mention *īśvara*'s role (i.e., as a material cause) in the creation, preservation, and destruction of the world, implying thus an absence of a creator God in Yoga. *Īśvara* is also not the kind of universal Absolute taught in the Upaniṣads and envisaged by many thinkers within the tradition of Vedānta. Nor is *īśvara* intended as a type of enlightened superbeing such as the transcendent *bodhisattva*s of Mahāyāna Buddhism. *Īśvara* is defined by Patañjali as a Self *(puruṣa) sui generis,* whose distinctiveness from the "ordinary" *puruṣa* is explained largely in negative terms. *Yoga-Sūtra* I.24 states: "*Īśvara* is a distinct Self *(puruṣa)* untouched by the afflictions, actions or their fruition or their latent residue [in the mind]."[228] The distinctness or specialness of *īśvara* consists in that at no time can *īśvara* become embroiled in the domain of *prakṛti,* whereas all other "*puruṣa*s" at one time or another will have been entrenched in the illusion of being a misidentified entity within *prakṛti* and thus enslaved to prakṛtic existence. *Īśvara* does not abandon "His" perfect condition of transcendence as pure consciousness and infinite existence. The Lord's freedom is eternal.[229] This view has led to theological difficulties since Patañjali also regards *īśvara* as being of positive relevance for humankind in that *īśvara* is: (1) that Being in whom "the seed of omniscience is unsurpassed";[230] (2) the first teacher *(guru)* of all former yogins because not limited by time;[231] (3) whose expression is *praṇava [Om];*[232] and (4) following from the recitation of *praṇava* and realization of its meaning,[233] one realizes the "inner consciousness" *(pratyak-cetanā)* and obstacles no longer arise.[234] The above statements (*YS* I.25–29) are meant to be understood in conjunction with the concept of *īśvara-praṇidhāna* or "devotion to *īśvara.*"[235]

One might ask: How is it possible that a wholly transcendent *puruṣa* can intervene in the spatial, temporal world? In his commentary (*YB* I.24) Vyāsa elaborates on this issue explaining *īśvara*'s teaching role in terms of the 'Lord's' appropriation of a perfect medium, which Vyāsa terms *sattva* ("beingness").[236] Vācaspati Miśra reasons that out of compassion for the individuated selves the 'Lord', as it were, reaches "down" and "touches" the pure *sattva* of *prakrti,* the power of *sattva* excelling beyond the reach of *rajas* and *tamas*. *Īśvara* "touches" this *sattva* as it prevails in the mind *(citta),* thus asserting a definite proprietorship (i.e., lordship: from the root *īś*: "to own, be master of" and *vara:* "choicest") over this aspect of *prakrti.*[237] But unlike the empirical selves, *īśvara* does not become subject to spiritual ignorance *(avidyā)* and bondage. This is comparable to the role played by an actor/actress who, while identifying with the part nevertheless remains aware that he or she is not identical with the character of his or her role. The 'Lord', unlike the individuated selves, does not identify with *avidyā* on the "stage" of a *sattva*-dominated mind.[238] This is made possible because the 'Lord's' unblemished *sattva* is devoid of any contamination of *rajas* and *tamas.*[239] All *purusa*s (assuming there are a plurality of *purusa*s) are of course intrinsically free but only the 'Lord' has been forever aware of this truth. According to *Tattva-Vaiśāradī* I.24 *īśvara*'s power of knowledge and "action"[240] continues to bestow "favor" to the mind of the devoted yogin all for the purpose of liberation. *Īśvara* therefore "acts" non-saṃsārically, in the spirit of what the *Bhagavadgītā* calls "ego-transcending" or "trans-action" *(naiskarmya)* action—acting without attachment to the fruits of action—whereby no binding, karmic fruition *(vipāka)* could ever accrue, nor could any afflictions ever arise. Vyāsa declares that *īśvara* appropriated such an untainted vehicle of *sattva* in order "to confer favor to living beings,"[241] and also insists that the proof for this conviction is located in the sacred scriptures, which are manifestations of *īśvara*'s perfect *sattva.*[242]

Īśvara was undoubtedly more than a mere concept to Patañjali and the yogins of his time. It makes sense to assume that *īśvara* corresponded to an "experience" they shared. Considering the distinctly pragmatic orientation of his Yoga, it is doubtful that Patañjali would adopt the concept *īśvara* for merely historical reasons or simply in order to make his philosophy acceptable to orthodox Hinduism. The idea of "grace" or divine recompense *(anugraha, prasāda)*[243] has been an integral element of Yoga since the rise of the theistic traditions as seen in the Pāñcarātra tradition—for example, as epitomized in the *Bhagavadgītā.*

If one were to classify Yoga as being a radical dualistic perspective thereby focusing on the purely transcendent nature of *īśvara,* that is, *īśvara*'s role as a teacher being viewed as entirely passive and disengaged from any relation to the mechanism of *prakrti,* it is possible to see *īśvara*'s role as *guru* in purely metaphorical terms. The practical significance of the 'Lord', which the classical exegetes see in terms of *īśvara*'s related existence to empirical selves entangled in the prakṛtic realm, can also be understood passively, namely as the utter formless transcendent teacher, the archetypal yogin who "guides" by "His" mere presence or sheer being.[244] Mircea Eliade speaks of this as a "metaphysical sympathy"[245] between *īśvara* and the aspiring yogin made possible by the ontological co-essentiality of *īśvara* and the spiritual essence of a human being *(puruṣa)*. To view *īśvara* as something not absolutely identical with *puruṣa* is of intrinsic value. Not only does it enable yogins of a more devotional disposition to advance along the "path" by way of *praṇidhāna* or "devotion," but also warns those with a more intellectual outlook not to think of themselves in terms too autonomous, thus falling prey to dangerous pride *(abhimāna)*, a quality of the ego-consciousness. It should not be overlooked that *īśvara* might have met primarily psychological and pedagogical needs rather than providing a purely ontological category. In other words, the term *īśvara* was used by Patañjali largely to account for certain yogic experiences (e.g., *YS* II.44 acknowledges the possibility of making contact with one's "chosen deity"—*iṣṭa-devatā*—as a result of personal, scriptual study—*svādhyāya*).

If there are many transcendent *puruṣa*s, then how exactly are they related to one another and to *īśvara*, singly and collectively? For the purpose of this study it suffices to say that the status and relationship of *īśvara* to the *puruṣa*s and the *puruṣa*s one to another is an open question. Empirically, however, the relation of *īśvara* to the yogin can be described as "a one-way affair in which the believing yogin emulates *īśvara*'s condition, which is co-essential with the condition of his inmost Self."[246] However, there can be no question of the intrinsic nature of the transcendent Self—whether *īśvara* or not—ever being affected in the literal sense by the afflictions (*avidyā, asmitā,* etc.) or any other saṃsāric phenomena. Notwithstanding some of the problems inherent in Patañjali's concept of *īśvara*, this term is of considerable importance for Patañjali's Yoga. Indeed, original Yoga within Hinduism always was *sa-īśvara* or "with God" (cf. *MBh* XII.300.3). However narrow and even unacceptable to some the conception of "God" in classical Yoga may appear, the devotional element in it cannot be ignored or denied. Even though Patañjali's *Yoga-Sūtra* appears to designate "devotion to the Lord" as an alternative "path," or only one of several ways that combine together to achieve a liberating transformation of consciousness, there can be no question of *īśvara*'s integral role in Patañjali's system.

It is of interest to note that neither Vyāsa nor Vācaspati tackle the issue of whether *īśvara* is an additional principle (implying a twenty-sixth *tattva*) of Patañjali's Yoga. It is entirely possible that being a particular kind of *puruṣa, īśvara* is not intended to be an additional principle. If this be the case, it can further be speculated that although *īśvara* and the so-called innumerable *puruṣa*s (or *puruṣa*) are formally differentiated as a numerical multiplicity, one can assume that at the absolute level of existence *īśvara* coincides with the *puruṣa*(s). It might then be possible that at the transcendent level *īśvara* and the "liberated" *puruṣa*(s) (the twenty-fifth principle) merge ontologically as one Being, that is, are qualitatively one in eternity; or even can be said to "intersect" as separate Self-monads whereupon they enter into a state of pure intersubjectivity. But speculation at this highly abstract level, however difficult it may be, does not seem to represent the spirit of the Yoga school, which is much more practical and experiential in character. The nature of *īśvara* as experienced in the liberated state of "aloneness" *(kaivalya)* is not a topic in the *Yoga-Sūtra*. What seems crucially important, however, is for the yogin to know that the existence of *īśvara* is clearly admitted. Unlike any other conscious "being" or "principle," *īśvara* can function as a transformative catalyst or "guide" for aiding the yogin on the "path" to spiritual emancipation. Thus, whether one asserts that Patañjali's descriptions of *īśvara* constitute a theistic stance or not, the concept of *īśvara* must be taken seriously as an authentic and dynamic aspect of Patañjali's philosophical platform.[247]

Paradoxically it appears that *puruṣa* is both aware of its transcendent nature as the "seer" (*YS* I.3) and yet is *seemingly* and mysteriously "entrapped" in *prakṛti* whereby human identity experiences itself to be a finite entity through a process of "conformity" (*sārūpya, YS* I.4) to the nature of the modifications *(vṛtti)* of the mind *(citta)*. What we normally call the mind or ordinary consciousness is due to the conjunction *(saṃyoga)*[248] between the "seer" and the "seeable"—that is, between pure consciousness and the complex of the body and personality. *Puruṣa* is, however, distinct from phenomenal consciousness *(citta)* and therefore is not to be confused with empirical selfhood and its turbulence or "whirls" of thoughts and emotions,[249] these all being a form and product of the three *guṇa*s. The *puruṣa*'s proximity to the highly evolved human organism "solicits" the phenomenon of consciousness.[250] The connection between *puruṣa* and *prakṛti* is made possible because at the finest, most subtle level of *prakṛti* is found a predominance of the *sattva* component *(guṇa)* wherein *prakṛti,* in the form of the mind *(citta),* is transparent enough to "reflect" the "light" of consciousness (of *puruṣa*) and create the appearance of sentience as well as an autonomous sense of intelligence in its evolutes or manifestations.

Patañjali effectively draws on the key yogic concept of "mind" *(citta)* in order to articulate the human "predicament" of mistaken identity. In the chapter that follows we will be exploring how Patañjali and his main commentator, Vyāsa, make use of the Sāṃkhyan *triguṇa* doctrine and present a study of the mind—its nature, structure, and functioning *(vṛtti)*—that is ineluctably and integrally linked to Yoga epistemology.

chapter three

The Mind (Citta):

Its Nature, Structure, and Functioning

This chapter will focus on Yoga epistemology and psychology by examining the nature, structure, and functioning of the mind *(citta),* the mind being the locus of consciousness through which we "know" and "experience" ourselves and the world. Yoga offers an acute analysis of the role played by the mind in the act of cognition and accounts for the decisive influence that the psyche exerts over human perception, cognition, and behavior, ethical or otherwise. Following from some of the questions raised in the last chapter regarding Yoga metaphysics and issues of an ontological nature, this chapter attempts to lay a foundation for understanding definitions and explanations of key terms in the *Yoga-Sūtra* with an epistemological emphasis rather than the ontological emphasis normally given to them.

In Yoga, the purpose of the human mind is not limited simply to the production of concepts that "correspond" to or are distinct representations of a presupposed external reality, as in the Western Cartesian model of understanding. Neither is the mind, according to Yoga, restricted to the role of imposing its own order on the world, as is the case, for example, in the Kantian epistemology, which states that all human knowledge of the world is in some sense determined by subjective principles. As we will see, in Yoga both of the above epistemological dualisms—themselves the product of spiritual ignorance *(avidyā)*—are understood and transcended in a larger and subtler understanding of the human mind. The truth of the world is realized within and through the human mind.

Sāṃkhya posits an analysis of human awareness *(buddhi, vṛtti)* or mental processes that Yoga more or less incorporates and that involves the principles *(tattva*s*)* of *prakṛti*. Human awareness functions through the "inner instrumentality" *(antaḥkaraṇa)* comprised of the following three principles:

1. The mind-organ *(manas),* which assimilates and synthesizes sense impressions acting as a conveyor of information and bringing the awareness in contact with external objects;
2. The "I-maker" *(ahaṃkāra)* or principle of individuation, which acts as a locus of self-identity; and
3. The intellect *(buddhi),* the finest or most subtle aspect of human awareness, the faculty of judgment or decision that determines overall perspective and intentionality and makes understanding possible.[1]

Puruṣa provides the "frame" for the above mental processes,[2] and though omnipresent, *puruṣa* remains "unseen" and transcendent of *prakṛti*'s activities.

In the consensus reality of egoic states of identity, *puruṣa* is as if "covered over,"[3] "veiled," or eclipsed by the dominance of the mental functions of the mind. Such states of mind define one's normal perception of reality and perpetuate in the individual the sense that the existence of an objective world is a presupposed or given static "entity" in opposition to one's notion of self. The unbridgeable gap between the individual subject or atomistic ego and object or world presupposed in the Cartesian-Kantian paradigm, a polarization that is itself part of the afflicted condition described in Yoga, can be effectively "bridged," "remedied," or "healed" according to Yoga. To be sure, Patañjali's Yoga is by no means a "Cartesian dichotomy":[4] it does not articulate the experience of an autonomous subjective self as being fundamentally distinct and separate from an objective external world of nature that it seeks to understand and achieve a mastery over. The Sāṃkhyan dualism that Yoga utilizes is quite distinct from the Cartesian dualism that bifurcates reality into mental and material aspects. Sāṃkhya's dualistic perspective—comprised of pure consciousness *(puruṣa)* and *prakṛti* as everything else including the mental and the material—asserts that psyche and the external world are not ultimately different. Both are forms of insentient or nonconscious *prakṛti*—termed the "seeable" *(dṛśya)* in Yoga. In order to place Yoga (or Sāṃkhya) within the context of Cartesian duality, *puruṣa* would then have to be reduced to the level of Descartes' "cogito," which in yogic terms is equivalent to the *asmitā-mātra* (i.e., *ahaṃkāra*)-*manas* level of *prakṛti* and in fact totally alienates human being from intrinsic self-identity *(puruṣa)*. Such a Cartesian-like subject is, from Yoga's perspective, a delusion or incorrect understanding of ourselves, an underlying misconception that is the very source of our suffering and dissatisfaction *(duḥkha)*.

In ancient and classical Hindu models of reality, the human mind takes on a more participatory and creative dimension. The Hindu view of the mind's highest potentialities is expressed in both the early and later Upaniṣads[5] where, far from advancing "an unsophisticated idealism," the emphasis is on the crucial role of the mind in gaining access to the world, thereby "exposing a complementarity between the perceived and the means of perception. Without the mind no world could be known nor could any action be accomplished."[6] Moreover, the mind becomes the instrument through which either enslavement to worldly existence, or spiritual freedom is cultivated.[7]

Patañjali's Yoga deals first and foremost with the human mind. In the *Yoga-Sūtra* the relationship between *puruṣa* (*draṣṭṛ*, the "seer") and *prakṛti* (*dṛśya,* the "seeable") can be viewed as a dynamic interplay manifesting itself through the instrument of the human mind. The mind—as is the case in the Upaniṣads and Sāṃkhya—is thus of great significance for determining how the world and self are "experienced" and "known," and finally, for "attaining" liberation from the saṃsāric enterprise of misidentification and ignorance. The pivot of the predicament of *puruṣa*'s "entanglement" with *prakṛti* is, I suggest, epistemological and it is here that we should look for an opening into the meaning of Patañjali's Yoga.

CITTA

Citta, which will be translated as "mind," is the perfect past participle of the verbal root *cit,* meaning: "to observe," "perceive," "to appear," "to shine," "to be conscious of," "to understand," "to know," "to attend to."[8] The term *cit* is widely employed in Yoga and Vedānta scriptures to denote the transcendent consciousness or pure awareness of the Self *(ātman)*. The term *citta* can mean: "thinking," "reflecting," "imagining," "thought," "intention," "wish," "the heart," "mind," "intelligence," "reason."[9] *Citta* is used in the *Ṛg Veda* and the *Atharva Veda*[10] besides the more frequently employed terms *asu* ("life" or "vital force") and *manas* (variously translated as "mind-organ" or "lower mind"), and it appears occasionally in the Upaniṣads[11] often translated as "thought." Feuerstein writes: "It is applied wherever pyscho-mental phenomena connected with conscious activity are to be expressed."[12]

By the time of the *Mahābhārata* the word *citta* gained more popular usage as can be seen in the *Bhagavadgītā.*[13] Unlike *manas* (which is used by most other orthodox schools to denote the concept "mind" in the loose sense mentioned earlier) the technical term *citta* is more specifically at home in Yoga and refers to phenomenal consciousness including both the ordinary level of awareness involving the conscious processes of the mind and the deeper level of the unconscious mind or psyche. The *citta* itself is not sentient.[14] Only *puruṣa* or pure consciousness is Self-luminous and "shines forth" unalloyed and unabated. Its "light" can be understood as being "reflected" or "mirrored" in insentient *prakṛti* (i.e., in the human mind), creating various self-reflective stages of the mind. This imagery is used by Vācaspati Miśra, who, in his gloss on *Yoga-Sūtra* II.20, states concisely: "The casting of the *puruṣa*'s reflection into the mirror of *buddhi [citta]* is the way in which *puruṣa* can know the *buddhi.*"[15] When the higher transcendent consciousness *(citi)* assumes the form of the mind, the experience of one's own intellect (and therefore of ideas, cognition, intention, and volition) becomes possible (*YS* IV.22).[16] Thus the mind becomes "consciousness-of" or is "conscious of" objects and can know all purposes (i.e., the purpose of objects is to provide experience and liberation for each being) and perceive all objects. The mind is in a way a function of *puruṣa* and *prakṛti* combined.[17] *Citta*'s consciousness[18] functions in the form of various modifications *(vṛttis)*[19] or "whirls" of consciousness often construed as cognitive conditions or mental processes that are constantly undergoing transformation and development *(pariṇāma).* Ordinary human consciousness is therefore an impermanent, fleeting or "whirling" state of consciousness. Therefore it is possible to decipher clearly between two radically different modes of consciousness as used in the *Yoga-Sūtra:* (1) pure, immortal consciousness, our intrinsic identity as *puruṣa* (Self); and (2) empirical consciousness or mind *(citta)* including mental activity *(vṛtti)* through which our perceptions and experiences inform and build a sense of person and self-identity. The latter is figuratively called "consciousness" because it is pure consciousness reflected in, or conditioned by, the mind.

In *Sāṃkhya-Kārikā* 33 the so-called synonym for *citta*—*antaḥkaraṇa* ("inner instrument")—is found, which is understood to be made up of *buddhi, ahaṃkāra,* and *manas.* In the *Yoga-Sūtra* the term *citta* can refer to these three manifest principles *(tattvas)* of *prakṛti,* namely: the intellect, sense of self, and mind-organ respectively. *Citta* can be viewed as the aggregate of the cognitive, volitional, affective activities, processes, and functions of human consciousness, that is, it consists of a grasping, intentional, and volitional consciousness, and functions as the locus of empirical selfhood. Outside the purview of classical Yoga *citta* is generally employed in a less technically precise sense and mostly refers to mind in general. This tendency is present in the commentarial literature on the *Yoga-Sūtra* where *citta* is often equated with *buddhi* or *manas,* these terms being used interchangeably.[20]

A variety of translations has been suggested for *citta* such as: "mind,"[21] "mind-stuff,"[22] "mind-complex,"[23] "consciousness,"[24] "awareness,"[25] "die innere Welt,"[26] "psyche,"[27] "psychic nature,"[28] "thinking principle,"[29] and "internal organ."[30] Even though the term is not defined explicitly by Patañjali, its meaning can be ascertained from its occurrences in the *Yoga-Sūtra.* S. Dasgupta states that the *citta* stands for "all that is psychical in man."[31] Koelman asserts that *citta* is "surely not a separate prakṛtic evolute,"[32] meaning that it is not distinguishable from its component factors, those being *buddhi, ahaṃkāra,* and *manas,* whose emergence from primordial *prakṛti* is the theme of the Sāṃkhyan ontological scheme. Feuerstein calls *citta* "an umbrella term comprising all the functionings of the mind."[33] The sixteenth-century commentator Vijñāna Bhikṣu supports the notion that *citta* comprises all of the above three prakṛtic principles and their internal functioning (including a volitional, grasping, and intentional nature) by explaining that the word *citta* does not signify only one of the above faculties but the entire *antaḥkaraṇa.*[34]

Whereas Īśvara Kṛṣṇa appears mostly concerned with showing the various components of the "inner world"—of the psyche—separately and in their evolutionary dependence, Patañjali, by his concept of *citta,* emphasizes the homogeneity or integral psychological constitution of the human personality as well as the processes (e.g., cognitive, affective, etc.) of empirical consciousness. Patañjali is only secondarily interested in an analytical categorization of the inner states. *Citta,* which is used a total of twenty-two times[35] in the *Yoga-Sūtra,* is a comprehensive concept that can be seen as embracing the various functionings of the ontological categories of *buddhi, ahaṃkāra,* and *manas,* and yet as reflected consciousness in total it is a nonstructural or ahierchical concept and cannot be equated or reduced to any one or more of the above evolutes in themselves.

The term *manas* ("lower mind" or "mind-organ") occurs only three times in the *Yoga-Sūtra. Yoga-Sūtra* I.35 and II.53 make use of the more traditional Hindu association of *manas* with the sense capacities that are to be controlled through sense withdrawal *(pratyāhāra)* and concentration *(dhāraṇā)*.[36] *Yoga-Sūtra* III.48[37] speaks of the speediness *(javitva)* of the *manas* that arises from the "conquest of the senses" (*indriya-jaya, YS* III.47). The consistent use by Patañjali of *manas* in conjunction with the senses is no accident and certainly reflects preclassical usage. Whereas Sāṃkhya asserts that *manas* is the size of the body, Yoga asserts that *manas* is all-pervasive.[38] In Vyāsa's exposition the word *manas* almost always is associated with some external activity such as speaking, shaking, the breathing process, and even sleep.[39] The term *buddhi* (intellect) is used only twice in the *Yoga-Sūtra* (IV.21 and 22)[40] and appears to be given a cognitive emphasis, although the dimension of *citta* as "will"—so crucial in Yoga (and as if absent in Sāṃkhya)—is included as an aspect of *buddhi*.

Hindu philosophical schools quite often distinguish two aspects of mental life called *manas* and *buddhi*. While *manas* assimilates and synthesizes sense impressions and brings the sense of self into contact with the external objects, it still, however, lacks discrimination furnishing the empirical sense of self *(ahaṃkāra)* only with precepts that must in turn be transformed and acted upon by a higher mental function, the intellect *(buddhi)*. The intellect can forget its inherent discerning power by either attending to *manas* and reifying or absolutizing its sense interpretations, or it can become free—functioning as a vehicle of liberation by attaining knowledge *(jñāna)*, which is in fact its own finest and most subtle nature as *sattva*.

Neither of Īśvara Kṛṣṇa's terms: *liṅga*—"the essential core" (*SK* 40)—a prerequisite for experience and comprising the thirteen evolutes (i.e., *buddhi, ahaṃkāra, manas,* and the ten *indriya*s), or the "set of eighteen" (*liṅgaśarīra* or *sūkṣmaśarīra* [*SK* 39], the subtle body comprising the above thirteen evolutes plus the five subtle senses), are able to convey the essentially dynamic interaction among the psychic structures or functional unity that the term *citta* connotes. In classical Yoga (see below), the Sanskrit commentators argue that because the *citta* is all-pervasive, the postulation of a subtle body is unnecessary.

Although *citta* is not treated as a separate ontological category *(tattva)*, it is nevertheless a part of insentient *prakṛti* and thus consists of the three *guṇa*s.[41] Moreover, *Yoga-Sūtra* IV.23 states :"[Due to] the mind being colored by the seer and the seeable, [it can, therefore, know] all purposes."[42] *Citta* is in a sense the product of the transcendent consciousness or seer and the perceived object, the seeable, inasmuch as it is said to be "colored" or tinted by both; however, it does not appear to be a derivation of either. It can be characterized as a function of the mysterious relation between *puruṣa* and *prakṛti* and plays a crucial epistemological role in Patañjali's Yoga as *Yoga-Sūtra* IV.22 (see n. 16 above) and IV.23 (see n. 17 and n. 42 above) clearly illustrate. Rather than being viewed as "substance" per se, *citta* can be seen as a heuristic device for understanding the dynamic interplay between pure consciousness *(puruṣa)*—the seer *(draṣṭṛ)*—and *prakṛti*—the seeable *(dṛśya)*—in the form of a reflected state of consciousness.

The philosophy of classical Yoga, in contrast to that of Sāṃkhya, recognizes the cosmic or root *citta;* it is the "one mind" that impels the many individualized minds. The root *citta,* becoming operative in a single personality, appears individual. This important point can be clarified as follows. In *Yoga-Sūtra* IV.4 the numerous fabricated, individualized minds *(nirmāṇa-citta*s*)* are said to arise from *asmitā-mātra*—the ontological principle denoting the exclusive sense of I-am-ness.[43] According to Vyāsa, *Yoga-Sūtra* IV.4 is alleged to have been composed in reply to the question: "(Opponent:) Well, when a yogin projects several bodies, do they have one mind between them or a mind each?"[44] The question arose from the treatment of powers *(siddhi*s*)* mentioned in *Yoga-Sūtra* IV.1[45] as to whether the multiple bodies that the yogin can produce at will are also endowed with a distinct consciousness. Vyāsa's answer to the above question is that the artificially created bodies do each have a mind.[46] Yet how could the activities of several minds wait on the purposes of a single mind?[47] The answer is given in *Yoga-Sūtra* IV.5: "[Although the multiple individualized minds are involved] in distinct activities, it is the one mind of [this] many that is the initiator."[48]

At this point in our analysis we take issue with Feuerstein's understanding when he states that, "the 'one consciousness' [mind in *YS* IV.5] is none other than the primary I-am-ness *(asmitā-mātra)* of aphorism IV.4."[49] Elsewhere Feuerstein has suggested[50] that *asmitā-mātra* is equivalent to the Sāṃkhyan term *ahaṃkāra,* an equation with which our study agrees. However, Feuerstein then goes on to equate the "one mind" *(cittam-ekam)* of *Yoga-Sūtra* IV.5 with *asmitā-mātra,* thereby reducing *citta* to a separate prakṛtic evolute and contradicting all that he has previously said about *citta* (i.e., that *citta* is an "umbrella term" and is "distinct from its component factors" such as *buddhi, ahaṃkāra,* etc.).[51] If the "one mind" of *Yoga-Sūtra* IV.5 were the equivalent of *asmitā-mātra* (*YS* IV.4), then Patañjali could have repeated the term *asmitā-mātra* in *Yoga-Sūtra* IV.5. Would it not be more accurate, and in keeping with Patañjali's consistent vocabulary, to assert that the "one mind" gives birth to individual minds (i.e., distinct personalities) through the medium of the bare

I-am-ness *(asmitā-mātra)? Asmitā-mātra* in turn would give rise to the individual, subjective sense of self or ego; this it does in conjunction with the reflected consciousness of the *puruṣa* located in the *citta*. The root *citta* illuminates *asmitā-mātra* with the reflected consciousness that it has "borrowed" from *puruṣa*. Here the "one mind" can be conceived ontologically as *liṅga-mātra* or *mahat* (in Sāṃkhya), and epistemologically as *buddhi* or intellect in its purest and subtlest form of *sattva* or knowledge *(jñāna)*. In Yoga, the discriminating discernment (*vivekakhyāti, YS* II.26) between *puruṣa* and the *sattva* takes place in the *sattva* of the mind. Being comprised of the three *guṇa*s, the mind is in some sense active but in its subtlest state the "one mind" is said to be like *puruṣa,* for at this finest degree of subtlety the mind has reached a state of purity analogous to that of the *puruṣa.* The coexistence of the purity of both *puruṣa* and *prakṛti* (as the mind) is associated in Yoga with the liberated state of "aloneness" *(kaivalya)*.[52] However, under the influence of spiritual ignorance *(avidyā)* the reflected consciousness, misidentified as *puruṣa,* appears as the affliction *(kleśa)* of "I-am-ness" *(asmitā),* which permeates the prakṛtic or empirical realm of selfhood and can include both the cosmic *(mahat* or *mahān ātmā)* and individual sense of self *(ahaṃkāra)*. Both levels of "I-am-ness" are, in the above, to be understood as being permeated by the reflected consciousness of *puruṣa* under the influence of ignorance or misidentification.

Patañjali does acknowledge that there exists a multitude of individuated minds and personalities (not to be confused with *puruṣa*s) and appears to reject the pure idealist view that the objects of experience are merely products of the mind and having no existence in themselves. This idealist perspective tends ultimately to negate the reality of the manifest world. In *Yoga-Sūtra* IV.14 Patañjali states: "From the homogeneity in the transformation [of the *guṇa*s] there is the "thatness" of an object,"[53] implying, it seems, a refutation of the idealist view that objects are merely projections or imaginings of the mind and thus are deprived of having ontological status in themselves. Patañjali continues: "Since there is difference of minds, while the object is the same, the two must be distinct levels [of existence]." "It [the object] does not depend on one mind; this is unprovable: then what could it [i.e., such an object] be?"[54] An external object, or any object for that matter, is composed of the three constituents *(guṇa*s*)* of *prakṛti* and has a real existence; therefore, it is not simply the product of a single mind.[55] Vyāsa interprets Patañjali as refuting the Buddhist school of Yogācāra,[56] which has often been understood (or misunderstood) as pure subjective idealism, implying a sheer negation of the external world.

AN INTRODUCTION TO *KARMA, SAṂSKĀRA,* AND *VĀSANĀ*

A key philosophical doctrine outlined in the *Yoga-Sūtra* is that of *karman (karma).* The word *karman* denotes action in general. The *Bhagavadgītā* (XVIII.23–25), for example, distinguishes three fundamental types of acts, depending on the agent's inner disposition:

1. *Sāttvika-karman,* which stands for actions that are prescribed by tradition, performed without attachment by a person who is nonobsessed or no longer egoistically consumed by the results or "fruit" *(phala)* of action; it is said to be of the nature of "purity" or "benevolence";
2. *Rājasa-karman,* which is generated out of a self-centered mentality or ego-sense *(ahaṃkāra)* in order to experience self-gratification or pleasure; it is said to be of the nature of "desire" or "passion";
3. *Tāmasa-karman,* which is performed out of a confused or deluded mentality in which one is unconcerned about the moral or spiritual consequences of his or her actions; it is said to be of the nature of "evil" or "dullness."[57]

Karman also means "ritual act."[58] But more specifically *karman* (or *karma*) refers to the moral dynamic behind one's intentions, volitions, thoughts, and behavior. In this sense, *karma* often corresponds to deterministic forces or fate as determined by the quality of one's being, including past lives and one's present embodiment. One's accumulated *karma* is often pictured as a "bank" or "store" consisting of good and bad stock that combine to mature in particular and unpredictable ways in one's life. In Hindu tradition, one's karmic "storehouse" has been distinguished generally as consisting of three types of *karma:* (1) *saṃcita-karma,* or the already accumulated "stock" of karmic residue or deposits *(āśaya)* that is not being activated and is therefore awaiting fruition; (2) *prārabdha-karma,* which has begun to mature in this life (e.g., related to our sex and genetic makeup); (3) *āgāmin-karma,* which is *karma* acquired during the present lifetime, that is, *karma* in the making, the fresh storage of merit or demerit that will bear fruit in the future.[59] *Karma* is often thought to stand for a mechanism that maintains worldly existence *(saṃsāra)* rooted in spiritual ignorance of the intrinsic, immortal nature of Self, implicating us as confused, egoic identities in a beginningless cycle of birth and death leading to suffering and dissatisfaction *(duḥkha).* Yet, however negatively portrayed the doctrine of *karma* may be, there is clearly room within Hindu tradition for a more nondeterministic, creative, and emancipatory dimension to the doctrine of *karma* that, from an ethical and soteriological perspective, takes into account the crucial role played by free will as either positively or negatively effecting one's life. Moreover, as we have seen in the *Bhagavadgītā*, the process of *saṃsāra,* conceived of as an inherently egoistic and therefore selfishly binding state of affairs, can be remedied—brought to a halt—through a form of nonegoistically motivated action sometimes called *niṣ-kāma* ("desireless" or "noncovetous"). Action, freed from all "attachment" to its results, need no longer bind one by generating further *karma*. Later on I will argue that, from Patañjali's standpoint, the yogin does not succumb to fatalism, but exercises the will to be free from the binding effects of all action. *Yoga-Sūtra* III.22 distinguishes between *karma* that is "in motion" *(sa-upakrama)* and "not in motion"/ "deferred" *(nirupakrama).*[60] Vyāsa imaginatively likens *karma* that is "in motion" or activated to a wet cloth that is spread out to dry quickly, and the later type to a wet cloth rolled into a ball, which only dries very slowly.[61]

In the *Yoga-Sūtra* the mind is the receptacle for the effects of *karma*. *Yoga-Sūtra* II.12–14 deal with the basic dynamics of *karma* and its fruits within the context of saṃsāric notions of self and activity. The central premise in these *sūtra*s is that insofar as *karma* is under the grip of spiritual ignorance *(avidyā),* it is associated with affliction *(kleśa),* including a misidentified or egoic sense of self. The five afflictions as outlined in *Yoga-Sūtra* II.3, namely: spiritual ignorance *(avidyā),* "I-am-ness" or egoity *(asmitā),* "attachment" *(rāga),* "aversion" *(dveṣa),* and "desire for continuity" *(abhiniveśa),*[62] provide the cognitive and motivational framework for the ordinary person enmeshed in conditional existence *(saṃsāra)* and unaware of *puruṣa*. As *Yoga-Sūtra* II.12 states, these *kleśa*s are the root of the residue of *karma,* the "action-deposit" *(karma-āśaya)* in the subconscious mind. The effects are felt not only in one's "seen" existence or present life, but they also determine the quality of one's "unseen" existence or future lives.[63] Rooted in ignorance *(avidyā),* afflicted action causes the repeated fruition *(vipāka)* of situations or births *(jāti)* and life span *(āyus),* furthering saṃsāric experience *(bhoga).*[64] Depending on whether acts are meritorious *(puṇya)* or demeritorious *(apuṇya), karma* produces joyful *(hlāda)* or painful/distressful *(paritāpa)* results.[65] Vyāsa notes that under the influence of the afflictions experiences of pleasure are pervaded with attachment *(rāga),* resulting in the latent residue of actions *(karma-āśaya)* due to that attachment; thus one can easily dwell on, or become obsessed by, pleasure and its objects.[66] When upon aversion to pain and its causes, one is unable to overcome painful experiences, one thus accumulates a residue of actions due to aversion *(dveṣa).*[67] When one desires pleasure and upon acting on this desire for pleasure causes favor to some and harm to others, thereby accumulating both merit and demerit, the latent deposit generated is said to be due to greed *(lobha)* and delusion *(moha)*.[68] Attachment and aversion, it is to be noted, are conceived in the context of a selfish or self-centered mentality, the basis of which is a misidentified sense of self *(cittavṛtti)* caused by ignorance.

Every action *(karman)* leaves an impression *(saṃskāra)* in the deeper structure of the mind, where it awaits its fruition in the form of volitional activity. The most general meaning of *saṃskāra* is "ritual" or "forming well, . . . making ready, preparation";[69] but in addition it also conveys the idea of "embellishment," "purification," "making sacred," "any purificatory ceremony."[70] The root *saṃs-kṛ* means to cleanse and perfect.[71] In Hindu tradition *saṃskāra*s can refer to the rites of passage such as birth rites *(jātakarma)*, marriage rites *(vivāha)*, and death rites *(antyeṣṭi)*, rites that are all intended to purify and transform the individual at specific phases in life. In the context of the *Yoga-Sūtra,* however, the most significant translation that can be extracted from Monier-Williams' list of meanings on the term *saṃskāra* is "mental impression or recollection, impression on the mind of acts done in a former state of existence."[72] In earlier scholarly works on Yoga, *saṃskāra* has often been translated as "impression"[73] and in more recent scholarship as "karmic impulse,"[74] "subliminal impression,"[75] "habitual potency,"[76] and "subliminal activator."[77] In this study, I have translated the term *saṃskāra* as "impression."

Yoga-Sūtra IV.9 tells us: "Because memory and impressions have a sameness of form, there is a causal relation even among births, places, and times that are undisclosed."[78] The various impressions have a "sameness of form" or "uniformity" *(eka-rūpatva)* with the "depth-memory" of a particular person. Even though we may not remember our past karmic involvements, they nevertheless continue to affect our present actions. Vyāsa states: "Memories *(smṛti)* are from *saṃskāra*s, distanced as to birth, place, and time. From memory again there are *saṃskāra*s, so that these memories and *saṃskāra*s are manifested in a concentration of power from the going-into-operation of the karmic residue."[79] Under the influence of the afflictions *(kleśa*s*)*, the impressions and memories of a person then form a "subset" of *saṃskāra*s known as the karmic deposit or residue *(karmāśaya)*, which in turn becomes operative.[80] It is because of the uniformity of the impressions and memory pertaining to a specific individual that one person does not experience the fruition of the *karma* of another person. Patañjali explains that the mind is suffused with beginningless latent impressions (*YS* IV.10)[81] left by action that form or combine into a great store of habit patterns, traits, or subtle traces *(vāsanās)*[82] that dictate personality: how one perceives and reacts or morally responds to the world. In a helpful passage, G. Larson suggests that "the 'causal' or 'active' *saṃskāra*-s of one's present embodiment are one's *karmāśaya* . . . which will largely determine one's future new experiences and memory experiences in this present embodiment and the next embodiment yet to come, whereas one's *vāsanā*-s or subtle traces . . . are the 'effect' or 'passive' *saṃskāra*-s from all of one's previous embodiments . . . not only of our prior embodiments in the human species but in numerous other species as well."[83]

Pertaining to the individual person, *saṃskāra*s are responsible for the production of various psychomental phenomena, in particular the five types of modifications *(vṛtti*s*)* of the mind that are described in the first chapter of the *Yoga-Sūtra*.[84] The functioning of the mind *(citta)* takes place through these *vṛtti*s, which give form to perceptions, thoughts, emotions, and so forth. The *vṛtti*s are empowered to produce *saṃskāra*s and vice versa. Vyāsa states: "The modifications *(vṛtti*s*)* produce their own kind of impressions; and in turn, the impressions produce corresponding modifications. Thus the wheel of modifications and impressions revolves."[85] The wheel to which Vyāsa refers can be taken as being none other than the "six-spoked wheel" of *saṃsāra,* the cycle of "suffering" and "misidentification" referred to earlier.[86]

In Patañjali's Yoga, *saṃskāra* has an obvious psychological significance and "stands for the indelible imprints in the subconscious left behind by our daily experiences, whether conscious or unconscious, internal or external, desirable or undesirable. The term *saṃskāra* suggests that these impressions are not merely passive vestiges of a person's actions and volitions but are highly dynamic forces in his or her psychic life. They constantly propel consciousness into action."[87] The *Yoga-Sūtra* (III.9) distinguishes between two varieties of *saṃskāra*s. The first variety refers to those that lead to the externalization *(vyutthāna)* or emergence ("centrifugalization") of empirical consciousness which prevents the realization of *puruṣa;* this set of impressions generates or sustains an extrinsic and afflicted sense of self-identity based on reified and fabricated notions of selfhood. The second variety of *saṃskāra*s refers to those impressions that cause the centripetalization or cessation *(nirodha)* of the *vyutthāna* processes of the mind and lead to the realization of intrinsic identity as *puruṣa* and therefore spiritual emancipation. Patañjali states: "[Regarding] the impressions of emergence and cessation, when that of emergence [i.e., extrinsic self-identity] is overpowered, there follows a moment of [the condition of] cessation in the mind. This is the transformation [termed] cessation."[88] "From the impression *(saṃskāra)* of this [moment of cessation] there is a calm flow [in the mind]."[89] *Saṃskāra* has not only psychological significance but also has a soteriological role in Yoga. The yogin must cultivate the *nirodha* type of *saṃskāra*s in order to achieve a calm flow or tranquility of mind wherein *samādhi* can arise and prevent the renewed generation of impressions of a *vyutthāna* nature. As we will see, the process of *nirodha* cultivates within the mind the condition of liberating knowledge *(jñāna)* or insight *(prajñā)* that counteracts the former condition of affliction and allows for the "aloneness" of the *puruṣa* to take place.

The fact that *saṃskāra*s are impressions of previous mental activity can be inferred from *Yoga-Sūtra* III.18,[90] which announces that by means of the direct perception *(sākṣāt-karaṇa)* of the impressions *(saṃskāra*s*)* the yogin can acquire knowledge of former (past life) embodiments. Moreover, whatever *saṃskāra*s remain at the end of one's present life will determine future experiences in a subsequent embodiment. *Saṃskāra* is thus "an active residuum of experience."[91] The concept of *saṃskāra* is illustrated in the notion of *bīja* or "seed" as used in *Yoga-Sūtra* III.50 (as *doṣa-bīja*).[92] In classical Yoga, *bīja* can denote the afflictions *(kleśa*s*)*, also called "seeds of impediments," which refer as well to the impressions *(saṃskāra*s*)* based on misconceptions of authentic identity *(puruṣa)* and manifesting in the form of afflicted action. Those impressions must become, in one of Vyāsa's favorite metaphors, "like burned seeds of rice."[93]

Thus, the impressions have internal currents or a "flow" of their own, currents that clearly influence or effect a person's intentional and volitional nature. When certain impressions, through the repeated practice of certain actions or by constant addition of like-impressions, become strong enough, the propensities they create impel a person in a certain direction. The choices or decisions that one makes produce pain leading to aversion *(dveṣa)*, or pleasure leading to attachment *(rāga)*, in the process of transmigration: "Attachment is clinging to pleasant [experiences]."[94] "Aversion is clinging to sorrowful [experiences]."[95] Vyāsa writes: "What is the painfulness of *saṃskāra?* From experience of pleasure there is a saṃskāric residue of pleasure; from experience of pain a saṃskāric residue of pain. So the maturing of *karma* is experienced as pleasure or pain, and it again lays down an action-deposit or karmic residue."[96] To the discerning yogin the saṃsāric enterprise of afflicted identity and its *saṃskāra*s is ultimately suffused with dissatisfaction and suffering (*YS* II.15). The substratum of this process within the mind is called the *karmāśaya* or residue of *karma*. Vācaspati Miśra elaborates on how, in the present lifetime, experiences arise appropriate to each person's individual condition:

> The result of the karmic residue is pleasure and pain, and, insofar as both birth and life span have the same purpose (viz., pleasure and pain) and are a necessary consequence of this (pleasure and pain), birth and life span too are propagated. Moreover, pleasure and pain correspond to attachment and aversion. And these are the necessary conditions (for pleasure and pain), since pleasure and pain are not possible in the absence of these (attachment and aversion). So this soil of the self sprinkled with the water of the afflictions becomes a field for the propagation of the fruits of the determined actions.[97]

Vāsanās are the various subtle traces in the form of personality traits or habit patterns that the strength of *saṃskāras* produces.[98] In *Yoga-Sūtra* IV.8 the origination of these habit patterns is to be linked up with the fruition *(vipāka)* of one's activity.[99] Feuerstein writes: "We can either say that a given volitional activity leaves behind a . . . trait *[vāsanā]* which, in conjunction with other similar . . . traits, will (given time) have certain consequences for the individual, or we can say that by a given volitional activity the individual accumulates merit or demerit."[100] Vyāsa tells us that, "The corresponding habit patterns [to the fruition of *karma*] are from the residue of action."[101] The *vāsanās* lie dormant in the mind until the fruition of *karma*. The impressions *(saṃskāras),* that combine into habit patterns *(vāsanās),* are thus the very substance of the karmic residue. The action one performs proceeds according to the residue of past actions. The presence of a *saṃskāra* begins to produce certain mental tendencies, attitudes, thoughts, desires, images, and so forth even before the fruition of *karma*. Thus *saṃskāras* provide a certain momentum toward the external decisions one makes. These decisions—which appear to be conscious, but are in fact propelled by the dominant and unconscious residue of action—expose one to situations that are then credited with or blamed for one's fortune or misfortune, merit or demerit. Past actions stored in the residue of *karma* continue to affect present actions even if those past actions are not remembered.[102] Within the *vāsanās* inhere the qualities of past action and of the fruits that are to ripen in due time, that is, in the present or a future life. In the following simile Vyāsa portrays the saṃsāric mind as a kind of "crystallization" or cemented network of *vāsanās*, "like a fishing net with its knots." He explains: "Propelled by experiences of afflicted actions and their fruition [which form] habit patterns, this mind has been crystallized from time without beginning, as it were variegated, spread out in all directions like a fishing net with its knots. These *vāsanās* have many lives behind them."[103]

Yoga-Sūtra II.12[104] points out that the notion of reincarnation or repeated births is one of the axioms of Patañjali's philosophy. The dynamics of saṃsāric re-embodiment is thought to operate on the simplest formula that meritorious action results in impressions *(saṃskāras)* of a positive quality leading to pleasant experiences in life, whereas demeritorious action produces impressions of a negative or painful sort that have adverse effects in a person's life.[105] The ongoing life-cycle of our conditioned self as person can be understood as beginning with the afflictions that color our action as world-experience, creating impressions which form the residue of action and out of which various personal traits or habit patterns are "cemented" in the mind. *Karma* thus conceived is the mechanism by which saṃsāric existence (i.e., egoic identity) maintains itself. For the ordinary person rooted in afflicted action and its residue or latent deposit, life is an unending accumulation and fruition of actions caused by craving, dissatisfaction, and ignorance. The yogin, on the other hand, recognizing the inherent suffering involved, does not succumb to this seemingly fatalistic state of affairs. Patañjali offers a way to transcend the nexus of "suffering" and its causes. Through the study and practice of Yoga, the *saṃskāras* of action as dictated by the afflictions of human weaknesses are lessened to the point where the yogin, yet active, can enjoy an established state of internal calm[106] no longer enslaved by what otherwise appears to be worldly existence *(saṃsāra)*.

Patañjali asserts: "The action of a yogin is neither 'black' nor 'white'; of others it is of three kinds."[107] While the activity of the adept yogin is stated to be neither "white" *(śukla)* nor "black" *(kṛṣṇa)*, that of the average person is threefold. Ordinarily, every action causing its fruition can be classified as either impure/demeritorious, pure/meritorious[108] or "mixed." Patañjali's fourfold classification of *karma* is explained by Vyāsa as follows:

> There are four classes of *karma*. [*Karma* may be] black, white and black, white, or neither-black-nor-white. The white and black category is effected through external means so that the karmic residue is strengthened by way of harming or benefiting others. The white belongs to those who practice ascetic [internalized] endeavor *(tapas)*, study *(svādhyāya)*, and meditation *(dhyāna)*. For these, being a matter of the mind alone, are not concerned with outer means, nor do they harm others. The neither-black-nor-white *karma* is that of the renouncer *(saṃnyāsin)*, whose afflictions have dwindled away, whose misidentification with the body is overcome. In that case, because of renouncing the fruits of action the not white belongs only to the *yogī*; it is not black because there is no cause for that. But all other living beings have the three kinds, as explained previously.[109]

In order to become disengaged from the binding effects of *karma* and all attachment to mundane existence one has to transcend the very empirical consciousness that generates afflicted mental and physical actions and modes of being. In other words, one must go beyond the boundaries of ego-personality and its self-centered mentality: the mistaken identity of one being essentially an empirical agent *(kartṛ)*. In contradiction to the three ordinary types of *karma* outlined above, the yogin, whose mind has become increasingly purified through *samādhi,*[110] does not generate any action that could be thus typified. Action here, noting that the yogin still "acts" at this finer level of awareness, is said to be "neither-black-nor-white" because the yogin has transcended the relative field of action insofar as it no longer wholly defines the yogin's self-identity, and thus the yogin is freed from any tendency to misidentify with prakṛtic existence (the "see-able" or *triguṇa* process) and its effects/affects. At this advanced stage, the yogin remains established in the true nature and identity of the *puruṣa* and has ceased to be attached to any empirical identity as authentic selfhood. Through a progressive purification of the body, mind and indeed all karmic influences, the yogin's action culminates in a state of "renunciation" meaning nonegoistic or noncovetous *(niṣ-kāma)* action[111] that does not produce further *karma* (i.e., karmic bondage). The yogin is no longer motivated, for example, by the merit *(puṇya)* or demerit *(apuṇya)* generated by the good and bad observance of traditional ritualistic religion including meditative practices that are performed for sheer personal gain or self-gratification and that merely result in pride and self-righteous attitudes.[112]

In *Yoga-Sūtra* IV.24 the mind *(citta)* is declared to be ultimately geared toward the liberation of human beings: "From action having been done conjointly for the purpose of another, it [the mind] is speckled with innumerable habit patterns."[113] The mind, like all manifestations of *prakṛti,* exists for the purpose of the *puruṣa.*[114] Not being self-illuminating because it is itself something perceived (*YS* IV.19), the mind and its modifications are known by the unchanging *puruṣa* (*YS* IV.18), that is, the mind is composed of the three *guṇa*s and due to its changing nature has an "object-character." Patañjali asserts that the mind is a composite process; it does not exist for its own sake (nor does the sense of self: *ahaṃkāra*) but must necessarily serve "another's purpose." Vyāsa writes: "With its commitment still unfulfilled, the mind is the repository of the habit patterns and personality traits *(vāsanā*s*)*. For when the mind has fulfilled its commitment, the *vāsanā*s have no repository and cannot maintain themselves."[115] He later adds: "The mind, being a conjoint activity, (what it effects) is done for itself. For a happy mind is not for the purpose of knowledge. Both are for the purposes of another. That other, which has as its purposes experience and liberation, is *puruṣa* alone . . . ."[116]

The teleology of the mind and its contents all have a purpose beyond themselves, namely the twofold purpose of world-experience and liberation. In fact, it is the *raison d'être* of the conjunction *(saṃyoga)* between the seer and the seeable, *puruṣa* and *prakṛti,* to be of assistance in the liberating process of the awakening of selfhood to its true identity.[117] The subservient role given to *prakṛti* is often understood in Sāṃkhya and Yoga scholarship as signifying an asymmetry of relationship between spirit and matter: all that is prakṛtic ultimately exists in the service of *puruṣa,* in the service of soteriology. As a counteractive to spiritual ignorance and bondage in the form of misidentification and suffering, *prakṛti* does indeed serve the purposes of *puruṣa.* What, however, is *prakṛti*'s status in the context of the enlightened state of *puruṣa?* Does *prakṛti* merely cease to exist for the liberated yogin? Can *prakṛti* be understood to play a more integral role here, implying, in the final analysis, an engagement of *puruṣa* and *prakṛti* in the "aloneness of seeing"? These and other questions relating to the meaning and place of *prakṛti* in the liberated yogin's life will be dealt with in a later chapter. For now, it suffices to say that the level of instrumentation of the mind *(citta)* is explicitly acknowledged by Patañjali in the above *sūtra* (*YS* IV.24), which asserts that even though the *citta* may be colored by innumerable *vāsanās* it still, however, retains its fundamental characteristic of serving the purpose of *puruṣa* (i.e., experience and liberation).[118]

The Sanskrit commentators on Yoga discuss at great length whether the mind corresponds to the size of the body (which is the Sāṃkhyan view) or whether it is all-pervasive *(vibhu).* They settle for the latter alternative. Vyāsa reiterates the Sāṃkhyan perspective, according to which the mind contracts or expands, and follows with the view offered by the teachers *(ācārya)* of Yoga: "Others hold that the mind, like the light of a lamp, contracting when put in a jar and expanding when placed in a palace, assumes the size of the body; and that transmigration becomes possible because of an intermediate state. Only then is it possible to explain its absence in between (the time of dissolution) and its worldly existence. But the teacher (Patañjali) says that it is only the modifications of this all-pervading mind which contract and expand."[119] Vyāsa proclaims that Yoga holds it is only the modifications of the mind—the mental processes or *vṛtti*-aspect of consciousness—that can be said to contract and expand, depending on efficient causes such as virtue.[120] The authorities in Sāṃkhya, however, admit of an intermediate stage (of a subtle body) in order to explain how transmigration takes place. In Yoga the mind is understood to be all-pervasive *(vibhu)* so there can be no question of the need for a subtle body (*sūkṣmaśarīra,* see *SK* 39). Vācaspati explains that there is no proof for the existence of a subtle body as posited in Sāṃkhya. The mind is neither atomic nor of medium size nor of the size of the body; the mind has the same entitative extension as prakṛtic existence itself.[121] The all-pervasive *citta* contracts or expands only in its manifestation or actualization as modifications or mental activity *(vṛtti).* "There is, therefore, no need in Yoga for a migratory subtle body."[122] Perhaps one other way to understand the above issue is that Patañjali saw no real pedagogical usefulness in talking about a subtle body. Patañjali's practical and pragmatic orientation emphasizes that spiritual emancipation can take place in this very lifetime and can be understood as an embodied state of freedom. Therefore, the need to posit a subtle body—which is itself a further limitation of identity—seems superfluous.

G. Koelman offers the following helpful explanation regarding the aspatial dimension of *citta:* "Since it is non-spatial and without extension, its contraction and expansion should not be conceived as spatial. Its expansion would mean rather its intentional extension to its object, which can be situated at any point of space. The mind also can shift in a moment from one object to another that is at the other extreme of space. Mind is, therefore, something immaterial and subtle, remaining however prakṛtic and undergoing change."[123] Defining mind more epistemologically, H. Āraṇya tells us: "Mind is not all-pervading like the sky, because the sky is only external space. Mind . . . is only power of knowing without any extent in space. Its connection with external things is always existing and they may become clearly knowable when properly brought to the mind, that is why it is everywhere as the faculty of knowing and is limitless. Only the modifications of the mind contract and expand. That is why the mind appears as limited."[124] As mentioned earlier, rather than being conceived as "substance" per se, *citta* can be viewed as a heuristic device for understanding the nature and functioning of consciousness in Patañjali's system.

The Yoga school formulated a doctrine of an all-pervasive mind to explain the very possibility of knowledge of all things or omniscience *(sarva-jñātṛtva)* and sovereignty over all states of being *(adhiṣṭhātṛtva).* Both of the above-mentioned yogic abilities or powers are made available and credited to the yogin who has attained the discriminative discernment between *puruṣa* and the rarefied *sattva* of the mind, the finest quality or constituent of *prakṛti.*[125] Vācaspati Miśra introduced the distinction between "causal consciousness" *(kāraṇa-citta)* and "effected consciousness" *(kārya-citta),* arguing that the former is infinite (all-pervasive), which can be understood to approximate Patañjali's concept of the cosmic or root *citta* (*YS* IV.5).[126]

INTRODUCTION TO YOGA EPISTEMOLOGY

One of the special features of Patañjali's Yoga system is that it elaborates a primary response to the epistemological problem of the subject-object relation—an issue that is fundamental to any metaphysical system and is especially crucial for any philosophy that purports to explain the state of spiritual enlightenment. In the *Yoga-Sūtra,* liberation *(apavarga)* or "aloneness" *(kaivalya)* implies a complete sundering of the subject-object or self-world relation as it is ordinarily known, that is, as a fragmentation or bifurcation within prakṛtic existence. Our normal experience and everyday relations function as a polarization within *prakṛti:* the self as subject or experiencer that as an empirical identity lays claim to experience; and the objective world as it is perceived and experienced through the "eyes" of this empirical self. The conjunction *(saṃyoga)* between *puruṣa* and *prakṛti* gives birth to phenomenal (empirical) selfhood or identity and its content of consciousness. However, this process, which is largely enmeshed in ignorance *(avidyā)* and egoity *(asmitā)* or affliction, actually entails utterly mistaken notions of who we are as our authentic being. What is needed, according to Yoga, is a total purification of the subject-object relation so that the spiritual nature of selfhood can be fully disclosed and the yogin, established in the true form and identity of *puruṣa,* no longer becomes misidentified with prakṛtic existence. Yet despite an overwhelming adherence to what normally amounts to being a mental array of confused human identity and its concomitant "suffering" *(duḥkha),* Yoga philosophy tells us that *puruṣa,* our true identity, is necessarily "present" to ordinary human experience in that without *puruṣa* all experience and knowledge would not be possible.[127] Based on this perspective—that *puruṣa* is simultaneously transcendent and immanent—Patañjali formulated a practical and transformative "path" of Yoga in which knowledge *(jñāna),* as an integral aspect of Yoga theory and practice, can have profound implications for human life in this world.

Despite Sāṃkhya's unique distinction between pure consciousness and human awareness, which allowed it to preserve its fundamental dualism in the face of monistic arguments—and thereby avoid the metaphysical problems attending monistic views—it could not avoid one fundamental philosophical question: What is it to say that *prakṛti* is dynamic because of the presence of *puruṣa?* To say that *prakṛti* reflects the presence of *puruṣa,* or that *puruṣa* is reflected in *prakṛti* preserves a rigid distinction between the two, for neither an object reflected in a mirror nor the mirror is affected by one another. In Sāṃkhya, liberation is the result of discernment *(viveka),* the highest knowledge. The process of attaining it suggests either an intention on the part of *puruṣa*—which, some would argue, is impossible considering that *puruṣa,* as pure consciousness, is contentless and nonintentional—or a response on the part of *prakṛti,* if not both. How then can *puruṣa* be said to have no relation, including no passive relation to *prakṛti?* Even Īśvara Kṛṣṇa's enchanting metaphor (*SK* 59) of the dancer before the host of spectators does not answer the question, for there is a significant relationship between performer and audience. In an effort to elucidate a proper response to the above questions from the perspective of Yoga, the remainder of this chapter will address among other related topics: (1) how cognition and knowledge take place in Patañjali's system; and (2) how cognition and knowledge inform our understanding of the relationship between *puruṣa*—the pure seer or knower—and *prakṛti*—the seeable or knowable.

In order to grasp how Yoga philosophy can be lived on a practical level, one must: (1) understand how *puruṣa* and *prakṛti* "relate" to one personally and in pragmatic terms, and (2) see that these two principles—"spirit" and "matter"—are not merely understood in the abstract thereby overemphasizing their metaphysical and impersonal dimensions. With the above consideration in mind, Patañjali translated what appears to be a universal macrocosmic philosophy—heralding some of the main ideas of Sāṃkhya—into microcosmic, subject-oriented, and practical terms that apply to human life, such as, for example: perception, cognition, and ethical sensibilities. The necessity of *puruṣa*'s presence to human experience notwithstanding (see above), it must also be emphasized that without the manifestation of psychophysical being that includes our personhood—the material source and cause of which in classical Sāṃkhya is said to be *prakṛti*—liberation would not "take place" in Yoga. Without *prakṛti, puruṣa*-realization would not be possible and the yogin could not "become" liberated. As *Yoga-Sūtra* II.23 spells out, it is by virtue of the conjunction *(saṃyoga)* between *puruṣa* and *prakṛti* that the essential nature of the "seer" *(puruṣa)* and the "seeable" (prakṛtic identity) can eventually be grasped.[128]

Throughout the *Yoga-Sūtra,* Patañjali's main contention is that *puruṣa*—pure, immortal consciousness—is our true nature and being and therefore the real foundation or ground of authentic identity and livelihood. However, due to spiritual ignorance *(avidyā)* human awareness mistakes the Self or "seer" *(puruṣa)* for the "seeable." In this state of misplaced identity brought about by the conjunction *(saṃyoga)* of *puruṣa* and *prakṛti,* and defined by Patañjali (*YS* I.2) as the misidentification with the modifications of the mind, the cognitive error of mistaking extrinsic (material) identity for intrinsic (spiritual) identity is continually reinforced. With the above "teaching" having been properly considered and through an appropriate form of pedagogy, Yoga seeks to establish our identity as the seer, and in the process to "dismantle" the mechanism of misidentification (*sārūpya, YS* I.4) due to which we remain deluded, confused, and dissatisfied.

VṚTTI

One of the most important terms used in the *Yoga-Sūtra* is *vṛtti.* The word *vṛtti* stems from the root *vṛt:* "to turn, revolve, roll, proceed."[129] *Vṛtti* can mean: "mode of life or conduct," "behavior (esp. moral conduct)," "mode of being," "disposition," "activity," "function," "livelihood," "mood (of the mind)," "nature," "character," "addition to," and "occupation with."[130] In the context of *Yoga-Sūtra* I.2 *(yogaś cittavṛttinirodhaḥ) vṛtti* has been translated as: "fluctuations,"[131] "modifications,"[132] "'acts' and 'functions',"[133] "Bewegungen,"[134] "activities,"[135] "processes,"[136] "transformations,"[137] and "mode."[138] I have adopted the general term "modification" for *vṛtti.* The functioning of the mind takes place through various modifications *(vṛtti*s*)* that give form to our perceptions, thoughts, emotions, and so forth.

Like all other aspects of "insentient" *prakṛti,* the mind undergoes continual change, and from the viewpoint of Yoga its most noteworthy modifications are of five kinds outlined by Patañjali as follows: the means of knowing or valid cognition *(pramāṇa),* error *(viparyaya),* conceptualization *(vikalpa),* sleep *(nidrā),* and memory *(smṛti).*[139] These *vṛtti*s must be clearly understood and witnessed in order for finer states of awareness to arise. The five kinds of modifications listed above are described in the first chapter of the *Yoga-Sūtra.*[140] The first, the means of knowing or valid cognition *(pramāṇa),* allows for the understanding of something that is fully manifested and is verified through one of the three avenues: perception *(pratyakṣa),* inference *(anumāna),* and valid testimony *(āgama).*[141] The experience of objects such as: people, animals, plants, buildings, and so forth, whether by direct perception, inference, or reliable testimony belongs to the modification called *pramāṇa.* I will be saying more on *pramāṇa* especially in its form of perception *(pratyakṣa)* in the last section of the present chapter.

The remaining four types of *vṛttis* explain other ways in which the mind operates. The second is "error" *(viparyaya),* that is, when one's understanding or a thought does not correspond with reality[142] and one apprehends something as other than what it is. Vyāsa (*YB* I.8) treats *viparyaya* as a synonym for the term *avidyā* (ignorance), *avidyā* being the principal among the five afflictions *(kleśa).*[143] The *vṛtti* of *viparyaya* is the fundamental error due to which we misinterpret or misconceive existence itself! Vyāsa writes of *viparyaya:*

> Why is this not valid cognition? Because it is sublated by valid cognition. The object of valid cognition is a thing as it is, and the fact of not being valid cognition is shown by the fact that valid cognition cancels it. For example, seeing the moon as double is refuted by seeing that it is in fact a single moon.
>
> This ignorance is fivefold, namely, the afflictions *(kleśa):* ignorance, I-am-ness, attachment, aversion, desire for continuity. These very five bear their technical names: darkness *(tamas),* delusion *(moha),* extreme delusion *(mahāmoha),* gloom *(tāmisra)* and utter darkness *(andhatāmisra).*[144]

For Patañjali the conjunction *(saṃyoga)* of the seer and the seeable, *puruṣa* and *prakṛti,* is the cause of all suffering and dissatisfaction *(duḥkha)*[145] because it gives rise to the incorrect understanding that one's identity is defined within the limits of the individuated psychophysical being or personality complex and not according to the unbounded nature of the *puruṣa* or spiritual Self. The conjunction is caused by spiritual ignorance *(avidyā),*[146] the primary affliction that is the origin[147] of all other afflictions including our mistaken identity as a finite, egoic self or "I-am-ness" *(asmitā). Asmitā* constitutes the major affliction that permeates the principle of individuation, thus leading to the ongoing misidentification of selfhood with the modifications of the mind. Ignorance is also at the root of three other afflictions: attachment *(rāga),* aversion *(dveṣa),* and the desire for continuity or the instinctive fear of death *(abhiniveśa).*[148] In attachment and aversion the emotive core of the concept of affliction *(kleśa)* comes into play, thereby signifying an obvious affective dimension to *vṛtti.* The impressions *(saṃskāras)* centered around the experiences of pleasure are operative in and supportive of *rāga* or attachment/attraction. The modifications are said to take the form of *gardha, tṛṣṇā,* and *lobha,* which may be translated as longing, thirst, and greed respectively.[149] Metaphorically speaking, the seeds *(bīja)* of *sukha-saṃskāras* or impressions of pleasurable experiences germinate and will give rise to a state of attachment leading to effort directed toward the attainment of the object of pleasure or desire. In a seeming opposition to attachment, the emotive core of the phenomenon of aversion *(dveṣa)* or revulsion is provoked by the seed recollection of pain. The states that arise are said to be those of retaliation *(pratigha),* malice *(manya),* revenge *(jighāṃsā),* and anger *(krodha).*[150] Thus, attachment and aversion dwell upon the *saṃskāra*s of pleasure and pain. In general terms the mind is not repelled by that which is pleasurable, nor does it desire that which is painful.

The description by Vyāsa that the *kleśa*s are prime examples of erroneous cognitions is especially noteworthy as it cuts through the stereotyped opposition between the emotive/affective and the rational/cognitive. This brings forth an integral view of the mind *(citta).* It is in this frame in which a picture emerges that saṃsāric identity (and its reified notions of self and world, i.e., worldly existence) is not possible without I-am-ness, attachment, aversion, and the desire for continuity or fear of extinction, and that these afflictions govern the mind of the individual and perpetuate the wheel of *saṃsāra.* The compulsive forces of attachment, aversion, and desire or fear cannot be uprooted and discarded unless *asmitā* is subdued, weakened. Thus the attenuation and ultimate transcendence of all the afflictions is the objective of Yoga praxis. The importance of the theory of the five afflictions has been emphasized by I. K. Taimni, who correctly notes that this theory is the foundation of the system of Yoga outlined by Patañjali.[151]

The function of Yoga is to oblige the yogin to "awaken" to the true status of *puruṣa* through progressive stages of removing any misidentification with the forms of *prakṛti,* of uprooting and eradicating ignorance *(avidyā),* the primary affliction defined in *Yoga-Sūtra* II.5. Here, Patañjali states: "Ignorance is seeing the noneternal as eternal, the impure as pure, dissatisfaction as happiness, and the nonself as self."[152] Interestingly, Patañjali seems to be admitting in the above that there is a special kind of happiness *(sukha)* that is intrinsic to freedom ("aloneness") in Yoga and that, far from resulting in a lonely or aloof nature or association with the world, implies that one of the fruits of Yoga can be experienced as an exalted sense of well-being that embraces our emotional/affective as well as our cognitive dimension.

Vyāsa correlates the five afflictions outlined by Patañjali (see n. 144 above) with the five categories of fundamental misconception or error *(viparyaya)* of classical Sāṃkhya.[153] The correlation of the five *viparyaya*s with the five *kleśa*s of Yoga is also made by Vācaspati Miśra[154] and Vijñāna Bhikṣu.[155] Ignorance is said to fall within the category of *viparyaya* and is a factor common to all the afflictions. Therefore, the other four afflictions are considered its segments.[156] Vijñāna Bhikṣu calls the *vṛtti* normally termed "error" (the fivefold *avidyā*) the seed of the calamity called *saṃsāra;* it is a special kind of misapprehension in which there is a superimposition of cognition in the object. Doubt *(saṃśaya)* is also included under this *vṛtti.*[157] It is, thus, the *kleśa*s manifesting in the form of the *vṛtti* of error or misconception *(viparyaya)* that control the network or web of saṃsāric existence. Vyāsa describes the domination of the *kleśa*s over empirical identity: "The word 'afflictions' means the five errors *(viparyaya)*. When active they confirm the involvement with the *guṇa*s, impose change, bring about the flow or current in the body and senses by mutually reinforcing each other, and bring on fruition of *karma.*"[158] The divisions of ignorance *(avidyā)*—which Vyāsa equates with the *vṛtti* of error *(viparyaya)*—can be explained[159] as follows:

1. *Avidyā* (*YS* II.5) means spiritual ignorance itself, sometimes called *tamas* ("darkness"), and is described as being eightfold: the error of mistaking as Self or *puruṣa (ātman)* the eight *tattva*s that are: (i) *avyakta:* unmanifest *prakṛti,* (ii) *mahat* or *buddhi* (intellect), (iii) *ahaṃkāra:* sense of self, (iv–viii) the *tanmātra*s: the five subtle senses. Spiritual ignorance *(avidyā)* is sometimes defined as "darkness" in that it veils liberating knowledge *(jñāna)*. It includes the error of misidentifying the physical body and psyche with *puruṣa* because body, and so on, are the products of the eight *tattva*s listed above. *Viparyaya*s—such as mistaking a seashell for silver—are not included in this category. *Sāṃkhya-Kārikā* 44 says that bondage *(bandha)* is caused by *viparyaya.* Hence *avidyā,* the major cause of bondage, is included here and not the other four "delusions."[160]
2. *Asmitā* means I-am-ness/egoity (*YS* II.6) or "delusion" *(moha)* and is eightfold: the error of considering the eight powers or accomplishments (*siddhi*s, *YS* III.45) as though they were something benevolent and belonging to, or an essential property of, the Self *(ātmīya).*[161] This preoccupation with one's prakṛtic identity occurs when finite beings seek to overcome their limitations by pursuing the eight well-known omnipotent or supernatural powers. According to Vyāsa these powers include: *aṇimā,* the power of becoming minute; *laghimā,* the power to become light; *mahimā,* the power to become enlarged or greatly expanded; *prāpti,* the power to reach or touch the most distant things (e.g., the moon); *prākāmya,* the power of an irresistable will to accomplish its tasks; *vaśitva,* mastery over all elements and elementals (their nature) not impeded by any; *īśitṛtva,* sovereignty, the ability to will the production, absorption, and disposition of the elements and the elementals; *kāmāvasāyitva,* implying that whatever one's purposive idea is becomes true for that person.[162] I-am-ness/

egoity and self-possession are synonomous[163] and therefore the above divisions apply; the *siddhis*, misunderstood as an end in themselves, are a form of possessive or obsessive power in that the attachment to their pursuit only furthers egoic states (i.e., pride, greed, fear, etc.).

3. *Rāga* means attachment (*YS* II.7) or "extreme delusion" *(mahāmoha)* and is classified as being tenfold: one becomes attached to the five subtle elements (e.g., sound, sight) and the five gross elements. The attraction is for the attainment of the eightfold *siddhis* through Yoga, thereby becoming a powerful or "perfected" being *(siddha)* and gaining sovereignty over nature. Thus it is thought that the yogin will enjoy the objects of the senses.[164]
4. *Dveṣa* means aversion (*YS* II.8) or "gloom" *(tāmisra)* and is said to be eighteenfold: when one is fixed upon the above pursuits [i.e., in (2) and (3)] and some impediment prevents the attainment of *asmitā* (the eight *siddhis*) and *rāga* (the ten enjoyments of the senses), then the anger arising with regard to that failure and toward its cause is gloom *(tāmisra)* or aversion *(dveṣa)*.[165]
5. *Abhiniveśa* means desire for continuity (*YS* II.9), a mode of clinging-to-life or instinctive fear of death. This state is referred to as "utter darkness" *(andhatāmisra)* and is eighteenfold: *asmitā* and *rāga* have been attained, yet there comes the realization that this attainment will one day perish as, for example, at the end of a cycle of creation *(kalpa)*. This fear is said to be the fear of death or "utter darkness" and the "darkness" or "night" refers to the period of dissolution in a single cycle of creation.[166]

In the above order of five, each succeeding affliction *(kleśa)* is considered from the perspective of Yoga pedagogy to be more undesirable and of an inferior "grade" than its predecessor, indicating progressively deluded or impure levels of attainment. It is interesting to note that the above definitions seem to be of concern only to the so-called advancing yogin whose attainment of powers, ironically, can equally result in an inflated sense of ego rather than liberation from the ego. The general definitions of the afflictions as provided under *Yoga-Sūtra* II.5–9 are wider and are applicable to the worldly-minded who are living more conventional states of awareness. U. Arya[167] has conceived the following scheme (see below), which shows *viparyaya* from *(a)* the "common view" or ordinary (worldly) person's viewpoint as compared with *(b)* the novice and "imperfect" yogin's viewpoint. While the yogin's consciousness is said to be more refined and subtle, it is clear from the scheme outlined below that the yogin, not yet having reached the fully liberated state of "aloneness" *(kaivalya),* can still be prone to a selfish mentality where attachment to the attainment of power diverts the yogin away from the true spiritual "goal" of Yoga:

Kleśa	Common View	Imperfect Yogin's View
avidyā	I am the body, male or female, with resultant pleasures and attachments.	I am *prakṛti* and its evolutes.
asmitā	I have an identity dependent on possessing the objects of experience. I desire worldly success, power and wealth.	I desire powers *(siddhis).*
rāga[168]	I desire the objects of my immediate pleasure.	I will appropriate my power to obtain refined pleasures.
dveṣa[169]	I have an aversion to specific objects, persons or situations that have caused me pain.	I am angry at causes, persons or situations that have prevented my fulfillment of *siddhis* and resulting enjoyment.
abhiniveśa[170]	I fear my death, that is the death of this body that I am.	I fear that all my powers and resulting pleasures and enjoyments of *prakṛti* will cease.

The above scale may be understood as constituting the range of misidentifications in the context of phenomenal selfhood. Under the dominating and delusive power of *viparyaya,* the yogin is in need of the guidance of a spiritual preceptor or *guru:* one who has transcended the compulsive need to identify with prakṛtic existence. In the *guru,* or "accomplished one," has awakened the "knowledge born of discernment" *(vivekajaṃ jñāna)* that, endowed with the power of liberating *(tāraka),*[171] enables one to "cross over" the limitations of saṃsāric identity. As the yogin progresses on the journey toward authentic identity, the influence of the afflictions progressively lessens. Vyāsa makes it clear that it is the *vṛtti* of misconception or error *(viparyaya)* that underlies our mistaken notions of selfhood and their attendant dissatisfactions and sorrows *(duḥkha).* According to Vyāsa (*YB* I.8), *viparyaya* encompasses the source-affliction of ignorance *(avidyā)* in which the karmic residue *(karmāśaya)* of *saṃskāras* and *vāsanās*, and the resultant fruition *(vipāka)* of afflicted action, are generated and sustained. In short, our afflicted identity rooted in spiritual ignorance functions through *viparyaya.* Curiously, this important insight, which can be attributed to Vyāsa, has not been clearly noted by scholars.[172]

The Sāṃkhya and Yoga systems hold divergent views on the nature of *avidyā.* The Sāṃkhya system proper uses the term *a-viveka,* "an absence of discerning knowledge" of the nature of *puruṣa,* which the teachers of formal logic place under the category of "nonapprehension" *(a-khyāti).* It appears that the Yoga system differs in this regard. Yoga considers ignorance to be a misapprehension *(anyathā-khyāti),*[173] the definition of ignorance being: mistaking the noneternal and the "nonself" for the eternal and the Self, and so forth, as in *Yoga-Sūtra* II.5.[174] Vyāsa states that although *avidyā* is a negative compound, it should be known as a positive existent, like the compound *amitra,* which signifies not the absence of a friend *(mitra)* but the contrary of friend, namely an enemy. Likewise, *avidyā* is neither valid cognition nor the absence of valid cognition, but is a cognition of a different kind, contrary to both of them.[175] In Yoga, therefore, *avidyā* is not *akhyāti,* that is, the nonapprehension of the nature of *puruṣa* as in Sāṃkhya, but *anyathākhyāti,* that is, a particular kind of cognition that mistakes *puruṣa* for prakṛtic existence. As the Sāṃkhyans (*SK* 44) hold that bondage is due to "the opposite of *jñāna*" *(viparyaya),* liberation occurs through the central expedient of discriminating knowledge (referred to in *SK* 2 as *vijñāna*). In the philosophy of classical Yoga, *avidyā* is a type of cognition, however invalid, that can be remedied by various methods such as the cultivation of faith *(śraddhā),* energy *(vīrya),* mindfulness *(smṛti),* cognitive *samādhi,* and clear insight *(prajñā)*—all outlined in *Yoga-Sūtra* I.20—or devotion to the Lord (*īśvara-praṇidhāna, YS* I.23). *Avidyā* can be completely overcome only through the realization of *puruṣa*—an "attainment" that takes place in the high-level state of *samādhi* termed *asaṃprajñāta* (*YB* I.18).

The third type of *vṛtti,* conceptualization *(vikalpa),* is defined by Patañjali (*YS* I.9) as the apprehensions arising out of verbal knowledge only but whose referents are words and ideas but not things.[176] *Vikalpa* involves a notion, not necessarily an error, that does not correspond to an object or thing, but that may in fact serve as a useful function as in a metaphor or simile. A *vikalpa* can be an imaginary cognition. The term *vikalpa* has been understood in the sense of "fancy"[177] or "hallucination,"[178] but these are insufficient meanings. In states of meditation, the engagement of *vikalpa* is considered important in strengthening and focusing the mind.

Vikalpa is that modification *(vṛtti)* of the mind that follows language, knowledge of words, and the knowledge provided by words, and is productive of the same where no actual thing is its referent. Yet, being verbal knowledge, why could it not be included under valid testimony (*āgama pramāṇa, YS* I.7)? According to Vyāsa (*YB* I.7), there has to be an actual object *(artha)* that is corroborated by an accomplished teacher *(āpta)* in order to qualify under *āgama.*[179] *Vikalpa* relates to no "objects" as such.

Nor is the *vṛtti* of conceptualization formally included under error *(viparyaya)* because in the latter (*YS* I.8) there is an "object" that is at first wrongly cognized, but when the error is corrected, the true form of the "object"—such as the moon, to use Vyāsa's example—is seen clearly. There is no succession of error and refutation, and one word does not replace another (e.g., the word "seashell" replacing "silver" in the case of an oyster). In *vikalpa* there is no real external object at all, the referent being language itself rather than things.

Paraphrasing Vyāsa, conceptualization does not amount to valid cognition or to error. As there can exist a certain satisfaction or sense of exaltation about the use of language and knowledge of words, people bring words into usage even when there is no actual substance or object signified or designated by the words and their definitions. For example, the statement, "Consciousness *(caitanya)* is the nature of *puruṣa,*" is ultimately meaningless or fallacious. When the actual position of Yoga philosophy is that consciousness itself *is* the *puruṣa,* what consciousness, other than the very *puruṣa,* could be designated as the nature of that *puruṣa?* Otherwise, as Vyāsa tells us, it is as though one were talking of a cow belonging to a person called Caitra, who—as the owner—is other than his possession. Similarly, to assert that, "*Puruṣa* being inactive is a denial that it has the attribute of a thing," is making no positive statement about any object. Only the the attributes of *prakṛti* as pertaining to *puruṣa* are denied.[180] The adjective "inactive" *(niṣkriya),* denying any possible activity in the case of *puruṣa,* expresses no qualification. The negative (psuedo) adjective is false, has no substance and is a mere verbal expression of the *vṛtti* called *vikalpa*. It is an absence, conceptualized as though a positive state, then attached to *puruṣa* as though it is its attribute, yet it expresses no attribute of *puruṣa*. However, the modification of *vikalpa* is by no means worthless and can serve a practical and pedagogical purpose. *Vikalpa* has, for example, a greater practical value than has *viparyaya:* "For unless we have a concept of a 'higher Self' or a 'path,' we cannot exercise our will to overcome the limitations of conceptual thinking and to break through to the level of the . . . Self."[181]

The fourth modification or *vṛtti* is sleep *(nidrā)* and is defined as: "the modification based upon the apprehension of non-becoming/absence."[182] It is a kind of rudimentary awareness, the awareness of "absence" *(abhāva).* That sleep is not simply the "absence" of experience, cognition, or apprehension is, according to Vyāsa, demonstrated by the fact that when one wakes up one can recollect that one has slept well or badly.[183] *Yoga-Sūtra* I.38 states that attending to the knowledge derived from sleep (or dreams) can help to bring about clarification of the mind.[184]

The last modification is memory *(smṛti)* defined thus: "Memory is the recollection of contents (conditions/objects) experienced."[185] Memory operates exclusively on the level of the inner organ *(antaḥkaraṇa),* wherein the contents of a previous experience are returned to consciousness (i.e., remembered) via thought, although there are no longer any corresponding objects (on the gross level). Although not a means of knowledge *(pramāṇa)* in Yoga, memory nevertheless does play an important role in cognition and in determining the nature and range of cognition. Regarding *smṛti,* Vyāsa asks: "Does the mind remember the process of apprehension of an object (e.g., a vessel) or, rather, the form of the object experienced?"[186] To which he then replies: "The cognition, colored by the experience of the object known, shines forth in the forms both of the knowledge (or content or the object) and the cognition itself, and generates a latent impression that conforms to the above process."[187] A cognition *(pratyaya)* is "colored" *(uparakta)*[188] or influenced by the object experienced. Therefore a cognition carries the form *(rūpa)* or representation of the object as well as the representation of the process or the fact of that apprehension. It contains both the representations of the *grāhya* (the object of experience) and the form or representation of the *grahaṇa* (the instrument and the process and the fact of the experience), that is, it resembles the various features and natures of both of these and manifests them.

The cognition then generates a *saṃskāra* in which both features are represented: (1) the fact that the person cognizes the content or object, has gained experience through the process of apprehension of the object, and (2) the content or object as it actually is. Memory does not arise by itself. An experience first becomes a *saṃskāra,* an impression in the stored karmic stock *(āśaya)* in the mind. From the impression the memory arises again as a mental function or modification *(vṛtti).* The object itself therefore ceases to be present, but the impression produces the memory. Vyāsa further states, "That impression, being activated when similar or cognate cognitions occur, brings forth the memory experience. This memory also consists of the representation of the content or of the process of cognition."[189] The cause of the *saṃskāra*'s activation is the original cognition. When it reproduces the experience in the form of memory, the memory also is "identical" to: *(a)* the *saṃskāra,* as it manifests, shows itself to be "identical" with the original experience, and *(b)* the experience itself that was the manifesting cause of the *saṃskāra* (although the memory has now been triggered by some other manifesting cause, such as a similar cognition or an appropriate time).[190] The memory, just like the original cognition and the *saṃskāra* it had formed, consists both of the representation of the object apprehended and the knowing experience or process of cognition. The chain of causation is as follows: *(a)* the experience, from which is produced *(b)* the *saṃskāra,* which generates *(c)* the memory, each with the twofold process: (1) the process of cognition that makes possible the awareness that "I know the object," and (2) the cognition of the nature of the object itself. Obviously, unless the mind "knows that it knows," it cannot reproduce as memory the experience of the original object. In this process the faculty of determination or ascertainment *(buddhi)* plays its part. Vyāsa tells us that the representation of the process of cognition relates primarily to the *buddhi.*[191] The expression "I know the vessel" is a particular type of apprehension *(anuvyavasāya)*:[192] the awareness the intellect *(buddhi)* has that it cognizes or experiences. It is an important part of the process of memory in which the other part of the cognition is the object, the vessel. However, when one sees the vessel a second time and says, "This is that vessel," this is not, in Yoga, technically included under the *vṛtti* of memory. In the cognition "I know the vessel," one apprehension—of "the vessel"—is the subject matter *(viṣaya)* of the other apprehension—"I know." "Knowing," here, is the primary feature. Vyäsa adds: "Memory has primarily the representation of the content or object known."[193] Even though the type of apprehension termed *anuvyavasāya* is an important part of the process of memory, the memory proper is a single apprehension: "the vessel." Here, the awareness "I know" is secondary.

In the list of five *vṛtti*s (*YS* I.7-11), memory has been placed last because, in Vyāsa's words, " All those memories arise from the experiences or apprehensions that come forth from [the other *vṛtti*s of the mind, i.e.] the means of knowing, error, conceptualization, sleep, or of other memories."[194] "Experience" in the above refers to the *buddhi*'s *(citta*'s*)* first ascertainment of or involvement with the remembered object;[195] thereafter it becomes the awareness of the cognition that *buddhi* has *(anuvyavasāya)* as explained earlier. It is also clear from Vyāsa's passage that a memory may be remembered, as the first-time experience of that memory. Thus there may occur the memory of a memory. As cognition (in the process of apprehension) generates impressions *(saṃskāra*s*),* so do the impressions serve to activate the memory experience by assisting the process of knowing and providing the content of the memory experience.[196] Insofar as the *saṃskāra*s and resulting memories are said to ensue under the influence of the afflictions, an afflicted latent deposit or karmic residue is formed and becomes operative. Thus the link between the *vṛtti*s, *karma,* and saṃsāric identity is established.

Vijñāna Bhikṣu informs us that *buddhi* is the "raw material" from which all *vṛtti*s are shaped, as images are shaped from gold. The *vṛtti*s are the specific transformations *(pariṇāma*s*)* arising from the intellect or *bud-*

dhi,[197] which, as we have seen, is located in the mind *(citta)*. Because *buddhi* is a form of *prakṛti,* which consists of the three *guṇa*s, Vyāsa says: "Also, all these modifications *(vṛtti*s*)* are characterized by pleasure, dissatisfaction (pain) and delusion and are to be understood as being under the sway of the afflictions."[198] The afflictions which correlate with pleasure, dissatisfaction (pain) and delusion are attachment *(rāga),* aversion *(dveṣa),* and ignorance *(avidyā)* respectively.[199]

Obviously, the above five categories of *vṛtti* do not offer a comprehensive list of all psychomental states. By classifying the *vṛtti*s into five categories, the totality of innumerable modifications that can actually take place can be seen generally as derivatives of these five. However, in the context of yogic praxis the five types of *vṛtti*s are all significant in that they contribute to the mechanism of our karmic identity and its "entanglement" within *prakṛti* and, as we will soon see, our spiritual liberation as well. It is therefore quite natural why those modifications that keep the yogin bound in misidentification and are of an afflicted *(kliṣṭa)* nature, and those modifications that are conducive to liberation and are of a nonafflicted *(akliṣṭa)* nature,[200] should be a topic of great concern in Yoga. We must keep in mind that according to Yoga, "knowledge" is not simply the ratiocinative process or reasoning, but correlates with the all-pervasive principle of *mahat (liṅga-mātra)*—the first principle of manifestation in *prakṛti* out of which everything else manifests and is activated.

The five types of *vṛtti* comprise the normal range of human functioning, encompassing three modes of everyday transactions, including things (as registered in *pramāṇa*), mental content or objects whether remembered *(smṛti),* conceptualized *(vikalpa),* or erroneous *(viparyaya),* and sleep *(nidrā).* Each of these states is related directly to a sense of self or subject who appropriates and lays claim to the experience. The experiences of discrete objects or mental content or thought are filtered through and referenced to an afflicted identity of self that permeates the mind. When this happens, *puruṣa,* the pure witness or knower of *vṛtti,* is forgotten or veiled/concealed; the ego-sense possesses the experience, thinking it to be its own. *Puruṣa* (seemingly) becomes as if reduced to the finite realm, of limitation, of the "me" and "mine" of worldly, empirical existence. As described by Patañjali (*YS* II.6), the unseen seer *(puruṣa)* becomes as if "mixed" with the seeable *(dṛśya)* in the process of *saṃyoga,* the congenital conflation of *puruṣa* and *prakṛti.* The result of this "mixture" or "conjunction" of "spirit" and "matter" is the emergence of reified notions of the world and self (egoity) rooted in ignorance, attachment, aversion, and fear and functioning in the mind in the form of *vṛtti* (i.e., *cittavṛtti*).

The *vṛtti*s may be described as being cognitive, conative, and affective considering the nature that Patañjali and Vyāsa attribute to them. As its general translation of "modification" indicates, *vṛtti* incorporates both a mental content as well as an activity, a function, an act of mind. Vijñāna Bhikṣu provides a helpful definition of *vṛtti:* "A *vṛtti* of the intellect, like the flame of a candle, is the foremost point of the mind whereby the mind's one-pointedness is experienced. This foremost point, contacting external objects through the senses, is transformed into replicas of objects like melted copper in a crucible."[201] The author of the *Sāṃkhya-Pravacana-Sūtra* (V.107) states: "The *vṛtti* is a principle different from a member or a quality; it reaches out to make a connection and glides forth [among objects, senses and the mind]."[202] In his commentary on the above text, Vijñāna Bhikṣu explains that the mind naturally forms *vṛtti*s that are real "psychic" transformations taking place through mental processes.[203] *Vṛtti* is not specifically defined by Vyāsa. Vācaspati Miśra understands the five modifications as "change into the form of an object."[204] Bhoja Rāja states: "The *vṛtti*s are forms of modification which are parts of the whole [the mind]";[205] and elsewhere he says, "the *vṛtti*s are particular modifications of the mind."[206] Even the discriminative discernment *(vivekakhyāti)*[207] that takes place in the *sattva* of the mind, as well as the five afflictions—understood as parts of the *vṛtti* of error *(viparyaya)*[208]—can all be classified under the category of *vṛtti*. *Vṛtti* is employed by Patañjali in a more general sense as "function" or "movement" or "mode of being,"[209] and as a technical term implying any mental content that falls into the five categories of *vṛtti*s (*YS* I.5; II.11; IV.18). In the latter sense it is often used in the plural.

By rendering *vṛtti* as "modifications," our study means to include the cognitive conditions, mental, emotive, and affective content, processes and activities, in fact any act or content of consciousness, self-identity, or mode of consciousness operating in the mind itself. Unlike the term *pariṇāma* (transformation, development), which implies serial change (of *prakṛti*), *vṛtti* in Yoga is an "occurrence," which implies a more local human (temporal) activity inextricably linked to self-identity.[210] A secondary meaning of *vṛtti* is "means of livelihood," as in "*vṛtti*s are the means for the mind (empirical selfhood) to attain its livelihood." As appropriated by limited self-consciousness, the *vṛtti*s are like individuated "whirlpools" metaphorically signifying "whirls" of consciousness or an existence that appears separate from the water (but is not really); the *puruṣa* "as if" conforms to an identity extrinsic to itself and takes on the appearance of a changing, finite, psychophysical being, rather than abiding in its true nature as pure consciousness.

We have seen that in the realm of empirical selfhood the law of *karma* operates if and only if the modifications of the mind are rooted in afflictions (*YS* II.12). Vyāsa (*YB* IV.11) likens this bound state of affairs to the wheel of *saṃsāra,* which turns due to the power of ignorance with its six spokes, namely, virtue *(dharma)* and nonvirtue *(adharma),* pleasure *(sukha)* and pain/dissatisfaction *(duḥkha),* as well as attachment *(rāga)* and aversion *(dveṣa).*[211] The five afflictions *(kleśas)* provide the dynamic framework through which mistaken identity of Self is maintained urging the psychophysical organism to emerge into activity, to feel, to think, to desire, and so forth. As the basic emotional and motivational forces, they lie at the root of all delusion, dissatisfaction, or pain. In Yoga, misidentification *is* suffering. As long as we live out of a deluded understanding of authentic identity, we remain subject to sorrow and conflict. Hence, Vyāsa labels the afflictions as "errors" or "misconceptions" *(viparyaya).* Thus the normal human situation can be characterized as the product of a cognitive error, a positive misconstruction of reality and an apparent loss or concealment of intrinsic identity. The correction of this error or misunderstanding of the world and the true nature of selfhood is contingent upon the full recovery or realization of *puruṣa.* What role, if any, does *vṛtti* actually play in the "recovery" process through which the disclosure of our authentic identity as *puruṣa,* the seer, takes place?

KLIṢṬA- AND *AKLIṢṬA-VṚTTI*

Patañjali understands the five types of *vṛttis* as being either "afflicted" *(kliṣṭa)* or "nonafflicted" *(akliṣṭa).*[212] Vyāsa explains:

> The afflicted *[vṛttis]* are caused by the five afflictions and are causes of the afflictions *(kleśa-hetuka);* they become the seed-bed for the growth of the accumulated residue of *karma.* The others [nonafflicted] have discernment *(khyāti)* as their object and oppose the sway of the *guṇas.*[213]

The compound word *kleśa-hetuka* used in the above by Vyāsa to explain *kliṣṭa* may be translated as "caused by the *kleśas*" and "causes of the *kleśas.*" Vācaspati states that the *kleśas* such as *asmitā* (egoity) are the causes that bring about the advent of (afflicted) *vṛttis.* Or, as Vācaspati adds, it may be said that as *prakṛti* serves *puruṣa,* only its rajasic and tamasic *vṛttis* are the cause of *kleśa.*[214] According to Vijñāna Bhikṣu, the word *hetu* (cause) can also mean a purpose as well as referring to the effects of the *vṛttis.* Bhikṣu states that *kleśa* should be taken mainly to mean suffering/dissatisfaction *(duḥkha),* which is the effect (e.g., greed) produced by the *vṛtti*s that take the form of objects experienced; hence it is said to be *kliṣṭa* ("afflicted").[215]

Feuerstein understands Vyāsa's explanation (see above) of *kliṣṭa* as making little sense in that "*akliṣṭa* would consequently have to be understood as 'not caused by the *kleśas,*' which is absurd, since all mental activity is *ex hypothesi* engendered by the *kleśas.*"[216] Feuerstein's claim in the above amounts to a tautological and reductionistic explanation of *all* mental activity as being engendered by the afflictions; it fails to take into account the soteriological purpose of *vṛtti* in the form of subtler mental processes leading to liberating knowledge (*jñāna, YS* II.28) or what I will refer to as the "sattvification" of the mind and its *vṛtti*-processes. The process of sattvification takes place in the *sattva* of consciousness, the most refined aspect of the mind *(citta),* and its effect is such that it opposes the afflictions by purifying and illuminating the yogin's consciousness thereby dissolving the barriers to spiritual liberation.

Bhikṣu interprets Vyāsa's exposition on *akliṣṭa* by paraphrasing it thus, "resulting in *akleśa,*"[217] meaning that *akliṣṭa-vṛtti*s do not result in afflictions. Through cognitive error or misconception, the *kleśa*s both generate and arise from the activity and changes of the *guṇa*s in the saṃsāric condition of self-identity, a condition that continues up to the discernment *(khyāti)* of *puruṣa* and *prakṛti.*[218] According to Vācaspati Miśra, *khyāti* (used by Vyāsa in the sense of discriminative discernment or *viveka-khyāti*) means "clarity of insight" *(prajñā-prasāda)* and occurs when the sattvic component of *buddhi* (intellect), having been cleansed of the impurites of *rajas* and *tamas,* flows tranquilly.[219] Any yogic "methods" that lead to the discernment of *puruṣa* and the mind (i.e., *sattva*) can be included under the clause "have discernment as their object."[220] Soteriologically, the unafflicted *vṛtti*s are helpful in bringing about discernment and reducing the power of the *guṇa*s (i.e., in the form of ignorance) over the yogin until the *guṇa*s (the seeable) have finally fulfilled their purposes, that is, of providing experience *(bhoga)* and facilitating liberation *(apavarga).* They do so by opposing or blocking the activation of ignorance in the form of egoity, its desires and attendant actions *(karma).*[221] In his commentary on Vyāsa *(Maṇi-Prabhā),* Rāmānanda Yati (sixteenth century CE) states that the result of *kliṣṭa-vṛtti*s is bondage *(bandha-phala),* whereas the result of *akliṣṭa-vṛtti*s is liberation *(mukti-phala);*[222] but this is technically incorrect. *Akiṣṭa-vṛtti*s only lead up to and include discernment (a quality of the *sattva* of the mind), which in turn must be transcended in higher *samādhi (asaṃprajñāta).*[223] Only then can final liberation *(kaivalya)* from misidentification with *all vṛttis* and their effects/affects take place.

Bhoja Rāja interprets *kliṣṭa* and *akliṣṭa* as "with *kleśas*" (in the technical sense: ignorance, etc.) and "without *kleśas*" (in the technical sense), or as "affected by *kleśas*" and "nonaffected by *kleśas*" (both in the above technical sense).[224] Hauer[225] agrees with Bhoja's interpretation. Many scholars understand *kliṣṭa* as "with *kleśas*" (in the general sense)—as in "painful," and *akliṣṭa* as "without *kleśas*" (in the general sense)—as in "not painful."[226] *Yoga-Sūtra* I.5 also appears in the *Sāṃkhya-Sūtras* (II.33) attributed to Kapila. In his commentary *Sāṃkhya-Pravacana-Bhāṣya ad locum,* Vijñāna Bhikṣu interprets *kliṣṭa* as the *vṛttis* that are proper to saṃsāric existence and produce suffering, and *akliṣṭa* as the *vṛttis* that arise through the practice of Yoga and are contrary to the *kliṣṭa-vṛttis*.[227] In his commentary on the same work, Aniruddha (fifteenth century) explains *kliṣṭa* as being united to the *kleśas* and composed of *rajas* and *tamas,* and *akliṣṭa* as being made of *sattva* wherein the *kleśas* have been destoyed.[228]

Based on the above analysis, and for the sake of clarification, I am suggesting that *kliṣṭa-vṛtti* refers to mental activity that helps to maintain the power and influence of the *kleśas*; and *akliṣṭa* refers to mental activity that facilitates the process of the dissolution of the *kleśas*. The "afflicted" modes of the mind refer to the ordinary intentional consciousness of everyday life. Referring earlier to Bhikṣu's (*YV* I.5) understanding of *akliṣṭa* as "resulting in *akleśa,*" it does not seem inappropriate to designate *akleśa* as that condition in which the grip of the afflictions on the mind is partially or completely checked. Evidently, according to the commentators (and to counter Feuerstein), not "all mental activity is . . . engendered by the *kleśas.*" *Kliṣṭa-vṛttis* are brought about by the afflictions, but this is not necessarily the case for the *akliṣṭa-vṛttis*. By reducing all mental activity to being a product of the *kleśas*, Feuerstein has failed to differentiate between two radically different causes in Yoga: (1) *avidyā,* which is responsible for the misidentification of self or egoity *(asmitā)* leading to further affliction, and (2) the purposefulness of *puruṣa,* which is the final cause of the three differentiated states of *prakṛti*[229] and for which the mind ultimately serves the purpose of liberation.[230] *Vṛttis* of the nonafflicted *(akliṣṭa)* variety are engendered by the purposefulness of *puruṣa* and cannot be reduced to being a product of the *kleśas*.

The task of the yogin lies in the gradual overcoming of the impressions *(saṃskāras)* of "emergence" *(vyutthāna)* that generate an extrinsic self-identity or the externalization of selfhood in its worldly attached modes "away" from the *puruṣa,* and the simultaneous cultivation of the impressions of "cessation" *(nirodha)*[231] and the eventual establishment of selfhood in its intrinsic spiritual nature. Based on our discussion of *saṃskāra* and *vṛtti,* it can be inferred that: (1) From *saṃskāra*s of a *vyutthāna*-nature arise *vyutthāna-vṛtti*s, afflicted *vṛtti*s that generate or support a deluded understanding of reality. (2) From *saṃskāra*s of a *nirodha*-nature arise *vṛtti*s that are conducive to the process of "cessation" *(nirodha),* and that, being of the *akliṣṭa* type, aid in removing the *kleśa*s and their effects, thus leading to an enlightened understanding of self and world. These two "directions," which imply radically different understandings of selfhood based on *saṃskāra* and *vṛtti,* can be correlated to the guṇic dispositions of the mind, as the following statement by Vyāsa makes clear:

> The mind always tends towards three dispositions: illumination, activity or stasis, which leads to the inference that the mind is constituted of the three *guṇa*s. The nature of mind-*sattva* is illumination. Mingled with *rajas* and *tamas* the mind is drawn toward power and possessions. The same mind when pervaded by *tamas* becomes subject to nonvirtue, ignorance, attachment and impotence. Again, when the covering of delusion *(moha)* [correlated with *tamas*] has diminished from the mind, it [the mind] shines in its fullness; when this is pervaded by a measure of *rajas,* it turns toward virtue, knowledge, dispassion and power. When the last vestige of the impurity of *rajas* has been eliminated, the mind is established in its own nature, becoming simply the discernment *(khyāti)* of the distinction of the *sattva* and the *puruṣa.*[232]

The presence of *sattva,* the purest *guṇa,* draws one toward *dharma* (merit, virtue), *jñāna* (knowledge that arises from Yoga), *vairāgya*[233] (dispassion/detachment), and *aiśvarya* (supremacy, possession of power, sovereignty).[234] These four qualities, according to *Sāṃkhya-Kārikā* 23,[235] are the natural aspects of a sattvic "mind," that is, intellect or *buddhi.* For example, sovereignty implies an unthwarted sense of will power or determination whereas the loss of sovereignty denotes that one's will is weakened or thwarted by many impediments. The word *aiśvarya* is an abstract noun formed from *īśvara* ("master," "lord"), used here not in the sense of God, but rather as an exalted human sense of power, of lordship, a commanding presence, the ability to be effective, to be "in control." According to Yoga philosophy, one cannot be "in control of things" or in harmony with one's objective world without first being in control of one's mental faculties or "subjective world," personality traits, and so on. The word *īśvara* is derived from the root *īś,* meaning "to command, rule, reign,"[236] "to be the master of." The presence of *sattva* gives one the clearsightedness so as to exercise such autonomy and effectiveness in a morally responsible way. One in whom *sattva* is predominant can easily and readily become engaged in Yoga and lead an increasingly purified, virtuous and cognitively illuminated existence with a preponderance of *akliṣṭa-vṛtti*s.

The "absence" of *sattva* and dominance of *tamas* robs the mind of clarity, and, consequently, effectiveness in wielding power in a morally responsible way is lost. This does not mean that one who wields power in a manipulative egoic fashion, or in a nondiscerning way, is also endowed with *sattva.* Nonvirtue, ignorance, and attachment are all symptoms of the predominance of *tamas,* whereas only "meritorious" effectiveness in wielding power would mark the presence of *sattva.* When *sattva* is eclipsed by *tamas* one becomes weakened, overly dependent, no longer a "sovereign" person. One in whom *tamas* predominates (mis)identifies with *kliṣṭa-vṛtti*s and is ensnared in the network of afflicted consciousness and identity.

In Vyāsa's statement that "the mind always tends to illumination *(sattva),* activity *(rajas)* and inertia *(tamas)*" as a result of the presence of the three *guṇa*s, it must be understood that the above list of qualities of the *guṇa*s is far from being an exhaustive one. *Sattva* in its form of moral and mental activity implies other luminous qualities such as clarity of mind, serenity, insight, kindness and compassion, benevolence, forgiveness, pleasantness of character, and so on. In the case of rajasic qualities, not only energy and will (volition leading to action), but passionate moral and mental activity, anguish, anger, and pleasure and pain of different kinds (joy, anxiety, dissatisfaction, conflict) are to be understood. The word "inertia" *(sthiti)* or "stasis," used to express the attribute of *tamas,* means both "stability" and "stagnation," and refers as well to other tamasic qualities such as dullness, confusion, stupidity, indolence, dejection, heaviness, sloth, and so forth. All forms of *prakṛti* carry within themselves all three *guṇa*s,[237] and nothing within *prakṛti* exists that does not include all the three *guṇa*s together. Variances in the nature of all phenomena, entities, attributes, self-identifications, tendencies and inclinations, personalities, choices, relationships, and acts depend on the dominance and preponderance of the *guṇa*s. In fact, the *guṇa*s are used to characterize almost all aspects of life including the nature of faith, knowledge, action, agency, intellect, and foodstuffs.[238]

Upon further analysis of the *guṇa*s it would appear to be the case that the mind can undertake an initiative only because of *rajas.* Through *tamas* it can be drawn to "negative" or irresponsible states such as malevolence toward others. *Sattva* brings to the mind serenity, clarity, pleasantness, and lucidity. What impels the mind to move in the direction of virtue? It is the presence of *rajas.* The mind, being a composition of the tripartite process, can never be without *rajas* and *tamas*. It is not, therefore, that in Yoga *rajas* and *tamas* are to be negated or abolished; rather, they are to be purified so that their presence as well as their effects (and affects) no longer obstruct the natural illuminating power intrinsic to *sattva*. In their natural state, *rajas* and *tamas* are essential and their measure is ideally sufficient to fulfill the purpose of *sattva*. When present within the limit of this measure, *rajas* initiates virtue, and so forth, and *tamas* imparts stability. What is initially intended by the discipline of Yoga is simply purification of mind so that *rajas* and *tamas* may be brought under the power of *sattva*. As such, *sattva* is then no longer dominated by the moral and mental processes of *rajas* and *tamas*. Vyāsa shows (*YB* I.2) the subtlety and the superiority of the *sattva* of consciousness, which functions as a "bridge" on the "path" to the untainted consciousness of *puruṣa*. The way and journey in Yoga from a tamasic or rajasic disposition to a sufficiently sattvified one thus involves a highly moral process; it is not, as one scholar puts it, an "*a-moral* process."[239] Yoga does not succumb to an antinomian perspective but seeks to integrate, through an embodiment of being, an enlightened consciousness with an affectively and morally matured sense of identity and personhood.

It is clear from the above analysis that tamasic *vṛtti*s are afflicted modifications of the mind and sattvic *vṛtti*s are nonafflicted ones. Vijñāna Bhikṣu regards rajasic *vṛtti*s[240] as mixed, both *akliṣṭa* and *kliṣṭa*. In classical Sāṃkhya the function of *rajas* is always to impel both *sattva* and *tamas*.[241] Without the initial impelling force of *rajas* the other two *guṇa*s are ineffective and inefficacious. In this sense the rajasic element may be considered to be mixed with either *sattva* or *tamas,* whichever is dominant, and therefore *sattva* or *tamas* is served or supported by *rajas*. The progress of the mind toward pure *sattva* is not possible without the operational capacity of *rajas*.

How do the different qualities of *vṛtti* interrelate in the system, that is, in the mind? Given our prevalent habit patterns of thought and misidentification and their proneness for generating and sustaining turbulence, affliction, and conflict—both within ourselves and in the world—how do nonafflicted states of mind survive in the midst of ignorance and suffering? One could, as does Vācaspati Miśra, pose an argument as follows: It is understood that all beings, with the exception of liberated embodiments (i.e., a "descent" *[avatāra]* or a *jīvanmukta*), bear afflicted *vṛtti*s and have various attachments, aversions, fears, and so forth. It would be rare if nonafflicted *vṛtti*s were to arise in the constant stream or "whirling" of such afflicted mental and emotional content. Moreover, even if nonafflicted *vṛtti*s were to arise among the afflicted ones, they would be powerless, having fallen among innumerable powerful opponents. Therefore, it could be deemed illogical that afflicted *vṛtti*s could be overcome through nonafflicted ones, and that even by cultivating dispassion *(vairāgya)* toward any manner or type of *vṛtti,* however sattvic,[242] the afflicted patterns of *vṛtti*-identification would in the end prove to be insurmountable. To counter this kind of pessimism, Vyāsa assuredly and optimistically replies: "They [nonafflicted *vṛtti*s] remain nonafflicted even if they occur in a stream of afflicted ones. In intervals between afflicted ones, there are nonafflicted ones; in intervals between nonafflicted ones are located afflicted ones."[243] In Yoga, practice *(abhyāsa)* and dispassion *(vairāgya)* can arise from *akliṣṭa-vṛtti*s, for example, from *āgama:* reliable testimony—one of the means of knowledge or valid cognition *(pramāṇa);* or from *anumāna:* inference, which is another *pramāṇa* and through which can take place spiritual upliftment or inspiration, or perhaps the instruction of a teacher resulting in contemplation and greater understanding.[244] When practice and dispassion cause a break in the flow or movement of afflicted patterns of thought, the *vṛtti*s leading to a "higher good" or "purpose" *(paramārtha)* arise.[245] Even though, as Vyāsa states, these latter *vṛtti*s arise in the stream of afflictions and afflicted *vṛtti*s, they nevertheless remain untouched by them and are not corrupted. The same applies to nonafflicted *vṛtti*s that appear in intervals between afflicted *vṛtti*s. Similarly, when nonafflicted *vṛtti*s are generated or activated, their stream is often interrupted by afflicted *vṛtti*s. However, these impure *vṛtti*s have no power to alter the purer ones; rather, as the purer *vṛtti*s grow in strength through repeated practice, their *saṃskāra*s gradually mature, and the impure *vṛtti*s and *saṃskāra*s lose their hold over the mind. Attention then need no longer be monopolized by afflicted states of identity. The mind and its modifications become progressively infused in the nature of *sattva,* the *guṇa* that predominates in the makeup of *akliṣṭa-vṛtti*s and *saṃskāra*s of "cessation" *(nirodha).* The yogin's identity becomes increasingly sattvified. As dispassion *(vairāgya)* toward forms of misidentification *(sārūpya)* matures into higher dispassion *(para-vairāgya),* even the dependency on sattvic *vṛtti*s—previously so necessary for the yogin's growth and spiritual development—falls away. The soteriological point to be made here is that any attachment to *vṛtti,* whether that *vṛtti* is afflicted or nonafflicted, must be transcended in Yoga. By fostering the *akliṣṭa-vṛtti*s, one masters the *kliṣṭa-vṛtti*s, and then, in turn, one dissolves any attachment to the *akliṣṭa-vṛtti*s through higher dispassion.[246]

Examples of the "nonafflicted" type of *vṛtti*s can be alluded to. A valid cognition of the *pratyakṣa* type can be deemed nonafflicted when it leads to higher perception of the true nature of both *prakṛti* and *puruṣa.* A conceptualization *(vikalpa)* is beneficial when one conceives of, or imagines, greater states of yogic awareness. For example, after having read the "great sayings" *(mahāvākyas)* of the Upaniṣads such as *tat tvam asi*—"That [the all-pervasive Self] you *are*" (*Chānd Up* VI.12.3.)—one can be left with a purificatory impression in the mind even if the sayings have not been fully understood. *Nidrā* (sleep) can be of value when a particular image in a dream acts as a catalyst for meditation (*YS* I.38). A memory *(smṛti)* is helpful when, for example, upon viewing "objects" in the world of nature such as a blue sky, one is reminded of the all-pervading nature of *puruṣa* or of descriptions of appearances of one's favorite "descent" *(avatāra)* or embodiment of the deity (e.g., Kṛṣṇa, Rāma, Śiva, etc.).[247]

Yoga-Sūtra I.33 states: "The mind is made pure and clear from the cultivation of friendliness, compassion, happiness and equanimity in conditions (or toward objects) of joy, sorrow, merit or demerit respectively."[248] Thus the sattvic *vṛtti*s or attitudes of friendliness *(maitrī)*, compassion *(karuṇā)*, happiness *(muditā)* and equanimity *(upekṣā)* replace the rajasic and tamasic ones based on more self-centered orientations or egoic modes of being and relating in the world. This is done in the spirit, as it were, of dispassion toward the moral and mental states of others. Vyāsa writes on the above *sūtra:* "Such devoted cultivation produces *dharma,* and thereby the mind is made pure and clear. When it is clear it attains the state of one-pointed stability."[249] Obviously, not the entire emotive and affective dimension of human nature can be subsumed under the traits of afflicted identity as the above attitudes make clear. The sattvic qualities that adhere within our emotive/affective dimension can be understood as positive (i.e., nonafflicted) aids on the yogin's journey.

Once an aspirant has begun to practice is success in Yoga definitely assured? Do the *vṛtti*s associated with affliction *(kleśa)* then cease to have power over the aspirant? The above questions may be answered in two ways: (1) Vyāsa (*YB* I.1) rejects those with distracted *(vikṣipta)* minds as being unworthy of consideration as serious yogins[250] and is, therefore, not talking about them. (2) The wording of the Sanskrit commentators (e.g., Vācaspati Miśra, H. Āraṇya) suggests that nonafflicted *vṛtti*s have to be strengthened through practice and dispassion until they cease to be intermittent and thus create a flow *(pravāha)* in the yogin's consciousness. As a result, afflicted *vṛtti*s arising intermittently lose their power over the yogin and are therefore mastered. The yogin is no longer enslaved by the afflicted modes of thinking and acting. This is the essence of what Vyāsa says: "It is only by the modifications *(vṛttis)* that the impressions *(saṃskāras)* corresponding to them are generated, and by the impressions are generated new *vṛtti*s. Thus the wheel of *vṛtti*s and *saṃskāra*s revolves."[251] The *vṛtti*s both generate and strengthen the *saṃskāra*s, the latter in turn facilitating the rise of the former. There is no conception of mind as *tabula rasa* to be found here. The only way the saṃsāric wheel of *saṃskāra*s and *vṛtti*s can cease, implying an end to mistaken identity and the experience of suffering, is through the process or practice of "cessation" *(nirodha)* itself.

Epistemologically, *vṛtti* refers to any mental "whirl," "wave," or modification. It is, thus, the medium through which a human being understands and experiences: whatever we know is based on the functioning of *vṛtti.* Our total apprehension of a conscious self/person is only by way of observing and recognizing the *vṛtti*s, intentions, ideas *(pratyaya),* and thought-constructs that arise in the mind. In other words, in ordinary human experience the existence of consciousness without an object in the mind is not suspected. *Citta* may be described as a network of functions that allows for the relay of information to the uninvolved experiencer *(puruṣa).* These functions include the inner organ *(antaḥkaraṇa)* composed of *buddhi, ahaṃkāra* and *manas,* in conjunction with sense and motor organs (*buddīndriya*s and *karmendriya*s) and their objects. The *citta* is regarded as the vehicle for perception (wherein the contents of experience take form for presentation to the *puruṣa*) as well as the receptacle for the effects of *karma*. The *citta* takes on a karmic shape or mentality due to the arising of each *vṛtti* that pervades it in the form of various perceptions, thoughts, emotions, and so on, and as referenced to a prakṛtic sense of self. In ordinary experience, *citta* is thus experienced as a series of particular mental states. However, according to Yoga, the *citta* is not capable of functioning by itself; it derives its semblance of consciousness through the proximity of *puruṣa* (*YS* IV.19 and 22–23) in a manner analogous to that in which the moon is illuminated by the light of the sun. As the sun shines on the moon, so the *puruṣa* "shines" its "light" upon the *citta* and thereby knows all that passes in the mind by observing *vṛtti*s, thoughts, and emotions as a witness (*YS* II.20; IV.18). Hence *puruṣa* is the true experiencer (*bhoktṛ*, *YB* II.6) and knower. However, the capacity to witness or observe the ongoings of the mind is not available to the empirical selves bound as they are to the identity of the body, mind, and its modifications, that is, psychophysical being.

Human consciousness, due to misidentification, experiences selfhood according to the changing modes *(guṇa*s*)* of *prakṛti.* All our "knowledge" as misidentified selves is structured in the prakṛtic realm of *cittavṛtti* and functions as a masquerading consciousness of phenomenal selfhood. In *Yoga-Sūtra* I.3[252] the seer *(puruṣa)* is said to be established in its true form, that is, in its unchanging, ever-wise, ever-pure nature. In the next *sūtra* (*YS*

I.4)[253] *puruṣa* appears to be misidentified with *prakṛti (cittavṛtti),* our self-identity having conformed to the changing nature of *vṛtti.* Does *puruṣa* have two natures? The total and permanent incorruptibility and unchangeability of *puruṣa* is the fundamental tenet of Yoga philosophy. If any of the "attributes" of *puruṣa* were to increase or decrease, the entire tenet would have to be rejected. In that case *puruṣa* would not be transcendent, pure, or free at all because it would be subject to factors outside of itself, namely, alteration, delusion, and suffering. There would simply be no point in pursuing Yoga because it would only lead to a series of temporary states of change and development *(pariṇāma)* rooted in egoity, attachment, aversion, fear, confusion, and conflict, and that ineluctably fuel further afflicted identity. But how and why does conformity *(sārūpya)* of self-identity with *vṛtti*s take place?

SAṂYOGA

The existence of empirical identity or self enveloped in spiritual ignorance *(avidyā)* does not mean that *puruṣa* deviates from its essential intrinsic nature of unconditioned freedom and purity. The starting point of the search for liberation in Yoga must be an inquiry into the nature of the "conjunction" *(saṃyoga)* between the seer *(draṣṭṛ)* and the seeable *(dṛśya),*[254] that is, of the congenitally conflated realms of *puruṣa* and *prakṛti.* Although the Yoga system has no qualms about expressing the shortcomings of mundane existence, to the discerning one (*vivekin, YS* II.15)[255] all identity contained within the saṃsāric realm is seen to involve dissatisfaction and suffering. Yet Yoga does not conclude on a note of existential despair by seeking, for example, to negate mundane existence or take flight from the world. From Patañjali's perspective, *saṃyoga* provides an experiential basis from which the yogin can then go on to apprehend the natures of *puruṣa* and *prakṛti* (*YS* II.23)[256] through a rigorous spiritual discipline for overcoming attachment to the modifications of the mind and thereby abiding in one's true identity or "own form" (*svarūpe'vasthānam, Yoga-Sūtra* I.3). Patañjali maintains that in the condition of *saṃyoga* the "contact" between the seer and the seeable is merely an apparent junction, since both the seer (intrinsic identity) and the seeable (extrinsic identity) are held to be utterly distinct.[257] He does not explicitly analyze this epistemological problem further. This has led to a great deal of speculation in the commentarial literature on the *Yoga-Sūtra.*

To explain the cognitive processes, Vyāsa resorts to various metaphors and analogies comparing, for instance, the mind to a magnet[258] that attracts the objects, and elsewhere (*YB* I.41 and IV.23)[259] compares it to a crystal that reflects the color of the object near it. Through the "contact" (explained below)[260] with *puruṣa,* the mind takes on a semblance of awareness and cognizes the objects just as a crystal receives the form of an object and appears identical with that form:

> Mind is colored by an object cognizable to the mind, and by the fact of being an object, it is bound up with the subject, *puruṣa,* by a mental function of belonging to it. It is this very mind alone that is colored by the seer and the seeable. It assumes the appearance of object and subject, the insentient ("nonconscious") becoming sentient ("conscious"). The mind, being insentient, essentially an object—conscious as it were, on the analogy of the crystal—is said to comprehend everything.[261]

Due to the association of the mind with *puruṣa, puruṣa* then appears to be an empirical state when knowledge and experience are attributed to it. Drawing on the philosophical teachings of both Patañjali and Sāṃkhya (*SK* 20), Vyāsa contends that it is through the conjunction of *puruṣa* and *prakṛti* (i.e., the mind) that consciousness "takes on" the role of an empirical identity or knower. He understands the "contact" to be in the form of mere proximity *(saṃnidhi).*[262] Yet how can there be "proximity" between these two eternal all-pervasive principles (that is, *puruṣa* and *prakṛti*)? The proximity, however, does not mean proximity in time and space because both *puruṣa* and unmanifest *prakṛti (pradhāna)* are beyond time and space, engaged as it were, in a beginningless relationship *(anādiḥ saṃbandha).*[263]

Finite categories of time and space would thus seem particularly inappropriate in any description of this "union." However, *saṃyoga* is an effective relation through which *prakṛti* is influenced by the presence of *puruṣa,* understood here as a transcendent influence.[264] This means that *prakṛti* can neither *be* nor *be understood* without reference to *puruṣa,* the realm of the *guṇa*s ultimately serving the purpose or "goal" of spiritual emancipation (*puruṣa*-realization). It is paradoxical that *prakṛti* manifests and is activated because of the transcendent influence of *puruṣa,* and yet *puruṣa* is revealed as being intrinsically free by nature—never really lost, forgotton, or acquired—by observing or "contemplating" *prakṛti.* Consciousness learns, from experiencing the manifestations of *prakṛti,* that it *(puruṣa)* is not contained within *prakṛti.* It is even more of a paradox to observe that both *puruṣa* and *prakṛti* are realized and recognized as what they truly are only after they have appeared to be what they are not: the mind itself appears conscious and *puruṣa* appears as if to be the empirical agent of activity (cf. *SK* 20). Vācaspati sees the nonspatial and nontemporal connection between *puruṣa* and *prakṛti* as a kind of "preestablished harmony." He speaks of their enigmatic relationship in terms of a special "fitness" or "capacity" *(yogyatā)* and explains the "proximity" *(saṃnidhi)* between the two principles as a "capacity" or juxtaposition of two complementary powers. The "proximity" of *puruṣa* and *prakṛti,* consisting of this "capacity" *(yogyatā),* is qualified by Vācaspati as the "power of being experienceable" *(bhogyaśakti)* belonging to *prakṛti* and the "power of being the experiencer" *(bhoktṛśakti)* belonging to *puruṣa.*[265] *Puruṣa* thus has the capability of being the "experiencer" and *citta* has the capacity of being an object of experience. What is, therefore, the mysterious "union," termed *saṃyoga,* between *puruṣa*—the "seer" *(draṣṭṛ)*—and *prakṛti (citta)*—the "seeable" *(dṛśya)?* Vyāsa considers the "union" to be a projection or superimposition *(adhyāropa)*[266] of the contents of consciousness we are aware of as given real existence with respect to *puruṣa,* that is, they reflect *puruṣa*'s existence. They appear real because of the reality of *puruṣa.* As Vyāsa explains, this superimposition results in a confusion of identity between *puruṣa* and the mental processes wherein *puruṣa* is not distinguishable from the process of the emergence or extraversion *(vyutthāna)* of consciousness that generates an extrinsic sense of self-identity,[267] that is, mistaken identity or misidentification.

In *Yoga-Sūtra* II.23[268] the terms "possessor"/"owner" *(svāmin)* and "possessed"/"owned" *(sva),* referring to the seer and the seeable respectively, epitomize well the nature of the conjunction between *puruṣa* and *prakṛti. Puruṣa* is the possessor who is "joined" to its own seen object for the purpose of apprehending or seeing. A *felix culpa,* a confusing temporary misidentification, appears almost a necessary prelude to the realization of yogic wisdom and true identity. Why should there be this apparant "loss" or "fall" of self-identity *(puruṣa)* from its pristine and unencumbered existence into a state of change and enslavement to the prakṛtic realm, only then to be followed by strenuous efforts for liberation? Patañjali's reply seems to be that the conjunction *(saṃyoga)* takes place so that the essential nature of the seer and the seeable can be grasped and discernment arises. Awareness of the seeable object arising from that conjunction is worldly experience *(bhoga).* Awareness of the nature of the seer, however, is liberation *(apavarga).*[269] Vyāsa explains:

> Insofar as the conjunction comes to an end and there is seeing *(darśana)* and its result, seeing is said to be the cause of disjunction, and failure-to-see as the opposite of seeing is said to be the cause of the conjunction. . . . Seeing, namely knowledge *(jñāna),* is said to bring about aloneness *(kaivalya)* only in the sense that in the presence of seeing there is annihi-

> lation of the failure-to-see which is the cause of bondage. What then is this failure-to-see *(adarśana)?*[270]

Vyāsa's commentary on *Yoga-Sūtra* II.23 becomes an exposition of various definitions of the "failure-to-see" *(adarśana)* or ignorance *(avidyā)*. He lists several alternatives for understanding the ignorance that lies at the root of a person's sense of worldly involvement and selfhood.[271] According to Vyāsa the present conjunction *(saṃyoga)* is caused by *avidyā* producing a mentality or "mind" of its own kind.[272] Patañjali states in *Yoga-Sūtra* II.24: "The cause of it [i.e., *saṃyoga*] is ignorance."[273] Vyāsa's commentary makes it clear that it is *avidyā*, understood as the subliminal traits or habit patterns *(vāsanās)* rooted in erroneous knowledge *(viparyaya-jñāna)*,[274] that is the cause of "contact" and the resulting bondage of self-identity. This is the theory of the nature of *avidyā* as favored by the Yoga school. Throughout his commentary (*YB* II.23), Vyāsa uses the word *adarśana* as a synonym for *avidyā*. The other terms commonly used for *avidyā* in the Yoga system are *viparyaya* (*YS* I.8 and *YB* I.8) and *mithyājñāna* (*YS* I.8). Vyāsa stresses that it is the particular conjunction of *avidyā* in relation to the inward individual consciousness *(pratyak-cetanā)* and not simply the impersonal, abstract conjunction of *puruṣa* with *guṇas* metaphysically conceived (which is the same for all beings) that is specifically being pointed to here.[275] This is in line with Yoga's more psychological and epistemological approach to reality in contrast to a metaphysical (ontological) approach. It would be misleading to impute to ignorance a cosmogonic function that would be more appropriate in the context of Advaita Vedānta. One scholar, for example, states: "In the Yogasūtra the reason given for the emergence or the evolution of the manifest world is *avidyā* ('ignorance')."[276] This appears to be a misunderstanding of the precise viewpoint of Patañjali and Vyāsa.

Vyāsa asserts that through the proximity *(saṃnidhi)* of spirit and psychophysical being (matter) the mind becomes the property of *puruṣa,* that is, is "owned" by *puruṣa:* "The mind is like a magnet, serving by mere proximity, by the fact of being seen. It is the property of its owner, *puruṣa.* There is a beginningless connection and this is the cause of *puruṣa*'s cognition of the mental processes."[277] *Saṃnidhi* (proximity) is a technical term used to describe the immanent association between *puruṣa* and the mind by virtue of which it is possible for the unchanging *puruṣa* to perceive the cognitions of the changing, finite mind. The service that the mind performs for *puruṣa* is to be of the nature of the "seeable" *(dṛśya)* so that cognition may occur and consequently *puruṣa*'s capacity to be the "owner" or "master" *(svāmin)* of the "owned" *(sva, prakṛti)* may be developed and actualized. To serve as the "seeable" means to be *puruṣa*'s object of experience when the mind registers the forms of the objects it encounters within the "objective" world. For example, a sight or sound presented to the mind is refined into a *vṛtti*. In the process of cognition, this *vṛtti* "commingles" with the reflected light of *puruṣa* in the mind and serves *puruṣa* by its proximity without actually affecting it. However, as Vyāsa clarifies, just as victory and defeat encountered by the soldiers are attributed to the ruler (because the ruler experiences the effects of them), so bondage and freedom happening in the mind alone are attributed to *puruṣa* because their effects are experienced.[278] That is to say, one experiences sorrow or dissatisfaction *(duḥkha)* in the case of bondage, and liberating knowledge *(jñāna)* in the case of freedom. However, any "change" in the *puruṣa* is only apparent.

Puruṣa has always been the "owner" or "possessor" and *prakṛti* has always been *puruṣa*'s possession *(sva)*. Their relationship is beginningless and natural. No other relationship between them is possible because of their respective natures. Referring to the relationship of *puruṣa* and *prakṛti*, Koelman writes: "the two terms, which *de facto* are in relation, are permanent; yet the relation itself, though without beginning, is not permanent. Hence the relation must be rooted in something over and above, in something additional to the very essence of *prakṛti*."[279] The afflictions experienced by each individual are present as modifications in *prakṛti* yet do not wholly belong to the prakṛtic essence. Furthermore, as Vācaspati Miśra informs us: "insofar as the originating of (i.e., the conjunction) is concerned, ignorance is its cause, but insofar as its stability (i.e., its continued existence and activity) is concerned, the purpose of the Self is the cause, since the stability of that (conjunction) is due to this (purpose) of the Self."[280] But how is ignorance the cause of the origination of the conjunction *saṃyoga?* Patañjali's answer is: by considering empirical selfhood to be the true experiencer and by mistaking the Self to be the active agent—however effected or altered—in the process of cognition and experience. Egoity is neither the pure root-cause, nor *puruṣa*, but rather is the distorted reflection of *puruṣa* in the form of ignorance as the root-cause.

Prakṛti does not plan for either deceptive or liberating knowledge, for *prakṛti* does not intrinsically possess the necessary capacity to be conscious *(cetana)* in herself. Any act of cognition will have a binding effect/affect if the mind is governed by the afflictions *(kleśa*s*)* and afflicted *(kliṣṭa-) vṛtti*s, or a liberating effect/affect if the nature of the experience is predominately of the nonafflicted *(akliṣṭa-vṛtti)* type leading one to the discriminative discernment *(vivekakhyāti)*. *Prakṛti* has only to show herself as she is, as the dancing girl image in the *Sāṃkhya-Kārikā* (59) illustrates. *Prakṛti*'s essentially ambivalent nature can lend its activity to both alternatives, can serve both purposes, but has only the capacity to collaborate according to the degree of understanding or misunderstanding which, located in the mind, informs our decisions,[281] intentions, volitions, and therefore how we experience the world and others.

THEORY OF REFLECTED CONSCIOUSNESS IN YOGA

The saṃsāric condition of self is the result of the failure to distinguish between the pure experiencer or seer *(puruṣa)* and the seeable or "experienced," thereby making "a mental self out of delusion."[282] The "mental self" referred to by Vyāsa is simply a *vṛtti*-accumulated sense of being and identity, the result of an afflicted condition or deluding process of selfhood called *asmitā.* Any attempts to claim the power of consciousness by way of identifying *puruṣa* within *prakṛti* amount to no more than reified notions or concepts of self and, from Patañjali's perspective, are clearly misguided; for the Self, not being an object of experience, can never be seen, can never be turned into a thing or entity to be experienced, can never be "thing-ified." Yet, to whatever extent the "coverings" or "veils" of *vṛtti*-identification *(sārūpya)* eclipse our identity as *puruṣa, puruṣa*'s power as the pure experiencer remains constant, for

> the power of the experiencer *(puruṣa)* does not change. Unmoving it has as it were passed into the changing object, conforming to its function. The assumption of its form of borrowed consciousness by mere resemblance to the mental process, and not distinguished from it, is what is called the [normal] mental process of knowing.[283]

In the above, Vyāsa is describing how the immutable *puruṣa,* without essentially undergoing modification, appears to conform to the mental state that has assumed the form of an object or content of consciousness and experiences that object or content through a self-refexive activity.[284] By definition the *puruṣa* is not the prakṛtic agent of activity and experience, yet it appears to be; although free from ignorance it appears to possess ignorance; and even though as pure awareness *puruṣa* is said to be transcendent of both the mind and the need to discern itself from the mind (which takes place in the *sattva* of the mind), nevertheless it appears to be dependent upon and illuminated by the mind. Vyāsa further explains (repeating the above analogy of the magnet in n. 277 above) that the qualities of the mind become attributed to *puruṣa* because of the condition of their conjunction or *saṃyoga,* just as the qualities of the magnet are induced in a piece of iron placed close to it.[285] When not properly discerned from *puruṣa,* the mental processes are said to be "the secret cave in which is hidden the eternal *brahman*."[286] Misidentification with the form and nature of *vṛtti* conceals our true identity; removing our misidentification reveals our true identity. Thus, a thorough understanding and insight into the mental processes located in the "secret cave" of the mind may be, in Yoga, the key to revealing the knowledge of our true nature and identity.

One of the central theories in Yoga philosophy that attempts to illuminate our understanding of how cognition and perception function in the mind is that of the theory of the "reflection" of consciousness. The notion of "reflection" *(pratibimba, bimba)* is a technical term in the epistemology of classical Yoga especially as interpreted by Vācaspati Miśra. I will now examine this key notion and see how it correlates with an analogical understanding of consciousness in Yoga. Later I will clarify the analogy of "reflection." "Reflection" denotes the "reflection" of the transcendent Self-awareness *(caitanya)* in the most lucid aspect of the mind, namely the *sattva* or *buddhi,* that is, the faculty of decision making and discerning. Vācaspati Miśra (*TV* I.7)[287] speaks of the mind as a mirror *(darpaṇa)* in which *puruṣa*'s awareness is reflected. While the *Yoga-Sūtra* itself makes no direct reference to a theory of "reflection," Vyāsa mentions the term *pratibimba* twice (*YB* IV.23) and understands it as the "reflection" of the object in the mind. Vyāsa uses the simile of the reflected image to explain the "tinging" of the mind by the object. Vācaspati, writing several hundred years after Vyāsa, makes a distinction (*TV* II.17) between *bimba,* or the mirroring of the object in the mind, and *pratibimba,* or the reflection of that content of consciousness back to the Self *(puruṣa)*. However, Vācaspati frequently uses both terms interchangeably and the simile of the reflected image "becomes almost a philosophical explanation and is applied chiefly to the imaging of the *[puruṣa]* in the *[buddhi],* while the tinging of the mind by the external things is generally rendered by the expression 'configuration' *(ākāra)*."[288]

The "reflection" theory is also referred to by Vācaspati as the "shadow of transcendent consciousness" *(citi-chāyā)* and seeks to explain how knowledge is possible given the fact that the mind (including the *buddhi* aspect) is an evolute of insentient *prakṛti.* Vācaspati subscribes to the *cicchāyāpattivāda,* which can be described as knowledge taking place due to the reflection of *puruṣa* in the intellect.[289] The *buddhi* coupled with the sense of self or *ahaṃkāra* becomes as it were an agent of knowledge due to the reflection of *puruṣa* in it. *Puruṣa* seemingly becomes "possessed" of knowledge, pleasure, and so on, knowledge taking the form of an object through the intelligized *buddhi*. The result is the apparent identity of the two: *puruṣa*—which comes to be erroneously associated or mixed with experience and knowledge[290]—with an empirical agent or sense of self that lays claim to or (mis)appropriates that experience and knowledge.

Reflected consciousness is a borrowed state of consciousness, borrowed as it were from *puruṣa*. Moreover, reflected consciousness becomes the locus of selfhood as an empirical identity. It is simultaneously: (1) not real, because it is merely a "reflected" state, of extrinsic value, and in spite of it being derived from the sustaining power and presence of the unchanging transcendent spirit, appears to reduce *puruṣa* to prakṛtic existence; and yet, can be said to be (2) real, because it is actually experienced as human awareness although it is understood that, for all but enlightened persons, this state of reflected consciousness constitutes a more or less confused or deluded and dissatisfying sense of self-identity. In Patañjali's central definition of Yoga (*YS* I.2 states: *yogaś cittavṛttinirodhaḥ*), *cittavṛtti* can refer to an analogical understanding of consciousness in that the consciousness reflecting in the mind, and functioning in the form of the modifications of the mind *(cittavṛtti)*, is analogous to the consciousness of *puruṣa*. As has already been established (see n. 198 in chapter 2 on *YS* IV.19), *cittavṛtti* has no self-luminosity because of its nature being that of the "seeable." Yet *puruṣa* (as if) becomes like the mind, as the locus of the congenital conflation of *puruṣa* and *prakṛti*. *Saṃyoga,* the cause of suffering or dissatisfaction, is a false "union" of sorts and refers to the pure Self as if becoming something other than itself. *Saṃyoga* is the state of the misidentification of the "seeable" (*cittavṛtti,* empirical selfhood) with *puruṣa;* and the misperceived identity of Self with the psychophysical being or ego in *saṃyoga* is merely a construct of the mind, a product of *vṛtti* and *saṃskāra,* which, unlike *puruṣa,* is not the authentic "center," "core" or spiritual "essence" of being. The above analogy is alluded to in *Yoga-Sūtra* II.20, where Patañjali describes the nature of the seer as follows: "The seer is seeing only; though pure, it appears in the form of a cognition (idea, apprehension)."[291] Vyāsa explains:

> "Seeing only" means the power of the seer alone, untouched by any qualification. This *puruṣa* is the witness of the mind. It is not like the mind, and not absolutely unlike it. To some extent it is not like the mind. In what way? Because mind is changeable in that an object is [sometimes] known to it and [sometimes] unknown. Its object, whether [for example] a cow or a jar, is known to it and also unknown, which shows its changeability. But the fact that the object of *puruṣa* is always known shows clearly the unchangeability of *puruṣa*. Why so? Because mind, which is by definition the

> object of *puruṣa*, could not be [sometimes] known and [sometimes] unknown to it; hence the unchangeability of *puruṣa* is established in that its object is always known to it.[292]

However, *puruṣa* is not absolutely unlike the mind, "Because though pure, it *[puruṣa]* appears in the form of a cognition (i.e., is intentional in the form of an idea, mental construct, apprehension). Looking on, it appears as if it were of the mind's nature, though it is not."[293] *Puruṣa*'s intrinsic, unchanging nature as the pure seer has an innate capacity to witness the thoughts, ideas, and apprehensions in the mind without any binding identification with or misappropriation of them; that is, *puruṣa* is the unaffected seer, not enslaved to the "things" of the mind. However, due to ignorance *puruṣa* appears to take on an extrinsic, changing nature of selfhood characterized by a binding identification with the mind: *puruṣa* appears to waver from its unchanging nature. There are, it seems, two very distinct possibilities resulting from the transcendent connection *(saṃbandha)* between *puruṣa* and *prakṛti:* (1) Due to epistemological distortion *prakṛti* takes on a "false" identity or misidentification with *puruṣa* in *saṃyoga;* the reflected consciousness of the mind takes on a confused, deluded nature of selfhood in the process of *vyutthāna*. (2) Through Yoga the yogin's identity is established in the ever-free, ever-pure nature of *puruṣa,* the reflected consciousness of mind having been purified through the enlightened disposition of knowledge leading to discriminative discernment (*jñāna-dīptir ā viveka-khyāteḥ, Yoga-Sūtra* II.28) in the process of *nirodha*. Patañjali does not go into a metaphysical explanation of the beginningless connection between *puruṣa* and *prakṛti.* His emphasis is on epistemological and psychological concerns relating to consciousness in the system.

The mind's changing nature consists of the three *guṇa*s, which, tending to illumination, activity, and inertia (stasis), are said to produce ideas of basically three kinds: peaceful *(śānta),* violent *(ghora),* and deluded *(mūḍha).*[294] Each *guṇa,* when predominant in operation and manifesting as an apprehension *(pratyaya),* cognition, or idea, clashes with the predominance of the others; but when unmanifest, they cooperate with the predominant one.[295] Thus, the three *guṇa*s "come to form ideas of happiness, dissatisfaction and delusion respectively, through the support of the other two, each one having the form of all. However, the distinction is made between them according to which *guṇa* is then in the principal place. The seed *(bīja)* which produces this great mass of suffering is ignorance."[296] The idea of happiness *(sukha)* is formed in the *sattva* through the support of *rajas* and *tamas;* in the state of *rajas* is formed the idea of dissatisfaction or frustration through the support of *sattva* and *tamas; tamas* comes to its deluded ideas through the support of *sattva* and *rajas*. The various human dispositions will depend on whichever *guṇa* is predominant, the other two being subsidiary and subservient. *Śānta* (peaceful), *ghora* (violent), and *mūḍha* (deluded) are the three major personality dispositions, depending on the "weight" being accorded to each *guṇa* and the quality of the intentions, inclinations, thoughts, words, and acts of each person. Any appearance of these attributes "in" *puruṣa* is a temporary condition of appearance *(aupādhika)* arising from a superimposed condition *(upādhi)*.[297]

Vācaspati takes recourse to the analogical theory of reflection in order to elucidate the nature of empirical experience illustrating it by the similes of the crystal and the moon. Using the analogy of a crystal and a hibiscus flower, Vācaspati explains that on account of the conjunction of the seer with the mind, we ascribe our mental states to the *puruṣa* by reflecting, "I am peaceful," "I am violent," "I am deluded." The pure consciousness of *puruṣa,* understood analogically as empirical selfhood, takes the function of the mind as its own just as there is redness reflecting in the clear crystal due to the proximity of the hibiscus flower.[298] It is like a man thinking his face is dirty when looking into an unclean mirror.[299] Vācaspati takes as another example the reflection of the moon in the water. The reflected form of the moon in the water appears as a shining object. Similarly, the intellect *(buddhi)* acts as an agent of cognition with the "light" of pure consciousness reflected in it. The movement of the water around the reflected light of the moon is superimposed upon the moon. Just as the full moon, although "stationary" and round, appears to to be moving and ruffled without any activity on its part due to its reflection in the clear water, so *puruṣa,* without any activity or attachment on its part, appears to possess activity or attachment on account of its reflection in the mind.[300] In this way, *puruṣa* is erroneously understood to be the locus of the functions of the *buddhi.* The transcendent *puruṣa,* however, is only indirectly related to the process of knowledge as an onlooker or witness and does not experience or know as would the prakṛtic agent in the process of experience.

While Vyāsa consistently describes the locus of knowledge as *puruṣa* since the intellect *(buddhi)* or mind is the property of *puruṣa* (see, for example, n. 277 above), in the *cicchāyāpatti* theory adopted by Vācaspati, the locus of knowledge is shifted to the intellect. Vācaspati makes it very clear that there is knowledge only because of the reflection of *puruṣa* in the mind (i.e., intellect) and the empirical consciousness *(cittavṛtti)* is not an object of *puruṣa* as in the empirical or phenomenal subject-object relation.[301]

We can say that the *sattva* aspect of the mind contains a reflection of *puruṣa* that, under the influence of ignorance, then yields the illusions, misconceptions, or errors *(viparyaya)* of the empirical consciousness *(citta-vṛtti)*. As Vyāsa implies, the empirical consciousness, wrongly understood as constituting intrinsic selfhood, *is viparyaya*. Vyāsa is thus describing the mechanisms of the *guṇa*s in the context of an analogical theory of consciousness, that is, as applied to thought-constructs, ideas, or relative states of self-understanding and their different levels or degrees of confused or deluded identity resulting in reified notions of self/personality and as appropriating action. In this regard, the *guṇa*s are modifications of consciousness of the mind and are governed by ignorance; they come to form ideas or concepts of reality based on the fundamental error of mistaking *puruṣa* for what amounts to being an afflicted sense of self-identity *(asmitā)* that permeates human consciousness. In other words, the *guṇa*s are being understood with an epistemological (and moral) emphasis, the various combinations of *sattva, rajas,* and *tamas* forming ideas pertaining to a deluded (in which *tamas* is predominant), violent/aggressive (in which *rajas* is predominant), or happy (in which *sattva* is predominant) nature. The predominance of *sattva* signifies more illuminated degrees of self-understanding that more "closely" resemble the true nature of *puruṣa*. Unlike classical Sāṃkhya, in Yoga the *guṇa*s do not appear to be given an ontological emphasis (i.e., as relating to categories of existence). We see, therefore, that in Yoga our psychosomatic organism involving thoughts, ideas, relationship, and so on, is primarily an integral part of the prakṛtic world as consciousness, albeit a reflected and changing consciousness. The *guṇa*s therefore apply to the world of phenomenal consciousness and (self-) understanding as much as to the world of things or categories of existence.

While Vijñāna Bhikṣu agrees with Vācaspati that the presentation of the object of cognition to an unchanging Self is not possible except in the form of a reflection, he states that cognition arises through the reflection in the spiritual Self of the mental state that has assumed the form of the object. Bhikṣu speaks of a "mutual reflection" *(anyonya-pratibimba)*[302] and offers a different hypothesis called the "double reflection theory" *(bimba-pratibimbavāda)*.[303] He maintains that not only does the *puruṣa* reflect in *buddhi* (as in Vācaspati's theory), but a second reflection of *buddhi* into *puruṣa* takes place. Having the reflection of both the *puruṣa* and the object, the *buddhi* is then reflected "into" *puruṣa*. Bhikṣu states: "This conformity with the objects is in the intellect in the form of an alteration . . . and is also 'in' the *puruṣa* in the form of a reflection."[304]

According to Bhikṣu, the first reflection intelligizes the content of the mind *(buddhi)* and the second reflection makes *puruṣa* the agent of the particular knowledge.[305] Bhikṣu brushes aside the objection—that this would make *puruṣa* subject to change—by arguing that a reflection is merely an appearance of change, as in the case with the reflection of the red flower reflected in a crystal, and is not a substantial change.[306] He justifies his "double reflection" as the correct view and points to the mutual reflection of each in the other as expressed in the *Sāṃkhya-Kārikā* (20) by the use of the two "*iva*-s." In the *Sāṃkhya-Kārikā* (20), Īśvara Kṛṣṇa states that through the conjunction *(saṃyoga)* of *puruṣa* and *prakṛti,* the nonconscious intellect appears *as if* conscious, and *puruṣa* appears *as if* it is the performer of action, that is, the prakṛtic agent of activity. Vācaspati Miśra's interpretation is perhaps "cleaner" in the sense that all transactions of experience occur only in the intellect after it has been "intelligized" by *puruṣa.* Vijñāna Bhikṣu's interpretation has the merit of ascribing experience to *puruṣa* (because the contents of intellect-awareness are reflected back on *puruṣa*).[307]

Bhikṣu's hypothesis, if understood literally, makes *puruṣa* changeable and subject to development or alteration *(pariṇāma-rūpa)* through the proximity or influence of psychophysical factors (including satisfaction, suffering, confusion, knowledge, etc.) or limited adjuncts *(upādhi)* outside of itself. This goes against the tenets of Yoga philosophy and destroys the very foundation of the doctrine of the eternal purity of *puruṣa.* Probably Bhikṣu hoped to avert a literal interpretation of his theory by citing the analogy of the crystal and using phrases like "semblance of mutability" and "*as if puruṣa* were undergoing a change, but *in reality* remaining unchanged like the crystal." Of course, Bhikṣu can be understood to be speaking analogically: The reflection of a red flower in a crystal does not mean to imply a change in the crystal nor in the substance of the crystal; rather, any change occurs merely in the (distorted?) "eye of the beholder" of the crystal.

As a result of the process of reflection, *puruṣa* and *prakṛti* appear *as if* united. They "appear" "one" in *saṃyoga* (*YS* II.17 and 23) as congenitally conflated realms even though they are distinct. One is not converted into the other though their proximity causes them to seem as one. How is it possible that the formless *puruṣa* reflects in the *citta,* which, though composed of the "material" of *prakṛti,* is so subtle as to appear formless? The analogy of reflection needs to be clarified. It does not mean an *actual* reflection like that of the sun into a pool of water. In ordinary perception, the reflection can be seen as being twofold: (1) through the proximity of *puruṣa* some natural change or alteration occurs in the mind enabling it to cognize; and (2) a certain other modification occurs in the mind upon the proximity of an object or content whereby the mind takes on the very form of the object or content perceived. That change is called a *vṛtti.*

Vṛtti serves the purpose of causing a connection between the mind and the object or content of perception.[308] *Vṛtti* gives to the mind a power of knowledge, a "consciousness-of" objects, content, persons, and so on. *Vṛtti* is meant to "ooze out" the knowledge of any object or experience, but its function is not to provide a direct realization or identification as *puruṣa,* for as the the true "subject" or experiencer *puruṣa* can never be the object of any experience, can never be known or experienced as can *prakṛti* and her manifestations.[309] The active agent in the process of the rise of knowledge is *citta*—the locus of the affliction *asmitā,* the false I-am-ness. The role of *puruṣa,* insofar as *puruṣa* is concealed throughout this process of masquerading consciousness, is said to be that of a passive witness through its mere presence. Thus Yoga emphasizes practices that can help to disclose the presence of *puruṣa* through the *sattva* of the mind. The immutability (*YS* IV.18) and unaffected nature of *puruṣa* is retained throughout the modifications occurring in the mind regardless of any misidentification taking place.

The crux of the problem of *puruṣa*'s appearance of changeability lies in the explanation of the *citta-puruṣa* relation. I suggest the following summary as a clarification of Patañjali's position on this matter. It is against the intent of Patañjali to consider *puruṣa*'s intrinsic nature, pure immutable consciousness, *as though* impure, changeable and therefore subject to suffering/dissatisfaction *(duḥkha).* It is not *as though puruṣa* mimics the *vṛtti*s of the *citta* and exclaims "I am impure." *Puruṣa*'s luminosity must remain constant and unaffected. It is the *citta* (and its modes) that, after having been activated by the luminous presence of *puruṣa* and under the grip of ignorance, masquerades as *puruṣa* as if to say, "I am spirit. Though I am pure, I appear as impure. Though not subject to pain and suffering, I appear to suffer." In other words, the locus of misidentification *(sārūpya)* is within the mind.

All the repetitions of the particle *iva* ("as if," "as though") and similar words and phrases employed by the commentators do not literally apply to *puruṣa.* They apply to the afflicted I-am-ness *(asmitā)*—the affliction of egoity being the true explanation of *sārūpya* (*YS* I.4). It is in the *sūtra* (II.6) defining *asmitā* that Patañjali uses the word *iva:* "as if" the two principles—the power of the seer and that of the mind—had assumed an identity appearing as a single self. Any superimposition *(adhyāropa)* goes only this far and does not literally extend to include *puruṣa.* Any assumption of false identity *(abhimāna)* is an act of the misidentified ego-consciousness *(cittavṛtti)* or egoity *(asmitā)* and to attribute this extrinsic form of self-identity to *puruṣa* is contrary to the understanding of authentic identity in Yoga philosophy.

A CLOSER LOOK AT "PERCEPTION" IN THE *YOGA-SŪTRA*

Both classical Sāṃkhya and Patañjali's Yoga accept three means of knowledge or categories of valid cognition *(pramāṇa):* perception *(pratyakṣa),* inference *(anumāna),* and valid testimony *(āgama).*[310] Because the mind *(citta)* is constituted of the three *guṇa*s, all of its operations such as the processes of logic, modifications *(vṛtti)* such as valid means of cognition *(pramāṇa),* and acceptance or rejection of a postulate or a conclusion do not in themselves possess consciousness. Being insentient or nonconscious *(jaḍa, acetana),* it is only through the presence of *puruṣa* that the mind and its processes can function and are intelligized.[311]

A *pramāṇa* is an instrument, means, or method for reaching a valid apprehension *(pramā)* of a state, condition, fact, object, or principle *(tattva)* previously not obtained.[312] Vyāsa states that following from the act of perception *(pratyakṣa)*—of internal and external objects, there results (i.e., in *saṃyoga*) an apprehension by *puruṣa* of the *vṛtti* of perception and not distinguished from it.[313] *Puruṣa* appears to become identical with the *vṛtti*s of the mind. In *Yoga-Sūtra* IV.17 Patañjali states: "An object is known or not known due to the requisite coloration of the mind by that [object]."[314] What is this ordinary act of perception? Vyāsa informs us that

> the mind is colored *(uparāga)* by an external object through the channels of the senses. With that as its object, a modification *(vṛtti)* is produced in the mind; this *vṛtti* is the valid cognition called perception. It takes as its "field" the determination mainly of the particular nature of the object, which has, however, the nature of the universal. The result is an apprehension by *puruṣa* of the mental process, not distinguishable from it.[315]

An external object *(vastu)* is a requisite in perception so that the type of apprehension that occurs in the *vṛtti* of conceptualization *(vikalpa)* may be excluded. The senses must consistently confirm the reality of the object. Such "proof" contradicts any "perception" of lesser validity (i.e., invalid cognition) and would prove the latter to be an error *(viparyaya).*

We can assume that when one person is attracted to another person, or the mind is drawn toward the experience of an object, the same process of "coloring" *(uparāga)* or "influencing" takes place with the qualities of the person or object reflecting in the mind. In the case of *pratyakṣa,* the qualities of the object of experience pass through the channels of the senses. We can also assume that Vyāsa's phrase *tad-viṣaya* (see n. 315 above): "With that as its object," refers to the entire process of coloring the mind in this way, with the mind taking on the form of the *vṛtti* that is being produced. If it were only a mental perception without contact through the senses, the realist philosophers of Sāṃkhya and Yoga would not classify it as a valid perception (of the ordinary *pratyakṣa* type). When the mind is presented certain information by the senses, a modification occurs in the mind whose object is the sense data. A doubt may arise regarding the actual properties of an object, particularly in the case of an object that shares certain of its properties with other objects. The determinative process *(avadhāraṇa)* helps the mind to eliminate general shared properties so that it focuses on the specific. For example, one can take the question, "Is that a person or a post?" In this question the general shared properties of the person and the post (e.g., tallness, thinness) are eliminated, and by focusing on the specific properties, one determines the visible object to be either a person or a post. This *vṛtti,* which chiefly determines the specifics, is a valid cognition called direct perception.[316] A perception is made possible because the origin of the awareness is *puruṣa*. Through its very presence as the witness or knower of the process of apprehension,[317] *puruṣa* gives to the mind its capacity to perceive. *Puruṣa*'s presence makes possible our processes of perception, which consist of the following: The "light" of *puruṣa* reflects in the pure *sattva* of the mind and enables the mind to perceive objects and experience sensations, and so on. The mind thereby perceives these objects as they also reflect into it. The reflection of *puruṣa* and that of the objects mingle in the mind generating *vṛtti*s (perceptions) and the mind in turn can reflect on these perceptions. In ordinary perception the mind does not distinguish between its experience of the object from the external world and the awareness generated by *puruṣa*. A person's mental processes are mistaken as being processes within and of *puruṣa:* the objects, the experience, the *vṛtti,* the mind, and *puruṣa* all being conceived to be as if identical.[318]

The above realism presents a problem because within the major schools of Indian philosophy "yogic perception" (*yogi-pratyakṣa,* see below) is often considered to be the supremely valid type of perception. The ordinary person's perception definitely requires the presence of external objects and the mind's contact with them through the functioning of the senses. But does Patañjali intend to include the process of *yogi-pratyakṣa* under *YS* I.7? Even a cursory reading of Vyāsa's words leads us to understand that *yogi-pratyakṣa* is not meant to be included here. The finer perceptions of the yogin are in fact described by Patañjali elsewhere.[319]

Yogi-pratyakṣa is another term for direct apprehension *(sākṣātkāra)*[320] which involves the yogin's conscious identification with an object. This is the basis of the practice of "unification" *(samāpatti),* and constraint *(saṃyama)* through which various yogic powers *(siddhi)* can be acquired (e.g., the yogin's perception of past lives, *YS* III.18). If we take our cue from *YS* IV.17 (see n. 314 above), it appears that Vyāsa's use of the phrase *uparāga* ("coloring") is for the purpose of stating the cause and process of the *vṛtti*s produced in the mind from merely external sources. The above description of perception should not be taken as part of the definition of yogic perception, otherwise, as Vijñāna Bhikṣu points out, the realization of the Self and *īśvara* could not occur,[321] not being a product of, and not having been induced through the contact between external objects and the senses. Nevertheless, Bhikṣu[322] and others (such as Vācaspati Miśra and Rāmānanda Yati) have attempted to classify *yogi-pratyakṣa* (under *Yoga-Sūtra* I.7) as a type of direct perception.[323] This seems to be in conformity with and supported by Patañjali's philosophy in general. It should be noted that ordinary cognition or perception is subject to distortion due to various karmic factors in the mind (that is, *saṃskāra*s and *vāsanā*s) that affect or color how we perceive and appropriate the objects we encounter, as is implied in *Yoga-Sūtra* IV.17 (see n. 314 above). Whether classified as being ordinary or yogic, perception is made possible because the origin or root-consciousness is *puruṣa* by which the mind obtains its capacity to perceive[324] and identify with the objects or content of experience.

Patañjali and Vyāsa acknowledge the superiority of perception over inference and valid testimony. Why? Both inference and testimony are concerned only with the general qualities *(sāmānya)* of an object and not with its particularities *(viśeṣa).* Words themselves are incapable of producing knowledge of particulars. Although the generic qualities of an object are also brought to consciousness in perception, still the special "field" of the latter is the ascertainment of particularities. Thus perception is seen to carry with it more conviction than knowlege derived from inference and testimony. Moreover, according to Yoga, the authority and efficacy of *anumāna* (inference) and *āgama* (reliable authority, i.e., *śruta*—tradition, that which is heard) is ultimately transcended in higher perception. As Patañjali makes clear in *YS* I.49: "The condition of that insight [which is Truth-bearing, *ṛtaṃbharā*] is of a particular purpose, and is different from the insight gained by tradition or from inference."[325] Direct perception gives knowledge of anything particular, but the yogic perception of "truth-bearing insight"[326] that arises in *samādhi* is entirely different in scope from that of heard (cf. *BG* II.52-53) or inferred knowledge as well as sensory perception in the ordinary world. Vyāsa writes:

> Scriptural authority and the teaching received orally are the same as the knowledge within the category of valid testimony *(āgama)*. The area is generalities. Valid testimony cannot communicate the particular. Why not? Because the particular does not have the conventional association with a word. Inference too has only universals for its object. Furthermore, inference leads to a conclusion through a generality. . . . Ordinary perception gives no knowledge at all of some subtle, remote or hidden object, but we should not think that the latter is not demonstrable and has no existence. A particular relating to subtle elements or to *puruṣa* is only perceptible through the insight [attained in] *samādhi* alone.[327]

Ordinary valid cognition as understood in the *Yoga-Sūtra* is therefore a sort of knowing wholly different from yogic "insight" *(prajñā)*. In its conventional usage, valid cognition is knowledge *about* reality *(puruṣa* and *prakṛti)*. Insight *(prajñā)* is direct yogic perception *(yogi-pratyakṣa, sākṣātkāra)*, and its purpose is to disclose knowledge of *puruṣa*.[328] It may be concluded therefore that ordinary perception, inference, and valid testimony (authority) can produce correct knowledge *about* reality. But in Patañjali's system the above means of knowing *(pramāṇa)* are merely instruments of conventional understanding, rational knowing, or even metaphysical knowledge, all of which can function as a buffer separating one from insight-by-direct-experience. Ordinary valid cognition is a mediated knowledge of *puruṣa* and *prakṛti;* yogic insight or *prajñā* (attained in *samādhi*) is immediate.

Pedagogically, it may well have been the case that Patañjali initiated disciples into yogic disciplines that, although including reasoned investigation *(tarka)* or discursive thought (*vitarka, YS* II.33–34), transcended the limitations of reasoning and discursive thinking.[329] Moreover, whereas the valid cognition of *Yoga-Sūtra* I.7 has the limited capacity to bring about intellectual conviction, yogic "insight" *(prajñā)* has the power to effect spiritual emancipation *(apavarga)*. Both levels of perception *(pratyakṣa)* are communicated in a pedagogical context in the service of soteriology. Therefore, the mind—the vehicle of perception—performs a crucial role in Patañjali's soteriological methodology. When, from textual sources such as scripture and the teachings of spiritual preceptors or *guru*s, as well as exercising our own processes of rational analysis and understanding, we have learned of and contemplated upon the culminating state of liberation in Yoga, there nonetheless can linger doubts (*saṃśaya, YS* I.30) about any existence subtler than that of the obvious world we "see" and "know," a world comprising the "things" of our daily perceptual experience. Perception, as defined in *Yoga-Sūtra* I.7 and the *Yoga-Bhāṣya* (I.7), therefore needs to be extended and expanded to include the direct experience of the subtler aspects *(sūkṣma)* of *prakṛti* through *yogi-pratyakṣa*. Having attained yogic insight directly through the vehicle of one's body and mind, the experience reinforces the faith (*śraddhā, YS* I.20) that what one had previously arrived at through inference, and based upon what teachers and texts have propounded, is true. Such perception strengthens one's resolve[330] to proceed to the subtler "invisible" reality and seek that identity (i.e., *puruṣa*), which one has not yet "experienced" and which alone can result in a state of freedom and lasting satisfaction. In Yoga epistemology, reality is accurately "seen" only by the seer who alone can "see" without any epistemic distortion caused by ignorance *(avidyā)* and the intervention of egoic states or egoity *(asmitā)*.

The mind can be understood as having a twofold faculty of perception. On the one hand, there is an "outward facing" capacity of the *citta* which, directed toward the object of perception, functions in a rational and conceptual mode and issues in a reflective cognition and discerning power of the intellect (equivalent to *adhyavasāya* in *Sāṃkhya-Kārikā* 23). On the other hand, the mind has an "inward facing" capacity "toward" *puruṣa* where it is temporarily disengaged from the external world of things and objects of the senses, and can function as a vehicle for liberating knowledge of discriminative discernment *(vivekakhyāti)*. Perception of the ordinary kind *(pratyakṣa)* as studied in *Yoga-Sūtra* I.7 functions by way of the "outward facing" power of the mind to perceive objects through the senses. Yogic perception *(yogi-pratyakṣa)* takes place through the "inward facing" power of the mind. The volitions of reasoned investigation *(pramāṇa)* and the higher knowledge called "insight" *(prajñā)* arise in the mind and both are types of mental content presented to *puruṣa* for its viewing. However, it is yogic perception that eventually leads to the mind's complete purification, sattvification, and liberation. Yogic perception—liberating insight—is soteriologically the most efficacious means in Yoga. At no time is the former lower level of perception to be confused with yogic perception and the discriminative discernment (between *puruṣa* and the mind or *prakṛti*) that occurs in the higher stages of *samādhi* and culminates in the realization of *puruṣa*. Rather, perception in its "outer facing" mode is initially to be understood in the context of the apparent identity of the mind and *puruṣa* wherein extrinsic selfhood in the situation or mode of "emergence" *(vyutthāna)* is mistaken for *puruṣa*.

Patañjali explains the mind's epistemological limitations. *Yoga-Sūtra* IV.20 tells us that the mind (i.e., *vṛtti*) and the "object" cannot in one circumstance (i.e., simultaneously) be clearly ascertained.[331] The mind cannot ascertain itself and the "object" at the same time; the mind's function is to cognize objects while its processes are witnessed by the self-luminous *puruṣa*. Also, if one mind were to know another mind, this would result in an unending series of minds each perceived by another. This infinite regress or overextending of the intellect from the intellect (from one cognition to another) would result in a confusion of memory.[332]

Unlike empirical selfhood, which is part of the "seeable" *(dṛśya)*, *puruṣa* can never be made an object, nor can *puruṣa* be realized through the ordinary processes *(vṛttis)* of valid cognition (*YS* I.7). Patañjali tells us (*YS* IV.18) that *puruṣa* is transcendent of the object-oriented realm of the "seeable" as the knower (witness) of the content and intentions of the empirical consciousness or mind. In *Yoga-Sūtra* III.35, however, it *appears* that *puruṣa* can be made an object of knowledge. Patañjali states: "Since it is for the purpose of the other *[puruṣa]*, experience is [based on] the idea that there is no distinction between the *puruṣa* and the *sattva*, though they are absolutely unmixed; from *saṃyama* (the practice of constraint) on the purpose being for itself (serving its own purpose), there arises knowledge of *puruṣa*.[333] In his commentary, Vyāsa surmises that *puruṣa* cannot be known in the ordinary way and cannot be made an object of constraint *(saṃyama)*: "It is not that *puruṣa* is known through the *sattva*-intellect which has the idea of *puruṣa*. It is *puruṣa* that sees the idea supported by its own self. Thus it is said [*BĀ Up* IV.5.15): 'By what indeed would one know the knower?' "[334] Why is it that *puruṣa* cannot be known or seen in the ordinary way? It is not that all distinctions necessarily collapse in some absolute realm; rather, it is that as pure experiencer and knower, *puruṣa* can never be made an object of experience and knowledge. *Vṛttis* and *puruṣa*'s awareness of them are two separate factors. The final goal is not one of knowledge as a mental state or activity, nor could it be a subjective state of being. In Yoga one cannot "find" true identity for *puruṣa* is not an entity or object to be found, that is, "there is no one there to find; the witness cannot be witnessed."[335]

Puruṣa as pure "subject" is both transcendent and immanent, uninvolved yet present and necessary to ordinary experience. The reality of *prakṛti* (and hence of *citta* and *vṛtti*) is not denied. However, what are normally held to be real independently existing "things" *(vastu)* or categories of existence (*tattvas*, as in Sāṃkhya) are seen in Yoga to be linked to the perceptual processes of the mind and as appropriated by empirical selfhood. The "world" thus experienced becomes an egoically referenced reality based on reified notions or ideas *(pratyaya)* of self and world that, having formed as sediments in the mind, limit human identity within the confines of a distorted way of "seeing" (i.e., a "failure-to-see") and "relating" to the world (i.e., how the sense-of-I relates to the "things" of the world). Psychologically, in such a fractured or fragmented state of selfhood *(cittavṛtti),* the network of impressions *(saṃskāra*s*),* habit patterns *(vāsanā*s*),* and *vṛtti*-identifications continues to sustain and reinforce a predominantly afflicted human nature. The power of consciousness potentially present to all is forgotten and concealed within this framework or "wheel" (or "whirl") of misidentification and spiritual ignorance. Life is experienced through a repetitive or seemingly unending generation of habit patterns *(vāsanā*s*)* rooted in dissatisfaction *(duḥkha)* and affliction *(kleśa).* Yet mistaken identity and its self-centered misappropriation of the world can, according to Yoga, be ended.

We have seen that cognition and knowledge play a crucial role in Patañjali's system, and are structured and function in the mind due to a reflection (understood analogically) of the presence of *puruṣa.* Without *puruṣa* or pure consciousness, ordinary "knowledge" and experience would not take place. Based on yogic insight into the nature of human identity, Patañjali was then able to communicate a "path" of Yoga through which the afflictions *(kleśa*s*),* so fundamental to the human condition of struggle and conflict in *saṃyoga,* can be uprooted and overcome. But the "path" from *saṃyoga* to Yoga (liberation) requires, as we have seen, a thorough study of the mind, for it is only by way of the transformation of the *mind* and its "modifications" (i.e., mental processes) that the key to success in Yoga becomes evident. Therefore, the concept of the mind *(citta)*—its nature, structure, and functioning—is an essential component or building block of Patañjali's philosophy. Along with the content of the previous chapter (chapter 2) focusing on classical Yoga's metaphysical perspective, a solid albeit theoretical foundation for understanding and appreciating Patañjali's presentation of Yoga has, it is hoped, been achieved.

Yoga has, not inappropriately, been described as a "theory-practice continuum,"[336] a philosophy, including a discipline, that unites theory and practice. With this idea held in mind, we will now go on to examine closely Patañjali's soteriological methodology and praxis-orientation beginning with an analysis of the meaning of "cessation" *(nirodha)* in Yoga, and then moving on to look at central methods of Yoga discipline showing how Yoga can be seen to culminate in an embodied and integrated state of liberated consciousness and identity.

chapter four

Nirodha, Yoga Praxis, and the Transformation of the Mind

NIRODHA: THE FOUNDATION OF YOGIC PRAXIS

The saṃsāric identity of self—ineluctably locked into an epistemological and ontological duality with the objective world—is ingeniously captured by Patañjali in the expression *cittavṛtti.* Being by nature an extrinsic identity of self and fraught with affliction *(kleśa), cittavṛtti* is rooted in ignorance *(avidyā)* and as such can be characterized as impermanent *(anitya),* impure *(aśuci),* dissatisfaction *(duḥkha),* and nonself *(anātman)* (*YS* II.5).[1] Clearly, then, the yogin must learn to distinguish between extrinsic and intrinsic identity of self, between *cittavṛtti* and *puruṣa.* By locating the cause and functioning of affliction within the mind *(citta)* itself, Yoga asserts that there is a way to overcome misidentification with the modifications *(vṛtti)* of the mind and "achieve" emancipation from the afflictions that permeate our everyday modes of perception, experience *(bhoga),* and livelihood. For example, Patañjali tells us that the modifications arising from the afflictions are overcome through meditation *(dhyāna).*[2] Our true form *(svarūpa)* or identity *(puruṣa)* is not intrinsically predisposed to the influences and affects of habit patterns *(vāsanā*s*),* latent impressions *(saṃskāra*s*),* and afflicted mental processes or modifications *(vṛtti*s*)* that perpetuate actions *(karma)* rooted in ignorance *(avidyā).*

How is the purpose of Yoga—the very ending of mistaken identity, suffering and dissatisfaction *(duḥkha)*[3]—to be brought about? The cessation of misidentification and its concomitant dissatisfaction is effected through a process of purifying and mastering the *vṛtti*-generating complex: the mind and the activity to which it gives rise. The foundation of yogic praxis, the mastery of mind, takes place through the process of *nirodha* as stated in *Yoga-Sūtra* I.2: "Yoga is the cessation of [the misidentification with] the modifications of the mind."[4] Through a study of the meaning of "cessation" *(nirodha),* the theory-praxis unity so central to Yoga philosophy can be better understood and appreciated. The process of "cessation" incorporates many forms of practice depending on the needs of the practitioner and includes the physical, moral, psychological, and spiritual dimensions of our being. As the cornerstone of all Yoga practice *nirodha* can be seen to encompass a wide range of methods—cited throughout the *Yoga-Sūtra*—that can be applied in a variety of situations.[5] In comparison, classical Sāṃkhya prescribes essentially one practice for the release from sorrow and dissatisfaction: the cultivation of knowledge *(jñāna).* Yoga, by contrast, offers over twenty practices that can be undertaken to prepare the mind for the event of spiritual liberation wherein *puruṣa* is allowed to shine forth in its pristine purity.[6]

However, rather than being "any ascetic technique or any method of meditation"[7] (as in Eliade's broad definition of Yoga), Patañjali's Yoga involves a serious inquiry into the structures and contents of the mind along with an analysis of how the mind—including the empirically rooted sense of self—differs from *puruṣa.* The human dilemma of misidentification is such that with each *vṛtti* the consciousness reflecting in the mind becomes that *vṛtti* and identifies with it, just as the sun reflected in a lake appears to be modified according to the nature of each wave in the water. To whatever takes place in the mind, the reflected I or ego says, "I am this wave, I am this experience," or "This is me, this is my experience." The *vṛtti*s of the ordinary person carry with them the influence or "coloring" and "seed" of misidentification (*vṛtti-sārūpya, YS* I.4) in the perceptions and experiences taking place resulting in a confusion of identity in the condition of *saṃyoga,* the seer being mistaken for the seeable. Vyāsa gives a dramatic portrayal of the underlying process of misidentification involving the empirical sense of self and the way out of this dilemma through right vision *(samyag-darśana):*

> that other [i.e., empirical identity] is subjected again and again to dissatisfaction brought on by [it]self, casting it off and then subjected again to what has been cast off . . . with the mental processes from beginningless time infected so to say with the various habit patterns, taking on what should be avoided, namely "I" and "mine," born again and again—(on

> that empirical self) the three-fold suffering, with causes both objective and subjective, flood down. Seeing that other one, and himself, and all beings, carried away by the beginningless stream of pain, the yogin takes refuge in right vision, destroyer of suffering.[8]

Vyāsa's above description notwithstanding, it is essential to note here that in Yoga the power of identification with the mind and *vṛtti* is not intrinsically problematic and without purpose. Identification involves potentialities of power (*sva-swāmi-śaktyoḥ, YS* II.23). When it is misdirected and misappropriated, identification remains confined to a particular person and what that person calls "I" and "mine." From this egoic perspective, the world and other persons are viewed as being separate from oneself. However, when the power of identification is properly directed and concentrated through Yoga, it can be transformed into illuminating and expanding states of consciousness and one can ultimately know one's identity as *puruṣa.* Identification is thus a power to be accessed and harnessed in Yoga discipline *(sādhana).* The average person is born with a limited power of identification. It is, as it were, a constitutional defect *(doṣa)* caused by *avidyā* and is not one's "personal" fault; nor is it ultimately the fault of one's parents, teachers, education, or society as a whole. For Yoga, the human dilemma of mistaken identity *(sārūpya)* is generated by ignorance or a profound misconception of authentic identity *(puruṣa).* This impure consciousness or confused state of selfhood is actually "built into" the unenlightened human apparatus, is a congenital infection located within our psychophysical being. Yet as the vehicle or catalyst that ousts one from one's complacency in the condition of ignorance by the sheer uneasiness, pain or affliction it creates, it can be said to be purposeful. Moreover, Patañjali informs us that wrong cognition or error is a momentous problem that must be tackled if one is to be free from ignorance and the turmoil it creates. Our authentic identity is *puruṣa,* pure consciousness. As a reflection of *puruṣa,* however, consciousness has two basic modes in which it can function: (1) as the consciousness (mind) that is under the sway of ignorance and is propelled in the direction of affliction; and (2) as the consciousness (mind) that due to increasing purification and illumination is propelled in the direction of liberation from ignorance. As will be later argued, "cessation" *(nirodha)* can be understood: (1) as a process through which ignornance is counteracted, temporarily preventing the afflictions' domination or hold over the mind and thereby checking the distorted or wrong functioning of *vṛtti,* that is, *vṛtti*s as appropriated in the condition of *saṃyoga;* and (2) as a process through which knowledge *(jñāna)* or insight *(prajñā)* is revealed, which can be called the "sattvification of consciousness," and which, grounded in knowledge of *puruṣa (puruṣa-jñāna),* allows for the corrected or right functioning of *vṛtti,* that is, *vṛtti*s as appropriated through the illumination and purification of mind. At the highest level, the process of *nirodha* culminates in the goal of Yoga—*kaivalya.*

NIRODHA (CESSATION): ANNIHILATION/NEGATION OR TRANSFORMATION OF THE MIND?

Nirodha (cessation) is one of the most difficult terms employed in the *Yoga-Sūtra* and its meaning plays a crucial role for a proper comprehension of Patañjali's system of Yoga. The "attainment" of liberation in Yoga is dependent upon the destruction of impurity (*aśuddhi-kṣaya, Yoga-Sūtra* II.28) and the increasing light of knowledge (*jñāna-dīpti, Yoga-Sūtra* II.28) both of which take place in the process of *nirodha.* Since, as I shall now argue, the misunderstanding of this process has been fundamental to the misapprehension of the meaning of Patañjali's Yoga, there is a need to clarify it.

The word *nirodha* is derived from *ni* (down, into) and *rudh:* "to obstruct, arrest, stop, restrain, prevent."[9] In some well-known translations of *Yoga-Sūtra* I.2 *(yogaś cittavṛttinirodhaḥ) nirodha* has been rendered as "suppression,"[10] "inhibition,"[11] "restriction,"[12] "cessation,"[13] "restraint"[14] and "control."[15] These meanings,[16] I suggest, are highly problematic, erroneous, or misleading if understood, as is often the case, with a view that emphasizes *nirodha* as an ontological negation or dissolution of the mind and its functioning. I am suggesting that any attempt to interpret Patañjali's Yoga as a practice that seeks to annihilate or suppress the mind and its modifications for the purpose of gaining spiritual liberation distorts the intended meaning of Yoga as defined by Patañjali. In regard to the process of *nirodha,* the wide range of methods in the *Yoga-Sūtra* indicates an emphasis on the ongoing application of yogic techniques including meditation, not a deadening of the mental faculties wherein the operations of consciousness, including our perceptual and ethical natures, are abandoned or switched off. By defining *nirodha* as "cessation," I mean to imply the "undoing" or "dissolution"[17] of the conjunction *(saṃyoga)* between *puruṣa*—the "seer" *(draṣṭṛ)*—and *prakṛti*—the "seeable" *(dṛśya),* the conjunction that Vyāsa explains as a mental superimposition *(adhyāropa)* resulting in the confusion of identity between *puruṣa* and the mental processes.[18] Our sense of self becomes misidentified with the mental processes *(vṛtti*s*)* thereby creating, in the words of Vyāsa, "a mental self out of delusion."[19] *Nirodha,* I am suggesting, refers to the cessation of the worldly, empirical effects of the *vṛtti*s on the yogin's consciousness, not the complete cessation of *vṛtti*s themselves. *Nirodha* means to cease the congenital, epistemological power of the *vṛtti*s over the yogin, that is, *nirodha* is the epistemological cessation of *vṛtti*s in the form of the congenital ignorance (*avidyā, YS* II.3–5) of our true spiritual identity and ultimate destiny.

To understand *nirodha* one needs to comprehend the entire Yoga scheme of the process of manifestation or "evolution" and the "return to the origin," especially the latter. The last *sūtra* of the *Kaivalya-Pāda* (*YS* IV.34) defines the liberated state of "aloneness" *(kaivalya)* as: *puruṣārtha-śūnyānāṃ guṇānāṃ pratiprasavaḥ kaivalyaṃ,* "Aloneness is the return to the origin of the *guṇa*s, now without any purpose for *puruṣa*."[20] The important term, *pratiprasava* (see discussion in chapter 2), refers to the "involution" or "counterflow" of the *guṇa*s into their source or state of "equilibrium. " It is of interest to note the one earlier context (only) in which Patañjali uses this term. *Yoga-Sūtra* II.10 states: "In their subtle form, they [the *kleśa*s] are to be overcome by a return to the origin or source *(pratiprasava)*."[21] In the above *sūtra* the term *pratiprasava* refers to the dissolution of affliction in the mind implying a purification and illumination of consciousness. Scholars have often interpreted *prasava* with an ontological emphasis signifying the "streaming forth" of the ultimate building blocks *(tattva*s*)* of *prakṛti* into the myriad forms of the cosmos in all its dimensions, including the human organism.[22] *Pratiprasava,* by the same token, is often understood to denote the process of the dissolution of those forms relative to the microcosm of the yogin who is about to win liberation.[23] Is this ontological dissolution of manifest existence—where the *guṇa*s are recalled back to their unmanifest condition of equilibrium—the intended meaning of *pratiprasava* as the term is used in the *Yoga-Sūtra?* Koelman refers to *pratiprasava* as the "inverse generation," the definite return of a given prakṛtic organism to its ultimate substrative cause.[24] He goes on to describe this process as follows:

> Everything has been exhausted or burnt out so that no living seed is left to enable a new energisation in the shape of a living prakṛtic organism.[25]

> Like a tree that slowly withers away for want of any moisture or contact with the soil, however rich that soil may be, the prakṛtic organism tends to dissolution, to the disintegration and suppression of our empirical personality. [The yogin] has induced a state of psychomental anaemia by starving his psychical life.[26]

These are, according to Koelman, some of the effects of Yoga discipline, and obviously imply the decomposition or death of the psychophysical organism of the yogin.

I would like to suggest that the term *pratiprasava* can be more appropriately rendered with an epistemological emphasis rather than (as in the above) an ontological one. Epistemologically, *pratiprasava* denotes a return to the source, withdrawal, or dissolution of the afflicted state of the *guṇa*s, that is, insofar as the constituents of matter/nature have been under the influence of *avidyā* (ignorance) and have fulfilled their purpose for *puruṣa* in the context of saṃsāric experience and liberation from the bondage of the afflictions, *karma*s, and their fruition. *Puruṣa* is therefore "disjoined" or "disengaged" from the *guṇa*s in the condition of *saṃyoga* implying here a state in which there is no longer misidentification with the mind and its modifications as in the empirical mode of selfhood.[27] *Pratiprasava* can be further understood as "withdrawal from the epistemological power of the *guṇa*s over the yogin." Vyāsa uses the term *pratiprasava* in the context of the elimination of the *kleśa*s (afflictions)[28]—a process in Yoga that involves a cognitive and moral cleansing or purification of the body and mind (i.e., *prakṛti*) leading to a state of liberating knowledge. This need not imply the ontological negation or dissolution of prakṛtic or manifest (i.e., human, embodied) existence. *Yoga-Sūtra* IV.32[29] also supports the view that the ultimate state of the *guṇa*s arrives when the tripartite process *(triguṇa)* has already served its purpose for experience *(bhoga)* and liberation *(apavarga)* and is of no further use soteriologically. By this is meant that the causative operations of the afflictions come to an end and there is the cessation of afflicted action.[30] The eternality *(ānantya)* of knowledge *(jñāna-sattva)* is no longer veiled[31] or concealed.

What has been stated as the final goal in the *sūtra* explaining the culmination of Yoga (*YS* IV.34) is linked to and supported by Patañjali's central definition of Yoga (*YS* I.2). Part of the intent of this study is to show how *Yoga-Sūtra* I.2 can be seen as "threading together" and integrating the text of the *Yoga-Sūtra* as a whole. The "cessation of the [misidentification with] the modifications of the mind" *(cittavṛttinirodha)* integrates the already interrelated concerns in Yoga of practice *(sādhana),* the "return to the origin" *(pratiprasava),* and the highest state of *samādhi* where the yogin embodies a state of equilibrium, equipose, and freedom *(kaivalya).* In this, *nirodha* can be seen to encompass a plurality of practices as well as descriptions of culminating states of Yoga providing a "thread" of continuity throughout the *Yoga-Sūtra* in which theory and practice are unified, of a piece.

The mind *(citta),* which incorporates the entire "inner instrumentality" *(antaḥkaraṇa),* is the "substratum" or arena of the *vṛtti*s and *saṃskāra*s in which all the modifications arise, all the cognitive, affective, and emotive processes take place. It is also that very "substratum" into which the yogin's *misidentification* with the mind dissolves, that is, where *saṃyoga,* for that particular yogin, goes into permanent dissolution *(laya).* Such dissolution *(laya)* is considered to be Yoga. Vijñāna Bhikṣu is correct to point out that Yoga does not result in the nonexistence of *vṛtti*s because that does not fit the idea of the special state of the "substratum" in Yoga.[32] Unlike Nyāya philosophy, for example, Yoga does not admit of the existence of a specific category called "absence" *(abhāva),* "absence" referring to the special state of the "substratum" itself. In Yoga philosophy, dissolution means that the karmically binding *vṛtti*s and their effects (and affects) dissolve, not the existence of *vṛtti,* that is, all *vṛtti*s, in total. The state of *nirodha* or *laya* need not imply the ontological negation of *vṛtti*s.[33] Bhoja Rāja comments: "Yoga means 'cessation,' that is their [i.e., the *vṛtti*s] dissolution *(laya)* into their cause when their outward transmutation ceases and the process of mutation is reversed."[34] Bhoja appears to give an ontological emphasis to the meaning of *nirodha,* thereby implying a definitive dissolution of the existence of the modifications in total. Our understanding sides more along the lines of Vijñāna Bhikṣu's interpretation, which alludes to the process of the effects of the *guṇa*s (all *vṛtti*s being composed of the three *guṇa*s) in the form of misidentification being dissolved back into their cause—ignorance *(avidyā);* and ignorance, no longer having a hold on the mind, disappears from the yogin's view, ceases to function due to the enlightened state of consciousness. The gradual process of *nirodha* leads the guṇic-identified consciousness of self toward a state of dissolution into the original pure *sattva* of the mind—a state of utter lucidity or transparency of consciousness (mind) wherein no epistemological distortion can take place, yet *vṛtti*s (e.g., valid cognition, memory, etc.) can still arise, can still function.

A word of caution must be given in order to avoid confusing the concept of "cessation" or "dissolution" of *vṛtti*s (in the sense that we have used it in the above) with the idea of rendering the *vṛtti*s nonexistent. The key to understanding the dissolution of *vṛtti*s into their cause lies in the Sāṃkhyan theory of causation known as *satkāryavāda,* which was explained earlier (see chapter 2). In this foundational theory all states of matter-energy including our psychophysical being are transformed according to the attributes within them, but there is never any amount of energy or material existence more or less than there was or will be. Nothing that ever exists goes into nonexistence;[35] it simply becomes unmanifest, the form returning to dwell as an attribute hidden in its cause, where it originally arose and from which it may emerge again. The temporary disappearance of any "entity," form, thought, or idea is not its extinction. Patañjali would not accept that whatever disappears is ontologically destroyed. Manifest existence does not become merely empty or extinct *(śūnya),* but identification with it is temporarily suspended, submerged, dissolved, or absorbed *(laya).* Modern interpreters of Yoga, however, often speak of the nonexistence or deadening of the *vṛtti*s in *nirodha,* implying, as it were, an anaesthetization of human consciousness, the view that is here being countered.

The meaning of *nirodha* as the cessation of the misidentification with the modifications of the mind (or the dissolution of the misperceived identification with the *vṛtti*s of the mind) is confirmed by the intent implicit in statements throughout the *Yoga-Sūtra* and more explicitly in Vyāsa's *Bhāṣya.* For example, *Yoga-Sūtra* II.27 mentions seven "grounds" or "stages" of knowledge that the yogin attains. This "sevenfold-insight" *(saptadhā-prajñā)* is described as following from the unwavering discriminative discernment *(vivekakhyāti),* the means whereby the misalliance or distorted conjunction *(saṃyoga)* of the seer and the seeable is progressively ended.[36] *Yoga-Sūtra* II.27 states: "Therein [for the one who possesses the unfaultering discriminative discernment] the last stage of transcendent-insight (wisdom) is sevenfold."[37] Patañjali does not explain what is meant by the "sevenfold-insight," however, though Vyāsa offers a very probable elucidation. Summarizing Vyāsa, the first four stages or "fourfold release" are: (1) that which is to be prevented *(duḥkha, saṃyoga)* has been identified, known; (2) that which is to be discarded [i.e., the cause of *duḥkha* or dissatisfaction] has been abandoned; (3) through the attainment of unification (in *samādhi*) also termed "cessation" *(nirodha),* freedom has been attained; (4) the means of discarding the conjunction *(saṃyoga),* that is, the practice of discriminative discernment, has been perfected.[38] Vyāsa tells us that the last three stages of the "sevenfold-insight" are known as "release of the mind" *(citta-vimukta).* Vyāsa informs us that having attained the fifth stage of the "sevenfold-insight," described as the intellect having fulfilled its role of providing experience and liberation, a sixth stage ensues whereby: "The *guṇa*s, like rocks dislodged from the top of a mountain peak finding no more resting place, are inclined toward dissolution *(pralaya)* into their own cause. Together with that cause *(saṃyoga, avidyā),* they are no longer produced into effects again since there is no further purpose for them."[39] The mind has accomplished its purpose of providing experience and liberation resulting in the cessation of mistaken identity. By this Vyāsa means that the *guṇa*s are of no further purpose insofar as they have fulfilled their purpose as a vehicle for the yogin's liberation.[40] Thus, the seventh and final stage takes place—the stage of the "aloneness" of the pure identity of *puruṣa* that is beyond any superimposed connection with the mind.

For the sake of clarity, however, we must attempt to pinpoint what Vyāsa means when he asserts that the *guṇa*s are no longer produced into effects. Discriminative discernment, the nature of which is *sattva-guṇa,*[41] is the expedient by which the discarding or abandonment (*hāna, YS* II.26) of *saṃyoga* and ignorance is brought about. As *Yoga-Sūtra* II.25 makes clear, without ignorance (as cause) there is no conjunction *(saṃyoga);* the overcoming of misidentification brings about the freedom of pure identity as *puruṣa,* the "aloneness" *(kaivalya)* or "goal" of Yoga.[42] Vyāsa asserts that ignorance specifically refers to the complex network of habit patterns *(vāsanā*s*)* and personality traits based on erroneous or misconceived knowledge *(viparyaya-jñāna)* and its *saṃskāras:*

> Under the influence of the habit patterns based on erroneous knowledge (misidentification of self), the mind does not attain fulfillment of what it has to do, namely "to know" *puruṣa*. While it [the mind] has that involvement, continuously it [the mind in its afflicted nature] revives. But in the culminating knowledge of *puruṣa* it attains fulfillment of what it had to do. With its [former] involvement at an end, and the failure-to-see terminated, there is no cause of bondage and it [the mind under the influence of *avidyā*] does not revive again.[43]

Vyāsa's statement (see n. 39), that the *guṇa*s are no longer produced into effects, can be understood to mean that the mind has been released from the binding mechanism of afflicted identity in *saṃyoga;* the mind does not revive or generate *vṛtti*s in the former afflicted and misappropriated mode of mistaken identity *(asmitā),* that is, as self-referenced to an egoic sense of identity. The mind is no longer anchored in the epistemological distortion of the failure-to-see *(adarśana),* and this removal of ignorance results in the yogin's release from bondage, dissatisfaction, and further suffering. *Puruṣa,* thus, is said to be established in its "own form" or nature *(svarūpa).*[44] Unlike the changing, ego-centered world of empirical selfhood, *puruṣa,* whose nature is uncaused, is no longer misconstrued as being under the influence of or subservient to the three *guṇa*s as mental consciousness and whose nature is cause and effect,[45] that is, changing. Based on our interpretation given in the above and as evidenced by other statements in Vyāsa's *Bhāṣya,* it seems reasonable to suggest that Vyāsa's description (in *YB* II.27) of the dissolution of the *guṇa*s refers to the dissolution of the *guṇas in the form of ignorance or affliction,* that is, of the worldly, empirical effects of the *guṇas* on the yogin's consciousness, thereby altering self-identity. "Dissolution" or "cessation" in Yoga need not be understood to mean the "disintegration and suppression of our empirical personality."[46] Rather, "dissolution" is of the (mis)perceived identification with the *vṛttis* of the mind. Yoga involves a radical deconstruction of a positive misconstruction of self and world caused by *avidyā.*

For the sake of clarification, I will now take issue with what I consider to be a popular misconception centered around the intent of Yoga praxis. In Swami Vivekānanda's (late-nineteenth-century) philosophical perspective,[47] *nirvikalpa-samādhi*—understood by Vivekānanda to be the spiritual goal of Vedānta—is equated with the goal of liberation as experienced in Patañjali's Yoga. The system of *rāja-yoga,* based primarily on Patañjali's *Yoga-Sūtra,* is proposed by Vivekānanda as a method for enabling one to attain direct perception of religious truths. In particular, he contends that *samādhi,* as the culminating experience of Patañjali's system, is the self-valid and only satisfactory authoritative source of all religious knowledge or *brahmajñāna.*[48]

Vivekānanda contends that *nirvikalpa-samādhi,* resulting in the liberating realization of the Self *(ātman),* finds its equivalent meaning in Patañjali's central definition of Yoga (*YS* I.2). He often describes the goal of *rāja-yoga* as the total suppression of all thought forms.[49] Since he understands that the prerequisite for *nirvikalpa-samādhi* is an inactive mind, the aim of Yoga is defined by him as follows: "Yoga is restraining the mind-stuff *(citta)* from taking various forms *(vṛtti)*."[50] "Yoga is the science in which we stop *citta* from assuming, or becoming transformed into several faculties . . . only when the 'mind-stuff,' the *citta* is controlled to absolute calmness is the Self to be recognized."[51] Vivekānanda speaks of the necessity to curb each thought as it enters into the mind, thereby making the mind a kind of vacuum,[52] and repeatedly asserts that the knowledge of the Self *(ātman)* spontaneously follows the extinction of the mind. In the above quotation he actually presents Self-knowledge *(ātmajñāna)* as being dependent on this extinction; *samādhi* is characterized by the definitive or final absence of all mental modifications.[53] Vivekānanda therefore proposes that the goal of spiritual practice *(sādhana)* is attained by the complete cessation of mental modifications. On this basis he has put forward several noteworthy injunctions regarding the aspirant's attitude and efforts in relation to the mind:

> We have to exclude all thoughts from the mind and make it blank; as fast as thought comes we have to banish it.[54]

> Control the mind, cut off the senses, then you are a *yogi.*[55]

> The mind has to be killed.[56]

> The rascal ego has to be obliterated.[57]

> So when the mind will end, be broken into pieces entirely, without leaving any *saṃskāra,* we shall be entirely free, and until that time we are in bondage.[58]

One must seriously question the logic behind this approach to human consciousness and the mind as it relates to Yoga philosophy.

One will naturally ask how practitioners who attempt to obey any teachings resulting in death to their minds would have the capacity to comprehend or carry out any further instructions. Perhaps, more importantly, how could one function practically as a human being without the faculties of thinking, memory, discernment and reason, and an individual sense of self with which one can distinguish oneself from other people and the world? Surely such a person would have to be mad or unconscious. If all the great Yoga masters of the past had obliterated or so thoroughly suppressed their minds in order to attain spiritual liberation, how did they speak, teach, reason, remember, empathize, or even use the word "I"? The mind and the body are the only vehicles in which to attain liberation. It is the mind, as Yoga readily admits, that must be utilized for study and to listen to the spiritual adept or *guru;* it is the mind that is needed to follow a spiritual path to liberation; and it is equally the mind that is required by the aspirant in order to function as a human being in day-to-day life.

By advising or explaining that the mind and its various faculties are to be negated, suppressed, abolished, or severed from consciousness, scholars, teachers, and writers on Yoga have, I would like to suggest, missed the point of practicing Yoga. For, in Yoga philosophy, it is not the *mind,* but rather the exclusive identification with material existence—including our various forms of egoity—as one's true identity that is the source of all human difficulties, sorrow, frustration, and dissatisfaction *(duḥkha)*. It is a specific state of consciousness or cognitive error evidenced *in* the mind and not the mind *itself* that is at issue. In other words, it is the condition of misidentification *(sārūpya)*—the saṃsāric condition of self and its self-referenced world—and not the mind in total that must be discarded in Yoga. Any advice or teaching that suggests the destruction or negation of the mind in Yoga is, it seems to me, detrimental to a human being and to the practice of Yoga and is representative of a fundamental and pervasive misunderstanding and misinterpretation of Patañjali's Yoga. How could progress on the path of Yoga be made with such an approach? What would the ethical ramifications be? The belief that mental annihilation or negation leads to spiritual emancipation has become a popular and unfortunate teaching of modern representatives or interpretations of Yoga. Despite the fact that it is neither truly yogic, practical, logical nor appealing, and furthermore may be destructive for aspirants, recent teachings and works on Yoga have often prescribed or assumed the negation or suppression of the mind, ego, and thoughts as the primary means to self-emancipation.[59] This stance, I submit, is a gross misrepresentation of Yoga; a confused, misleading and, at best, naïve attempt at conveying the depth and profundity of the yogic process that Patañjali refers to as *nirodha*. As will be explained in chapter 6, Yoga does involve levels of insight in which the ordinary mental processes and identification with *vṛtti* are temporarily suspended. This process culminates in enstasy *(asaṃprajñāta-samādhi):* a state where the pure experiencer or knower—*puruṣa*—is "alone" and the yogin is left with nothing more to experience or know for the sake of liberation. This advanced and crucial stage of yogic practice is for the purpose of the final elimination of ignorance; but it need not be understood as resulting in a definitive or permanent cessation or suspension of the mental processes of the mind in total.

I am arguing that it is misleading to view *nirodha* as a process of repression, suppression, or inhibition. *Nirodha* does not refer to a forced cessation, coercion, or restriction or to the nonexistence of *vṛtti*s, as many modern translators seem to imply.[60] I am suggesting that Yoga (*YS* I.2) is not such a manipulation or control of the mind, nor is it a "blank" or unconscious state of mind or a "thoughtless" or "mindless" state of being. One recent commentator on the *Yoga-Sūtra* aptly writes:

> *Nirodha* does not mean and imply a willful control of *vṛtti*s, or their suppression or repression. Willful control, suppression, and repression must necessarily result in a derangement, if not the destruction of the human psyche. Because any egocentric act of [a human being], already caught in *vṛttisārūpya* ["conformity" of self-identity to the nature of *vṛtti*], which has conditioned [one's] mind, will be tantamount to exercising [one's] mind in the same old way. . . . This can never bring about *nirodha,* but only the death of the psyche, if the pressure of willful control, suppression or repression is persisted beyond the point of endurance.[61]

Could efforts to achieve a willful control of the mind (as mentioned in the above) be the result of a fanatical, ascetical, imbalanced approach to Yoga, a misguided attempt to transcend ego and to go beyond the enterprise of dissatisfaction and affliction? Does psychic closure—a compulsive shutting out/down or switching off of the psyche, constitiute an authentic opening to true identity? A careful examination of the mind and its functioning in the context of Yoga philosophy suggests that any form of psychic suppression or repression runs counter to the underlying principles on which Yoga practice is based. Ego-transcendence is not something that can be forced or ultimately willed. The ego itself must give way or let go into the illuminating power of *sattva,* which, located in a subtler dimension of the mind (the *buddhi*), eludes the ego's grasp and its self-centered efforts as well as other afflicted modes or attitudes generating action or inertia (stasis) as mediated through *rajas* and *tamas* respectively. In short, self-transcendence is only possible as a voluntary gesture, a gesture that is often misunderstood by seekers resulting in a perversion of praxis leading to forms of self-denial or self-indulgence that can surreptitiously inflate the ego and even cause harm to the psychophysical organism and to others.

The "willful control" referred to in the above quotation (n. 61) must, therefore, be qualified in the context of those personality types in which *rajas* and *tamas* are predominant and *sattva*-knowledge is covered over (*āvaraṇa, YS* IV.31). Such willfulness leading to suppression, and so forth, is simply a form of misguided effort based on rajasic and tamasic *vṛtti*s and predispositions in the form of aggressive *(ghora)* or deluded *(mūḍha)* ideas[62] *(pratyaya)* or intentions—in order to achieve a state of *nirodha.* For example, *nirodha* cannot be equated with a state of inertia or stasis *(tamas)* wherein the mind and its modifications are suppressed or forcibly stopped, rendered inoperative. It is misleading to assert, as has S. Dasgupta,[63] that *nirodha* is a complete (final) stopping of the movements of the mind. According to Vyāsa (*YB* I.2), such an inert state of the mind, far from being an experience of yogic illumination, merely constitutes a state of *tamas,*[64] implying a confusion of sorts or delusive mentality leading to dullness or static vacant states of mind, perhaps even mistaking what are nonvirtuous qualities in Yoga for being virtuous ones. The disempowerment of *avidyā* over the mind is not to be confused with the *guṇa* of *tamas!* The mind's highest disposition is sattvic, *sattva* or "illumination" *(prakāśa)*[65] being the purest and most lucid aspect of *prakṛti. Sattva* is inclined to ideas of a peaceful *(śānta)* nature[66] and supportive of the practice of Yoga. As a moral, psychological, and epistemological state, *tamas* is not supportive of the practice of Yoga, is not Yoga proper. The nonafflicted *(akliṣṭa) vṛtti*s, intentions, and ideas *(pratyaya)* pertaining to a sattvic nature are morally and cognitively drawn upon or attuned to, serve the soteriological dimension of Yoga, and are part and parcel of the sattvification of the will or intellect—the faculty of discernment and decision making. *Vṛtti*s return to their source of pure *sattva* and can then arise in a purified and illuminated mode when that purpose is fulfilled, as for example, in the form of yogic perception and moral virtues. Thus the cessation of *vṛtti*s in the process of *nirodha* refers to the "undoing" or dismantling of the yogin's misidentification with *vṛtti* in *saṃyoga. Avidyā*—the cause of the erroneous appropriation of *vṛtti*—is dispelled, and the purified mind, in its subtlest nature as pure *sattva* (knowledge or insight) can give rise to the right functioning of *vṛtti* in that *vṛtti*s are no longer appropriated by a mistaken identity of self.

Explaining the Sāṃkhyan view of causation in terms of yogic praxis, Patañjali shows how, through direct experience and perception *(yogi-pratyakṣa),* we can see that our mind and sense of self continuously change depending on the nature and type of *vṛtti*s, cognitions and ideas *(pratyaya),* in the process of apprehension, that we are entertaining at any given moment. This changing sense of identity, which continuously wavers from authentic identity, must be transcended in Yoga. Thus, Yoga discourages any clinging to ideas or perceptions of *puruṣa* experienced along the way; whatever idea one arrives at through the process of *vṛtti* will never be the actual liberated state itself. Only by breaking through the barriers imposed by the relative states of consciousness or the mind can one enter into the domain of the knowledge of *puruṣa (puruṣa-jñāna)* and experience life in the light of yogic awareness rather than the limited awareness in the situation of *saṃyoga.* The Sāṃkhyan theory of *satkāryavāda* takes on a highly experiential dimension in the actual practice of Yoga. The experiential element consists of: *(a)* putting into practice a method or methods that lead one to experience yogic perception in *samādhi* wherein *cittavṛttinirodha* will be "attained" and matured; and *(b)* the transformative processes—including the physical, ethical, and psychological—that occur while the process of "cessation" is taking place.

Primarily, Patañjali takes the Sāṃkhyan theory of causation and applies it to understanding states of mind or "shapes" the mind takes when left to its own karmically derived momentum. The modifications *(vikṛti*s*)* of the mind are its *vṛtti*s, all the mental functioning, processes, and content. Insofar as we are ensconced in a worldview generated by *avidyā* and are ineluctably programmed within the circumscribed patterns of afflicted identity *(asmitā)*—a mere product of the *guṇa*s in the form of misidentification—our self-referential center of awareness and its compulsive attachment to *vṛtti* must be severed in order for the mind to be transformed into finer states of perception and understanding. What is *pralaya* or *prati-sañcara* (the dissolution of the universe and its phenomena) in the cosmological context of Sāṃkhya[67] becomes in the *Yoga-Sūtra* respectively *nirodha* or *pratiprasava* (the cessation or dissolution of the misperceived identity with *guṇa*s as they manifest in the form of *vṛtti*s). This can only happen through the experiences in *samādhi* that culminate in "aloneness" *(kaivalya).*

In the *Yoga-Sūtra* the principles *(tattva*s*)* of existence are of special relevance with regard to their relation to the individual yogin, including the intellect, ego, mind-organ, senses, and body. One needs to know their origin and processes of manifestation and actualization so as to cease from any misidentification with them. Not only does the empirical sense of self identify with the body and the nature of the mind and everything about which one says "I am"; it even becomes identified with the objects and persons one calls "mine," and experiences dissatisfaction or enjoyment according to the changes that take place in relation to the objects of experience, including our *vṛtti*s. Patañjali asks us to learn to discern the difference between our true identity as Self *(puruṣa)* and our self as a mistaken identity—the congenital conflation or mixture/conjunction *(saṃyoga)* of the "seer" and the "seeable"—by observing the processes of identification and cognition taking place within our own minds. Thus Patañjali describes the nature of the "seeable" *(dṛśya)* with an epistemological emphasis focusing more on its manifestations as psychological and cognitive phenomena rather than as ontological essences (as in Sāṃkhya). *Puruṣa* appears to take on or conform to *(sārūpya)* an identity which, based on the changing nature of the *guṇa*s, is contained within *prakṛti* and defined and given shape according to the nature of the mind and its modifications *(vṛttis).* This reflected albeit deluded I-consciousness, as human consciousness, appears in the form of a body-mind and in the nature of the elements *(bhūta*s*)* and the sense-organs *(indriya*s*),* and is for the purpose of experience and eventual emancipation[68] from the saṃsāric condition of self in *saṃyoga.*

In Yoga, even ignorance and misidentification ultimately serve the highest purpose of liberation through a fundamental transformation of the mind. The various categories of the "seeable" should not be reified,[69] but rather should be understood as interconnected and interdependent dimensions of human experience. The descriptions of the "seeable" outlined in *Yoga-Sūtra* II.18-19[70] can be understood as descriptions of the situation of the seer *(puruṣa) as if misidentified with* the seeable *(prakṛti). Prakṛti*'s various levels of manifestation are correlated in the *Yoga-Sūtra* with states of consciousness, self-understanding, and identity analogous to *puruṣa,* and, I suggest, are to be understood with an epistemological emphasis; through *prakṛti,* the yogin comes to realize authentic identity as *puruṣa.*

The ultimate significance of *prakṛti* is seen in very definite, positive terms, wherein, from at least a provisional point of view, *prakṛti* has meaning, metaphysically speaking, in the service of soteriology: the metaphysical dualism of *puruṣa* and *prakṛti* can be taken as a provisional perspective and as one that has been abstracted from yogic experience. As I have suggested in chapter 2, this provisional approach to the existences of *puruṣa* and *prakṛti* can serve important pedagogical purposes. In fact, the whole concept of the mind *(citta)* in Yoga can be seen primarily as a heuristic device, rather than as a substance per se, whereby the yogin comes to understand the functioning of consciousness and discerns the difference between the mind *(citta)* and *puruṣa.* The essence of the "seeable" to which Patañjali refers and whose reality is for the purpose of *puruṣa*[71] translates into being a form of *vṛtti*-identification, that is, identification and experience referenced to an egoic center of consciousness with its mental content in the form of thoughts, intentions, or ideas *(pratyaya)*. Ego-identity is essentially a *vṛtti*-accumulated sense of self, which as a false "center" of consciousness, has become dependent on the activity of *vṛtti* for its existence. Egoity is thus an *activity* of misidentification of self constituted of the three *guṇa*s. The yogin must ultimately be identified as the auto-transparent knower (*YS* IV.18) or seer of *vṛtti*s—free from any misidentification with and misappropriation of *vṛtti*—in order to discern permanently the difference between mistaken identity in *saṃyoga* and authentic identity as *puruṣa*. It is here that a clear understanding of the difference between *puruṣa* or pure consciousness (our intrinsic identity as the "seer") and *prakṛti* or matter (the "seeable," including all modifications of the mind or processes of identification that give form to an extrinsic nature and identity of selfhood) is essential.

In his commentary on *Yoga-Sūtra* I.1 Vyāsa defines Yoga as *samādhi (yogaḥ samādhiḥ)*.[72] He goes on to state the two divisions of that Yoga as: (1) *saṃprajñāta,* the *samādhi* of cognition consisting of four types (outlined in *YS* I.17), and in which sattvic *vṛtti*s persist and can still arise in the context of *sārūpya,* "conformity" to or misidentification with the nature of *vṛtti;* and (2) *asaṃprajñāta,* the supracognitive *samādhi* in which all the *vṛtti*s, including the sattvic ones, are mastered and all attachment to *vṛtti* and its resultant effects in the form of sorrow and dissatisfaction *(duḥkha)* is overcome, transcended. In (2), ignorance no longer masks authentic identity for the yogin. The power of misidentification has been temporarily removed and *puruṣa,* left "alone," abides in its true form *(svarūpa)* and identity.[73] Vyāsa elaborates on the meaning of Patañjali's definition of Yoga (*YS* I.2), pointing out that because the word "all" is not included to suggest the "cessation" of all misidentifications with *vṛtti*—which reduce *puruṣa* to some form of prakṛtic existence, however subtle, thus reifying *puruṣa*—it implies that *saṃprajñāta* is also included in Yoga.[74] In *saṃprajñāta* or cognitive *samādhi* the rajasic and tamasic *vṛtti*s—all of which are of an afflicted *(kliṣṭa)* nature—are mastered by resorting to the sattvic, nonafflicted *(akliṣṭa) vṛtti*s.[75] If *Yoga-Sūtra* I.2 had said all *vṛtti*s in total, then the definition would have been limited to *asaṃprajñāta*—the supracognitive *samādhi*—and the cognitive *samādhi* would not be included in Yoga. The term *nirodha* is therefore ambiguous. It refers to both the *process* of cessation of the misidentification with the modifications of the mind *and* the culmination or "goal" of Yoga, that being spiritual liberation. There is a similar ambiguity in the terms *samādhi* and Yoga.

If *nirodha* were seen as the restriction, suppression, repression, or the ontological negation of *vṛtti*s, then Yoga would have to be defined as a particular condition of the substratum of those *vṛtti*s, the substratum being a state somewhere within the mind. But *samādhi,* it must be emphasized, is not such a state within the mind. As I later argue, in the actual experience of *samādhi* the mind is not made blank or is not in a state of void, nullification, or the permanent absence of *vṛtti*. The mind may continue to function according to its own nature but as a purified instrument of *sattva*-intelligence that is capable of perfectly reflecting the light of *puruṣa*. The *vṛtti*s of the mind become transparent to the knower *(puruṣa)* of *vṛtti*s, whereas in *saṃyoga* the *vṛtti*s are "colored" in affliction—egoity, attachment, aversion, and so on—constantly altering and fragmenting one's sense of self. *Nirodha* means to take away or discard the empirical limitations, including all "restrictions" and suppressions located in the mind; *nirodha* is the removal of the *kleśa*s and karmic barriers only to reveal the full-blown nature of *puruṣa*. The yogin therefore is not a mindless, inactive being. Rather, the mind has become an instrument of consciousness under the yogin's direction. The modifications of the mind may continue in day-to-day life but they no longer enslave the yogin, no longer divert the yogin's attention away from authentic identity. Ultimately the yogin attains to the status of a *jīvanmukta*—one who is liberated while yet embodied[76]—and can use the body and mind out of benevolence and compassion for the spiritual benefit of others. The presence of the enlightened being, adept, or spiritually wise person is confirmed in the historical tradition of Yoga through the *guru-śiṣya* relationship, a relationship made possible by the grace of the *guru* or liberated being *(jīvanmukta)*.

What therefore is the *"cittavṛtti"* that must cease through the discipline of Yoga? Based on the argument put forward in this study—that mental activity, cognition, feelings, emotions, and thoughts are not incompatible with Yoga praxis or the final goal of *puruṣa*-realization—I will now attempt to clarify Patañjali's definition of Yoga. No doubt addressing an audience primarily composed of Yoga aspirants, it seems logical to suggest that Patañjali defined Yoga in *Yoga-Sūtra* I.2 with a strong pedagogical intent so that his listeners would be able to grasp (and be sufficiently disillusioned with) their present understanding of themselves and the world. *Nirodha* implies that it is the worldview born of ignorance "located" within one's own psychophysical being that is to be abandoned or discarded, not *prakṛti* herself. *Yoga-Sūtra* I.2 is in part a teaching and a heuristic device that is aimed at devaluing the level of understanding based on misidentification with the body and mental processes and that sees identification with or attachment to thought-constructs or mental content as bringing ultimate satisfaction. *Nirodha* is not the denial or renunciation of *prakṛti in total;* it is a negative affirmation of the reality of *puruṣa*. Initially one could say that *nirodha* actually is a recommendation to the practitioner to develop meditational practice. Yet on the other hand, Patañjali had to inform seekers who had incorrectly assumed a subjectively idealist viewpoint that the mind and the objects perceived through it are real and are not to be negated or denied. As noted earlier, many people see the external, "objective" world and therefore it is does not arise from the mind itself (*YS* IV.15–16). *Prakṛti* is real; the external world is not denied or renounced. All effects are preexistent in their cause. However, the concern of Yoga is not merely to describe, categorize, or explain the "outside" world, but rather is to show various means by which the practitioner may obtain direct access to empirical reality without the interference of *avidyā*'s network of confused and impure identity patterns that veil a clear, direct perception of the world. Yoga "undoes" the world of misidentification, *cittavṛtti* or fractured selfhood and corrects a basic misalignment between the seer and the seeable so that life as a whole, and on the basis of an unfractured self-identity, is revealed. Clearly, *cittavṛtti* does not have the capacity to see and experience life from the perspective of Yoga *darśana,* which discloses the full integrity of life. The cultivation of an ever-deepening process of "cessation" in Yoga serves to dismantle the habitual tendency to reify one's self and the world by unfolding an awareness that reveals the transcendent yet immanent seer *(puruṣa)*.

The yogin does not need to force, struggle with, or push away the mind, *vṛtti*s, and thoughts as is usually recommended in discussions on *nirodha*. Any attempt at a forced removal of *vṛtti* or coerced "identification" with *puruṣa* is merely a perpetuation of the rajasic and tamasic tendencies or habit patterns *(vāsanās)* of the mind. The yogin's need is to contact and connect with more *sattva*-intelligence, which is concealed in the mind. However, due to the afflictions present along with their karmic investment, this innate sense of *sattva* is covered over[77] and obscured from entering fully into consciousness. Through Yoga discipline, one learns to recognize and identify with purer, sattvic, and subtler forms of *vṛtti*s and is relieved from the former identification with *vṛtti*s of a rajasic and tamasic nature that were predominant. The mind can then more easily settle into its finest nature of *sattva;* the yogin's understanding becomes sattvified. Similarly, by identifying as *puruṣa,* in *asaṃprajñāta,* the yogin overcomes the need to identify with sattvic *vṛtti*s for the purpose of steadying and stabilizing self-identity. Cessation *(nirodha)* implies a process of "subtilization"[78] or sattvification of consciousness, of a gradual de-identification with *vṛtti* to the point of being unmistakably one-in-identity as *puruṣa.*

Thus the cessation of the misidentification with the modifications of the mind involves a progressive "interiorization," "subtilization," or "sattvification" of consciousness, of one's focus of attention, wherein initially the congenital perceived misidentification with the tamasic and rajasic *(kliṣṭa-) vṛtti*s constituting one's mental apparatus ceases (in *saṃprajñāta-samādhi*). Eventually (in *asaṃprajñāta-samādhi*) the congenital perceived misidentification with sattvic *(akliṣṭa-) vṛtti*s also ceases. Yet *vṛtti*s themselves do not cease to exist. Even in the enlightened yogin there are tamasic, rajasic, and sattvic dimensions constituting his or her prakṛtic apparatus but these guṇic qualities no longer obscure the yogin's perception of reality. The yogin is, however, detached from any identification with the *guṇa*s, is no longer enslaved to the *vṛtti*-generating complex of the mind.

Summarizing this section, it has been strongly suggested that *nirodha* denotes an epistemological emphasis and refers to the transformation of self-understanding, not the ontological cessation of *prakṛti* (i.e., the mind and its modifications). *Nirodha* is not, therefore, as many have explained, an inward movement that annihilates or suppresses *vṛtti*s and thoughts, nor is it the nonexistence or absence of *vṛtti*s; rather, *nirodha* involves a progressive expansion of perception that eventually reveals our true identity as *puruṣa.* Taking another angle and clarifying further our interpretation of Patañjalis central definition of Yoga (*YS* I.2), I suggest that *cittavṛtti* (from the definition of Yoga as *cittavṛttinirodha*) describes the very basis of all the empirical selves: under the influence of *avidyā* the unenlightened person's mental processes *(vṛtti)* both generate and are ineluctably driven by[79] deeply rooted impressions *(saṃskāras)*[80] and habit patterns *(vāsanās)*[81] sustaining a sense of I-am-ness or egoity *(asmitā)* that is by definition afflicted. Seen in the above context, *cittavṛtti* can be understood as a generic term standing for a misconceived knowledge *(viparyaya-jñāna)*[82] that, although seeking to ground empirical selfhood, amounts to no more than an error that is structured in the network of our psychological makeup and veils our identity as *puruṣa*. The epistemic distortion or erroneous knowledge *(mithyā-jñāna)*[83] functioning as the *vṛtti* of *viparyaya* (*YS*/*YB* I.8) acts as the basis for all misidentification with *vṛtti*s in the unenlightened mode (*vyutthāna, YS* III.9) of perception and extrinsic identity. Thus, after questioning why the knower is released while still alive, Vyāsa tells us: "Because erroneous cognition *(viparyaya)* is the cause of rebirth. When *viparyaya* has vanished no one is ever seen to be born anywhere."[84] That is, the liberated yogin does not see *puruṣa* as an entity misidentified as body, mind, intellect, ego, and so forth, that is reborn or comes into being. Unlike ordinary, empirical identity, the yogin's identity is no longer diverted into the prakṛtic dynamic of cause and effect including birth and death. *Puruṣa* is never born and as such is not subject to death; *puruṣa* is immutable, immortal. Ignorance claims its foundational support or agent *(asmitā)* in the mind and forms a mind of its own kind[85] through the *vṛtti* of *viparyaya*. In short, our afflicted identity rooted in spiritual ignorance functions through *viparyaya*. Oddly enough, this fundamental insight, which can be attributed to Vyāsa,[86] has not been clearly noted by scholars. I have attempted to clarify Vyāsa's position, and furthermore suggest that Vyāsa's insight into the nature of *viparyaya* has profound implications for our understanding of Patañjali's whole system.

Accordingly, *cittavṛtti* does not mean all modifications or mental processes in the mind—cognitive, affective, or emotive—but is the very seed *(bīja)*[87] mechanism of the misidentification with *prakṛti* and from which all other *vṛtti*s, thoughts, intentions, or ideas arise and are (mis)appropriated in the unenlightened state of mind. There are therefore many *vṛtti*-identifications (*YS* I.6) that can come from and modify the seed mechanism of *cittavṛtti*.[88] *Cittavṛtti*'s nature is dualistic and functions as a polarization within *prakṛti:* a masquerading consciousness of selfhood conceived as being separate from the world. It is this dualistic, afflicted sense of self or ego as separate from the world and other human beings that must, according to Yoga, "dissolve" or "cease." The yogin learns to witness this subject-object dichotomy within *prakṛti* (or worldview born of *avidyā*) as constituting the "seeable" *(dṛśya)*. Spiritual ignorance gives rise to a malfunctioning or misalignment of *vṛtti*—as appropriated or referenced to egoity—that in Yoga can be "corrected" thereby allowing for the right functioning or proper alignment of *vṛtti*. *Vṛtti* will then function as subordinate to the knower *(puruṣa)* of *vṛtti* rather than the sense of self in effect remaining subordinate to *vṛtti. Cittavṛtti* is an analogical understanding of consciousness in that the consciousness that has become the mind as a reflected state of *(puruṣa*'s*)* consciousness is analogous to pure consciousness, *puruṣa.* It is the *cittavṛtti* as our confused and mistaken identity of authentic selfhood *(puruṣa),* not our *vṛtti*s, thoughts and experiences *in total* that must come to a state of definitive cessation.

I am suggesting that the pivot of the predicament of *puruṣa*'s "entanglement" within *prakṛti* is epistemological and it is here that we should look for an opening into the meaning of Patañjali's Yoga. Our analysis thus far views the conjunction *(saṃyoga)* of *puruṣa* and *prakṛti* much as a state of epistemic distortion, a mental superimposition (*adhyāropa, YB* II.18) caused by ignorance (*YS* II.24) and resulting in the confusion of identity—located within the mind itself—between *puruṣa* and the mind. There is no real evidence to the effect that *saṃyoga* constitutes a definitive association or ontological alliance between *puruṣa* (the seer) and *prakṛti* (the seeable), or that any *direct* or *truly aligned* association of *puruṣa* and *prakṛti* is intrinsically binding. A closer examination of the *Yoga-Sūtra* and Vyāsa's commentary suggests that *saṃyoga* involves a misalliance between spirit and matter, a misalignment that, as the cause of suffering and dissatisfaction *(duḥkha),* needs to be corrected. The condition of ignorance "creating a mind of its own kind" and the resulting mistaken identity in *saṃyoga,* which fundamentally *is* a misguided relationship to and misappropriation of the world, does not grant direct insight into the nature of the perceived world. This in turn leads to problematic, obfuscated, or karmically binding involvements in the world. *Saṃyoga* is a failure to gain sufficient access to the world of the "seeable," in short, a "failure to see" *(adarśana),* an alienation from authentic identity, which alone has the power "to see." Yoga corrects the misalliance inherent in the condition of *saṃyoga* and allows for a full participation in the world to the point of "uniting," in *samādhi,* with the objects of experience. *Saṃyoga* is an incorrect way of viewing the world. Yoga is clear seeing (*YS* II.20) of the true nature of *puruṣa* and world; Yoga purifies and establishes our identity and the mind in a state of equilibrium, balance—a "sameness" of purity between *puruṣa* and the mind[89]—that is "aloneness" *(kaivalya)* or freedom as a state of embodied knowledge and nonafflicted action.

Through Yoga, the mind can be transformed, purified, and liberated from the bound state of affairs in *saṃyoga. Nirodha* is to be sought because its pursuit implicates the yogin on a path of liberating knowledge or "right vision" (*samyag-darśana, YB* II.15) that ultimately culminates in the realization of our true identity as *puruṣa.* The cessation of the misidentification with *cittavṛtti* in our day-to-day existence does not, however, imply the cessation of our personal identity: mind, body, personality, relationships, career, and so forth; rather, "cessation" results in our consciousness remaining unbound, nonenslaved, and transparent to things of a worldly nature while yet being thoroughly engaged in practical life.

ABHYĀSA (PRACTICE) AND *VAIRĀGYA* (DISPASSION)

The central means given in the *Samādhi-Pāda* for the attainment of *nirodha* are practice *(abhyāsa)* and dispassion *(vairāgya)*. Patañjali states: "Cessation arises through practice and dispassion."[90] This *sūtra* refers to the cessation of the *vṛtti*s insofar as they arise from the seed mechanism *(cittavṛtti)* of ignorance *(avidyā)* and misidentification with *prakṛti (vṛtti-sārūpya)*. *Cittavṛtti* is an analogical understanding of consciousness and is our primary analogue of empirical discourse wherein *puruṣa* and the mechanism of *cittavṛtti* become indistinguishable, resulting in the misappropriation by ego-consciousness of those *vṛtti*s that, Vyāsa tells us, basically consist of pleasure, pain, and delusion.[91]

The yogic "path" formulated by Patañjali can be (and has been) appropriately described as a bipolar process of gradual "interiorization"[92] resulting in an expansion and liberated state of self-identity. Vyāsa illustrates the functional interdependence of *abhyāsa* (the positive pole of "practice") and *vairāgya* (the negative pole of "dispassion") in a helpful metaphor:

> The stream of the mind flows both ways. It flows to the good and it flows to evil. The one commencing with "discrimination" and terminating in aloneness flows to the good. The one commencing with failure to discriminate and terminating in conditioned existence flows to evil. Through dispassion the current towards conditions/objects [extrinsic identity] is dammed, and by practice of the discriminating vision the current of "discrimination" is made to flow. Thus the cessation [of the misidentification with] the modifications of the mind depends on both [practice and dispassion].[93]

The "stream" metaphor used by Vyāsa helps us to understand how closely the psychological, ethical, and soteriological aspects are interwoven into the Yoga view of the incessant modifications of the mind. The imagery of "both ways" (i.e., "two directions") transforms the flow of mental life into something more than a mere psychological description. "Both ways" are initially characterized as flowing toward all that is: (1) good, auspicious, beautiful and benevolent *(kalyāṇa)*, and (2) evil/"demeritorious" *(pāpa)*, which in Hindu thought has both a naturalistic and moral dimension. Later, Vyāsa specifies that the direction that flows toward "discrimination" and emancipation is "to the good," whereas the direction commencing with a failure to discriminate resulting in an afflicted identity of selfhood is "to evil," clearly indicating a soteriological concern. The metaphor acquires a specific technical significance in the *Yoga-Sūtra* as the stream of modifications *(vṛttis)* that can flow in both directions are, as we have already seen, classified as being either afflicted *(kliṣṭa)* and leading to further suffering and dissatisfaction *(duḥkha)* in the condition of *saṃyoga,* or nonafflicted *(akliṣṭa)* and leading to discernment *(khyāti)*[94] and the liberated state of "aloneness" through Yoga. The stream of the mind—encompassing the nature and functioning of *vṛtti*—refers to the movement (of attention) either toward liberating knowledge in the process of *nirodha* or toward ignorance in the process of misidentification. "Both ways" have not only a cognitive direction denoting what is good and bad epistemically, but also have a moral direction.[95] The term *vṛtti* incorporates both cognitive and moral content and refers to cognitive and moral conditions as interrelated aspects of our being. As well as referring to moral *ends* (i.e., of good and evil), liberating knowledge *(jñāna)* and ignorance *(avidyā)* are also value terms and point to the moral *condition* of the yogin or knower. The moral and epistemological dimensions are thus interrelated in Yoga. It is crucial to take note of this integral aspect of Yoga. Feeling, emotion, and volition are intimately bound up with our modes of cognition. Liberating knowledge "flowing to the good" implies purity and clarity of mind and is a condition arising from *sattva,* the illuminative constituent or power of the mind. Spiritual ignorance "flowing to evil" implies a confused or delusive sense of identity rooted in various impurities of mind (and body) and is predominately a condition arising from *tamas*—seen here as the deluding constituent or power of the mind. Such a range of qualities constitutes the moral and cognitive extremes of the mind and indeed our empirical identity. There is, I submit, no need in Yoga to divorce cognition from ethics and the world of human relations. For example, the "inner" illuminative experiences that can take place in Yoga are indeed related to the "outer" world. They inform the nature of our relationships (cf. *YS* I.33) by purifying/sattvifying them and serve to illuminate our understanding of and participation in the world.

The practitioner is being advised to choose not just one of the two methods, either practice or dispassion, but the two together. Each of the two fulfills an essential part of the purpose of Yoga, as Vyāsa makes clear. Unless practice is accompanied by an attitude of dispassion, the whole enterprise of Yoga, which implies a balance, will be offset—the yogin therefore inflating rather than transcending the egoic modes of consciousness. Furthermore, dispassion without practice is as well inefficacious for self-transcendence: "The psychosomatic energies released through dispassion are not channelled appropriately and thus may lead to confusion and possibly delusion instead of liberation."[96] Both means are interdependent in Yoga. Practice and dispassion transform randomly generated thoughts or distracted states of mind (see next section below) into one-pointed, concentrated states or responsible intentions and ideas, thus propelling one on in the process of "cessation" *(nirodha)*. Practice includes a wide range of techniques to stabilize the mind, while the cultivation of dispassion prevents the yogin from misappropriating the results of such practice, that is, in an egoic, selfish, or irresponsible manner. The bipolarity of the yogic path is already highlighted in the *Bhagavadgītā* (VI.35), which uses the same terms adopted by Patañjali to designate the two poles. Kṛṣṇa tells his disciple, Arjuna: "Doubtless, O mighty-armed, the mind is unsteady and difficult to restrain; but O son-of-Kunti, it [the mind] can be held (mastered) through practice and dispassion."[97]

Even though in *Yoga-Sūtra* I.2 *nirodha* has already been defined, the term occurs again in *Yoga-Sūtra* I.12 as the stated result of practice and dispassion. The *Yoga-Sūtra* (I.13–14) asserts: "Practice is the effort toward stability in that [process of *nirodha*]."[98] "That practice, however, is firmly grounded when properly attended to for a long time and without interruption."[99] Yoga practice needs the three qualifications stated above. It must be observed: with proper attentiveness (i.e., care), for a long time, and without interruption. In other words, the practice must be consistent, regular, and persistent over a long time and with careful attention, and one might add, a positive and devout attitude. The above qualifications are supplemented by Vyāsa with the cultivation of austerity *(tapas),* sexual restraint *(brahmacarya),* knowledge *(vidyā),*[100] and faith *(śraddhā)*.[101] When practice becomes firmly established, the yogin cannot be swayed from it even by the strongest adversity *(dveṣa)* or pain, nor can the yogin be allured away from practice by the subtlest pleasures or attractions *(rāga)*. The yogin must have the necessary vigor, enthusiasm, and will power to undertake the discipline "to the end" in order to realize its spiritual effects and "attain" fulfillment.[102] In short, the yogin must be utterly committed to practice.

It is noteworthy that Vyāsa qualifies the word *sthiti* (stability) in *Yoga-Sūtra* I.13 to mean the tranquil flow of the mind, the ordinary patterns of *vṛtti*s having subsided.[103] Practice is the effort towards stability or steadiness of mind. This does not mean, however, a complete transcendence of *vṛtti*s.

As Vijñāna Bhikṣu surmises, the usage of the term *sthiti* in *Yoga-Sūtra* I.13 implies that the mind is free of any kind of *vṛtti* other than that which is involved with the object in a state of one-pointed contemplation. One does not begin even the practice of the lower forms of cognitive *samādhi* until after this stability is established.[104] In the context of *Yoga-Sūtra* I.13 Vācaspati Miśra asserts that "stability" here means a state free of the rajasic and tamasic *vṛtti*s implying a one-pointedness of mind wherein sattvic *vṛtti*s alone remain.[105] Certainly in the context of practice *(abhyāsa), sthiti* could not refer to a delusive state of *tamas:* a dullness of mind, or an overall lack of mental alertness. According to Bhoja Rāja (*RM* I.13), *sthiti* refers to a mental state that takes place when the mind is without *vṛtti*s and dwelling in its own nature.[106] However, Bhoja's definition would raise the meaning of *sthiti* to a state beyond the experience of cognitive *(saṃprajñāta) samādhi;* the path would then come after the goal, the effort would supersede its own purpose. The intent of the *sūtra* seems to be to state implicitly that the effort toward *abhyāsa* or meditational praxis denotes bringing the mind to stillness or stability, which implies freedom from the rajasic turbulences or tamasic delusions, the mind's one-pointedness on a single sattvic *vṛtti* remaining uninterrupted so that it flows in a calm, smooth stream "toward" liberation. Moreover, it can be suggested that, epistemologically, stillness or stability of the mind means that the former type of functioning of the mind (i.e., individual identification taking place exclusively in its rajasic or tamasic modes) has been "stilled" and the transformation into sattvic understanding has dawned. Again, the important theme in Yoga of the "sattvification of consciousness" is being underlined.

Vyāsa states that the purpose behind the effort to be firmly grounded in practice is that the yogin is then "not suddenly overpowered by a *saṃskāra* of extraversion or emergence *(vyutthāna),*"[107] which would exacerbate affliction and lead to further dissatisfaction *(duḥkha)*. In its full-blown sense, perhaps Dasgupta is not far off the mark when he writes: "Practice stands for the concentrated inner application to the realization of the [transcendent] being which constitutes the essence of all yogic operations. It consists of the careful discrimination between the real and the wholesome on the one hand and the transient and all that is unworthy of human motivation on the other. It is the inwardness and unification resulting from this enlightened discernment."[108] But one must be careful not to overemphasize the method of practice *(abhyāsa)* for it has intrinsic value in Yoga only in relation to dispassion *(vairāgya),* the meaning of which we will now examine.

Turning to the second method mentioned above to bring about "cessation," namely dispassion *(vairāgya),* Patañjali states: "Dispassion is the knowledge of mastery in one who does not thirst for any object either seen [i.e., of an earthly nature] or heard of [i.e., of the subtle worlds]."[109] The word *vairāgya* is derived from the verb root *rañj* "to color." Literally, *vairāgya* means the state of being devoid of, or free from *rāga,* the attachment that accrues, as it were, from the objects of attraction reflecting in and coloring or influencing the mind. Yet this is not a complete definition of *vairāgya* for the purpose of Yoga. Vijñāna Bhikṣu tells us that merely the absence of the "coloring process" or conditioning of the mind will not suffice, nor will even the freedom from attractions that is gained from seeing their faults; this form of *vairāgya* is not conducive to the goal that is implicit in the process of *nirodha.* Mere disinterest in or indifference toward objects of experience whether enjoyable or painful can be of no value for this purpose, as for example, a disinterest in "objects" or conditions that may bring about the event of an illness. Bhikṣu points out[110] that often an attraction toward objects or other persons remains even after one becomes aware of their attendant faults or imperfections. Therefore dispassion as defined by Patañjali in *Yoga-Sūtra* I.15 does not imply a simple turning away from or suppression of a craving, becoming perhaps indifferent in an apathetic way through some form of intermittent withdrawal; rather, dispassion means a knowledge *(saṃjñā)* of mastery *(vaśīkāra).*

Mastery—breaking free from the movement of misidentification with *vṛtti*—is an essential part of dispassion. If this were not so, one might mistakenly think one had attained *vairāgya* when one simply had not acknowledged and experienced the objects of one's desire or lacked the capacity to enjoy them. Seen here, the normally upheld translation of *duḥkha* as "suffering" in a way leaves much to be desired. In the present context under discussion, *duḥkha,* which can be translated as "dissatisfaction," refers to an *inability to be satisfied.* In Yoga (and Sāṃkhya, see *SK* 23) such a state of powerlessness or impotence refers to a state of *tamas. Duḥkha* is a state of dissatisfaction brought on by inner, psychological, subjective causes at least as much as external, objective causes. Nor could *vairāgya* entail a superficial abandonment of one's aversions *(dveṣa)* toward the world, other persons, and things. Any literal (physical) discarding of objects implying an outward mode of renunciation of what is essentially an inner afflicted condition of mind would simply result in the avoidance of, or inability to deal with, real life situations, thereby perpetuating the original affliction. For example, being attached to a state of impotence or helplessness *(tamas),* one could easily develop an aversion or negative attitude toward the world, internalizing one's anger or pain. Thus, having "given up" the world, perhaps including one's family and relationships, one has merely disempowered oneself from working through one's deep-seated pain. The ego-mechanism closes in on itself with nothing to blame but the world. The result of such an aversion or negative attachment may take the form of a compulsive struggle to "give up" or escape from the world by "practicing" aloofness or indifference toward it. But Yoga is not about the cultivation of *amoral* attitudes, nor does it imply an escape from one's own *saṃskāra*s, *vāsanā*s, and mental-emotional tendencies. To withdraw from the world out of a sense of fear, anger, greed, or pride, or simply to avoid social interaction with others as if such interactions were of little or no importance in Yoga, is to misunderstand profoundly the meaning and purpose of Yoga. To anesthetize our feelings, to fail to be responsible or accountable for our actions, intentions, or attitudes to others[111] and the world, is a sign of hubris rather than illumination.

Vaśīkāra ("mastery," see n. 109) is the capacity for direct perception of an object devoid of attachment or aversion.[112] Both *rāga* and *dveṣa* are based on a superimposition that incorrectly attributes or seeks for permanent happiness or fulfillment in either the attachment or aversion to objects including other persons. It is not, however, the sheer presence or absence of objects that releases one from attachment or aversion; one is released through the transformation of one's present state of understanding. The issue here is really epistemological (rather than ontological) and has to do with a metaphorical and attitudinal rather than a literal understanding of *vairāgya*—often understood as a "physical" detachment or movement away from the objects of experience. Dispassion is a knowledge of mastery wherein the yogin becomes increasingly disengaged from misidentification with the "seeable," that is, attachments and aversions based on a mistaken identity of selfhood *(asmitā)*. Mastery is not mastery over nature or the world, is not ultimately *puruṣa*'s mastery *over prakṛti,* but as I will later argue, implies a harmony with our embodied, relational existence, nature, and the world. Dispassion removes our self-inflicted forms of conflict and imbalance. Through dispassion, the *guṇa*s are allowed to function in harmony with self-identity, resulting in a nonenslavement to things prakṛtic, for instance, *vṛtti*. The path of Yoga is not to be reduced to a master-slave mentality, of "spirit" triumphant over matter/nature/energy. The knowledge of mastery implied in *vairāgya* corrects all former life-imbalances, all enslavement to prakṛtic existence. Thus, dispassion is an irreplaceable method for the removal of ignorance *(avidyā),* which, as we have seen, is the cause, in Yoga, of all dissatisfaction *(duḥkha)*.

Vairāgya is not so much an act of dispassion or detachment as it is a state of understanding and insight, dispassion being for Patañjali a knowledge of "mastery" resulting from a genuine persistence on the part of the yogin to disengage the mind from everything that is inimical to its steadiness in practice, thereby generating purification from affliction. Normally, the ordinary person's "mindstream" and thought patterns flow in the "outward direction" *(vyutthāna)* extrinsically motivated toward worldly experience in *saṃsāra.* The yogin breaks the momentum of that flow through dispassion and makes the stream progressively more subtle or sattvic through the practice of Yoga, leading to the discriminative discernment between the pure *puruṣa* and the mistaken sense of self that has become sedimented within the mind and that, due to ignorance, masquerades as true identity until all attachment to the *guṇa*s including *sattva* is transcended.[113]

Using Vyāsa's metaphor, it is through practice that the stream of discriminative discernment is opened up, releasing its flow from the saṃsāric blockages and "knots" of empirical self-identity. The predisposition of the *vṛtti*s to flow saṃsārically in the direction of extrinsic identity and fuel the seed mechanism of *cittavṛtti* is checked or prevented, at least temporarily. Through this bipolar methodology, the conjunction *(saṃyoga)* between the seer and the seeable, as if manifesting a real creation in the form of a polarization or bifurcation of the subject or "experiencer" (empirical selfhood) and the object or "experienced" (world), gradually ceases and ignorance loses its hold or sway over the mind.

Patañjali knows of two levels of dispassion. He asserts: "That superior [dispassion] is the thirstlessness for the *guṇa*s [which results] from the discernment of *puruṣa.*"[114] As we shall see, the lower or preliminary stage of dispassion *(apara-vairāgya)* defined in *Yoga-Sūtra* I.15 above falls within the practice of cognitive *samādhi* (*saṃprajñāta, YS* I.17), but it is external to the higher stage of dispassion *(para-vairāgya)* that is associated with the supracognitive *samādhi* (*asaṃprajñāta, YB* I.18). Vyāsa informs us: "One who sees the defects in objects perceptible and heard about is dispassionate. But one who from practising the discernment of *puruṣa* has one's mind purified and strengthened in discriminating knowledge is dispassionate toward the *guṇa*s whether with manifest or unmanifest qualities."[115] Through the lower form of *vairāgya* the yogin develops dispassion toward the objects and conditions of this world as experienced through the senses, such as the compulsive need or craving for sensual enjoyment (e.g., food, drink, sex) as well as worldly affluence, success, possession, and power.[116]

The yogin develops dispassion toward: *(a)* the manifest attributes of the *guṇa*s, those that constitute knowledge of, and consequent activity in, the gross *(sthūla),* visible world as well as the attainment of heavenly realms or the subtle *(sūkṣma),* invisible worlds; and *(b)* the unmanifest attributes as experienced by the the *videha* ("bodiless") yogins, and *prakṛti-laya* yogins—those "absorbed" or "merged" in unmanifest *prakṛti.*[117] It is this lower-level *vairāgya* that is said to be the means of reaching the *prakṛti-laya* state in the *Sāṃkhya-Kārikā.*[118] The yogins of the above categories do not go beyond the lower stage of dispassion to the higher form of dispassion; they have not mastered the higher level of *vairāgya* by attaining dispassion toward the unmanifest qualities of the *guṇa*s. They continue to seek permanence, happiness, purity and authentic identity within *prakṛti*'s domain, remaining, in a more subtle mode, under the spell of ignorance and its network of deeply rooted impressions *(saṃskāras),* habit patterns *(vāsanā*s*),* and modifications *(vṛtti*s*),* the basic fabric of afflicted selfhood.

Vyāsa continues: "Of these two [levels of *vairāgya*], the latter is nothing but clarity of knowledge."[119] Vācaspati Miśra understands the higher *vairāgya* as eliminating the effects of *rajas,* the mind now being clear and in a state of discriminating knowledge or *sattva.* On this basis Vācaspati Miśra states that the mind now requires no external objects, not even as objects of concentration.[120] This explanation is misleading. No matter how much the clarity of *sattva* may be emphasized, Vyāsa's passage cannot refer merely to a state of mind or guṇic consciousness, but rather it fits the definition of higher dispassion in which the effects or influences of all three *guṇa*s, including *sattva,* have been transcended and any dependence on *prakṛti* has ceased, at least temporarily. The knowledge contained by the primary constituents *(guṇa*s*)* is certainly not indicated here. A more accurate reading, it would appear, is that the passage refers to the pure state of Self-knowledge which is synonymous with that freedom from all craving *(vaitṛṣṇya),* the definition of higher dispassion given by Patañjali. This clarity of knowledge constitutes freedom from any compulsive attraction or enslavement to the manifest or unmanifest aspects of the *guṇa*s. When the purity of knowledge or higher dispassion unfolds, the yogin contemplates and observes thus: "Whatever was to be attained has been attained. The afflictions which were to be eliminated have been eliminated. The continuous chain of the cycle of being has been broken, without the breaking of which one is born and dies, and having died will be born again. *The ultimate limit of knowledge is dispassion* [italics mine]. After this very state of dispassion aloneness follows."[121]

It appears to be the case that without the higher dispassion liberation cannot be attained, at least not by discriminative discernment *(vivekakhyāti)* in itself. As Patañjali states: "Through dispassion toward even this [discernment of the distinction between *puruṣa* and the *sattva* of consciousness], the seeds of impediments are destroyed, and there is aloneness."[122] Attachment to the knowledge of the difference between *puruṣa* and *sattva*—the discernment *(khyāti)* that provides the yogin with omniscience *(sarvajñātṛtva)* and supremacy over all states of being *(adhiṣṭhātṛtva)*[123]—can yet bind the yogin to phenomenal existence and misidentification. Here it can be said that Yoga's higher dimension of *vairāgya* goes beyond the classical Sāṃkhyan *(SK)* adherence to discrimination *(viveka)* as the final means to liberation. An ongoing purification of the mind (from ignorance) takes place for the embodied yogin until *kaivalya* ensues. *Para-vairāgya* transcends discriminating knowledge and enables the yogin to achieve a clear, direct knowledge of *puruṣa*. It represents an act of will—along with its own transcendence—subsequently leading to *asaṃprajñāta-samādhi,* the state of supracognition through which *avidyā* and its effects (e.g., *saṃskāra*s) and affects *(duḥkha)* are finally laid to rest. As it is direct knowledge of *puruṣa,* Yoga's higher dispassion, by constituting a total disengagement from the superimposed condition of *saṃyoga,* is the final means to liberation. There must develop in the yogin an equanimity *(upekṣā)*[124] toward even the highly advanced stage of discriminative discernment *(vivekakhyāti);* a nonacquisitive attitude *(akusīda)* must take place at the highest level of yogic practice.[125] Vyāsa emphasizes that the identity of *puruṣa* is not something to be acquired *(upādeya)* or discarded *(heya)*.[126]

The highest state of dispassion concerns knowledge of *puruṣa* itself. Any dependency on or attachment to Yoga methods and techniques and the functioning of the mind for the purpose of experience and the pursuit of liberation is ultimately a bondage or form of enslavement to ignorance. Through *para-vairāgya* the yogin, as it were, becomes aware of knowledge of the knower-of-discernment *(vivekin)* that is revealed when no other thoughts or ideas arise in the mind because the coverings of impurity that veil true identity have been "washed away."[127] This transcendent knowledge arises because the mind has become detached even from its power of discernment;[128] all *attachment* to power including attachment to the (supreme) power over all beings as well as omniscience is finally discarded in Yoga.

It is of interest to note that the higher dispassion alone transcends the *vṛtti*-mechanism of empirical identity: its activities and appropriation including the various means of Yoga, which, as W. Halbfass observes, "may even turn into obstacles if the seeker becomes attached to their pursuit and believes that such 'result-oriented,' inherently dualistic and saṃsāric activities can bring about final liberation."[129] As has become evident by now, Yoga is acutely aware of the danger referred to in the above, namely that the yogin may remain only within the sphere of the mind *(citta)* or three *guṇa*s while making efforts to transcend the mind and "acquire" freedom or true identity. One is struggling to attain a freedom that one already intrinsically *is* and as such can never really acquire. This paradoxical situation can only be fully resolved through *samādhi.*

The three fulfillments or accomplishments given in Vyāsa's *Bhāṣya* (*YB* I.16; see n. 121) appear to be a general summary of the sevenfold *(saptadhā)* wisdom or insight *(prajñā)*[130] that follows from *vivekakhyāti* and culminates in the knowledge that *puruṣa* is "the light of its own form only, alone and pure."[131] It is *puruṣa* and not the mind or empirical sense of self that "sees" this knowledge in its sevenfold final stage.[132] This knowledge is "known" or "seen" only by *puruṣa* and can be claimed only by *puruṣa.* Moreover, though it is the mind that has been transformed and liberated through knowledge and the cessation of the seed-mechanism *(cittavṛtti)* of misidentification and ignorance, it is *puruṣa* that is said to be skillful and free because *puruṣa* has "become what it always was and is beyond the three *guṇa*s."[133] What takes place after this awareness of the ultimate limit of knowledge (i.e., dispassion) is the abiding of identity in its true form *(svarūpa)* as *puruṣa,* and this realization provides a foundational grounding for the permanently liberated state of "aloneness" *(kaivalya).*

A PRELIMINARY LOOK AT THE MEANING AND PRACTICE OF *SAMĀDHI*

A careful examination of the concept of *samādhi* is essential for understanding Patañjali's philosophical perspective, for it is based upon the meaning of *samādhi* that the arguments of Yoga, and in particular, Patañjali's soteriological methodology, derive their greatest strength and value. In classical Yoga, the term *samādhi* is generally conceived as being the last member and the consummation of the yogic path of self-transformation, referring to the eight-limbed *(aṣṭāṅga)* Yoga outlined in the *Sādhana-Pāda* (chapter II) of the *Yoga-Sūtra.*[134] *Samādhi,* and the meditative discipline that accompanies it, are the *sine qua non* in Yoga for the realization of the truth of existence. The importance of this stage is expressed in Vyāsa's definition (*YB* I.1) of Yoga: *yogaḥ samādhiḥ* ("Yoga is *samādhi*"). In effect, much of the first chapter *(Samādhi-Pāda)* of the *Yoga-Sūtra* constitutes a definition of the stages of *samādhi* in Patañjali's thought. A special feature of the *Yoga-Sūtra,* therefore, is the detailed analysis Patañjali proffers of different kinds of *samādhi,* which has often been misinterpreted and rarely done justice to. Patañjali's distinct stress on *samādhi* shows a deep insight of his own into the phases of meditational praxis that are encountered by earnest practitioners of Yoga.

Throughout our study of the concept of *samādhi* it will become apparent just how closely Yoga theory and practice are intertwined and how the culmination of Yoga—"aloneness" *(kaivalya)*—is made possible. In the experiences of *samādhi* the types of knowledge that arise and the methods by which that knowledge takes place form, as it were, an "inner" core of Yoga soteriology and inform us of the metaphysical basis of Yoga praxis as viewed in its pedagogical context.

Etymologically, *"samādhi"* is an abstract noun derived from the verb root *dhā*: "to put, place, or hold" (in its feminine, nominal form *dhi*) and joined with the verbal prefixes *sam* ("together") + *ā* ("unto") to form the stem *samādhā*, which literally means "putting together": "to place or put or fix together . . . ; to compose, set right, . . . put in order, . . . restore . . . , to add," are a few of the meanings given for the term *samādhā.*[135] Some of the meanings cited for the term *samādhi* are: "joining or combining with," "union," "a whole," "bringing into harmony," "intense application or fixing the mind on," "attention," "completion," "profound or abstract meditation," "intense absorption or contemplation."[136] Yet, as is evident from even a cursory look at various translations of the term, it may be misleading to translate the word *samādhi,* as it is used in the context of the *Yoga-Sūtra,* according to any one specific meaning as given in the above or elsewhere.

Suggested renderings of the term *samādhi* are: "trance,"[137] "meditation,"[138] "concentration,"[139] "absorption,"[140] and "enstasy."[141] "Ecstasy"[142] or "rapture," terms often used to convey a sense of exalted feeling, are also cited as general meanings for *samādhi.* But despite the multitudinous ways of construing the term, most attempts are either too restricting or too vague to be acceptable. For example, "trance" can refer to states of mind that are: half-conscious, sleeplike, catalyptic, hypnotic, or morbid—states of mind that are more indicative of a predominance of *tamas* rather than *sattva.* "Rapture" can convey the sense of being carried away by something or someone through a profound attraction or attachment to the desired object and having more to do with a state of mind in which *rajas* is predominant. "Concentration" can be interpreted to mean an exclusively mental process of fixing one's mind on something external to or utterly separate from oneself. "Meditation" is, from a yogic perspective, often misunderstood to mean the act of "thinking" or "pondering over." In fact, the terms "concentration" *(dhāraṇā)* and "meditation" *(dhyāna)* are given as the sixth and seventh "limbs" *(aṅgas)* respectively of the "eight-limbed" *(aṣṭāṅga)* Yoga (*YS* II.29) and are preparatory or preliminary stages to the eighth limb—*samādhi.* Therefore, to describe or explain *samādhi* only in terms of "concentration" or "meditation" is to miss the intent of Patañjali's usage of the term, which, technically speaking, designates the highest stage of practice and awareness in a semantic "hierarchy" of yogic discipline.

M. Eliade uses the Greek term "enstasis" or "enstasy,"[143] which attempts to clearly demarcate the phenomena of *samādhi* from that of "ecstasy," a term frequently confused or conflated with "enstasy." R. C. Zaehner[144] observes that enstasy "is the exact reverse of ecstasy, which means to get outside oneself and which is often characterised by a breaking down of the barriers between the subject and the universe around him." Patañjali does include *ānanda* (*YS* I.17), meaning "bliss" or "joy," as a state of cognitive *samādhi*. The Greek-derived word *ecstasy* means to stand *(stasis)* outside *(ex)* the ordinary (empirical) self, whereas *samādhi* ultimately signifies one's "standing in" *(en)* the Self—one-in-identity as *puruṣa*—as one's authentic being or intrinsic identity. In ecstasy, the experience entails at least a partial transcendence of the limited ego-identity or *cittavṛtti* mechanism accompanied perhaps by a sense of well-being. As normally conceived, ecstasy can refer to states of emotional rapture and mental exaltation. Since these characteristics do not appear to apply to or fully capture the typical yogic state of "mind-transcending" consciousness, Eliade and Feuerstein[145] have proposed to render the term *samādhi* as "enstasy." But the distinction is not always clear cut. Both interpretations are correct according to the stage or level of *samādhi* being experienced.

There are, in Patañjali's *Yoga-Sūtra, samādhi*-experiences that resemble more ecstasy than enstasy. These, I will be suggesting, refer to the stages of *saṃprajñāta-samādhi* (*YS* I.17), the object- or content-oriented *samādhi*s of cognition that are accompanied by degrees of mental "refinement" (in *vitarka-* and *vicāra-samādhi*), or perhaps intense joy *(ānanda),* or a subtler and more lucid sense of self-identity in *asmitā-samādhi*. By ordinary standards these states are extraordinary and constitute a significant shift in one's sense of self. They are ecstatic in that they shift one's normal focus of attention "outside of" or beyond the empirical self as it is normally experienced and perceived in the state of "emergence" (*vyutthāna, YS* III.9 and 37) or extrinsic self-identity, that is, saṃsāric existence. The above stages constitute part of the unfoldment of the "sattvification" of self-awareness in the process of *nirodha*. However, the experiences in ecstasy can be said to take place "outside" *puruṣa* in that they are associated with the subtler objects of prakṛtic existence as perceived in the mind and do not directly or consciously involve *puruṣa* as the pure, knowing experiencer; they are not *puruṣa*-centered. In this sense they may be understood as being ecstatic. *Asaṃprajñāta-samādhi*—the supracognitive *samādhi*—on the other hand is enstasy or true abiding "in" or rather *as* the *puruṣa*. It is not, as Zaehner would have it, a complete *reversal* of ecstasy, at least not in the context in which this study is proposing to use the term ecstasy. Ecstasy and enstasy are not mutually exclusive states. Rather, ecstasy is propaedeutic to enstasy: there is a continuum or continuity of experience that links the two in the process of "cessation" *(nirodha)*. Only in enstasy, however, is Yoga discipline fully matured, a maturation made possible through the cessation of any tendency to "see" (i.e., misperceive) *puruṣa* "outside" itself or to mistake or misidentify prakṛtic existence for *puruṣa*.

Therefore I will refer to *samādhi* as meaning both "ecstasy" (as in cognitive or *saṃprajñāta-samādhi, YS*/*YB* I.17) and "enstasy" (as in supracognitive or *asaṃprajñāta-samādhi* referred to by Vyāsa in *YB* I.18), bearing in mind the above distinctions and carefully noting that ecstasy is propaedeutic, and not inimical, to enstasy. Ecstasy refers to the process of *samādhi* in its cognitive (and affective) stages and results in illuminating experiences of *sattva* for the purpose of *puruṣa,* namely experience and liberation. Enstasy is the realization of *puruṣa* in its true form (*svarūpa, YS* I.3) and transcends all saṃsāric experience or misidentification with and identity-dependency on *prakṛti*'s realm. Enstasy is the awareness of one's experiencer as *puruṣa,* utterly "alone" and with nothing (or no-thing) left to experience for the sake of liberation. Positively conceived, enstasy is a state of supracognition as the ever-free knower of *vṛtti* (*YS* IV.18); or, negatively conceived, enstasy is the "a-cognition" of "seeing," that is, of falsely cognizing, *puruṣa* within *prakṛti,* and the termination of the "failure-to-see" *(adarśana)*. The yogin is then no longer implicated in the struggle and dissatisfaction inherent in the deluded or confused guṇic modes of consciousness or saṃsāric identity of self.

PREPARATION FOR *SAMĀDHI*

According to Vyāsa, two primary forms of Yoga are outlined by Patañjali. One, described in the first chapter *(Samādhi-Pāda),* is for the advanced yogin—one with a concentrated, engrossed mind. The other form of Yoga, described in the second chapter *(Sādhana-Pāda),* is for one not so advanced in yogic discipline in that it shows how one of an extroverted and distracted mind may become steady in Yoga.[146] For one whose mind is concentrated, the practice of *samādhi* is emphasized. For one whose mind is distracted, the practice of Yoga must involve a preliminary stage of purification. Vācaspati Miśra observes that in the *Samādhi-Pāda* practice *(abhyāsa)* and dispassion *(vairāgya),* which result in *samādhi,* are stated as the means of Yoga: "However," he goes on to state, " as these two do not come into being instantaneously for one whose mind is extroverted, that one is in need of the means taught in the second chapter in order to purify the *sattva* [of the mind.]"[147]

So long as the mind is ineluctably activated by inner saṃsāric drives, functions, disturbances, and agitations, it cannot be made pure and attain stability. It flows in the direction of affliction: to all that is evil and destructive in life. What is needed is a counterflow *(pratiprasava)* to the destructive tension of the mind, a return to its intrinsic clarity and purity through the process of *nirodha,* thereby counteracting the outward flow *(vyutthāna)* of worldly identification wholly fixed upon or obsessed by the objects of experience. *Vyutthāna,* the extroverted state of mind and extrinsic nature of self-identity, is a deluded and extrinsic sense of selfhood that contains an implicit desire to know the nature of an object that it holds separate from itself and to derive satisfaction or even permanent happiness through this knowledge. It is a compulsive, extraneous, emerging consciousness rooted in ignorance *(avidyā)* and appearing in the form of egoity *(asmitā).*

The word *vyutthāna* can mean "rising up," "swerving from the right course," "independent action."[148] A *vṛtti* of a *vyutthāna*-nature, which can arise from or generate a *vyutthāna-saṃskāra,*[149] is not merely a mental modification, fluctuation, "wave," or "whirl" of consciousness that goes outward to the world, but signifies the processes of cognition and experience that "arise" from and are appropriated by a mistaken identity *(cittavṛtti);* in effect, the *vṛtti*-generating power of *vyutthāna*[150] leads to a misidentification of self and misappropriation of the world, self-identity having been entangled in the network of *vāsanā*s and *saṃskāra*s—the "inner" wheel of *saṃsāra.* Thus one is "forgetful" of authentic identity and fails to recognize *puruṣa* as one's intrinsic identity. Due to thoughts and impressions of a *vyutthāna*-nature, one looks to and becomes dependent on others for meaning and identity, feels possessive and fearful, and is ignorant of the "knowledge" of one's true nature *(puruṣa).* Moreover, one's identification or thought patterns are conditioned in terms of a compulsive lack of "something" that one feels one needs in order to be fulfilled, yet a "some-thing" that is experienced as existing "outside" of oneself. The expression *vyutthāna* thus carries with it the sense of separation or alienation from authentic identity, incompleteness, compulsive desire and dependence on "objects" (that is, things, persons, wealth, and so on). It is only by a "reversal" of the usual centrifugal, de-centering "flow" of the mind and its extroverted impressions, traits and habit patterns that influences in the form of afflictions can cease *(nirodha)* and the mind and empirical identity—through a process of a centering or a centripetal "flow" of attention—can function correctly and "fit into" their proper place with respect to *puruṣa: that of the known or seeable rather than the knower or seer itself.*[151] *Vṛtti* will then be subordinate to the knower *(puruṣa)* of *vṛtti* rather than our selfhood being contingent upon and a product of the movement or functioning of *vṛtti* as in the previous condition of *saṃyoga* (that is, egoity and ignorance)—the *vyutthāna* (extrinsic) mode of identity.

The ground to be prepared in Yoga is the entire body-mind organism for it is through the psychophysical being as a whole that yogic insight *(prajñā)* arises and *puruṣa* is revealed as the true seer. In the *Sādhana-Pāda,* it appears that Patañjali offers two main Yogas by which the process of *nirodha* is effected. The counterflow to the usual afflicted tendencies *(kliṣṭa-vṛttis)* of the mind is attained, as indicated in *Yoga-Sūtra* II.1-2, through a practice called *kriyā-yoga* (the Yoga of "action," not to be confused with the *karma-yoga* of the *BG*), which has as its purpose the attenuation of the afflictions and the cultivation of *samādhi.*[152] *Kriyā-yoga* consists of: austerity *(tapas),* personal scriptural (i.e., self-) study (*svādhyāya,* see below), and devotion to *īśvara (īśvara-praṇidhāna).*[153] Vyāsa qualifies *svādhyāya* (literally, "one's own going into") as the recitation of purifying *mantras* such as the sacred syllable *Om,* or the study of scriptures on spiritual liberation.[154] The second Yoga, the eight-limbed Yoga (*aṣṭāṅga, YS* II.29), is the one most commonly identified with Patañjali[155] and an overview of this will be presented in the last section of this chapter. A comparative analysis of these forms of Yoga is not within the scope of this study.[156] However, it must be admitted that they both share a common praxis-orientation and purpose: effecting the cessation of afflicted identity—of the misidentification with the *cittavṛtti* mechanism—thus leading to the realization of *puruṣa.*

It is noteworthy that Patañjali includes a section in the *Samādhi-Pāda* on methods for purifying, clarifying, and stabilizing the mind prior to the practice of *samādhi. Yoga-Sūtra* I.33-39 give the *cittaparikarmas*: the ways of refining, purifying, and preparing the mind through diligent practice *(abhyāsa).* Thus the mind may reach a necessary degree of stability and attentiveness so as to be steadied for the attainments of *samādhi.* For example, *Yoga-Sūtra* I.34 informs us that by expulsion and retention of the breath *(prāṇa)* one attains stability of mind.[157] As well, Patañjali states (*YS* I.37) that by having as its object of concentration a mind (e.g., of a sage) that is in a condition free from all attachment, one's mind becomes stabilized.[158] Or according to Vyāsa, as in the case of enlightened sensory awareness *(divya-saṃvid)*[159] or directly perceived sensations, there arises the activity of involvement with an object that steadies the mind-organ (*manas, YS* I.35).[160] Another example, mentioned in chapter 3 (*YS* I.33), states that the mind is made clear and pure by cultivating friendliness, compassion, happiness, and equanimity in conditions or toward objects, be they joyful, sorrowful, meritorious or demeritorious.[161] Elsewhere (*YS* I.36) Patañjali suggests that one direct one's mental activity to bring about (meditative) experiences that are sorrowless and illuminating.[162] Each of these techniques requires a redirecting and restructuring of the thought process, a transformation from identification with distracted, afflicted, and self-centered mental activity in the condition of *cittavṛtti* to identification with responsible thought, intentions *(pratyaya),* attitudes, and volitions. All ethical virtues are explicitly mentioned by Patañjali with reference to the obtaining of the stability of mind for the purpose of furthering the yogin's practice and awareness. That he has not discussed the social implications of ethical virtues in Yoga does not mean that he was unaware of their importance for society. His purpose was not to explain the virtues as social virtues, but to point out their significance for Yoga soteriology. Cultivating the moral attributes in Yoga (as in *YS* I.33), one develops a transformed personality in which one's sattvic nature has increased resulting in a greater propensity toward purer (*YS* II.41), nonafflicted, and nonselfish attitudes and activity. One generates morally and cognitively purer virtues, including responsible, nonharmful, and creative mental activities (sattvic *vṛtti*s) that replace the more afflicted *(kliṣṭa)* or painful (rajasic) and stagnated (tamasic) types of *vṛtti*s. Due to its destructive and delusive nature, identification with the afflicted *vṛtti*s conceals or frustrates the potential within human nature for an enriched cognitive and moral development, individually and collectively, including the relational sphere of human existence.

When the effort is made to obtain stability of mind, the mind can then pass through five stages *(bhūmi*s*),* levels, or qualities. Vyāsa[163] lists these as:

1. *Kṣipta:* impulsive, restless, agitated, disturbed
2. *Mūḍha:* dull, somnolent, stupified
3. *Vikṣipta:* distracted, changeable
4. *Ekāgra:* one-pointed, concentrated
5. *Niruddha:* mastered, nonenslaved, transcendent

Vyāsa (*YB* I.1) has included *kṣipta* and *mūḍha* in his enumeration of the states of mind but throughout the rest of his *Bhāṣya* he has nothing much to say about them. These two states are of little practical interest to Patañjali and Vyāsa in the context of Yoga practice itself. Of the five states of mind listed in the above, the agitated, impulsive state *(kṣipta)* is dominated by *rajas* and is always unsteady, forcing one's mind (attention) to waver, scattering it from one object to another. The dull, somnolent state of mind *(mūḍha)* is dominated by *tamas*—a state that is also predominant in the state of sleep[164]—and is responsible for forms of stupor (e.g., as in states of inebriation) and dullness as well as cowardice, mental confusion, and an overall lack of alertness. There is not a definite boundary line between *kṣipta* and *mūḍha*. Often in a wakeful or active state of mind we may consider ourselves to be alert, but under the influence of *tamas* forget or neglect to do something.

There are other examples of the alternation between *kṣipta* and *mūḍha,* or between the dominance of *rajas* and *tamas*. According to Vijñāna Bhikṣu,[165] *rajas* draws us toward the objects of attraction, causing a mood called *rāga* in which the mind is colored or influenced by the object of attraction. When the desire to enjoy or possess the object of that attraction or attachment *(rāga)* is thwarted, a disappointment ensues. The mind becomes clouded with *tamas,* and consequently depression *(viṣāda)* sets in. One can similarly analyze the fluctuations of varying moods and emotional states (which have their cognitive counterparts) by observing the alternating dominance of *rajas* and *tamas*. *Avidyā* or spiritual ignorance is in its most dense form in the condition of *tamas* that, as a natural "staining" constituent of the mind, dominates the knowing mechanism. *Tamas* and *rajas* both, insofar as they veil the *sattva* component of the mind, lend themselves to immoral and amoral states that, as we have seen earlier, correlate with delusion, confusion, and various forms of selfish behavior.

Vikṣipta, the third state of mind, is subtler than, and an improvement upon, both *kṣipta* and *mūḍha*. On the journey toward clarity of knowledge and *samādhi, sattva* begins to assert its illuminative power. The mind now begins to find some sustained concentration, but its former habit patterns keep propelling it away from *sattva*. In this condition the mind is still under the influence of *rajas* and *tamas;* however *sattva* has begun to make its presence known and felt. When the mind—having attained a state of concentration—is unable to maintain it, that state is called "distraction" *(vikṣipta, vikṣepa)*.[166] In *Yoga-Sūtra* I.30 the term *vikṣepa* is used as a synonym for *antarāya* ("obstacle") and clearly suggests that the nine distractions *(vikṣepas)* given by Patañjali impede one from engaging properly in the practice of Yoga. The nine obstacles are listed as follows: sickness *(vyādhi)*, langor *(styāna)*, doubt *(saṃśaya)*, carelessness or negligence as in the lack of commitment to the means of *samādhi (pramāda)*, laziness *(ālasya)*, sense addiction (i.e., caused by past addiction to objects) *(avirati)*, false views *(bhrāntidarśana),* failure to attain the stages of Yoga (*YB* I.30) *(alabdhabhūmikatva),* and instability—as when a state has been attained but the mind is not able to remain established in it *(anavasthitatva).*[167] All of the above impediments are called *vikṣepa*s because they divert the mind from the path of Yoga.[168] Vyāsa asserts that the nine obstacles appear only in conjunction with their corresponding mental processes *(vṛtti*s*),* and that without the obstacles the latter do not arise. Only in *samādhi* is the mind truly stabilized.[169]

The natural accompaniments of the above distractions are: pain/dissatisfaction (*duḥkha,* which Vyāsa[170] says refers to the three types of pain: *ādhyātmika*—the physical and mental pain proceeding from oneself; *ādhibhautika*—pain caused by other beings; and *ādhidaivika*—pain proceeding from deities or natural forces), despair *(daurmanasya),* unsteadiness of the "limbs" of the body *(aṅgam-ejayatva),* and faulty inhalation *(śvāsa)* or exhalation *(praśvāsa).*[171] Vyāsa informs us that these natural accompaniments accrue to one whose mind is in the distracted state and not to one whose mind is concentrated or harmonized in *samādhi.* Vyāsa uses the word *samāhita,* which is the ordinary past passive participle of *samādhā,* expressing the fact that a harmonizing of the mind or resolution of the conditions of all conflict, including personal conflict, have been accomplished by reaching *samādhi.*[172] Only then are the nine obstacles and their five correlates overcome completely. Furthermore, as Vyāsa emphasizes, any state of *samādhi* subordinated and eclipsed by distraction (in the distracted state of mind) is not fit to be included within the category of Yoga.[173] The dominance of *rajas* and *tamas* in the first three states of mind implies that one is unable to focus properly on Yoga discipline; through the various distractions one can easily lose the necessary grounding or traction for further development or growth in Yoga.

Having dismissed the first three states as not being classified as Yoga (i.e., *samādhi*) proper, Vyāsa introduces the fourth state of mind: *ekāgra,* the one-pointed state of mind that attains its stability and matures in the practice of *saṃprajñāta-samādhi.* Thus begins Yoga proper. Koelman informs us that: "The first three psychological dispositions . . . must first undergo the discipline of the Yoga of action *[kriyā-yoga].* Only the last two psychological states are directly disposed for the purely mental discipline of *Rājayoga.*"[174]

Cognitive *samādhi* has as its foundation the "one-pointed" state or *ekāgra,* which refers to the one-pointedness *(ekāgratā)* of the mind on an object. Vyāsa describes *samādhi* in the one-pointed mind as having the power to: (1) fully illuminate an actual object as it is; (2) diminish the afflictions or impurities; (3) loosen the bonds of *karma;* and (4) bring about the possibility of total "cessation" *(nirodha)* into view.[175] In the state of *niruddha (nirodha)*—the most subtle state of the mind—the dependency on an objective "prop" or object of contemplation in *samādhi* comes to an end, and the yogin, liberated from mistaken identity and thus having transcended the effects (and affects) of *vṛtti* or cognition, is left "alone" as the auto-transparent knower, no longer under the influence of *avidyā.*

AN OVERVIEW OF THE *AṢṬĀṄGA-YOGA*

Here I will follow the more elaborated scheme (*YS* II.28-55 and III.1-8) of the "eight-limbed" Yoga *(aṣṭāṅga),* which consists of: *yama* (restraint), *niyama* (observances), *āsana* (postures), *prāṇāyāma* (control of breath, restraint of vital energy currents), *pratyāhāra* (withdrawal of the senses), *dhāraṇā* (concentration), *dhyāna* (meditation), and *samādhi* (ecstasy, enstasy).[176] Through the practices involved in *aṣṭāṅga-yoga* there results the destruction of impurity and an increasing light of knowledge up to the discriminative discernment between the seer and the seeable.[177] The disjunction from, or disengagement with, the condition of *saṃyoga*—implying the cessation of the seed-identification or misidentification with the seeable in the condition of *cittavṛtti*—can then take place.

Within these eight "limbs," the empirical world is dealt with aspect by aspect in a manner similar to the reversal of the Sāṃkhyan process of world manifestation and actualization. All actions, intentions, volitions, and thoughts are scrutinized and subjected to a purification or process of sattvification in which all attachment and aversion toward initially the grosser and later on the subtler manifestations of and identifications within *prakṛti* are discarded. One's actions and interactions in the world are first brought under control or harmonized through the application of ethical restraints and observances. The first limb, *yama* (*YS* II.30),[178] means "restraint" and includes five important moral obligations. These are: nonviolence *(ahiṃsā),*[179] truthfulness *(satya),*[180] nonstealing *(asteya),*[181] sexual restraint *(brahmacarya),*[182] and nonpossessiveness/greedlessness *(aparigraha).*[183] As abstinences in the practice of Yoga, they involve refraining from actions that generate negative impressions, and constitute the "great vow" that, as *Yoga-Sūtra* II.31 spells out, must be practiced irrespective of place, time, circumstances, or a particular person's social status.[184] These moral obligations are unconditionally valid and demonstrate that moral integrity is an indispensable aspect of successful Yoga practice.

The second limb, *niyama,*[185] requires the observance of particular activities that are conducive to the quest for spiritual liberation. These refer to rules for regulating life and consist in the observance of moral, physical, and mental purity *(śauca),*[186] contentment *(saṃtoṣa),*[187] austerity *(tapas),*[188] personal/scriptural (self-) study *(svādhyāya),*[189] and devotion to the 'Lord' *(īśvarapraṇidhāna).*[190] The last three observances are, arguably, the same that were said earlier to constitute *kriyā-yoga.*[191] Through these regulatory activities, applied in day-to-day life, one minimizes the distractions that arise due to interacting in the world, thereby stabilizing one's social intercourse.

If there is any obstruction to the practice of the *yama*s and *niyama*s brought about by the distraction of discursive thought in the form of contrary ideas, such as violence/harming, and so on, the yogin must be devoted to the cultivation of their opposite.[192] For, as Patañjali warns:

> Discursive thoughts like violence and the others, done or caused to be done or approved of, preceded by greed, anger or delusion [whether] mild, medium or intense—all result in endless dissatisfaction/sorrow and ignorance; thus the cultivation of their opposites [is prescribed].[193]

The above practice applies not only to *yama* and *niyama* disciplines but to various techniques or methods mentioned earlier[194] that prescribe purificatory and ethical practices.

The first two limbs, *yama* and *niyama,* regulate the yogin's social and personal life in an effort to reduce the production of unwholesome volition or intention, which would only add to the binding karmic residue *(karmāśaya)* already stored in the mind. The yogin's goal is to cease to be under the sway of *karma* in the form of ignorance including all the impressions embedded in the depths of the psyche. For this transformation of consciousness to be successful, the yogin has to create the right environmental conditions, within and without. *Yama* and *niyama* can be seen as the first necessary steps in this direction.

In Yoga the social dimension involving our emotive and ethical natures is seen in the background and attitudes of the yogin and includes an interpersonal context. The cultivation of positive, virtuous attitudes such as friendliness, compassion, and nonviolence imply a gradual eradication of other attitudes that are the companions of a disturbed state of mind enveloped in affliction. Obviously, the point of Yoga is not for the yogin to adopt various attitudes or modes of understanding that intentionally conflict with others and society at large. The point is *not* to shun or escape from the world or neglect our personal and moral responsibilities in society. The personal soteriological resolve of the yogin incorporates an understanding of person through which an affective, emotive, and moral core involving interaction and relationship with others is not seen as irrelevant in the pursuit of liberation. Virtues such as benevolence and compassion, for example, are essential to develop on the Yoga path *(yogadharma)* in order to eradicate any propensity to cause fear or harm in others.[195] Without the cultivation of higher virtues, one-pointedness or concentration of mind cannot be sustained leaving one unprepared to undergo further refining processes of purification and illumination and the arising of discriminative discernment. To strengthen the *akliṣṭa-vṛtti*s means to weaken the power of the *kliṣṭa-vṛtti*s. Thus, to describe the yogin's accomplishment as being "too selfish," the yogin being one who "uses insight and discipline to remain self-enclosed,"[196] simply ignores or fails to consider the important fact that Patañjali lists compassion *(karuṇā)* and friendliness *(maitrī)* as two of the virtues to be cultivated by the yogin.

Once the *yama*s and *niyama*s have been sufficiently grasped, practised and matured, the yogin can focus directly on the body (i.e., the most obvious aspect of one's immediate sense of self or identity) through the perfection of right posture *(āsana)*. According to *Yoga-Sūtra* II.46 one's posture should be firm and comfortable[197] making one both relaxed and alert.[198] The proper execution of posture makes the yogin immune to the impact of the "pairs of opposites" *(dvandva*s*)*[199] such as heat and cold, dark and light, quiet and noise, that is, external conflict. From *āsana* one develops regulation of the breath *(prāṇāyāma)*.[200] Patañjali mentions four movements or modifications of *prāṇāyāma*.[201] After the successful practice of the fourth form of *prāṇāyāma*—which transcends the internal and external conditions of the breath[202]—it is said that the "covering" of the inner light *(prakāśa)* ("covering" referring here to the karmic impulses that veil discriminative knowledge or *sattva*) disappears.[203] Furthermore, from the practice of *prāṇāyāma* the mind-organ *(manas)* is said to attain fitness for concentration.[204] Thus the practice progresses inwardly to deal with more subtle phenomena of the mind.

The fifth limb, *pratyāhāra,* is when the senses, disjoined from their respective objects, assume as it were the nature of the mind.[205] Withdrawn from their objects, the senses are freed of external stimuli and settle in their source, the mind. The mind is no longer distracted by external sources. Such an effort does not result in the destruction of the senses. The yogin is not in a coma or a catatonic or lifeless state. On the contrary, when the senses are inwardly settled, the mind generally becomes very active and it then becomes necessary to tackle the more subtle aspects of one's self-identity such as the impressions *(saṃskāra*s*)* and *vṛtti*s that govern the habituations of the mind. Attention can then be focused internally: on an internal object. *Pratyāhāra* is said to result in the supreme mastery or "obedience" of the senses,[206] which is the ability to "switch off" at will and allow for a state of inward-mindfulness. Vyāsa gives the following simile: "As when the queen-bee flies up and the (other) bees swarm after it, and when the queen-bee settles and they also settle: similarly, the senses are mastered when the mind is mastered."[207] The senses, following from the mind's withdrawal from sensory activity, also withdraw.

Dhāraṇā, the sixth limb, is concentration in which the yogin's consciousness as a purely mental process is focused on one place or a single locus,[208] which may be a particular part of the body (e.g., the tip of the tongue or nose; or a *cakra* such as the naval circle, heart lotus, or the light-center in the head), or an external object that is internalized.[209] The term *dhāraṇā,* which stems from the root *dhṛ,* "to hold, maintain," refers to the holding of one's attention, which is fixed on an internalized object. The underlying process is called *ekāgratā* (composed of *eka:* "one, single," and *agratā:* "pointedness"), which stands for the singleness of mind or unwavering (purely focused) attention—the very foundation of yogic concentration—which deepens and matures in *dhyāna* and *samādhi.*[210]

Dhyāna (*YS* III.2)—meditation—follows from *dhāraṇā* as a linear continuation of one-pointedness. Patañjali understands *dhyāna* as an unbroken, singular "extension" *(eka-tānatā)*[211] of one idea *(pratyaya),* cognition, or intention with regard to the object of concentration, an uninterrupted flow of attention from the yogin to the object of concentration. All arising ideas or cognitions revolve around the object of concentration. Meditation *(dhyāna)* is, however, a mental state with its own distinctive properties. T. R. Kulkarni writes:

> While in *dhāraṇā* the mind remains bound up, as it were, in a restricted space, its continuation in that bound up state in such a way that the experimental state corresponding to it remains uniformly and homogeneously the same despite variations in the internal or external perceptual situation, constitutes *dhyāna*. . . . In the state of *dhyāna,* the indeterminateness of perception disappears with the mind remaining unaffected by distracting stimuli.[212]

J. W. Hauer, known to have personally experimented with Yoga, describes his insights into the nature of meditation:

> *[Dhyāna]* is a deepened and creative *dhāraṇā,* in which the inner object is illumined mentally. The strict contemplation on one object of consciousness

> is now supplemented with a searching-pensive contemplation of its actual nature. The object is, so to speak, placed before the contemplative consciousness in all its aspects and is perceived as a whole. Its various characteristics are examined till its very essence is understood and becomes transparent. . . . This is accompanied by a certain emotive disposition. Although the reasoning faculty functions acutely and clearly, it would be wrong to understand *dhyāna* merely as a logical-rational process: the contemplator must penetrate his object with all his heart, since he is after all primarily interested in a spiritual experience which is to lead him to ontic participation and the emancipation from all constricting and binding hindrances.[213]

The British psychologist John H. Clark characterizes *dhyāna* as being a paradoxical process in that meditation "both empties the mind and, at the same time, encourages alertness."[214] By adding a depth and lucidity of consciousness in meditation, the yogin's alertness or sense of wakefulness is enheightened even though there can be very little if any awareness of the external environment. *Dhyāna* is a necessary condition for *samādhi* to ensue. The definition of *samādhi* in *Yoga-Sūtra* III.3 begins *"tad eva"*[215] showing clearly that *samādhi* is not separate from *dhyāna* but is a continuation albeit a deepening/flowering/maturing of the meditative process.

In *dhāraṇā* and *dhyāna* the mind *(citta)* is involved as a locus of empirical selfhood or self-appropriation, a cognizer or prakṛtic sense of self that claims to know and see the object and intensify or make subtle one's relationship with the object; the distinction between the subject, object, and cognition persists. However, through the practice of the eighth limb—*samādhi*—the mind of the yogin becomes so completely absorbed in the object that it appears to become the object, reflecting the object as it truly is: "That [meditation], when it shines forth as the object only, apparently empty of its own form/nature [as knowledge], is indeed *samādhi*."[216] *Samādhi* refers to the "oneness" or identity we must attain in order to know the true nature of anything. *Samādhi* involves a complete transformation of the usual mode of knowing or perceiving *(pratyakṣa)*. It is a transformation *(pariṇāma)* of the mind and consciousness from a state of "all objectivity" or "dispersiveness" into one-pointedness *(ekāgratā)*.[217] Prior to *samādhi* the mind received the impressions of the objects through the senses and imposed its own habit patterns and *vṛtti*s upon the objects. In *samādhi* the mind progressively acts as the arena or medium through which there is no subjective or egoic center of consciousness that can introduce any distortion of the object; there is only the pure grasping, knowing. No agency or organ interferes between the object and the knowing. Thus, the insight *(prajñā)* obtained in cognitive *samādhi* is not a mental projection, is not a self-referenced, indulgent (i.e., emotive, affective, wishful/imaginative, cognitive) projection onto the object. It is not individual (i.e., "my") knowledge, nor is it subjective. It refers wholly and exclusively to the object; it is clear insight into the object as it is without any violation or forcing from the yogin (observer), for, at the moment of the *samādhi* experience of knowing, the observer as a subject separate from the object does not come into play.[218]

The last three limbs of Yoga, namely: concentration, meditation, and *samādhi,* continually practiced and cultivated together, constitute what is called *saṃyama* ("constraint").[219] It is the application of *saṃyama* to any object that leads to the yogin's direct perception *(sākṣātkāra, yogi-pratyakṣa)* of it yielding suprasensuous knowledge or insight *(prajñā).*[220] The application of *saṃyama* and its mastery progresses gradually[221] wherein the mind becomes like a precious jewel taking on the true "color" of the object that fuses with it.[222] It is a unitive state of awareness in which the unification *(samāpatti)*[223] of subject, object, and means of perception is achieved. The special attention that prevails in the state of *saṃyama* can be brought to bear on any aspect of *prakṛti* encompassing all that can be known, however subtle, and extending to unmodified or undifferentiated *(aliṅga) prakṛti.*[224]

Each of the eight limbs, from the *yama*s—as, for example, the cultivation of nonviolence—to proficiency in *samādhi,* serves to lessen the influence of the afflictions on the mind and body and cuts away at the root cause—ignorance *(avidyā)*—that binds one in the condition of *saṃyoga* and the saṃsāric cycle of egoful thoughts, actions, habits, and their repetition. Of the eight limbs, the last three are said to be "inner means" *(antaraṅga)*[225] and the first five are said to be outer or external to the last three.[226] However, by comparison with the "seedless" *(nirbīja) samādhi* or enstasy—the perfected state of Yoga—the combined practices of the latter three limbs, though direct means (in the case of the former two limbs) to "seeded" *(sabīja)* or cognitive *samādhi* and (in the case of the later means) to the discriminative discernment *(vivekakhyāti),* are yet "outer" *(bahiraṅga)* means[227] on the journey to the realization of one's identity as *puruṣa.* The "seedless" *samādhi* (*nirbīja, YS* I.51) represents the climax of the path of Yoga, the culmination of the process of "cessation" *(nirodha).* The stages of cognitive *samāhi* are concerned, at very subtle levels of perception, with mistaken identity or selfhood still involved in the tripartite relationship of knower-knowledge-known and, as such, are experienced in the context of the mind *(citta)* and its modifications *(vṛtti).* In its supracognitive state, however, *samādhi (asaṃprajñāta)* refers to the "liberated" state of consciousness *(puruṣa)* or inalienable identity, the intrinsically enlightened Self left alone by itself; the yogin then has nothing further to experience *(bhoga)* or know for the sake of liberation *(apavarga)*.

Throughout the above analysis it can be seen how one "limb" builds upon and complements the other, leading from the more everyday, common life of virtuous forms of self-appropriation, restraints, and observances and their social significance to the more uncommon awakening to *puruṣa*-realization beyond the ego-personality. In this sense the "eight-limbed" Yoga can be depicted as a ladder entailing a spiritual progression that can be looked at from different perspectives. Viewed from one angle, the progression consists of a growing unification of consciousness or increasing light of knowledge; from another angle, it discloses itself as a matter of progressive purification.[228] As a means to spiritual emancipation, the whole system of Yoga takes off and gains, as it were, an effective momentum as the process of the sattvification of consciousness unfolds, preparing the yogin for ultimate self-transcendence.

However, it is obvious that not all practices in Yoga fit neatly into one particular "member" or category. Some of the earlier practices result directly in the attainment of, as well as preparation for, the later ones: "Thus, for instance the practice of purification *(śauca)* [one of the *niyama*s] may comprise a physical cleaning process, a psychic process of catharsis and also a moral act of pure intention."[229] In Hindu tradition, purification emphasizes: natural (physical and mental), moral, and ritual purification. In Yoga the ritualistic emphasis is transcended insofar as the yogin adopts a more disinterested or detached ethic in relation to the merit gained by faithfully practicing, for example, the *yama*s and the *niyama*s; such attainments would be, from the yogin's perspective, not unlike the virtues gained through traditional, ritualistic religion. The yogin downplays the importance of outer ritual and focuses instead on physical, moral, and mental purification. As in the early Upaniṣadic tradition, the earlier Vedic emphasis on the importance on external ritual—often intended for material gain and for "worldly" purposes—becomes "internalized" or spiritualized and experienced as a sacrifice *(yajña)* of misidentified selfhood or spiritual ignorance. This internalization of attention allows the yogin to "locate" ignorance within the mind and to sattvify or purify the psychophysical being as a whole.

Vyāsa distinguishes external *(bāhya)* cleanliness from internal *(ābhyantara)* or mental purity. The former is achieved by such means as earthy water (baths) and a pure diet, whereas the latter is brought about by a cleaning of the impurities of the mind[230] involving concentration and meditation. Mental purification is essential in order to transcend any self-centered ritualistic mentality. Ultimately, the mind in its *sattva* aspect must be so pure so as to flawlessly mirror or receive the light of *puruṣa* without any distortion.[231]

Patañjali also informs us that perfection in *samādhi* can be attained through devotion to *īśvara,*[232] another one of the observances *(niyama).* Vyāsa states that the *samādhi* of one who is fully devoted to *īśvara* is perfect. Through devotion the yogin comes to know unerringly whatever he/she desires even in other places, times, and bodies, and the knowledge attained from that *samādhi* reflects the object (desired) as it actually is.[233] Moreover, through this devotional *(bhakti)* and meditational disposition toward *īśvara,* the yogin's liberation is said to be near at hand. Vyāsa observes (*YB* I.23): "On account of the special devotion which is through the love of God, the Lord inclines toward the yogin and rewards the yogin according to his/her meditative and devotional disposition. By this disposition [i.e., approach] only, the yogin draws near to the attainment of *samādhi* and to its fruit [emancipation]."[234] In the above, Vyāsa allows for a psychic component of devotion, a meditative and devotional reorientation of the mind to the Lord *(īśvara).* Later in his commentary, Vyāsa supplements the meaning of devotion to *īśvara* by adding: "Devotion to the Lord is the offering-up of all actions to the supreme teacher, or the renunciation of their fruits."[235] This is practically a restatement of (or at the least is very close to) one of the fundamental doctrines of the *Bhagavadgītā,* namely, the "Yoga of action" *(karma-yoga),* where the spiritual devotee, Arjuna, sacrifices every action and thought to the Supreme Being by renouncing all selfishness or attachment to the egoic fruits of his actions. Thus *niyama* implies more than self-effort, because it entails the element of *īśvara*'s grace and favor.[236] However, according to *Yoga-Sūtra* I.23 devotion to *īśvara* is a possible, not a necessary means to the enstatic consciousness.[237]

It is also possible that the first five limbs outlined in *Yoga-Sūtra* II.29 need not be completely sufficient conditions in determining the last three. Cultivating and perfecting physical posture *(āsana)* or developing moral conduct may aid meditational practice but does not guarantee it. Ideally, the external behavior will reflect the internal development, "inner" and "outer" viewed as being intertwined with each other. For example, one does not necessarily attain to a clarity of mind by breathing or thinking in a certain way; one breathes and thinks in that way because one's mind is clear/pure. Nor does it seem appropriate that the earlier methods are to be discarded when the later ones are practiced, or that the latter should not be cultivated until the earlier ones are perfected. But some steadiness of mind is presupposed in the earlier stages before initiating the later methods, and the latter help to master the former. Meditation *(dhyāna)* and *samādhi* do have clear ethical implications. By overcoming *vṛtti*-patterns that arise from the *kleśa*s (*YS* II.11), meditational praxis[238] aids the yogin in the cultivation of virtues such as compassion, joyfulness, and so on (*YS* I.33). Perhaps the most fundamental of all moral injunctions—nonviolence *(ahiṃsā)*—denotes much more than a physical restraint of "nonkilling"; it can refer to non-harming in both thought and action, an attitudinal perspective and "inner" state of nonviolence where one is no longer embedded within and predisposed to the psychological matrix of inherent dissatisfaction and conflict both in oneself and in the world as was formerly the case in the condition of *saṃyoga*.[239] It can also be noted, therefore, that meditational praxis contributes to the "good life." The state of attentiveness or one-pointedness in Yoga is often overlooked as a virtue; yet it clearly plays a pivotal role in the development of other virtues. Moreover, as I later argue,[240] there is no sound reason why the virtues attained through Yoga discipline cannot be seen as an integral component of an embodied state of liberation in Yoga. The tendencies of the afflictions to assert themselves (*YS* II.10–11) are only fully recognized and overcome through meditation and *samādhi*. Similarly, the practices of posture and control of the breath[241] are not exclusively bodily acts but also have a psychic correlate.

Some of the apparent linear interpretation of the eight-limbed Yoga arises from the tendency to objectify, enumerate, and categorize the practices and attainments in Yoga, a tendency derived no doubt in part from the analytical and sequential nature of the eight-membered discipline. But these eight members could, from a somewhat different perspective, be seen not only as being complementary, but also as being integral, overlapping and sustaining, feeding into each other and giving rise to a transformed sense of identity, a nonfragmented (holistic) state of being. Having purified, "gathered together," and integrated one's physical, moral, psychological, and spiritual components, the yogin can live in the world not being enslaved by worldly perspectives and involvements. It is by the combined momentum and power of the methods and insight that the yogin progresses along the "path" of Yoga in the process of "cessation" *(nirodha)*.[242] It would, however, be incorrect to interpret the "limbs" as definitive stages[243] to be surpassed and even discarded along the way. The plurality of practices and stages of attainment in Yoga as illustrated in the eight-limbed Yoga (there being many other methods and descriptions of Yoga given throughout the *Yoga-Sūtra*) "coexist in complementarity, not competition."[244] Moreover, all practices and perspectives are an integral part of a continuum or continuity throughout the *Yoga-Sūtra* in that they are all supportive of and work toward a transformation of consciousness and identity as a whole that alone can bring an end to dissatisfaction, misidentification, and ignorance.

The disclosure of authentic identity *(puruṣa)* and the establishment of selfhood in its true form *(svarūpa)* is dependent upon the insights that arise in *samādhi*. I will now turn to an analysis of the stages of cognitive *samādhi*, examining further the process and meaning of "cessation" *(nirodha)* up to the attainment of the discriminative discernment *(vivekakhyāti)* between the seer and the seeable.

chapter five

Cognitive Samādhi

Patañjali distinguishes between two kinds of *samādhi:* the first covering all those ecstatic states connected with objects of cognition; and the latter being devoid of objects and thus transcending all mental content. The former, which can also be designated as the "seeded" *(sabīja)*[1] or "extrovertive" type of *samādhi,* is termed *saṃprajñāta-samādhi*[2] and constitutes a range of ecstatic experiences that have an objective "prop" *(ālambana)* with which the mind becomes identified and "united" and which are associated with yogic insight *(prajñā)*. The second kind, what can be called the "objectless" or "introvertive" type of *samādhi,* is termed *asaṃprajñāta,*[3] the "acognitive"[4] or rather supracognitive and "seedless" *(nirbīja) samādhi*. It is acognitive in that there is no longer any cognition of authentic identity *(puruṣa)* as existing in *prakṛti,* no longer *prakṛti*'s misidentification with *puruṣa*. As *saṃprajñāta* explicitly denotes illuminated yogic experiences that take place "outside of" or are "external to" *puruṣa*-realization, I will refer to it as ecstasy.[5] *Asaṃprajñāta* denotes the *puruṣa* being left "alone" by itself—the confused identity in the condition of *saṃyoga* having been discarded. The yogin is left with nothing more to experience or know for the sake of "liberation." I will refer to it as enstasy. Eliade renders the term rather conveniently as enstasis "without [mental or objective] support."[6] The main concern in the present chapter is with *saṃprajñāta-samādhi:*

those stages in Yoga where the yogin, as it were, comes to recognize more subtle forms of prakṛtic identity in a self-reflexive manner through the process of the subtilization of knowledge or sattvification of the mind, that is, through states of self-reflection. *Asaṃprajñāta,* however, transcends self-reflexive knowledge, that is, it is a transmental or transconceptual state of identity.

A general definition of *saṃprajñāta* is based on the derivations of the word from: (1) *"sam,"* meaning "together," "altogether," and as a preposition or prefix to verbs and verbal derivatives it can express "conjunction," "thoroughness," "intensity," "union."[7] (2) *"pra,"* a preposition meaning "before," "forward," in front," "forth";[8] the preposition *"pra"* joins with (3) *jñāta,* "known . . . perceived, understood" (from the verb root *jñā,* "to know")[9] to form *saṃprajñāta*. Some of the meanings for *saṃprajñāta* are: "distinguished, discerned, known accurately [as in the] Yoga-Sūtra."[10] *Saṃprajñāta* refers to the *samādhi* of cognition wherein one has the consciousness of an object or mental content.

In his *Bhāṣya,* Vyāsa introduces the *sūtra* on *saṃprajñāta-samādhi* by asking: "How is the *samādhi* defined which is cognitive and which follows when the [misidentification with] the modifications (mental processes) of the mind has ceased by the two means [*abhyāsa* and *vairāgya*]?"[11] Earlier (*YB* I.1) Vyāsa stated that "Yoga is *samādhi*." Now the specifics of that definition are being described. Vijñāna Bhikṣu qualifies the above statement by Vyāsa (n. 11), correctly explaining that cognitive *samādhi* refers to a stage of practice where the yogin has brought the rajasic and tamasic *vṛtti*s under "control."[12] This reinforces and clarifies the traditional understanding in classical Yoga that it is only in the supracognitive *samādhi* *(asaṃprajñāta)* that all the *vṛtti*s, including the sattvic ones, are mastered[13] and that any attachment to or soteriological dependence on *vṛtti* is finally overcome. *Puruṣa*—no longer misconceived as being attached to or dependent on knowledge and enjoyment (mind-*sattva*) as had previously been the case in the process of "cessation" *(nirodha)*—is "left alone" in its self-effulgent nature as the ever-free knower.

The stages of *saṃprajñāta-samādhi* are highlighted by Patañjali in *Yoga-Sūtra* I.17. He writes: "*Saṃprajñāta* [arises] from association with [the forms of] cogitation—i.e., having verbal association *(vitarka),* reflection *(vicāra),* joy *(ānanda),* and I-am-ness *(asmitā)*."[14] Vyāsa's commentary runs as follows:

> The mind's experience of a "gross" object of support/contemplation [in *samādhi*] is "cogitation." It is "reflection" when the object of support is subtle. "Joy" means delight. "I-am-ness" is the perception of the essential, unified nature of self. Of these [four forms of cognitive *samādhi*], the first

> *samādhi*—with "cogitation"—is associated with all four. The second one—with "reflection"—is without the verbal associations of the first. The third one—with associations of "joy"—is without the subtle associations of the second. The fourth, "I-am-ness" only, is without the association of joy. All these kinds of *samādhi* are with supportive objects/content.[15]

Thus the *Bhāṣya* proposes the following schema to understand the order of the four forms of cognitive *samādhi:*

1. *Vitarka* ("cogitation") actually includes all the other subsequent forms also, namely *vicāra, ānanda,* and *asmitā.*
2. *Vicāra* ("reflection") is without *vitarka* but also includes *ānanda* and *asmitā.*
3. *Ānanda* ("joy") is without *vitarka* and *vicāra* but includes *asmitā.*
4. *Asmitā* ("I-am-ness") is without *vitarka, vicāra,* and *ānanda.*

Feuerstein rightly comments that the systematic schema of Vyāsa "is a beautiful illustration of the *sat-kārya* axiom according to which the effect is preexistent in its cause. In this particular case, the lowest degree of . . . realization contains *in posse* the . . . cognitive elements typical of the higher forms [of cognitive *samādhi.*]"[16] In Yoga, contemplation on each "effect" leads to the direct perception *(sākṣātkāra)*[17] of the form and nature of that "effect."

The reason for the initial position of *vitarka-samādhi* in *Yoga-Sūtra* I.17 is given by Vācaspati Miśra. He writes:

> Just as an archer, when a beginner, pierces first only a gross and afterwards a subtle target, so the yogin, when a beginner, has direct experience merely of some gross object of concentration made up of the five gross elements, [such as] the Four Armed [i.e., Viṣṇu], and afterwards a subtle object. So with regard to the object of the mind the experience becomes a subtle one. Meditation has for its sphere of action the causes of the gross phenomena, the subtle elements, the five *tanmātra*s, the manifested and the unmanifested essence of matter *[prakṛti].*[18]

The experiences to be realized in the four stages of *saṃprajñāta* exist in everyone in potential form. The mind is not normally prepared to enter the subtler stages at once—at least it is not the common experience. It is not likely that an average practitioner could suddenly leap to the highest state of *samādhi* and understand the processes of the intermediate states as part of such an instantaneous development. If a development of this nature should normally occur, there would be no need for the order as described by Patañjali. As a rule, and as Vācaspati implies (see n. 18 above), only by starting from the grosser objects does the mind gradually harmonize or unite with the subtlest and settle there. Vijñāna Bhikṣu affirms that this application by stages is, however, only a general rule, "since by the grace of *īśvara* or by the grace of the enlightened teacher *(sad-guru),* [the yogin] finds his or her mind capable of abiding in the subtle stages at the very beginning [of practice]. Then the previous lower stages need not be practiced by the one desirous of liberation, [for this would be] a waste of time."[19]

SAMĀDHI: THE HEART OF PATAÑJALI'S SOTERIOLOGICAL METHODOLOGY

Throughout the *Yoga-Sūtra,* Patañjali's central concern is how to attain a knowing-oneness that is not merely a mental activity or self-reflective state of mind, but rather involves a tacit recognition, an uncompromising identity as the ever-free, unmodified *purusa.* Identity as *purusa,* recognizing one's true Self as pure, nonfragmented consciousness, is the primary concern in Yoga practice, wherein the seer is established in its authentic form (*YS* I.3): the aloneness of "seeing" (*YS* II.25). Without this realization, as Patañjali says, we can never be certain we are knowing other "things" clearly and not merely seeing "things" in a distorted manner (through an impure mind) that colors our perception and experience of them. In *samādhi,* contemplation on and unification with the objects of experience is not for its own sake but provides insight *(prajñā)* that leads to liberation. The main purpose of Patañjali's detailed analysis of four stages of cognitive *samādhi* is to help the yogin or "knower" who, having become sensitive "like an eyeball"[20] to the presence of pain and dissatisfaction within the mind and in the world at large, desires to be liberated from such suffering and its cause—*samyoga*—which arises from ignorance *(avidyā).*

The intent of the *Yoga-Sūtra* is primarily soteriological: How do we "attain" identity as *purusa* and "know" that clearly? The means offered by Patañjali can be understood to proceed through an analysis of different stages or levels of insight *(prajñā)* expressing a "deeper" and "clearer" understanding of oneself and the world. Through yogic ecstasy *(samprajñāta)* our attention is led to four related though distinct kinds of insight and associations with self ultimately leading, in the case of the discernment of *purusa (purusa-khyāti),* to enstasy or realization of *purusa.*

What then is the purpose of the various associations, identifications, and levels of self-understanding attained in *samprajñāta-samādhi?* It is to fulfill the soteriological purpose described in *Yoga-Sūtra* I.15–16: to develop a knowledge or consciousness of freedom, mastery, nonenslavement, implying detachment or dispassion *(vairāgya)* toward each level of identification with the objects of experience "either seen or heard of" culminating in a superior form of dispassion (*YS* I.16) toward the manifest and unmanifest existence of the *guṇa*s. At each stage of *samādhi* one may have a "conviction" that the next subtler level of experience is purer, more permanent, more joyful, and a closer "likeness" or resemblance to the real nature of *puruṣa*. However, by means of direct experience *(sākṣātkāra)* and insight *(prajñā)* the yogin discovers that the purity or virtues attained are only relative, at best derived from *sattva-guṇa*—the finest constituent of *prakṛti*. Each level of unification or identification that takes place in *samādhi* is successively found to be attended by or prone to affliction *(kleśa),* that is, mistaken identity and invariable dissatisfaction *(duḥkha)* rooted in spiritual ignorance *(avidyā)* and generating further karmic residue *(karmāśaya)*. The identifications or states of unity attained in *samādhi* are expedients to the realization of authentic identity *(puruṣa)*. Yet these high-level yogic experiences may in turn be misappropriated or self-referenced, claimed by an I-sense or egoity that is not *puruṣa,* and lead to further misidentification, confusion, and dissatisfaction. Dispassion toward all experiences in *samādhi* liberates the yogin from further attachment to the results or "fruit" attained through practice *(abhyāsa)*. Practice keeps the process of Yoga *(nirodha)* in a working condition and allows for subtler realizations and perceptions to take place.

According to *Yoga-Sūtra* II.4[21] the *kleśa*s exist in various states. They can be:

1. "Dormant" *(prasupta),* that is, exist in the form of latent impressions *(saṃskāra*s*)*[22] in the potential condition as a seed *(bīja),*[23] awakening when they confront their objects and generating various afflicted forms of psychomental activity;
2. "Attenuated" *(tanu),* that is temporarily prevented from taking effect by way of cultivation of their opposite (*pratipakṣa-bhāvana, YS* II.33) or other yogic techniques;[24]
3. "Interrupted" *(vicchinna),* which is the case when one kind of *kleśa* (e.g., attachment or *rāga*) in the form of desire temporarily blocks the operation of another (e.g., anger as associated with aversion, *dveṣa);*[25]
4. "Aroused" *(udāra),* meaning "fully active," in that "what possesses the mind in regard to an object is called aroused."[26]

According to Patañjali (*YS* II.2),[27] it is the purpose of *kriyā-yoga* to achieve the attenuation of these afflictions and bring about the cultivation of *samādhi.*

Vyāsa also declares that whatever is given form or influenced by spiritual ignorance, "that the afflictions inhere in. They are felt at the time of deluded apprehension, thought or ideas; when ignorance dwindles, they dwindle accordingly."[28] Through *samādhi* the mind is borne on toward the discriminative discernment *(vivekakhyāti):* the knowledge that *sattva* and *puruṣa* are different.[29] However, ego-centered apprehensions, intentions, or ideas such as self-appropriated notions of identity (e.g., "I-am-ness" or "It is mine") may continue to arise from the activation of previous *saṃskāras*[30] whose seed-power or cause in the form of the afflictions gradually fades away.[31] Patañjali informs us that the overcoming or abandonment of this self-centered mentality or thinking is like that of the afflictions,[32] a process referred to as *pratiprasava* (*YS* II.10 and IV.34): the "return" to the state of equilibrium or nonafflicted identity. Just as the afflictions are reduced to the condition of "scorched seed" (i.e., are made obsolete) through unfaltering discriminative discernment,[33] so the previous *saṃskāras*, having become "seeds" scorched by the fire of knowledge, can no longer generate attachment to ideas[34] or fixed notions of self rooted in ignorance.

Viewed from within the pedagogical context of the Yoga tradition, Patañjali emphasizes that a necessary detachment or dispassionate attitude toward each successive experience in the practice of *samādhi* must develop for the yogin. Simply perfecting a particular level of realization in *samādhi* and remaining at that level of understanding is not conducive to furthering one's spiritual growth. It is only when a complete detachment or dispassion *(vairāgya)* develops toward the present experience that the next step can be taken involving a yet subtler object of contemplation and support.

Since the mind must be purified and illuminated, and therefore brought to a gradual refinement or subtilization of understanding through the sattvification of consciousness, it must "move along" the scale of the various evolutes of *prakṛti* until it reaches an identification with the subtlest, finest possible state. Liberation lies in our becoming disentangled from the misidentification with the objects of experience, a form of identification involving a misguided sense of relation with the objects of experience and the world—understood in terms of "my" objects, "my" attainments or "my" world—that merely perpetuates a self-serving mentality. All the objects, including mental content, are evolutes, transformations or actualizations of *prakṛti.* If bondage and suffering are due to an enslavement to the *vyutthāna* mode or centrifugal tendency of consciousness—of mistaken identity and self-fragmentation, freedom can take place through a counterprocess of the *nirodha* mode or centripetalization of consciousness, an interiorization and centering of consciousness that transcends and heals the fractured consciousness of self, thereby correcting our mistaken identity. The process of *nirodha* can be broadly conceived as a de-identification with[35] and final dispassion toward the "seeable" *(dṛśya)* starting from grosser forms of manifestation (i.e., physical objects) up to and including unmanifest *prakṛti.* Through the process of "cessation" one can realize that *puruṣa* is distinguishable from everything with which one had been misidentified and through which self-identity had become shaped by the seeable in one way or another. The sattvification and ultimate liberation of consciousness has to be effected voluntarily by the yogin's efforts[36] and, as the pedagogical context of Yoga ascertains, under the guidance of a spiritual preceptor *(guru)* or perhaps through devotional surrender or dedication to *īśvara.*

The twenty-four principles *(tattvas)* with which the mind may identify and unite are divided fourfold by Patañjali. Patañjali's model[37] can be understood to include the following:

1. The "Particularized" composed of the sixteen *viśeṣas*—distinct, specific forms of *prakṛti* comprising : *(a)* the five gross elements *(bhūtas),* namely: earth, water, fire, air, space; *(b)* the five action organs or conative senses: hands, feet, voice, evacuation, and generation; *(c)* the five sense organs or cognitive senses: smell, taste, sight, touch, and sound; *(d)* the mind-organ *(manas).*
2. The "Unparticularized" or six *aviśeṣas*, the general material causes of the *viśeṣas*, namely: *(a)* the five subtle elements *(tanmātras)* that produce the five gross elements; and *(b) asmitā-mātra,* pure I-am-ness or ego *(ahaṃkāra),* the identifying or self-referencing principle by which the conflated self-identity of *puruṣa* and *prakṛti* or root composite sentience *(asmitā)* begins to identify itself as such-and-such a being particularizing itself into individual selves ("I's") or persons.
3. *Liṅga-mātra,* the "Designator" or first manifestation of the presence of *prakṛti,* referring to the subtlest evolute, *mahat* or the "great (self)" *(mahān ātmā),* which is also a synonym for the *buddhi.* This principle is the receptacle for the reflected consciousness of *puruṣa,* the point where a material evolute first appears to "unite" with *puruṣa* producing *asmitā*, "I-am-ness" (*YS* II.6), the root composite sentience not as yet self-conscious as a particular "I." It is at this junction or interface where *puruṣa* and the mind "meet" that our notion of person takes root and develops.

4. *Aliṅga,* the "Unmanifest," "Undifferentiate," or transcendent core of *prakṛti,* not manifest *(avyakta)* as the phenomena of the universe.

In cognitive *samādhi* the above states can act as the "objects" of experience and can be utilized as supportive factors for the aspiring yogin. This type of *samādhi* is based on the constitution of the empirical personality consisting of the mind (*citta,* which includes, as we have seen, *buddhi, ahaṃkāra,* and *manas*), the subtle elements, the action and sense organs, and the gross elements.

In the context of Yoga praxis, the cosmogonic model of Patañjali is not meant as a purely speculative construction. Rather, it is "a mixture of a priori theorizing and a posteriori explanation of concrete yogic experiences" (see n. 38 below) and, moreover, is to be used as a heuristic device for properly orienting the yogin on "his [her] inner odyssey."[38] As stated previously, this study understands Patañjali's metaphysical schematic as having been abstracted from yogic experience, whereas in classical Sāṃkhya it appears that all experiences are fitted into a metaphysical system that at the highest level posits a radical duality or severance between *puruṣa* and *prakṛti.* The model in Yoga is primarily a practical map comprised of contemplative directives that engage one in the process of sattvification or meditative interiorization, and realization of intrinsic identity. Secondarily, the model acts as a descriptive account of the processes of manifestation and actualization of *prakṛti.*[39] Thus, the yogin is progressively led toward the ultimate realization of *puruṣa* via a scheme not unlike that which is portrayed in the Upaniṣads and which denotes more and more causally subtle grades of self-understanding, identity, and being.[40] Eventually the yogin transcends the hierarchy of cognitive possibilities provided by *prakṛti* and becomes established in the identity of the knower, *puruṣa* alone.

Since the various levels of cognitive *samādhi* lead from the identification with grosser objects or content (as effects) to the identification with subtler objects or content (as causes), the lower-level *samādhi*s include (in potential) the subtler levels but at each level any attachment to the former and less subtle identification and experience is transcended. When the *vṛtti*s concerning any effect are mastered in the process of *nirodha,* the mind's "doors" of perception open to the material and efficient cause of that effect. The efficient cause does not actuate the objects or content of *prakṛti* but removes obstacles to their realization[41] as causally subtler grades of identification accompanied by progressively more subtle (sattvic) levels of self-understanding and cognitive clarity. By developing the capacity to locate, identify with, and be detached from more refined (and less afflicted) states of the reflected consciousness of *puruṣa,* the yogin gradually diminishes the impurities or afflictions *(kleśas)* within the mind. The result is an increasing "light" of *sattva*-knowledge or insight *(prajñā)* and refinement of experience that leads to discriminative discernment *(vivekakhyāti).*[42]

As a method, and when practiced together with concentration and meditation, *samādhi* refers to one of the disciplines used to attain the highest levels of yogic interiorization or constraint *(saṃyama).* In regards to content, cognitive *samādhi* refers to the ecstatic states of consciousness of the yogin who is yet dependent on objects *(prakṛti),* and to the types of knowledge and levels of self-understanding unfolded through its practice.[43] Like *nirodha,* the term *samādhi* alludes to both a *process* of purification and illumination and a *state* of consciousness and self-identity. In fact, the yogic insight *(prajñā)* gained from the mastery attained in the practice of *saṃyama*[44] can be none other than the full-depth of cognitive *samādhi,* that is, *nirvicāra-samādhi.*[45] The success of the method or practice presupposes a sattvified state of awareness and understanding. Liberating knowledge cannot be acquired, produced, or manufactured by the mind. Mechanical, repetitive approaches to practice involving the use of yogic technique cannot bring about or acquire insight or the desired goal of liberated selfhood. According to Yoga philosophy, insight already exists in the mind as a potential within nature *(prakṛti)* in the form of *sattva*-intelligence. Through the "beginningless" accumulation of the sedimentation of ignorance in the mind, liberating knowledge is covered over, concealed from consciousness. However, by means of the attenuation of the afflicted condition of the mind, insight and "goodness"—the sattvic nature of consciousness—is gradually revealed as being intrinsic to the mind. To repeat from an earlier chapter (3), it is the presence of *puruṣa* and its reflected "light" in the mind *(citta)* that makes the functioning of consciousness in the mind, including cognition, possible.

Cognitive *samādhi* obstructs the recurring manifestation of the afflictions in the form of *rajas* and *tamas* while simultaneously aiding in the direct experience of the pure *sattva* of the mind as being distinct from the *puruṣa. Samādhi* uncovers fully the light of *sattva* through which our misconceived identity and distorted cognition or error *(viparyaya)* dissolves and clear knowledge *(jñāna)* or insight *(prajñā)* is revealed. All barriers to the realization of *puruṣa* are thus removed.

While through ordinary perception *(pratyakṣa)* a tangible object can be seen, experienced, thought of, contemplated, yet its material cause may not be conscious, known, or obvious. Observing a clay pot, for example, one normally may not think of what the clay pot is made of. But when knowledge of the underlying nature of the pot (i.e., as clay) reaches a definite clarity or "fullness," the clay substance—the real "stuff" of the pot—becomes, as it were, more "real" or "permanent" and the pot is perceived as a subsidiary of the clay. A clay pot breaks easily; its durability and stability is minimal compared to that of its cause, the clay. Using a clay pot and its material cause *(upādāna)* as an analogy, we can say that it is for the above reason that the subtler objects in the practice of *samādhi* lead to a greater and more lasting stability and one-pointedness of mind. As the mind focuses on the normally experienced, conventional nature of an object, it slowly transcends its tangible or extrinsic nature and grasps the unobvious, the cause or intrinsic nature and value that was previously not known, seen, or experienced. In Yoga, the identification with the modification *(vṛtti)* of the effect is, through the process of *nirodha,* understood, mastered, and transcended, thereby disclosing the form *(vṛtti)* of its cause. The identification with *vṛtti* may take the form of a *pratyaya—pratyaya* referring to the significance or content of a *vṛtti* including fixed, egoic notions of self and identity that are cemented or crystallized in the mind (see discussion on *YS* I.41 below). Because a cause is always subtler, less tangible, and is located deeper within the mind-processes—closer, as it were, to the light of *puruṣa*—the next step in the practice of *samādhi* is invariably subtler. Thus, the process of the sattvification of the mind that leads the attention of the yogin from the grosser objects or content to the more subtle, and effects to causes, continues until the yogin reaches the most refined state of understanding and experience. This is the meaning of progress in cognitive *samādhi.* When the mind becomes as "unified" with the object as a red-hot ball of iron is with fire[46] (where there is no perceivable difference between the fire and the ball of iron), the former (familiar) ground is superseded and the next exercise to gain the yet subtler, finer ground begins.

The process of *samādhi* and its application in stages through *saṃyama* (*YS* III.6) leading to the progressive attainment of yogic insight does not entail an ontological negation or cessation of the "seeable," nor does it entail a denial, withdrawal, or "escape" from the phenomenal world. Rather *samādhi* suggests a fullness, completion, and transcendence of experience and its effects in the form of misidentification and attachment at each stage of practice. In *samādhi* transcendence implies a knowledge of mastery *(vaśīkāra),*[47] a dispassion toward, not a denial of or isolation from relative existence, thereby dispensing with the empirical *limitations* or prakṛtic *barriers* to the realization of *puruṣa*. What is involved here is not only a focusing of attention on a subtler object or rising to a higher realm that includes universalist values such as an ethical universal of purity or insight, but a "rising above" ("transcend" is from the Latin *trans* + *scandere:* to climb over or rise above) our normal perception and relation to the "given"—the "see-able" or experienced "object"—that allows the possibility of leverage over it, of changing the perception and relation to that "given." Transcendence involves a gradual shedding of the layers of ignorance and misidentification, the mental conditioning of *cittavṛtti.* What is transcended in Yoga is one's identity as it is given shape and functions within the framework of a bifurcation between self and world rooted within *prakṛti,* a consciousness of self that ineluctably holds itself to be separate from, yet craves satisfaction through, the objects of experience. The yogin becomes detached from the world of *saṃyoga* and its polarization of self and world—a subject-object dichotomy that governs and defines our self-identity as egoity. The failure-to-see, that is, the failure to distinguish between the true experiencer *(puruṣa)* and what is experienced, comes to an end and along with it the misidentification or affliction that had been responsible for generating a "mental self out of delusion" (*YB* II.6) is dispelled from consciousness.

I have noted in the last chapter that the practice of *samādhi* is not merely the concentration on an object or idea, nor is it getting lost in self-hypnotism. Nor has it to do with a relapse into unconsciousness or "drug-induced" experiences.[48] Having been released from its rajasic and tamasic functioning, the mind in the experience of *samādhi* is not made dull, inactive, incapacitated, thoughtless, or unconscious. *Samādhi* is accompanied by acute "wakefulness," alertness, and mental lucidity, in fact, an overcoming of the egoic limitations of consciousness. The possibility for a "trans-egoic" or an "egoless knowing" (as Yoga claims takes place in the state of *samādhi*) was rejected for instance by the twentieth-century psychologist C. G. Jung, who felt that the yogic claim to a deepening and fullness of knowledge and consciousness through ego-transcendence was a psychological impossibility. A total overcoming of ego-identity would result, Jung argued, in a state of unconsciousness, not in a perfected state of self-awareness. In fact, Jung held the opinion that Yoga technique was an exercise of the conscious ego that served to *increase* the ego's hold on consciousness.[49] In disagreement with Jung, our study suggests that the redirecting of attention through the yogic practices of concentration *(dhāraṇā),* meditation *(dhyāna),* and "unification" *(samādhi)* serves to disengage consciousness from egoic patterns of identification, thereby opening up consciousness to subtler levels of perception, understanding, and identity. Through meditative discipline in Yoga the mind can be purified and liberated from all mistaken identity of self, resulting in the illumination of consciousness for the yogin.

The essence of cognitive *samādhi* is the centering of our diversified, fractured being leading at its most profound or advanced level into an organic and spiritual reunification of our individuated sense of self with the universal matrix *(mahat)* of manifest *prakṛti. Prakṛti,* it is to be remembered, while being a multidimensional principle of existence, is yet in essence of one "piece." The main task of the yogin lies in the gradual overcoming of the power of the emerging *(vyutthāna)* ego-consciousness or extrinsic identity of selfhood and the simultaneous cultivation of the sattvification process in *nirodha* that counteracts the powerful tendency of human consciousness to become attached to and utterly shaped by the objects of experience. *Yoga-Sūtra* III.11 explains that the mind has two basic characteristics to which it conforms: (1) dispersiveness or the tendency of attention to be drawn into all-objectivity, and (2) one-pointedness.[50] The mind can become concentrated through the dwindling of its dispersive predispositions generated by the forces of attachment *(rāga)* and aversion *(dveṣa)* and the subsequent cultivation of one-pointedness wherein the transformation *(pariṇāma)* termed "ecstasy" (or "unification" in cognitive *samādhi*) takes place. At this concentrated stage the mind is favorably disposed toward illuminating insight and dispassion—qualities of its inherent sattvic nature—as the distractions *(vikṣepa)* or obstacles (*antarāya, YS* I.30) to such illumination are rendered inoperative. In *Yoga-Sūtra* III.12 Patañjali tells us, "Hence again, when there is similarity between the arising and the quieted (subsided) ideas, there is the transformation *(pariṇāma)* of one-pointedness *(ekāgratā)* of the mind."[51] In *samādhi* the mind—"like a precious jewel" (*YS* I.41: see discussion in next section)—equally assumes the form of both the subsiding and then the arising idea during the period in which *samādhi* takes place. The transformation *(pariṇāma)* that has taken place in the mind possessing this particular quality is referred to as "one-pointedness" *(ekāgratā)*.[52] During this period of *samādhi* the mind retains its state of one-pointedness whether an idea has subsided or another idea arises. This state of one-pointedness is the basis for yogic perception *(yogi-pratyakṣa)*. Both of the above transformations can be seen as a change in form (*dharma,* see discussion on page 61) or quality of the mind implying an increasing steadiness and sattvification of consciousness.

It could be argued that the levels of *samādhi* are more or less common to other schools of Yoga or Hindu thought. Yet the analysis of *samādhi* given by Patañjali, from the point of view of the depths of human existence, is centrally important and more illuminating than many of the others. In order to know the true nature of things, Patañjali tells us in no uncertain terms that it is necessary to experience states of *samādhi* and attain greater epistemic "oneness" with our objects of experience. Why, might we ask, is this "oneness" necessary in order to know the true nature of things? The answer Patañjali gives is that, otherwise, hindrances in the form of impurities (i.e., the afflictions) are bound to get in our way, to come between us, as knowers, and what we are trying to know. These hindrances, impediments to "oneness," can be seen to come from three places (*YS* I.41): (i) the nature of the knower or grasper *(grahītṛ);* (ii) the nature of what is being known or grasped *(grāhya);* and (iii) the nature of the medium between these two, the act of knowing or grasping *(grahaṇa)*.[53] Ian Kesarcodi-Watson aptly observes:

> If I perceive things through inner or outer veils—mental ones like biases, preconceivings, categories, memories; or physical ones like defective sense-organs—I will not perceive things properly. Or if these things do not present themselves properly to me, or are not allowed to present their proper selves by something intervening, like smog or a hessian screen, again, it will not be their true nature that I will perceive.[54]

How do we purge ourselves and situations of the preceding kinds of unclearness? Numerous questions may arise which can lead one to doubt the possibility for the kind of epistemic clarity Yoga is talking about. For example, one could ask: Is the world as object(s) in some essential sense only a construct? Is all knowledge radically interpretive? Is every act of perception and cognition contingent, mediated, situated, contextual, theory-bound? Is what one knows and experiences to an indeterminate extent a projection? To these questions and others like it Patañjali would reply with a final, emphatic "No." Human cognition is not so limited although, as we have seen, Patañjali admits that there are obstructions to clear "seeing," obstructions that, however, *can be removed, discarded or overcome* through yogic discipline. Kesarcodi-Watson makes the following incisive comment:

> In the end Patañjali declares, and I think rightly, that we escape these problems by being at-one-with the things we seek to know. Without this oneness we never can be quite sure that it is the *svarūpa* [true form/nature] of the thing we are acquainted with, and not some mere surrogate. This is, indeed, the central problem of perception. Many, especially in Western thought, have counselled despair; or fled to one or another of several forms

> of Idealism. Very few have had the courage to claim that we really can contact *svarūpas*. Yet this is what Patañjali does in his doctrine, or doctrines of *samādhi*.[55]

Even though the mind has the capacity for direct knowledge of things, or to register clear insight into the nature of our objects or conditions of experience, it fails to do so because of the afflictions *(kleśas)* and their intervening processes which generate misidentification with mental content or the objects of perception (i.e., through the *vṛtti*-generating complex). Only when their (i.e., the afflictions) interruption is finally prevented through the clarity attained in *samādhi* does the full realization *(sākṣātkāra)* of the objects of perception or contemplation occur. In Yoga, unmediated perception is possible and such clarity allows for insight into the true nature of any object. This is the direct perception of the yogin *(yogi-pratyakṣa)*. In Yoga philosophy these finer states of perception arise in *saṃprajñāta* and not in the "lower" concentrations (the *cittaparikarmas*, *YS* I.33–39), where the totality of the object of concentration cannot be fully grasped. Through the concept of *samādhi* Yoga has worked out the epistemological presuppositions necessary in order to connect the interiority of the inner viewer (observer) with the interiority of the objects viewed (observed).

In spite of the central role given it in the process of liberation in Yoga, one must guard against mistaking higher perception as an end in itself. It is not that the yogin's direct perception of a grosser object in *samādhi* automatically leads to the finer ground of a subtler object. A material object or mental content cannot in itself bring about spiritual realization or ego-transcendence. In perception only a *vṛtti* is generated. One must also develop a detachment or dispassion toward that *vṛtti* of perception. Insight into the true nature and form *(svarūpa)* of an object in *samādhi* only leads to the powers *(siddhis)* that are described in the third chapter (entitled the *Vibhūti-Pāda*) of the *Yoga-Sūtra*. The *Yoga-Sūtra* posits an ultimate goal *(kaivalya)* of Yoga that is decidedly not personal knowledge or power. The practice of *saṃyama* has also a soteriological purpose. Patañjali and Vyāsa view yogic power as instrumental to the attainment of *kaivalya,* but also as being without intrinsic value. Citing Adolf Janácek, C. Pensa points out that the powers in Yoga are presumed to be "a sign of correct Yoga procedure"[56] but are not the true aim of Yoga. G. Feuerstein correctly avers:

> the special gifts acquired through the practice of constraint *[saṃyama]* cannot possibly be stamped as unwanted side-effects which inevitably block the yogin's path to Self-realization. . . . The danger lies not in the extraordinary insight or powers which the practice of constraint is said to yield,

> but in the yogin's attitude towards them. For, like any form of knowledge or power, these super-normal results can be misused or become ends in themselves. The popular opinion that these yogic abilities are not part of the path to Self-realization is demonstrably wrong.[57]

According to *Yoga-Sūtra* III.37 certain supernormal powers—called *prātibha* (understood in *Yoga-Sūtra* III.36 as "vividness" or "intuitive illumination" in regard to hearing, touching or sensing, sight, taste, and smell)[58]—are to be looked upon as "impediments to *samādhi* but perfections in the state of extroversion or emergence *(vyutthāna)*."[59] These powers, which can be understood as a natural byproduct of the yogin's meditative practice, are accomplishments only from the point of view of the egoic consciousness. Indulging in them only serves to inflate the ego and prevents spiritual growth precisely because the deployment of them presupposes that we invest our attention in the sensorial world and the desire for power or control over it (reinforcing the subject-object duality within *prakṛti* that Yoga seeks to overcome). The powers are made available or accessed by means of an ascension through the *tattva*s (principles of existence) as enumerated in Sāṃkhya. The enhanced abilities, for example, to observe the subtle elements *(tanmātra*s*)* giving rise to the gross elements *(bhūta*s*)*—which is the import of *Yoga-Sūtra* III.36 and clearly follows the Sāṃkhyan scheme[60]—need not be a problem in Yoga. It is rather one's attachment to these powers or selfish manipulation of them that inevitably creates difficulties and confusion for oneself and others. Any clinging to or misappropriation of power means that we reinforce the habit of assuming we are ego-personalities rather than *puruṣa*. Clearly then the powers are detrimental if one had no higher goal or aspiration. On the other hand they can be supportive of the true "goal" of Yoga: "aloneness" *(kaivalya)*. *Siddhi*s can be understood as natural by-products or "fruits" of a disciplined mind properly cultivated in concentration, meditation, and *samādhi* and not utilized for selfish gain or control. The yogin is capable, through *saṃyama,* to attain a mastery over the elements (*bhūta*s, *YS* III.44) and develop the set of eight powers: of becoming minute, perfection of the body, and so on, (as mentioned in *YS* III.45 and *YB* III.45). It is noteworthy that the powers can be read as a progression from mastery of the elements, to mastery of the sense organs (*YS* III.47), mastery of the source of the manifest (*pradhāna, YS* III.48), and sovereignty over (i.e., non-enslavement to) all states of existence, as well as knowledge of all (*YS* III.49). Yet, in the final analysis, there is the need for a detachment or dispassion toward all power and knowledge (as *YS* III.50 clearly indicates, see n. 122 in chapter 4) in order for the liberated state of "aloneness" to arise. Even the "supreme" knowledge and power arising from the purified realm of the *guṇa*s can be no substitute for the immortal knower, *puruṣa.*[61] Vyāsa boldly advocates that although great powers can be accessed through Yoga, the true yogin does not venture to transgress the natural laws of *prakṛti.*[62] Patañjali was not opposed to the right use of *siddhi*s—which could serve to bring about a more insightful understanding of oneself and the cosmos—or else he would not have dedicated the entire third chapter of his work to these manifestations of power *(vibhūti*s*)*. Vyāsa maintains that the realization of the purity of *puruṣa* and the culminating stage of liberated "aloneness" *(kaivalya)* can take place whether the yogin has acquired power (that is, the powers or *siddhi*s) or not; for when the seed of all affliction has been "burned up" or purified out of the mind, the yogin has no further dependence on knowledge.[63]

AN ANALYSIS OF *YOGA-SŪTRA* I.41

When the modifications (*vṛtti*s) of the mind have diminished or subsided through practice *(abhyāsa)* and dispassion *(vairāgya)*,[64] the "barriers" between the mind and the object dissolve and both "coincide." This process is elucidated by Patañjali in *Yoga-Sūtra* I.41 as follows: " [The steadied mind] of diminished modifications, like a precious (flawless) jewel assuming the color (i.e., respective qualities) of the grasper, grasping, or grasped, has unification."[65] This *sūtra* describes the basic processes and mechanism of any form of cognitive *samādhi.* The term *samāpatti* has been translated as: "balanced-state,"[66] "engrossment,"[67] "transformation,"[68] "thought transformation,"[69] "illumination,"[70] "complete identity,"[71] "consummation,"[72] "Zusammenfallen,"[73] "coincidence,"[74] "intentional identity,"[75] "identification-in-samādhi,"[76] "unity."[77] According to Monier-Williams, *samāpatti* means "coming together, meeting, encountering."[78] In the context of the *Yoga-Sūtra, samāpatti* (herein translated as "unification") denotes the proficiency, accomplishment, and transmutation of the mind *(citta)* that takes place in *samādhi*. More specifically, *samāpatti* is the insight *(prajñā)* thus gained as derived from *saṃprajñāta* (*YS* I.17) signifying that the mind "breaks into" and coincides with the sphere of the "object" grasped, unifies or fuses with it, and reveals its innermost nature or "essence." This process of "unification" is elaborated upon by way of an example. Vyāsa writes:

> The analogy is given of a precious jewel. As a crystal, according to the things set near it, becomes tinged with their colors and appears to take on

> their respective forms, so the mind is colored by the object of contemplation, and through uniting with the object appears in the form of the object.[79]

Having extinguished, through practice and dispassion, the external impurities of the mind, the objects or supportive factors *(ālambana)* can more clearly and fully reflect in the mind and an identification or unification occurs. In the above analogy, both the crystal and the colored object—although they persist in actually remaining two separate, distinct "entities"—appear, from the moment in which the crystal is placed near the object, as a single thing: a colored crystal. Similarly, the mind and the object in *samādhi* are two different prakṛtic states that at the moment of the identification appear in the experience of the yogin *as if* they are the same "thing" (ontologically) due to the total absorption of the mind in the object. As the crystal does not undergo any permanent modification by having been colored by the object, likewise the mind, as the underlying "*dharma*-holder" *(dharmin)* of consciousness, is not intrinsically altered by being absorbed in, that is, assuming the form or characteristic *(dharma)* of, the object.

Patañjali and the Yoga school look upon the "one mind" (*cittam-ekam, YS* IV.5) as the primary "state" or "*dharma*-holder" *(dharmin)* that remains constant (as pure unblemished *sattva*) throughout the transformations *(pariṇāma)* that occur in ordinary life. All impressions (*saṃskāra*s, whether of a *vyutthāna* or a *nirodha* nature—*YS* III.9) and thought constructs/ideas/intentions (*pratyaya*—*YS* III.12) are considered as forms or characteristics *(dharma)* of the mind. Applying the *satkāryavāda* doctrine—that change affects only the form of a thing, not its underlying "substance"—we have seen how the three basic forms or states of an object, namely: its "subsided" *(śānta)* or past aspect, its "arisen" *(udita)* or present aspect, and its "undetermined" *(avyapadeśya)* or future aspect are related to the same *dharmin* that is constantly present, yet different from (i.e., is not to be reduced to), its forms or modifications.[80] For example, the mind is not annihilated or negated when the mental processes diminish or subside. Hence, throughout the changing modes of identity brought about by the impressions and mental processes, the mind does not intrinsically lose its finest, essential nature as pure *sattva* (i.e., clarity, knowledge) that reflects the pure light of *puruṣa*. Without the presence of this reflected illumination of *puruṣa* in the mind, the human personality in whatever mode could not function. The mind, however, extrinsically conforms or corresponds to its characteristics *(dharma*s*)* as in the case of, for example, its tendency toward either dispersiveness/objectivity or one-pointedness (*YS* III.11), extroversion or interiorization (*YS* III.9), these being transformations of the forms *(dharma-pariṇāma)* in which consciousness and cognition function. Each characteristic *(dharma)* is connected with the three aspects of time/designation *(lakṣaṇa-pariṇāma)* and has its own states or stages of development *(avasthā-pariṇāma)*.[81]

In his exposition of *Yoga-Sūtra* I.41 Vyāsa states: "When the modifications/mental processes have subsided means: when the ideas/intentions have diminished."[82] Based on Vyāsa's commentary (*YB* I.1), we have previously explained that the definition of Yoga given in *Yoga-Sūtra* I.2 does not only mean that Yoga is the cessation of the misidentification with *all vṛtti*s because the cessation with the misidentification with *all vṛtti*s takes place only in enstasy *(asaṃprajñāta)*, whereas cognitive *samādhi* or ecstasy *(saṃprajñāta)* is also meant to be included in Yoga. Since *Yoga-Sūtra* I.41 deals (at least provisionally) with *saṃprajñāta* or *sabīja-samādhi,* as *Yoga-Sūtra* I.46 suggests, Vyāsa (*YB* I.41) omits the word "all." In other words, Vyāsa's clause, "the modifications/mental processes have subsided" indicates that *vṛtti*s other than those[83] of the one-pointedness (*ekāgratā, YS* III.11–12) with the object in *samādhi* have been mastered and have therefore subsided because the identification/unification *(samāpatti)* defined in this *sūtra* is also a form of *vṛtti,* albeit one of knowledge, insight, or yogic perception *(prajñā, yogi-pratyakṣa)*. The subsiding of the *vṛtti*s in this context is limited to the rajasic and tamasic mental processes. Vācaspati Miśra therefore explains that the ability of the mind to function in a crystal-like fashion requires a *sattva* dominance within consciousness.[84]

Both Vyāsa and Vijñāna Bhikṣu explain *vṛtti* (as used in *YS* I.41) in the context of *pratyaya. Vṛtti* and *pratyaya* do not strictly refer to the same thing, *vṛtti* indicating an underlying mental process and *pratyaya* meaning the product/content (i.e., cognition, idea, intention) or significance of a *vṛtti* that, by means of this mental process, arrives at consciousness. However, for the purpose of the explanation that follows, the apparent identification of both terms seems acceptable.[85] Vyāsa and Vijñāna Bhikṣu acutely observe that when the *samāpatti* takes place the *pratyaya*s have not all been eliminated since there subsists one *pratyaya*—the *samāpatti* itself, which constitutes in itself a *pratyaya*.[86] It is evident that in the experience of *samāpatti* there occurs an act of perception/cognition in which something becomes present or is revealed to consciousness.

Yoga-Sūtra I.41 constitutes a phenomenological analysis of experiences in cognitive *samādhi* wherein the "seeable" *(dṛśya, prakṛti)* is described experientially. Concerning the objects, the "grasped" *(grāhya*s*)*, Vyāsa states:

> Colored by a gross object which is its supportive factor, the mind appears to take on the nature of that object. Similarly, when colored by contemplation on a subtle object, unified with a subtle object, it appears to have the nature of that subtle object. Colored by any particular thing (material object) and identified with that thing in *samādhi,* it appears as that particular form.[87]

The realm of the "grasped" in Yoga can be divided into three categories:

1. The gross objects of support and identification *(sthūla-ālambana),* comprising the five gross elements and involving the physical senses.
2. The subtle objects of support and identification *(bhūta-sūkṣma):* theoretically including all subtle principles from the subtle elements *(tanmātra*s*)* up to and including unmanifest *prakṛti.*[88]
3. The various material objects or particular "things" of the universe *(viśva-bheda*s*),* comprising the "sentient" and "insentient" entities and objects (such as cows and jars respectively).

It appears to be the case that the category of the "grasped" *(grāhya*s*)* in Yoga is structured to include the objects of *samāpatti* only in the *vitarka-* and *vicāra-samādhi*s: the lower forms of cognitive *samādhi.* This seems to be consistent with the approach adopted in *Yoga-Sūtra* I.17 and I.42–44. The gross and subtle objects of the category of the "grasped" refer technically to the external or "objective" world only and therefore could not be inclusive of the "subjective" or "interior" categories of ego *(ahaṃkāra)* and intellect *(buddhi),* and then on to the unmanifest *prakṛti (aliṅga).*[89]

Concerning the instruments of knowledge or "grasping" *(grahaṇa*s*),* Vyāsa says: "So also with the senses, which are the instruments of grasping. The mind, colored by the instruments of grasping, identified (unified) with them, appears to have the nature of the instruments of grasping."[90] "Grasping" refers to the perceiver's own senses and this may include the innermost senses, namely, *ahaṃkāra* and *buddhi.*[91] At this stage of our analysis it seems reasonable to suggest that because the physical senses have already been included in the gross elements (as *grāhya*s), only the "inner" senses need to be understood as *grahaṇa*s.

On the term *grahītṛ* ("grasper," "knower"), Vyāsa writes:

> Similarly, when the mind is colored by the self who is the prakṛtic agent of grasping (i.e., the empirical grasper) as its supportive factor, united with *puruṣa* as that grasper, it appears to have the nature of *puruṣa* as that grasper. Again, when the mind is colored by the liberated *puruṣa* as its

> supportive factor, unified with that liberated *puruṣa,* it appears to have the nature of that liberated *puruṣa.*[92]

Grahītṛ, explained by Vyāsa as the prakṛtic agent of experience, cannot be subdivided between gross and subtle and no such attempt, to our knowledge, has been made by the commentators. Vyāsa, however, differentiates between *(a) grahītṛ puruṣa—puruṣa* appearing as an empirical or prakṛtic agent, and *(b) mukta puruṣa*—the liberated Self. Vyāsa not only says *"grahītṛ"*—the prakṛtic, empirical, or knowing agent—but adds *"puruṣa"* so as to preclude *buddhi* alone[93] but to include *puruṣa* reflected in the mind as *asmitā,* totally "identified" with it, as *mahān ātmā* (the "great self") or *mahat.*[94] Vyāsa consistently describes the locus of knowledge with reference to *puruṣa* regardless of how *puruṣa*'s identity (or misidentity) is being conceived (e.g., as an analogical understanding of consciousness as in *cittavṛtti, asmitā*).[95]

The question arises: Are there indeed two kinds of *puruṣa*s? In Yoga, certainly not. There is no intrinsic difference between the *puruṣa* that appears to dwell in a bound personality and the *puruṣa* that appears to be liberated. *Puruṣa* is ever-free by nature *(nitya-mukta-svabhāva).* The subject of *Yoga-Sūtra* I.41 (at least provisionally) is not the intrinsic nature of *puruṣa* but the stages of cognitive *samādhi.* The final stages of cognitive *samādhi* may be divided into three levels: (1) the realization, mastery of, and unification with *buddhi*—the principle of intelligence—also referred to as *mahat,* where there is not yet the realization of *puruṣa;* (2) the realization of the reflection of *puruṣa* in the *buddhi* in *asmitā*—the principal constituent, the agent or "grasper" *(grahītṛ);* (3) the realization that the reflection is not itself *puruṣa. Puruṣa* is the ever-free principle of pure consciousness, the reflection of which is seen in *asmitā-samādhi* (*YS* I.17). Vyāsa therefore differentiates between the reflection of *puruṣa* (in *asmitā*) and the changeless *puruṣa* whose existence transcends the realm of the *guṇa*s.

As the constituents of an empirical personality the principles of *prakṛti* can be divided into a scheme of apprehension that can be formulated as follows:[96]

1. *Viśeṣa*s, the sixteen manifestations of the "Particularized," the objects *(grāhyas)* "grasped" by the "grasper" or knower-agent. Ego—the sense of self *(ahaṃkāra, asmitā-mātra)* or sixth *aviśeṣa*—is the instrument through which *asmitā* appropriates or claims the knowledge of the objects. *Ahaṃkāra* is *grahaṇa,* the instrument of grasping or cognizing.

2. *Aviśeṣa*s, in the form of the five subtle elements *(tanmātra*s*)*, are also objects "grasped" *(grāhya*s*)*.
3. *Liṅga-mātra (buddhi* or *mahat)* receives and reflects consciousness from *puruṣa,* thus creating *asmitā*—egoity or I-am-ness—the composite sentience, as if the seer and the seeable are a single self (*YS* II.6). This is where the potential for dissatisfaction *(duḥkha)* actually takes root. The division or polarization of "seeing" into "seer and seeing" and the subsequent conjunction *(saṃyoga)* based on the epistemological distortion enveloping the subject (subjectified self) and the objectified world can be dismantled and discarded. When the mind, fragmented by the power of ignorance, is assumed to be the locus of the seer, there results the afflicted I-sense *(asmitā),* a mere reflection of *puruṣa.* The reflected sense of I-am-ness, and not *puruṣa,* is the agent *(grahītṛ),* the one who attempts to grasp or apprehend.

The above scheme is important in the classification of *samādhi* in *Yoga-Sūtra* I.17: (1) *Grāhya*s are the supportive factors *(ālambana)* in the *vitarka-* and *vicāra*-accompanied ecstasies. (2) *Grahaṇa* is the supportive factor in the *ānanda*-accompanied ecstasy. (3) *Grahītṛ* is the supportive factor in the *asmitā*-accompanied ecstasy. How these states interconnect and are related will be dealt with later. The Yoga tradition states the above to be the purposeful factors of cognitive *samādhi.*[97] Any other objects are only parts or composites of these.

A note of caution should be given here regarding *saṃprajñāta,* especially those *samādhi*-experiences that focus on the sixteen *viśeṣa*s, and particularly the five gross elements. One may mistake these to be *samādhi*s on the external world, that is, the earth, physical forms, and so on, with all the gross elements. It should be remembered that: *(a)* a perception of gross elements in the ordinary world falls within the normal category of *pratyakṣa* (*YS* I.7), a *vṛtti* that has subsided, and *(b)* holding the perception in the mind is memory *(smṛti),* another *vṛtti* that has subsided. In *samādhi* the focus on supportive factors is internal, as they exist, operate and are cognized within the mind *(citta):* The locus for identification with the "grasped" *(grāhya)* is the *manas,* the locus for identification with "grasping" *(grahaṇa)* is *ahaṃkāra,* and the locus for identification with the "grasper" *(grahītṛ)* is the *buddhi.* It is within the mind *(citta)* that their nature is observed and mastered through a more refined process of perception *(yogi-pratyakṣa). Samādhi* consists of the convergence of the particular evolute as one of the subjectively inherent components of the mind with its correlate or counterpart in the objective world. For example, since mind *(citta)* is the "controller" of the senses (*YS* II.54–55 and *YB* II.54–55), the various powers of the senses are all included in the mind. The mind focuses on the objects and assimilates the *vṛtti*s arising through the experience of those objects. Thus, the lower-level agent of *samādhi,* the mind-organ *(manas)* and the object converge and merge establishing a "unification," fullness and perfection of the insight *(prajñā)* at that level. This applies not only to *vitarka* but to all the levels of cognitive *samādhi.*

In the process of *nirodha* there takes place an interiorization of attention, a necessary, inward movement or "flow" of consciousness in the mind, allowing for a retracing of consciousness and identity from a distorted, unsteady state of dispersion and emergence *(vyutthāna)* to a finer, concentrated state whereby experience, no longer frustrated due to epistemic distortion, is allowed to complete itself through a full merging or unification with the object of experience. This process involves as well a retrieval in consciousness of the formerly obscured and misappropriated source principles or subjective evolutes (e.g., *manas, ahaṃkāra, buddhi*) through which experience takes place. Only such a merging or "oneness" with the object will enable the yogin to transcend the mechanism of ignorance through which misidentification and dissatisfaction are perpetuated. At each stage in *samādhi* consciousness is focused so as to dispel the ignorance coloring the mind's perception. The yogin can then "see" and "know" the object as it actually is, in itself.

VITARKA-SAMĀDHI

Of the four states of cognitive *samādhi (saṃprajñāta)* outlined in *YS* I.17 the less refined or most impure state is called *vitarka.* We have seen that the stages of *samādhi* are graded according to the grossness or subtlety, tangibility/concreteness or intangibility/abstractness of the evolutes of *prakṛti.* It is more difficult to concentrate on the subtler "inner" principles within the mind *(citta)* than on grosser, "outer" objects. It is recommended, therefore, that one should start with gross forms and, as Vācaspati Miśra acknowledges,[98] then reach more subtle stages.[99]

Vitarka has been translated as: "deliberation,"[100] "reasoning,"[101] "supposition,"[102] "rationale überlegung,"[103] "philosophical curiosity,"[104] "consciousness of sentient,"[105] "cogitation,"[106] "analysis of gross object,"[107] "discursive thought."[108] I shall in the above context adopt the term "cogitation." *Vitarka,* in normal language, refers to a mental activity, a process of thought in which the various details of an object are examined. In Patañjali's Yoga *vitarka* has the technical sense of contemplation on the sixteen *viśeṣas*—including *virāṭ* (or cosmic form of the "godhead" as in *BG* IX.10-11) as well as the manifest or incarnate forms of a deity—with the goal of finally realizing the whole nature of the object. H. Āraṇya gives the following examples as objects of cogitation: cow, jar, yellow, blue.[109] R. Śarmā lists other objects under this category, which include the sun, moon, and stars, as well as Rāma, Kṛṣṇa, Śiva, Durgā, and other deities.[110] It is to be understood that the deities as objects of cogitation are the images of the deities or the same deities manifest or appearing in some form.

"Cogitation" refers to the spontaneous thought processes that occur in relation to a "gross" *(sthūla)* object/form or content for contemplation. There is no doubt that *vitarka* is a special form of mental activity. That is how it is interpreted by Vyāsa, Vācaspati Miśra[111] and Vijñāna Bhikṣu.[112] Vyāsa states: "The mind's experience *(ābhoga)* of a 'gross' object of support/contemplation is 'cogitation'."[113] The word *ābhoga* ("expansion," "fullness")[114] means the experience of insight *(prajñā)* in which the realization of—"making evident"/"effecting with one's own eyes" *(sākṣātkāra)*—the true form and nature of an object of support/contemplation has occurred. At the first level it is considered gross because the object is in its gross form, thereby giving to the mind the like *vṛtti,* the mind identifying and uniting with that modification of knowledge. Vijñāna Bhikṣu explains that all the details of the grosser form of an object including the past, present, and future manifestations, its near and remote (distant) features, and so on, are attended to with the goal of finally realizing the whole nature of that object[115] in an ensemble-type knowing outside the time-space dimension. As cogitation *(vitarka)* is refined, the next step comes into view and the formerly concealed nature of the object of support is gradually revealed. The cogitation should remain constant, continuously maintained, ascertained *(avadhāraṇa).*[116] Thus, the cultivation *(bhāvana)* then causes the perceived or object, the faculty of perception, and the perceiver or agent, to unify, become "one"—epistemologically. In the final realization of the nature of the object, the knowledge of all its aspects occurs at once, not in sequence, or in parts, or apart from the perceiving mind. Such a total, whole realization maintained without interruption is termed "the *samādhi* associated with *vitarka.*" It is *grāhya-samāpatti* (*YS* I.41); its area of mastery is *grāhya,* the objects grasped within the gross body. *Vitarka* is further divided into *savitarka* and *nirvitarka.*

The first division of *vitarka* is outlined by Patañjali as follows: "Unification is with cogitation *(sa-vitarka)* when it is commingled with conceptualization of word, object (signified), and knowledge."[117] *Savitarka-*

samāpatti is invariably accompanied by the names of the objects of contemplation. Hence, this *sūtra* centers upon the words, the objects denoted thereby, and the ideational knowledge that is the relationship between the words and the objects grasped. Vyāsa says:

> For instance, we can see that the process of knowing takes place without distinguishing between the word "cow," the object "cow," and the idea (knowledge) "cow," though they are all on different levels; for there are some characteristics distinguished as belonging to words and others to objects signified, and still others to ideas (knowledge).[118]

Vācaspati Miśra explains: "In ordinary life, although word, object, and idea are distinct, in the process of knowing they are not distinguished."[119] When there is the holding of a word in consciousness (in this instance "cow"), there arises the conceptual or imaginative cognition *(vikalpa)* that the object denoted (the cow itself) and the mental ideation (of the cow) are not distinct from the word. In other words, when a cow is held as an object, there arises the conception that the word and the ideation are not apart from the object. Similarly, when the mental content or idea of the cow appears, the conceptualization or *vikalpa* registers that the word "cow" and the external object perceived as cow (which was denoted by the word) are both indistinct or inseparable from the idea. On closer examination, however, it can be found that these components of the word-object-ideation complex named "cow" are all distinct, each with their own characteristics. For example, the word is formed of syllables or letters of the alphabet; the object "cow" has hardness, legs, a tail, and so on; the idea is more abstract and is devoid of apparent dimension and parts. In conceptualization *(vikalpa)* the error of nondistinction among these components appears, causing them to be identified or commingled with each other. Vyāsa continues:

> When, during insight attained in *samādhi,* the yogin achieves unification with an intended object such as a cow and this unification appears intertwined with the mental constructs of the word, object signified, and the knowledge derived, [then] that interspersed identification is called "the one associated with cogitation."[120]

In *savitarka* unification, the word, object, and the idea are commingled and confused, causing the *samādhi* to be mixed with the notions and ideations, the constituents of which are analyzed and consequently are several. Having many constituents as supportive factors superimposed *(adhyāsa)*[121] on each other as though they were the same thus prevents the true one-pointedness *(ekāgratā)* and unification from developing in its fullness.

The mental processes embedded in the confusion outlined above occur in patterns such as the following: In the process of experiencing the presence of a single word-object-idea such as "cow," the yogin does not at this stage distinguish among these three constituents. Therefore it is uncertain which one of these three constituents is being attended to, realized, or mastered. The understanding and mastery is thus incomplete. There remains a separation between the observing mind and the object (cow) so that there may appear the observation: "This is a cow I am viewing." Vijñāna Bhikṣu has adopted the expression *gaur-ayaṃ bhāsate,*[122] which means literally, "here this cow shines forth, appears, is being experienced." In this experience the occurrence of the thought "cow" comprises the superimposition of the word and the object. In the series of thoughts: "appears, is being experienced," it is the object and the idea that are confused. Since these superimpositions of word, object, and idea on one another—causing the appearance of a conceptual or imagined unity in a manifold reality—only present what, in effect, is unreal, all such superimpositions come under the category of *vikalpa.* Any superimposition as such does not aid the yogin to realize or fully master the reality of any of its constituents, just as water and milk mixed together cannot be classified separately either as one or the other.

The ideas that arise are called "cogitations" only as an analogy to the ordinary thought processes where thoughts come and go one after the other. One should not think that the experiences in *savitarka-samādhi* are merely a product of the ordinary perceptual processes, and therefore that they can be reduced to the category of discursive thought or reasoning. If this were the case, there would be no state of the absorption of mental activity. The ordinary mental process or *vṛtti* of perception *(pratyakṣa)* is, temporarily at least, suspended, but the identification/unification *(samāpatti)* "is in terms of and expressed in rationalizing and conceptualizing signs."[123] Ordinary thought processes lack the immediacy and lucidity of *savitarka,* of the spontaneous thought processes that occur in cognitive *samādhi.* Feuerstein writes: "There is no rambling of thoughts in *samādhi,* no vague conceptualization, but these . . . ideas constitute spontaneous acts of insight or knowledge, which although grounded in the concepts derived from ordinary experiencing, have a different quality or feel to them."[124]

Because of the presence of the analyzing and particularizing activity or cogitation *(vitarka)* of the mind, of the words *(śabda),* of the cognitive process, and of the conceptualizing activity *(vikalpa),* it can be said that in the yogin's mind is still taking place a perceptive process that has to do with what, in general, Indic epistemological theories call a "*savikalpa* perception."[125] As it is yet touched by epistemological distortion due to ignorance *(avidyā),* this stage of *samādhi* constitutes a lower category of perception *(apara-pratyakṣa)* in contrast with the higher perception *(para-pratyakṣa)*[126] of *nirvitarka* to be explained next.

In *YS* I.43 Patañjali informs us that: "Supra-cogitative unification is when memory is completely purified, as if emptied of its own form, and with the object alone shining forth."[127] In *nirvitarka,* all cogitation or association with "gross" thought has ceased. Vyāsa's commentary reads: "When, however, there is complete purification of the memory of verbal conventions in that insight attained in *samādhi* which has become empty of conceptualization of ideas heard or inferred, then the object stands out in the form of its real nature alone."[128] The expression *pari-śuddhi,* which is used by both Patañjali and Vyāsa, is not merely "purification" but may be taken to mean at this stage of the processes of *samāpatti* a "complete purification." It has been understood as denoting the abandonment and eradication of such memory altogether.[129] Based on our analysis in the preceding chapter, purification can be understood with an epistemological emphasis, meaning here the dissolution *(pralaya* or *pravilaya)*[130] of memory as referenced to an afflicted identity of selfhood: memory that has been rooted in or filtered through a confusion or error *(viparyaya)* within consciousness. Memory *(smṛti)* is a *vṛtti,* and its association with ignorance/misidentification (in the form of the superimposition of karmic residues onto the form of the object) is to be transcended in the process of "cessation" *(nirodha).*

This purification does not result in the yogin suffering a loss of memory of words and their meaning in practical life. Rather, it means the yogin no longer carries the former confused memory into *samādhi,* does not rely on words, and so on, as objects (mental content) of support for the mind. At this stage the practice becomes free of the attachment to names and verbal contemplation; the experience in *samādhi* is now dissociated from any dependency on speech and language. Not only does the yogin not resort to the memory of words and their denotations, but the entire cogitative process that was caused by the presence of words and indicative of the nature of universals is left behind. This includes the three categories of: (1) *āgama pramāṇa:* verbal testimony; (2) *anumāna pramāṇa:* inference [both (1) and (2) being categories of the *vṛtti* of valid cognition (*YS* I.7)]; and (3) the unification defined as *savitarka* that has a less subtle degree of realization *(sākṣātkāra)* and that can be described as impure and alloyed. Again, we read from Vyāsa:

> [The object then] excludes all else and remains distinctly in the form of its own nature. That is supra-cogitative unification and it is the higher direct perception. It is the seed of authority and inference; from it they both originate. That seeing (perception) is not associated with any knowledge from valid authority or inference. The yogin's perception, not interspersed and confused with any other source of valid cognition, arises out of this *nirvitarka-samādhi.*[131]

There is now not the slightest superimposition of the "erroneous" onto the object. The mind transcends the limitations of a "cogitative identity" of self, that is, cogitation as appropriated by or referenced to egoity, and moves on to a more complete unification or identification with the object at hand. The reality or true form of the object known *(grāhya)* is revealed. It is thus that the phrase from *Yoga-Sūtra* I.43 (see n. 127 above): *svarūpa-śūnya-iva,* "as if emptied of its own form"—with reference to the mind and to the *samāpatti,* becomes meaningful. "As if" *(iva)* indicates that the yogin does not become mindless, but that the locus of self-identity within the mind along with the cognition that "I know the object" no longer obscure clear perception of the object in *vitarka-samādhi.* In this experiential unification of grasper, grasping, and grasped, the subject—whose former level of self-understanding was limited to the mode of cogitation—is no longer ensnared by those epistemological limitations. Thus ensues a transcendence of the limitations of perception and self-identity misidentified with gross associations in the mind.

The cessation of the superimposition of karmic residue resulting from the purification of memory allows for a mode of cognition and experience that is no longer influenced by the misidentifications and projections of the past. The "grasper" no longer performs an obstructive role in the mode of being a "cogitator" of objects, that is, identified with the ideas or *vṛtti*s arising in *savitarka.* Although it does not seem to be the case, the stability of the mind "unified with" the object and its coloration by the object continue to occur. The extraordinary presence of the object monopolizing, as it were, the consciousness of the yogin, and as a consequence of it, the disappearance of the word, of the conventional knowledge and of the conceptualizations create the false appearance that the stability of the mind in the object and its coloration by it have also disappeared. The yogin is no more aware of the process of stabilization and coloring that has taken place in the mind; that is to say, it is as if this process did not exist for the yogin. But the word *iva* ("as though," "as if") is used to show that memory and, by implication, the mind's essential form/nature as *sattva*-knowledge, implying clear insight, are not destroyed. For this reason, Patañjali can say that the mind (in its functioning as memory) at this moment of the process appears *as if* devoid of its own form.

Koelman refers to the level of *samādhi* in *nirvitarka* as "refined sense-intuition shorn of its super-structures," which "cannot be communicated to others, it is eminently personal. To express it or explain it to others one has to resort to the universalizing and rationalizing way of thinking."[132] That is why yogins who have attained to a form of perception unhindered by processes of conceptualization *(vikalpa)* can make efforts to communicate, teach, and transmit that clarity of knowledge through the medium of concepts,[133] verbal testimony, and inference, even though these particular *vṛtti*s and their mental content or significance in the form of ideas *(pratyaya)* do not themselves constitute the direct experience. Rather, these *vṛtti*s and their significance can be used as a heuristic device to point beyond their meaning to the direct experience/perception itself that in the mode of supracogitation *(nirvitarka)* is the source and cause of cogitation. In *nirvitarka* the yogin's identity and perception are transcendent of and no longer dependent on the former functioning of *vṛtti* and the processes of apprehension in *savitarka*.

In Yoga, an origin or cause is not dependent on its effects. As Vācaspati Miśra explains, even though the perception of smoke leads to the inference that there is fire, the fire itself is not dependent on the smoke.[134] By way of the above analogy, it should be clear that the yogin attains higher perception through non- or rather trans-conceptual ecstasy and can then appropriate *āgama* and *anumāna* (which deal with abstract universals or generalities) heuristically for the purpose of aiding others in the study of Yoga and for clarifying the crucial element in Yoga of direct experience or unmediated knowledge. Even though liberating knowledge is taught in the revealed texts *(śruti)* or by a *guru,* it is impossible to experience it directly without entering into *samādhi* oneself just as one cannot experience the sweetness of sugar through mere description (of its sweetness) alone.[135] Nor in Yoga can the *guru*'s guidance be complete without proper initiation *(dīkṣā)* of the aspiring yogin into the direct experience of higher perception in which doubt and skepticism subside, thereby freeing up the yogin's energy and attention for the pursuit of the "goal" of liberation itself.

The real objects of the empirical, practical world are indeed the objects of contemplation and support in *vitarka-samādhi*. They are not merely the ideas of objects or their atoms, but rather the object as a complete whole *(avayavin)* to which all its parts *(avayavas)* belong.[136] That the true nature of a gross object—whether it be a cow, a stone, or any other object within nature—is realized internally in *samādhi* does not mean that its objective, external nature or form is considered to be less real or is even denied. Since the object's complete nature is perceived internally, the direct perception includes the existence of its grosser manifestations that are also understood, mastered, and transcended. On account of the purification of the *vitarka* activity of the mind that removes misidentification with, and misappropriation of, the mental processes at this level of *samādhi* (the cessation of the misidentification and attachment that normally accompanies the functioning of *vṛtti* in the form of *pramāṇa, vikalpa,* and so forth, already having been attained), it can be said that in the yogin's mind is taking place a perceptual or awakening process that has to do with what, in general, Indic epistemological theories call a "*nirvikalpa* perception."[137]

VICĀRA-SAMĀDHI

Seeing that *vitarka-samādhi* (in both its *"sa"* and *"nir"* forms) is involved with the *guṇas* and their manifestations/actualizations, the yogin develops dispassion *(vairāgya)* toward these experiences and opens up to a range of experiences in the next stage of cognitive *samādhi,* that stage being referred to as *vicāra-samādhi. Vicāra* is without the verbal, cogitative, or grosser associations of *vitarka.*[138] The level of *vitarka* refined, subtilized, becomes *vicāra*—"reflection," with subtle associations. The term *vicāra* has been translated as: "reflection,"[139] "discrimination,"[140] "clear vision,"[141] "sinnende Betrachtung,"[142] "consciousness of discrimination,"[143] "meditation,"[144] "analysis of subtle object."[145]

Vicāra, which will be translated by "reflection," is used by Patañjali in a sense specific to Yoga. The word *vicāra* is derived from *vi* + *car,*[146] expressing a progressive movement. In the context of the *Yoga-Sūtra vicāra* refers to the movement of the mind away from the gross objects to subtler objects of association. Having seen the defects and limitations of the involvement with gross objects and content, however clearly realized in *vitarka,* which confine the yogin's level of perception to "cogitation" *(savitarka)* or "without cogitation" *(nirvitarka),* the yogin looks at the causes of those objects and accompanying self-identifications. The yogin thus moves from the sixteen *viśeṣas* (generated from the *aviśeṣas*) to the six *aviśeṣas* themselves: the five subtle elements *(tanmātras)* and the ego-sense *(ahaṃkāra* or *asmitā-mātra).* The yogin contemplates these subtler essences of the elements and of the senses and brings before consciousness all the "subtle" particularities and constitutive parts of a "subtle" object. It is the making evident of, "effecting with one's own eyes" *(sākṣātkāra)* the subtle. The mind takes the form of the *vṛtti* of perception during *vicāra-samādhi* and becomes identified with it. According to Vyāsa, *vicāra* then becomes an expanded perception and experience *(ābhoga)* of the mind toward the subtle object of support *(ālambana),* awakening deeper insight *(prajñā)* in which the realization of the true nature of the object occurs.[147] It is the fullness and perfection of the mind with regard to subtle objects as has already been described with regard to the gross objects.

The (Sāṃkhya-) yogin H. Āraṇya suggests that *vicāra* is a refined analytical process.[148] The philosophical analysis of the relationship of the evolutes of *prakṛti* with *puruṣa* finally leads to the realization that "I am none of the evolutes with which I have identified myself." However, this type of analytical process seems more a part of the practice of intense *vicāra* contemplations on the path of *jñāna-yoga* as taught in the Vedānta lineage. It may also reflect an obvious Sāṃkhyan influence on Āraṇya's interpretation, that is, the classical Sāṃkhyan approach to liberation tends to present itself as an intellectual path based on an analysis of the evolutes of *prakṛti* (see discussion on Yoga and Sāṃkhya in chapter 2). In the context of Yoga, analytical thought is more likely to fall within the categories of: *(a)* the *vṛtti* of valid cognition *(pramāṇa),* specifically inference (*anumāna,* which prior to *samādhi* has been transcended), or *(b) svādhyāya,* "self-study" involving the personal recitation of *mantra*s and the study of scriptural injunctions leading to liberation, the fourth of the *niyama*s ("observances") that constitute the second limb (*YS* II.32 and 44) of the "eight-limbed" Yoga (see discussion in chapter 4). Both of these categories play a more preparatory role in Yoga and may be seen as being propaedeutic to, but not inclusive of, *samādhi.* The evidence suggests that *vicāra* is a technical term for the practice of yogic one-pointedness on objects with subtle associations in order to know their nature and, furthermore, to master their nature entirely through dispassion (*YS* I.15). It is possible that one-pointedness can be seen as an "analytical thought process" in that it deals with the sort of subtilization found in the processes of liberating knowledge *(jñāna).* However, to subsume *vicāra* under the category of an "analytical thought process" does not seem to do justice to the Yoga system at this level of experience in *samādhi.*

Among the subtle evolutes and according to the scheme adopted in this study (see chart on p. 77 referring to the categories of Sāṃkhya and their overlap with Yoga), the objects of this level of *samādhi* are: (1) the five subtle elements *(tanmātras)*—sometimes said to be located in the subtle body *(sūkṣma-śarīra)*—which are the cause of the five gross elements and are the five subtle essences of the five cognitive senses consisting of sound, touch, form-percept, taste, and smell; and (2) *ahaṃkāra* or *asmitā-mātra* (the sense of self, individualized I or ego). As the immediate cause of the subtle senses, *ahaṃkāra* begins to be mastered in this form of ecstasy, but primarily, as I will later suggest, it is the object of support in the next stage of ecstasy: *ānanda*. I have argued in chapter 2 that according to Yoga philosophy it is not correct to replace *ahaṃkāra* (i.e., *asmitā-mātra,* an ontological principle of *prakṛti*) with the term *asmitā* (the affliction of I-am-ness or egoity, a mistaken identity of self) or with the total "inner instrumentality" *(antaḥkaraṇa)* that is collectively subsumed under the term *citta* (mind) in Yoga and is threefold in Sāṃkhya: (1) *manas,* the mind-organ or lower mind, which is one of the sixteen *viśeṣa*s (the "Particularized"), the objects of support in *vitarka-samādhi;* (2) *ahaṃkāra,* ego—included by the classical commentators as being one of the six *aviśeṣa*s—and the object of support in the later stages of *vicāra-samādhi* and in *ānanda-samādhi;* (3) *buddhi* (*mahat,* intelligence) or *liṅga-mātra,* the first prakṛtic principle of manifestation and object of support/contemplation in *asmitā-samādhi.*

Yet, in the light of the above definitions of the various levels of *saṃprajñāta* that specify the different components of the *antaḥkaraṇa* involved, it would be clearly erroneous to assume that the entire *antaḥkaraṇa* is an object of support in *vicāra-samādhi,* that is, in the context of its technical usage in *Yoga-Sūtra* I.17. I will deal more with this issue in the discussion below on the *ānanda* and *asmitā* ecstasies. The *vicāra-samādhi* also correlates with *grāhya* (*YS* I.41); its field of mastery is *grāhya,* the objects grasped, not with gross associations, which is the field of *vitarka,* but with subtle associations.

Vicāra-samādhi appears to be further divided into *savicāra* and *nirvicāra*. *Yoga-Sūtra* I.44 states: "Similarly explained [as in the *savitarka-* and *nirvitarka-samāpatti*s], when it is on subtle objects, are the [unifications called] 'with reflection' *(savicāra)* and 'supra-reflection' *(nirvicāra)*."[149] In the *savitarka-* and *nirvitarka-samāpatti*s, the gross elements in various tangible forms grasped with the external senses and focused internally within the mind-organ *(manas)* are the objects of support. In the *savicāra* and *nirvicāra* identifications, the five subtle elements and the subtle senses of apprehension are the objects of support and contemplation. Vyāsa states: "Of these two, the *savicāra* unification refers to subtle elements whose qualities are manifest, and are delimited by the experience of space (location), time, and cause."[150] In *savicāra,* Vyāsa tells us, the object of *samādhi* is experienced with reference to a particular location, time, and cause. Even though the subtlest, minutest particles seemingly occupy no space, nevertheless a relationship in space (i.e., a location) is attributed to them, the detailed mechanism of which is an area of specialization within Vaiśeṣika philosophy as well as modern physics. The same applies to time.[151] Causation in the above refers to the fact of the subtle, atomic realities of the gross elements being products of the respective *tanmātras*.[152] Vyāsa clarifies the manifest characteristics of *savicāra,* asserting that: "The object of support is the subtle elements, characterized by the qualities which are now manifest, and it presents itself to insight in the *samādhi*. This is to be grasped as one single idea [i.e., grasped by a unitary intelligence alone and not divided up among several ideas]."[153] Vyāsa continues:

> That unification on the subtle elements is called "supra-reflection" (without subtle associations) when, corresponding to and being the essential nature of all of the qualities, there is in all ways and by all means no delimitation by any qualities subsided, arisen, or undetermined.[154]

The qualities of an object may be: *(a)* dormant, subsided, *(b)* manifest, arisen, or *(c)* undetermined (*YS* III.14). An object has many attributes that are manifested from time to time, while others may subside or are held in potential form. When certain qualities have already made their appearance, after some time they become dormant, submerged, and are of the past. Some qualities manifest in the present, and some—undetermined at the moment—will arise in the future. In *savicāra-samādhi* the direct realization of the nature of the object is limited only to those characteristics that are manifest, have arisen *(udita),* in the present. The insight thus gained is delimited. However, Vyāsa says that "this is to be grasped as one single idea,"[155] that is, as a state of one-pointedness (*ekāgratā, YS* III.11-12) in *samādhi*.

To summarize the rest of Vyāsa's commentary (*YB* I.44), it is made clear that in contrast to the imagery in *savicāra,* the awakening insight *(prajñā)* in *nirvicāra,* which is without imagery, comprises the entirety of the subtle object (e.g., the subtle elements or subtle senses of apprehension) of contemplation. The object here is not delimited by space, time, or causation, nor is it limited to those attributes that are apparent only in its present time. All of its possibilities and potentialities are grasped and realized in the one-pointedness of *samādhi;* not being divided up among many ideas, the object is grasped as a complete whole by a unitary (nonfractured) intelligence *(buddhi)*. Vyāsa is very emphatic in stating that the objects here are: (1) *sarva-dharma-anu-pātin:* such that they relate to all their qualities; (2) *sarva-dharma-ātmaka:* such that their self-nature comprises all their qualities; (3) *sarvathā:* in every possible way; (4) *sarvataḥ:* from whichever possible mode. Vyāsa emphasizes that at this stage the subtle object, in its true form alone, colors the mind by its proximity *(uparañj),* the mind (i.e., knowledge or *prajñā* in Vyāsa's commentary) understood here to be as though devoid of its own form, with only the object remaining.[156] Vācaspati Miśra is of the opinion that *savicāra-* and *savitarka-samādhi*s share the state of a *vikalpa*—of the divisions of the word-object-idea triad, and that *nirvicāra,* like *nirvitarka,* is free of such cognition.[157] In clear disagreement with Vācaspati, Vijñāna Bhikṣu argues that since the limitations of *vikalpa*-cognition have already been abandoned in *nirvitarka,* which is a lower (that is, less subtle) stage of ecstasy, how then can it continue to be pursued in the next higher stage, which is *savicāra?* Bhikṣu declares that the "error" that has already been abandoned in the previous stage cannot then find a place in the next stage.[158] Bhikṣu's understanding seems to be more in accord with Vyāsa, who states: "Thus by explaining *nirvitarka,* the absence of *vikalpa* in the case of both of these has been explained."[159] Based on Vyāsa's commentary, it is more technically correct to say that *savicāra* and *nirvicāra* are both extricated from the defect of the *vikalpa,* which has already been transcended in *nirvitarka.*

In *nirvicāra-samāpatti,* the yogin is completely "at one" (epistemologically) with the object, that is, the yogin knows its past states as well as its present moment and is fully aware of the various possibilities of the future. The last limitations of space and time attributed to the object are transcended. According to Vyāsa, an ecstatic state reaches both the supracogitative and suprareflective levels when the mind is, as it were, void of its own nature and is free to "become" the object itself. Whereas the "unification" *(samāpatti)* in *nirvitarka-samādhi* is a distinct perception limited to the gross object, in *nirvicāra-samādhi* the "unification" is expanded to include subtle objects. These so-called objects at the subtlest level are themselves the "seeds" of ignorance *(avidyā)* in the form of *saṃskāra*s—the deep-rooted impressions or karmic residue of affliction in the mind. These seeds of affliction are to be "roasted," are to become, in the words of Vyāsa, like burned *(dagdham)* seeds of rice.[160] Once scorched through meditative discipline by the "fire of knowledge" (*YB* IV.28) these "seeds" in the form of mistaken identity and attachment can no longer sprout. Through *samādhi,* the insight *(prajñā)* thus gained along with the increasing purification and refinement of the mind leads to a deepening of dispassion. From this detached perspective, neither subject nor object, perceiver nor world, can be seen as substantial or separate.[161] There is no longer any adumbration of interpretation as applied to the object or condition at hand. Yoga states that the object shines forth alone, nonseparate from the mind, which is as if empty of its own form.

The *"nir"* forms of ecstasy are indicative of a radically different knowledge from their *"sa"* forms. Both the *"nir"* types of *samādhi* are forms of knowledge that can be called "indeterminate" (as opposed to the "determinate" knowledge inherent in the *"sa"* forms). Indeterminate knowledge can be understood here as being knowledge, whether of gross or subtle objects, in which the distinction between the consciousness of the subject (the "grasper") knowing the object (the "grasped") is not present. As soon as the distinction is present, the other formations—like the word-object-idea triad (in *savitarka*) or space, time, and causation (in *savicāra*)—make their appearance and monopolize the yogin's consciousness. In more ordinary perception we are not aligned with and therefore do not "catch" or become aware of the stages and experiences of indeterminate knowledge; they remain concealed, "hidden" from our conscious view, existing merely in potential form as insight *(prajñā)* embedded in the *sattva* of consciousness. But the indeterminate knowledge of which Patañjali speaks is something attained through voluntary effort (cf. *YS* I.20–22) leading to purification of mind. Yoga maintains that we can and should recognize or become aware of these purer, more subtle levels of cognition if we want to progress to the supracognitive level of *samādhi* and on to the intrinsic identity as *puruṣa*. A conceptual, rational, and egoic understanding of oneself and the world is thus superseded by an immediate, transconceptual, transrational, and trans-egoic understanding. And to repeat a suggestion made in chapter 4, Yoga does not hold to an anti-intellectual or prerational/preconceptual perspective amounting to a regression in consciousness. Nor does Yoga discipline proper bring about a suppression or repression of *vṛtti*s. As argued earlier, such misunderstandings of the transformative processes leading to illumination and purification are more representative of tamasic (e.g., deluded/stagnated/escapist) states of mind and identity that are far removed from the purer states of awareness arrived at through Yoga.

In *Yoga-Sūtra* I.47 it is implied that *nirvicāra-samāpatti* is the highest stage of cognitive *samādhi,* which suggests the following progressive ("hierarchical") organization[162] in descending order from the purest, most subtle, and most sattvified to the least pure, least subtle, and least sattvified: *nirvicāra-samāpatti, savicāra-samāpatti, nirvitarka-samāpatti, savitarka-samāpatti.* Patañjali describes the *nirvicāra* ecstasy as culminating in a state of "supra-reflexive lucidity" *(nirvicāra-vaiśāradya)* that is coterminous with the state of clarity of the inner or authentic self/being known as *adhyātma-prasāda.*[163] At this finer level, knowing and knower "lose" their dualistic and independent status and states as well: the analogy of radiance or clarity extends to oneself *(adhyātma)*. The insight *(prajñā)* engendered in the highest stage of object-oriented *samādhi* is said to be "truth-bearing" *(ṛtaṃ-bharā)*[164] because it discloses the contemplated object as it is without any mental distortions: "there is no trace of erroneous knowledge in it" (*YB* I.48).[165] In addition to the aspect of cognitive clarity there likewise occurs in the lucidity of *nirvicāra* a clarity and ease regarding one's affective/emotive nature, thus incorporating, for example, the sense of "contentment" *(saṃtoṣa)* and "unexcelled happiness" obtained (*YS* II.42; see n. 187 in chapter 4) through the cultivation of the various "observances" *(niyamas)*. The cessation of the afflicted *vṛtti*s, as Vijñāna Bhikṣu suggests, simultaneously bears with it the subsiding of all afflicted and compulsive affective/emotive patterns of thought and behavior and any further karmically binding activity thus generated.[166] That is why clarity (implying serenity) becomes a characteristic of the yogin immersed in this stage of *samādhi.* Vyāsa writes:

> When the mind-*sattva (buddhi),* whose nature is luminosity, is freed from [the effects of] *rajas* and *tamas,* and has a steady flow without any veiling contamination of impurity, that is, the lucidity . . . has occurred, there is clarity in the inner being of the yogin, which is a progressively clearer and more brilliant light of knowledge of the object as it really is.[167]

Drawing on Vyāsa's metaphor (*YB* I.12, see discussion in chapter 4) of the "steady flow of the mind toward the good," there is implied in the above—and after a sufficient degree of purification has taken place—a momentum or movement in the "direction" of transcendence and liberation ("aloneness"). The yogin's identity is freed from the binding effects of *rajas* and *tamas,* thus bringing about a sattvification of consciousness. The yogin becomes cognitively, morally, and affectively purified, spiritually developed and uplifted as person, ushering the yogin into a different order of life from that of an egoic or selfish mentality rooted in *saṃyoga*—dissatisfaction and ignorance. Having attained to that insight *(prajñā)* which is "truth-bearing" (*ṛtaṃbharā*, *YS* I.48), "bearing the truth in oneself,"[168] the yogin apprehends the innate order *(ṛta)* of cosmic existence and is integrally linked with that order.

Adhyātma (*YS* I.47) refers to the disclosure of the clarity of the inner being, an awakening to one's spiritual identity as a reflection in the *sattva.* In cognitive *samādhi* it appears to be limited to the identification with mind-*sattva* and does not literally apply to *puruṣa*. This stage of *samādhi* reminds us of Vyāsa's description (*YB* I.1)[169] of *samādhi* in the one-pointed state *(ekāgra)* of mind that fully illuminates an object as it is, diminishes the afflictions, loosens the bonds of karma, and brings the state of the cessation of mistaken identity *(cittavṛtti)* into view. There ensues a transcendence of self as identified with subtle associations of the mind. The sense of self no longer acts as a vehicle that obstructs perception and misappropriates objects in the mode of "reflection," that is, one ceases to misidentify with the ideas (mind content) and *vṛtti*s arising in *savicāra*. In *nirvicāra* the mind is released from the binding associations and identifications that formerly accompanied the experience of subtle objects. A deepening detachment or dispassionate knowledge and mastery has taken place. The yogin is emancipated from the limitations of empirical identity ensconced within the "reflexive" mode of knowledge and self-understanding. Vijñāna Bhikṣu[170] makes the pertinent suggestion that although the "truth-bearing" insight *(ṛtaṃbharā-prajñā)* arises in the last stage of cognitive *samādhi,* the steps leading to it are through *vitarka, vicāra,* and so on. It follows that there is a "vertical" progression or continuum that implies some direct perception in the earlier stages as well and accounts for the interdependence and interconnectedness of the levels of perception in *samādhi*. The lower levels of insight gained pertaining to gross objects are not negated or abandoned but are integrated and reconciled in a manner that no longer references experience to a false center of consciousness laying claim to authentic identity. The first three stages of *saṃprajñāta* naturally lead to the fourth *(asmitā)* and the insights generated through the former may be incorporated in the later. Thus, the insight and mastery gained from the lower ecstasies is not extinguished or relinquished, rather it is included, consolidated, and integrated. At each level, the empirical limitations of a superimposed condition *(cittavṛtti)* of *puruṣa* or authentic identity are discerned and sifted out from the yogin's purview, allowing for a clearer understanding and insight into the true nature of *puruṣa*. *Avidyā* and misidentification are thus differentiated from liberating knowledge *(vidyā, prajñā)* and intrinsic identity. An unbroken continuum of perception can then take place through which all objects, gross or subtle, can be known in the light of the clarity of the inner being/self.

The yogin's experience in *nirvicāra* is far from being "misty," "vague," or "mysterious." It is as vivid and immediate as is possible for one who lives at the levels of ordinary awareness to imagine. The yogin's consciousness, although transcending the normal barriers of egoic identity, has not however been reduced, nor has it been negated or subsumed into the realm of the "unconscious." In *samādhi* a state of suprawakefulness is disclosed in which the yogin "comes face to face with the true nature of the object, which ordinarily remains hidden behind the outer forms."[171]

The subtle objects, as Patañjali points out, extend up to, and terminate their forms in unmodified *prakṛti*.[172] Vyāsa takes pains to emphasize[173] that the reference to the subtle objects of support *(sūkṣma-viṣaya)* in *Yoga-Sūtra* I.44 does not mean that only atoms (*paramāṇu*s or *aṇu*s) and the subtle elements constitute the limit of the subtle realm. A mistake of this nature could be made because objects of support in the *vicāra*-accompanied *samādhi* are the subtle elements and the subtle senses and *Yoga-Sūtra* I.44 speaks of *savicāra* and *nirvicāra* as being realizations of the subtle realm. The subtle realm does not, however, end there but extends all the way to the higher stages of ecstasy where *ahaṃkāra* and *liṅga-mātra (mahat/buddhi)* are realized. Thereafter *aliṅga* (unmanifest *prakṛti*) is understood and included.

It should be noted that even though the formal Sāṃkhya system considers unmanifest *prakṛti* to be beyond any cognition at all—too shy a "maiden" to show "her" face to *puruṣa* (*SK* 61)—in Yoga *prakṛti* is indeed "experienced" by the *prakṛti-laya*s—yogins who have merged their awareness into *prakṛti,* as Patañjali and Vyāsa explain.[174] Thus, the yogin's subtle realm extends all the way up to unmanifest *prakṛti*. There is nothing of a prakṛtic nature more subtle beyond *aliṅga*.[175] Yet, as Vyāsa is careful to state:

> Now *puruṣa* also is subtle, is that not so? But the subtlety of *puruṣa* is not in the same category as that of the unmanifest beyond the great principle/designator *(liṅga)*. Furthermore, *puruṣa* is not the cause which generates the designator but is the [indirect] cause. Thus the unexcelled subtlety as it is in *prakṛti (pradhāna)* has been explained.[176]

Puruṣa is not an object in *samādhi. Puruṣa* is "subtle" but is in an entirely different category from *prakṛti* and her evolutes. Whereas the levels of subtlety in *prakṛti*'s evolutes are comparative, *puruṣa*'s "subtlety" is not relative or subject to transformation, but is unchanging, absolute. Unlike *prakṛti, puruṣa* has no direct products as its effects. As pure consciousness, *puruṣa* is an indirect cause of the awareness *asmi,* "I am," that makes its appearance in the composite sentience—*asmitā*—when *puruṣa*'s presence passively reflects in *liṅga-mātra*. That is the extent of *puruṣa*'s "involvement."

Since the topic of these *sūtra*s is cognitive or object-oriented *samādhi* (i.e., ecstasy), and it is not until *asaṃprajñāta* (objectless *samādhi*) that the "aloneness" *(kaivalya)* of *puruṣa* can occur, the degrees of subtleness mentioned above only lead up to unmanifest *prakṛti*. Backtracking somewhat to the stages of cognitive *samādhi* (as outlined in *YS* I.17), a crucial question now arises. Bearing in mind that *Yoga-Sūtra* I.47–50 extol the perfection of *nirvicāra-samādhi* and that *Yoga-Sūtra* I.51 explains *asaṃprajñāta-samādhi,* where do the *ānanda*- and *asmitā*-accompanied ecstasies that were included in *Yoga-Sūtra* I.17 fit in to Patañjali's scheme? Although this has not been explicity mentioned by Vyāsa or by any of the major Sanskrit commentators, it appears that the term *nirvicāra* is not limited to being a variation of the *vicāra*-accompanied ecstasy alone. The term *nirvicāra-samāpatti* can be taken in a broader sense to include the other two ecstasies: *ānanda* and *asmitā,* which appear to have been left out or overlooked. Two reasons can be posited[177] why this is so: (1) The later two forms of cognitive *samādhi* are also in this sense forms of *nirvicāra-samāpatti* because the association with subtle objects as in *vicāra* has ceased. The experience in the *ānanda*-accompanied *samādhi* is "I am joyful," and in *asmitā-samādhi* it is simply "I am." These are neither discursive-like thoughts associated with *vitarka*-accompanied *samādhi,* nor subtle thoughts of the *vicāra* type of ecstasy, but are rather deeper, more subtilized, sattvified experiences in *nirvicāra-samāpatti.* (2) The subtle realm incorporated in *samādhi* extending up to and including unmanifest *prakṛti* clearly warrants recognition of the other two ecstasies.

Vyāsa does assume that *ānanda* and *asmitā* (*YB* I.17) constitute the contents of separate stages of cognitive *samādhi.* It would not be unreasonable to suggest that Vyāsa would take *ānanda*- and *asmitā-samādhi* to be instances of *nirvicāra-samāpatti* and that this can be seen as being in accordance with Patañjali's scheme. It would then follow that the *vicāra*-accompanied ecstasy referred to in *Yoga-Sūtra* I.17 is a specific category of cognitive *samādhi* that technically and structurally corresponds with *savicāra-samāpatti; vicāra* (*YS* I.17) thus is not intended to include the full depth of the *nirvicāra* levels.

ĀNANDA-SAMĀDHI

On the subject of the third form of ecstasy presented in *Yoga-Sūtra* I.17—called "joy" *(ānanda)*—Vyāsa writes: "Joy means delight."[178] The word for joy, *ānanda,* does not denote here a state of intrinsic, unconditional, transcendent "bliss," one of the familiar epithets of *brahman*—the Supreme Being as extolled, for example, in Upaniṣadic works and Vedāntic commentaries. In *Yoga-Sūtra* I.17 *ānanda* is initially the conditional and temporary property called *sukha:* the pleasure, well-being, or happiness inherent in the *sattva-guṇa.* In *ānanda*-accompanied *samādhi* the yogin grasps or captures the delight of *sattva* and identifies/unites with this exalted sense of happiness.

It is acknowledged in the Sāṃkhya and Yoga traditions that pleasure belongs to the *sattva* of the mind and is within the realm of the "experienced" or "seeable," that is, it is object-oriented. *Puruṣa*—the pure, unchanging seer—transcends the realm of the *guṇa*s and is by nature free of the binding influence of, or attachment to, *sattva*. This is related to the idea that pleasure, pain, and other experiences belong to the transformations *(pariṇāma)* of *prakṛti* and so *puruṣa*'s nature, although immanent as well as transcendent, maintains its immutable, unmodified, and nonfragmented identity throughout all the changes taking place within *prakṛti*. Even though the prakṛtic scheme includes the delusive power of *tamas,* the often turbulent nature of *rajas,* and the pleasurable states of *sattva,* human beings basically involve themselves with the world in pursuit of the pleasure of *sattva*. It is ultimately the *attachment* to the pleasure derived from *sattva* that causes misidentification, dissatisfaction, and bondage and that, even on the subtle levels of *prakṛti,* generates and sustains saṃsāric or mistaken identity.

In the *savitarka* and *savicāra* ecstasies, the insights attained show one the futility of pursuing happiness through the various objects of contemplation, starting with "cogitation" *(vitarka)* on the earth elements and going up to the "reflection" *(savicāra)* on the subtle elements and possibly the initial stages of the sense of self *(ahaṃkāra)*. As identification with the grosser evolutes/objects/content gradually dissolves or is transcended, and an identification with their subtler causes arises, in *ānanda-samādhi* identification dissolves or merges into *ahaṃkāra*. Koelman appropriately writes that after mastering the *vicāra* stage one sets oneself "to focus the subjective-objective entities" in order "to concentrate and achieve one-pointed attention on those entities which constitute [one's] own cognitive organism."[179]

Since tamasic *ahaṃkāra* generates the elements, and sattvic *ahaṃkāra* generates the mind-organ *(manas),* the sense organs and action organs, all with the aid of *rajas* (activity/motion),[180] it can be understood that a gradual refinement of awareness would lead the yogin to the more subtle "location" of *sattva* as it presents itself in *ahaṃkāra*. As is the case with the other evolutes of *prakṛti, ahaṃkāra* consists of all three *guṇa*s yet *rajas* and *tamas* are here subordinated to *sattva,* especially now that the yogin has ascended beyond the *vitarka* and *vicāra* levels. The locus of joy that was experienced and referenced through the grosser evolutes has its "fount" here. The yogin then concentrates on the pleasure of the *sattva* of *ahaṃkāra* and enjoys a temporary blissful state. To repeat, this temporary state of intense joy is not to be mistaken for the notion of the absolute bliss of *brahman*. In classical Yoga this elevated joy *(ānanda)* must also be seen in its parts and as a whole until the "unification" of the enjoyer and the enjoyed is perceived and the expanded sense of awareness attains to a greater fullness; that is, its nature (i.e., of "joy") is fully realized.[181] Vijñāna Bhikṣu explains that in *ānanda-samādhi* the only *vṛtti* that prevails is: "I am happy, joyful."[182] Even though *mahat* or *buddhi* proper is not reached until the next level *(asmitā)* of cognitive *samādhi,* it can be assumed here that the sattvic nature of *mahat* filters through into *ahaṃkāra (asmitā-mātra),* adding to the sense of joy.

Those yogins who attain this level of experience *(ānanda-samādhi)* may be temporarily absorbed in joyful states of contemplation or mystical ecstasy. Yet there is a danger at this stage in that the yogin may incorrectly consider the enhanced sense of well-being in *ānanda* to be the supreme attainment in Yoga. Having mastered the ego-principle—everything from the physical body made up of the *viśeṣa*s to the *ahaṃkāra*—powers *(siddhi*s*)* may attend upon the yogin. Remaining identified at this level of *samādhi,* one may be called *videha,* "bodiless" one, or a "bodiless shining god" *(videha deva).*[183] The root cause of the *videha*'s attachment and misidentification with the rapturous conditions of *ānanda* is of course ignorance *(avidyā),* which leads one to mistake the noneternal as eternal, the nonself as self, and so on, and thus keeps one engulfed within and enslaved to subtle forms of prakṛtic existence. The *videha*'s state is a possible stage along the way but if a dispassion toward it is not cultivated it merely results in a subtler form of pleasure addiction and misidentification in *saṃyoga*. Egoity *(asmitā)* itself has not yet been rooted out. From the enlightened perspective in Yoga this stage of attainment and identity is still within the guṇic realm of impermanence leading to further dissatisfaction.

The field of *ānanda-samādhi* is *grahaṇa,* the "grasping" or instrument of knowledge. Unlike the *vitarka-* and *vicāra-samādhi*s, it is not subdivided (for example, into *sānanda* and *nirānanda*) by Patañjali or Vyāsa. I therefore understand Vācaspati Miśra as having given an erroneous explanation of the cause and nature of the rapture in this ecstasy. He writes: "Because the nature of *sattva* is illumination . . . the experience of the sattvic pleasures inherent in the senses is the delight of this *samādhi.*"[184] This statement is incorrect in suggesting that the object experienced here is that joy inherent in the senses *(indriya*s*)*. Vijñāna Bhikṣu points out that the above suggestion confuses the *ānanda* ecstasy with *vitarka* and *vicāra,* in which the full realization of the nature of the senses has already occurred, the senses *(indriya*s*)* as objects of support having already been "left behind" as unworthy of further pursuit. If the pleasure inherent in the senses were the object of contemplation in this ecstasy, such experiences would generate the kind of *vṛtti*s in which attraction/attachment *(rāga)* and aversion *(dveṣa)* are implied. This would—like the *"sa"* and *"nir"* forms of the *vitarka* and *vicāra* ecstasies—necessitate two levels in the *ānanda*-accompanied ecstasy: (1) one with the *vṛtti*-identification centered on "joy," and (2) a subtler one without the *vṛtti*-identification of "joy." Neither Patañjali nor Vyāsa have suggested two categories for this ecstasy, and therefore Vācaspati Miśra's interpretation seems erroneous.[185]

For the purpose of furthering our analysis on *ānanda-samādhi,* it is necessary to focus the discussion somewhat on the next stage of cognitive *samādhi:* the *asmitā*-accompanied ecstasy. Vācaspati Miśra, stating the delight inherent in the senses to be the object of the *ānanda*-accompanied ecstasy, considers *puruṣa,* qualified by *ahaṃkāra,* to be the object of *asmitā-samādhi.*[186] This raises a question about *buddhi (mahat)*—the first and finest evolute in the order of manifestation and the last to be experienced, incorporated, and mastered. If *ahaṃkāra,* which arises from *mahat,* is the object in *asmitā-samādhi,* in what other ecstasy would *mahat (buddhi)* be mastered? Furthermore, in what ecstasy would *asmitā* be realized? There are no further stages of *samādhi* given by Patañjali after the *asmitā*-type with supportive factors (*ālambana*s) or objects of contemplation. Nor would this fit in to our present scheme of understanding, which for the sake of clarity, is repeated as follows: (1) sixteen *viśeṣa*s, the gross objects known *(grāhya)* in *vitarka-samādhi;* (2) five *aviśeṣa*s, the subtle objects known *(grāhya)* in *vicāra-samādhi;* (3) *ahaṃkāra* (the sixth and most subtle of the *aviśeṣa*s, the instrument of knowledge or "grasping"—*grahaṇa*), experienced in the later stages of *vicāra* and in *ānanda-samādhi* (note that *ahaṃkāra* is not the same as *asmitā*); (4) *liṅga-mātra (mahat/buddhi)* wherein *asmitā*—the agent of knowledge *(grahītṛ)*—is experienced in *asmitā-samādhi.* It must be pointed out that there is little agreement among the commentators with regard to the objects of contemplation in both the *ānanda* and *asmitā* ecstasies. Disagreements among the commentators notwithstanding, the above scheme can function as a heuristic device in Yoga by presenting a consistent and workable framework for formulating a careful classification relating the levels of cognitive *samādhi* in both a metaphysical/theoretical and experiential/practical way.

Vijñāna Bhikṣu's[187] view—that delight *(hlāda)* alone is the object of contemplation in *ānanda-samādhi*—does not sufficiently explain the source and nature of the rapture. He includes *ahaṃkāra* and *mahat* among the objects of *savicāra-samādhi.*[188] In this case, there appears to be a confusion between *grāhya* and *grahaṇa*. Since, as our study suggests, *ānanda-samādhi* has *grahaṇa* as its classification, delight *(hlāda)* alone cannot be the "object" of contemplation. Being the instrument of "grasping" through which knowledge is self-referenced/appropriated, the evolute *ahaṃkāra (asmitā-mātra)* must find a place in the practical scheme of Yoga.

H. Āraṇya[189] is of the opinion that the sense of happiness in *ānanda-samādhi* arises from the feeling of relaxation in the five organs of action, the five sense organs, and the three constituents of the inner senses: *manas, ahaṃkāra,* and *buddhi.* This may well represent the affective nature of the experience, but Āraṇya's view confuses the subtle scheme of understanding related to these ecstasies and therefore remains incomplete with regard to the ecstasy associated with joy. I agree, however, with Āraṇya's suggestion (below) that the object of contemplation in the *asmitā*-accompanied ecstasy is *buddhi* intent upon *puruṣa*. He writes: "The object concentrated upon in *asmitā samādhi* is not the real *puruṣa* but its imitation, the pseudo-seer. . . . It is *buddhi* shaped after the *puruṣa,* . . . a sort of feeling of identity between the pure consciousness and individual consciousness or *buddhi.*"[190]

Bhoja Rāja's view—that *ahaṃkāra* is the object of support in the *ānanda* ecstasy and *buddhi* being the supportive object in the ecstasy of *asmitā*—seems accurate. However Bhoja Rāja errs in that he considers the pleasure of the *ānanda* ecstasy to be the attribute of pure consciousness, or rather the power of consciousness *(citi-śakti),* which by definition (*YS* IV.34) transcends the realm of the *guṇa*s. Bhoja says:

> When [contemplation on the] *sattva* of the inner instrumentality somewhat penetrated by a residue of *rajas* and *tamas* is cultivated, then, there being no *guṇa*s located in the power of consciousness, the excellence of its (the *antaḥkaraṇa*'s) essence—whose nature is pleasure and illumination—thus cultivated, is called the *samādhi* associated with joy.[191]

Bhoja's entire statement seems self-contradictory. If the contemplation is still on the *sattva* of the *antaḥkaraṇa,* then the (pure) power of consciousness *(citi-śakti)* has not yet been realized. Furthermore, *sattva,* whose nature is pleasure and illumination, is a part of *prakṛti* and not an attribute of *citi-śakti* (i.e., *puruṣa*). The above statement by Bhoja can be stretched somewhat and understood to mean that one is now closer to *citi-śakti,* whose own bliss (*sukha,* happiness in the case of the *sattva guṇa*) and illumination (i.e., knowledge, *jñāna*) have begun to penetrate the *sattva* of the inner sense, causing the excellence of the latter's pleasure and illumination to expand, thus overcoming the residue of *rajas* and *tamas.* In any case, Bhoja's comment does aptly suggest that in *ānanda-samādhi* the *sattva* is still somewhat alloyed with a trace of *rajas* and *tamas* (as is the case with *ahaṃkāra/asmitā-mātra*).

Bhoja Rāja considers *asmitā* to be the counterpart of the *ahaṃkāra* evolute in Sāṃkhya philosophy. According to the understanding of Patañjali's system presented in this study, it has been suggested that *ahaṃkāra,* as the object of support in *ānanda-samādhi,* is purified and no longer performs an obstructing role in the realization of authentic identity. The *samādhi* associated with joy serves its purpose in that contemplation on—becoming aware of the limitations or temporary nature of—the *ahaṃkāra*-principle has been accomplished. I am arguing that if *asmitā* (not *asmitā-mātra*) and *ahaṃkāra* were at all identical, there would be no possibility, indeed no need for, the stage of *asmitā-samādhi*. Like many other commentators, however, Bhoja Rāja insists upon maintaining the identity of *ahaṃkāra* and *asmitā*, but he divides them by function, asserting:

> The identity of *ahaṃkāra* and *asmitā* should not be doubted. Where the inner sense referring to itself as "I" *(aham)* apprehends the objects of experience, it is called *ahaṃkāra*. When by turning inwards in the transformative process of dissolution or return to the source *(prakṛti)* there appears (in the mind) a mere reflection of "pure being," that is called *asmitā*.[192]

While it is accurate to say that *ahaṃkāra* is outward-going toward the mind-organ *(manas),* the senses, and the objects of the senses, and that *asmitā*—located in *mahat (buddhi)*—is a more subtle, internalized process that occurs in the "inner face" of the mind *(citta),* there is no real basis for asserting an identity of *ahaṃkāra* and *asmitā. Asmitā* occurs in *mahat (buddhi),* which is subtler than its product, *ahaṃkāra.*

Vācaspati Miśra as well equates *asmitā* with *ahaṃkāra.* Even though in Sāṃkhya the senses *(indriyas)* are an evolute of (i.e., directly arise from) *ahaṃkāra,* not of *mahat,* he writes: "The senses are products of *asmitā.* Therefore *asmitā* is their subtler form. That intellect *(buddhi)* unified with the self *(ātman)* is referred to as the perception of the essential nature of the self."[193] Here Vācaspati confuses *buddhi* with *ahaṃkāra*. The criticism directed at Bhoja Rāja also applies to Vācaspati Miśra in this regard.

ASMITĀ-SAMĀDHI

Having awakened to and fully realized *ahaṃkāra* in the *ānanda* ecstasy, the yogin sees the inherently flawed nature of guṇic identity at this stage (that is, the yogin observes here the guṇic limitations on self-identity), cultivates dispassion *(vairagya)* toward this state of identification, and moves to the yet subtler ground of the ecstasy associated with *asmitā.* Just as the products among the evolutes can be said to "dissolve" or are transmuted into their subtler and subtler causes, so the yogin's identification with *ahaṃkāra* "dissolves" *(nirodha)* and an identification with *buddhi/mahat* arises. The root-identification as *asmitā* ("I-am-ness") or afflicted (mistaken) identity of self (where ignorance takes root in the mind) denotes a cosmic, pre-individual or even trans-individual state of being within *prakṛti* and is referred to as *mahat* (*Yoga-Bhāṣya* II.19) or the "great self" *(mahān ātmā).* The identification as *asmitā* accompanies the yogin through the contemplation and unification that focuses on the mind-*sattva, mahat/buddhi,* the evolute of "intelligence." Since the previous identifications with the "less refined" evolutes, such as *ahaṃkāra,* have been transcended—meaning that the yogin is no longer misidentified with those phenomena—and *mahat (buddhi)* is the first evolute of *prakṛti,* there is no other object of contemplation or support but *mahat* itself. It is the "designator" *(liṅga-mātra),* the "first sign" that *prakṛti* gives of her presence. The principle of convergence and unification of the object and the agent of contemplation reaches its finest dimension here. Vyāsa asserts: "I-am-ness is the perception of the essential, unified nature of self."[194] Since the "inner face" of *citta (buddhi)* is the most sattvic and purest constituent of the evolutes of *prakṛti,* it most approximates—is analogous to—*puruṣa.* Pure consciousness "reflects" in *buddhi* as into a clear crystal. It is here and nowhere else that *puruṣa* and *prakṛti* "meet" in *saṃyoga,* taking on a single nature, as it were, which is defined as the affliction of "I-am-ness" (*YS* II.6 and *YB* II.6). It is in the reflected consciousness in the mind that ignorance and misidentification "begin" and are terminated, a process with which *puruṣa* is said to have no direct involvement.

At the interface or juncture of the seer and the seeable spring all notions or ideas of selfhood, the reflected consciousness being the primary ("sentient") constituent of our self as person. The growth of self as person is made possible through this conjunction; all the various projections, adjuncts, and instruments of selfhood arise from this "meeting place." Here the person first utters "I am," meaning: "I am this conditioned, contingent, delimited being, a composite of consciousness and insentience." In realizing the nature of *asmitā,* the yogin understands it as the final "break" between *puruṣa* (intrinsic identity) and *cittavṛtti* (mistaken or extrinsic identity) whereby the two constituents of "I-am-ness"—"insentience" in its finest essence of the mind-*sattva,* and the reflection of the *puruṣa* therein—dissolve or "undo" their "union" *(saṃyoga)* or superimposed condition of selfhood[195] that resulted in a confusion of identity between *puruṣa* and the mental processes *(vṛttis)*.

The stage of *samādhi* associated with *asmitā* means the realization of *mahat/buddhi/liṅga-mātra* in which the *guṇa* of *sattva* is predominant. In the previous ecstasy called *ānanda, sattva* is dominant, although, as Bhoja Rāja explains, at this stage of *samādhi* the experience of *sattva* is still somewhat penetrated by residual *rajas* and *tamas*.[196] In *asmitā-samādhi* the *rajas* and *tamas* have been completely subdued, but not expelled, and only the purity and clarity of *sattva* shines. In this experience the sattvic inward face of *buddhi* is "turned away" from its outward facing evolute, *ahaṃkāra* or ego. That is, ego-identification, the nature of which is, for example, to appropriate objects and experiences as being "mine" and not "yours," "ours," or "his"/"hers," and so on, is transcended, submerged, or rather transformed into the pure "am-ness" that is still first-personal but not egoistic. The normal, individual conditions and barriers imposed on consciousness are dissolved in the experience of pure *sattva,* but the *ahaṃkāra* as *grahaṇa* (the instrument through which intelligence asserts itself, experiences, and knows) is not destroyed or negated. Rather, the yogin now experiences a heightened form of perception and understanding that is freed from the misidentification with mere egoic identity. Ontologically, *mahat,* out of which the ego arises and is absorbed, is pure "am-ness" but not "is-ness," which is third-personal and may not have the significance of self-conscious being. The yogin realizes that by turning the mind "inwards" through the practice of *samādhi* the purity of the mind's *sattva* receives the reflection of *puruṣa*. It is due to the presence and power of consciousness *(puruṣa)* in its reflected state functioning through the mind, and not the mind itself, that all the life-processes of our psychophysical being are initiated and sustained.

The word *asmitā* does not refer merely to being, or to existence, but to the consciousness of being or existence, since the term *asmi* is specific to a subject ("I") that proclaims its existence. The concept of *asmitā* has a close relationship in Yoga with that of *sārūpya* (*YS* I.4). *Sārūpya,* implying a misidentification with or conformity to the nature of *vṛtti,* represents the objective aspect (the situation of *puruṣa appearing* to conform to the mental processes), and *asmitā* the root-subjective aspect (the consciousness of being, conditioned by an identification with the mental processes) of a single phenomenon: the superimposed limitation of selfhood in *saṃyoga* due to misidentification with the prakṛtic conditions of individual and cosmic existence, the congenitally conflated realm of *puruṣa* (the seer) and *prakṛti* (the seeable) constituting one's mistaken identity or conditioned being.

In a rare description of *asmitā-samādhi,* Vyāsa states: "'The mind that has reached the unification called *asmitā* becomes serene and infinite like a great (still) ocean."[197] Because *puruṣa* is an undisturbed, infinite existence—like a "still" ocean—the inward face of the mind *(buddhi)* receiving *puruṣa*'s "reflection" and as experienced in *asmitā-samādhi* appears like an infinite, calm ocean, without rufflement, that is, without distracting or disturbing mental "waves" or activity. The experience of this "reflection" of *puruṣa* is both expansive like the ocean and minute like an atomic particle. Vyāsa quotes from the Sāṃkhyan teacher, Pañcaśikha: "Having found that self which is minute like the atom, one realizes oneself only as 'I am'."[198] No contradiction need be implied in the description of the Self *(ātman)* or its reflection as being both minute and expansive. It is repeatedly described as being as subtle as, or more specifically in the Upaniṣads, as being more minute than an atomic particle.[199] It is also, however, referred to as being great/expansive *(mahān)*[200] or even as being both minute and great.[201] It is noteworthy that the descriptions of the realization of *ātman* (or *puruṣa*) and of its "reflection" in *asmitā* (correlating with cosmic being—*mahān ātmā*—or *mahat*) are very similar. It is as though one person were to describe the sky in its utter vastness and another speak of its clear reflection in a pond.

What needs to be emphasized at this point in our analysis is that the progression in *samādhi* from *vitarka* to *vicāra* to *ānanda* to *asmitā* results in experiences of an ever-increasing sense of I or self, *a continuously expanding sense of self-identity*. This expanding sense of identity, which incorporates the levels of person/individual and cosmic (trans-egoic/individual) being, arises due to the finer perceptions *(yogi-pratyakṣa)* or insights *(prajñā)* of the yogin that disclose the nature of the objects experienced (the seeable, *dṛśya*). As stated in chapter 2, Yoga ontology follows from epistemology. In *asmitā-samādhi* the yogin is identified with *mahat*[202] (cosmic or trans-individual being) or *mahān ātmā* (the great self), attains omniscience, and experiences self-identity as an undivided, nonfractured, unified self-nature or being.[203] Through *samādhi* one's identity has expanded to include the whole of manifest existence, a state that is transcendent of any subject-object (ego-world) bifurcation or fragmentation within *prakṛti*. The yogin knows "I am the whole, the all-pervading sense of self that gives rise to and permeates all manifest existence." In *asmitā-samādhi* the yogin is liberated from the idea of being a bound or limited identity dependent on being in association with joy or happiness *(sukha)* and attached to the pleasure of *sattva*. It is not until *asmitā-samādhi* that the insight attained is said to be "truth-bearing" *(ṛtaṃbharā)* disclosing the object as it is without any epistemological distortion. At this exalted stage of *samādhi,* rather than being deprived of the levels of knowledge, perception, and understanding gained previously, the yogin reconciles and incorporates these levels into the fullness and perfection of the "truth-bearing" insight.[204] Having discarded all *attachment* to the lower or grosser levels of perception, the yogin's capacity to experience, understand, perceive, remember, rationalize, and so on, far from being negated or abandoned, is transformed, purified, enhanced; the various mental faculties thus being properly harnessed can then function more effectively in the practical world. There is a recognition and purification of self-identity in relation to the world and nature culminating in a reunification and integration of the individuated sense of self *(ahaṃkāra)* with the trans-individuated, cosmic, or universal sense of "I-am-ness" or self as supported in *mahat/buddhi.*

Perception is not suppressed, flattened out, or destroyed through Yoga; it is transformed. The lower levels of realization are encompassed, not negated. By attaining increasingly subtler levels of perception through the sattvification of the mind, the yogin is more capable of embodying a richer affective life—one that is inclusive rather than exclusive of the practical, relational world—for prior to *samādhi* what had been held as ontologically and epistemologically separate from oneself is now seen for what it actually is, part of one corpus *(prakṛti)* of existence. The moral-affective dimension of Yoga that includes the cultivation of friendliness, compassion, happiness, and so on, toward others (*YS* I.33) is an indispensible part of the yogin's journey into subtler levels of realization and self-understanding and thus the overcoming of the selfish, contracted nature of ego. Through moral purification finer perception can arise, virtue thus acting as an efficient cause for removing nonvirtue (*YB* IV.3; see chapter 2), which in turn allows for greater concentration and meditative insight in Yoga. What is involved here is not a suppression but a reconciliation of past actions and a healing summation and transmutation of the human psyche. The moral, affective, and epistemological dimensions of Yoga are refined, and virtues, whether of an ethical or cognitive nature, are seen to converge in the *sattva* of the mind. By developing the capacity or power *(siddhi)* to "contact" or "locate" finer, clearer, and undiverted reflections of *puruṣa* within the mind, the yogin is purified of distorted perception, deluded self-understanding, and a host of other forms of nonvirtue. An increasing light of *sattva*—including liberating knowledge (*jñāna, YS* II.28), dispassion (*vairāgya, YS* I.15), and other virtues such as compassion (*karuṇā, YS* I.33)—pervades the yogin's consciousness, augmenting and spiritualizing the yogin's identity.

Yoga is not therefore a dissolution, negation, or rejection of psychophysical being—the purpose of which is to isolate the yogin from relational, embodied existence. By including subtler dimensions of consciousness, Yoga can mean "addition"[205] implying here a recognition of its much overlooked capacity to value, enhance, and vivify human embodied life: cognitively, ethically, physically, and so on. To repeat our claim from the last chapter, "dissolution" or "cessation" *(nirodha)* is of the deluding power of misidentification (in *saṃyoga*); "cessation" *(nirodha)* is not a complete relinquishment of the power of identification itself that enables one to give attention to, empathize, understand, and "unite" with objects, persons, and so forth. Yoga discards all ignorance and attachment, not knowledge *(vṛtti)* and relational existence in total. In order to be accomplished in Yoga, the yogin must be able to pinpoint or arrive at the cause of *saṃyoga*—namely, ignorance *(avidyā),* the mind in its unenlightened state as locus of selfhood. *Samādhi* uproots the afflictions as they manifest themselves within our prakṛtic makeup including the subtler levels of *ahaṃkāra* and *buddhi.* In *saṃyoga, puruṣa seems* to conform to the nature of the seeable, selfhood being experienced within the context of the afflictions implying a mistaken identity of self *(asmitā).* The world (of objects) is misperceived through the "eyes" of egoity or ignorance. The mind's *(citta)* nature is paradoxical in that: (1) In *asmitā-samādhi* the root-afflicted-identity *(asmitā)* is located where the seer and the seeable appear to be one (in the *buddhi*). Yet (2) the *buddhi* or finest instrument of the mind *(citta)* has the quality of *sattva* or illumination through which the yogin discerns the difference between the *puruṣa* and the *sattva* of consciousness and gradually uproots and eradicates the affliction of *asmitā.* There results a purification of self in relation to the world and nature. Thus, through a series of subject-object identifications in cognitive *samādhi,* the yogin succeeds in temporarily transcending the polarization of self and world, the subject-object dichotomy that had previously governed and defined self-identity in *saṃyoga.* In fact, Patañjali's main concern throughout his analysis of *samādhi* is not with the objects themselves but with the misidentifications, attachments, aversions, desires, and fears that accompany the experiences of objects.

Prakṛti and her various manifestations, including the concept of mind *(citta),* are ingeniously utilized by Patañjali for pedagogical purposes, that is, as states (or powers) of identification that, functioning positively as contemplative directives along the "path" of Yoga, can serve as heuristic devices for practitioners of Yoga. The practitioner must first discover or recognize aspects or evolutes of *prakṛti* that he or she is misidentified with, attached to, or has an aversion toward. By way of yogic technique and one-pointedness of mind the practitioner then learns to "undo" any misidentification with objects or mental content including thought constructs/ideas *(pratyaya)* and mental processes *(vṛtti)*. Through cessation *(nirodha)* brought about by practice and dispassion, including the unhinging of attention from its confinement to ego-consciousness, the power of identification or *vṛtti*-generating complex no longer functions under the influence of ignorance *(avidyā)*. All *enslavement* to the nature of the seeable *(dṛśya)* is eradicated. *Prakṛti* is not negated from the yogin's purview; she is more correctly aligned with pure consciousness *(puruṣa)* and therefore can be more fully incorporated. Through a deepening process of purification and illumination of the mind, misidentification dissolves. Thus in *samādhi, prakṛti*—on whatever level, gross or subtle—ceases to function as an obstacle to clear, liberating insight. Without *prakṛti* there would be no ontological backdrop, no levels of existence or vehicles through which knowledge could take place. It would be impossible for liberation to arise because there would be no forms of subject-object identifications from which to locate any semblance of pure consciousness, overcome attachment, and grow in one's understanding. The concept of mind *(citta)* is in part a heuristic device for understanding the nature and functioning of reflected consciousness. In its unenlightened mode *(vyutthāna)* under the sway of ignorance in the form of *vāsanā*s of misconceived knowledge (*YB* II.24) the mind—as reflected, impure (prakṛtic) consciousness—can be viewed as the cause and sustaining power of *saṃyoga,* bondage, and dissatisfaction *(duḥkha)*. Yet when *sattva*-knowledge is allowed to shine forth, the mind, as reflected albeit purified consciousness, can be seen as the efficient cause of liberation disclosing knowledge for the purpose of *puruṣa,* the final cause (*YB* II.19). Thus Vyāsa tells us that in the mind alone takes place both bondage and liberation.[206]

When *asmitā* has been examined (in *asmitā-samādhi*) its nature is fully realized. This corresponds to the state of "unification" *(samāpatti)* with the "grasper" *(grahītṛ),* (see discussion above on *YS* I.41); the "field" or focus of this ecstasy is the prakṛtic agent of knowledge. At this level "grasping" (knowing) and "grasper" (knower) lose their independent status: the analogy of radiance or clarity extends to one's inner being *(adhyātma)*.[207] Vyāsa[208] and Vācaspati[209] have understood contemplation on the "grasper" *(grahītṛ)* as being that mysterious intersection of the prakṛtic knower-agent (located in mind-*sattva* or *buddhi*) and *puruṣa,* the authentic knower-witness. Here unification with the "grasper" *(grahītṛ)* links up with *asmitā-samādhi*. The yogin concentrates on the reflected "knower" ("grasper") in *prakṛti;* the real knower (*YS* IV.18)—*puruṣa*—cannot be made an object of knowledge, a mental content *(pratyaya)* or modification *(vṛtti)*. What the yogin actually succeeds in realizing is *asmitā,* the mental stand-in for *puruṣa*. Koelman puts it this way: "By concentration on the knower we reach the awareness-light projected by the Self. We do not actually grasp the very essence of the Self, we gain access only to its liminal result, that is its illuminating participation in the *sattva* of the *[buddhi]*."[210]

I have translated Vyāsa's description of *asmitā: eka-ātmikā saṃvit*[211] (*YB* I.17) as "the perception of the essential, unified nature of self." This refers to the prediversified, undifferentiated (unified), or rather trans-egoic condition of reflected self-identity in *prakṛti*. The sattvic illumination of the mirror of *buddhi* and the reflected light of *puruṣa* are unified in *asmitā.* Vijñāna Bhikṣu[212] explains that the word *eka* ("one") here signifies "only one," that is to say: "Only one, the Self *(ātman),* is its object." He interprets this to mean that at this stage of *samādhi* there is only one object of support, the mind's perception of only the *puruṣa,* by which one realizes that "I am." As the object of contemplation merges here with the agent, the mind appears unified with *puruṣa*. In this view it is correct that the mind is seen to be unified with the Self, but it would be incorrect to assume that the pure, unreflected *ātman (puruṣa)* is the object of contemplation. If we understand Bhikṣu's statement literally, then it seems safe to say that Bhikṣu has erred by asserting that in *asmitā-samādhi* the yogin knows "I am thus—thus alone," that is, that there is nothing further to know, and that this is the ultimate ground (or height) of realization. The union in *asmitā* more likely expresses (as Bhikṣu would probably agree) an analogical understanding of consciousness. In Yoga philosophy, *asmitā* is the apparent unity in consciousness of two very distinct self-identities: the Self or intrinsic identity on the one side, and on the other side its most subtle prakṛtic conditioning, an extrinsic, empirical identity of self. It is then disclosed that what was taken for authentic identity, which is pure and unchanging, is really a composite and changing identity *(cittavṛtti), asmitā* being generated through the interplay of *puruṣa* and the mind under the influence of *avidyā.* Actually, the realization of the pure *puruṣa* does not begin until *asaṃprajñāta,* the supracognitive *samādhi.*

The only "passage" to authentic identity in Yoga seems to be through the exercise of a purified cognitive faculty.[213] The mind *in itself* does not form a link between *puruṣa* and *prakṛti*. Only an actual exercise of knowledge on the side of *prakṛti* is the "wire" (or "stream") that can convey the "current" (or "flow") within the mind that in turn leads to liberation (*Yoga-Bhāṣya* I.12). Knowledge *(jñāna)* becomes the efficient cause of spiritual "release." Due to the presence of *puruṣa,* the mind inevitably "undoes" its own saṃsāric entanglements as locus of mistaken identity *(cittavṛtti)* by means of the cultivation of knowledge. This process of the cessation *(nirodha)* of mistaken identity continues throughout the stages of cognitive *samādhi* up to the discriminative discernment *(vivekakhyāti).* At this level of perception *asmitā-samādhi* matures into the realization of *vivekakhyāti,* the re-cognition or illuminated cognition (*YB* II.26) of the distinctness of mind-*sattva* and *puruṣa.* Because of the unified, one-pointed awareness of *asmitā,* this ecstasy, as with the *ānanda* state of ecstasy, is not divided into *sāsmitā* and *nirasmitā.*

The ability of the yogin in the practice *(abhyāsa)* of *samādhi* to identify completely with the object of support/contemplation and yet cultivate dispassion or detachment *(vairāgya)* allows for the realization that the yogin's true being is not the same as, nor is it dependent on, the contemplated object. Moreover, the yogin is aware that the realization of *puruṣa* is still to take place. *Asmitā-samādhi* reveals insight into the nature of the original identification *(asmitā)* with the reflection of consciousness in the mind. With clear insight and understanding, its practice enables the yogin to cultivate dispassion toward the subtlest vicissitudes of *prakṛti.* Patañjali's use of the term "as if" (*iva, YS* II.6 and III.3) applied to this stage of "unification" indicates that even the "identification" of the seer—or power of seeing—with the seeable—or objects of experience—is only an apparent "as if" identification or union. In Yoga one becomes "as if" ontologically at one with the objects in the *"nir"* forms of *samādhi* because at this stage of practice there is as yet an implied ontological duality of seer and seeable. In cognitive *samādhi,* the actual oneness attained with our objects of experience can more accurately be understood with an epistemological emphasis. The knower-agent in *asmitā-samādhi* is nonseparate from the known, the power and potential of the whole of manifest existence *(mahat).* This can be seen to be the case because the reflection of the infinite *puruṣa* received by the mind is and has to be as vast or all-pervading as manifest *prakṛti*[214] herself, just as the consciousness of our being a person is at least as extensive as our physical body. The "I" that identifies itself with the physical body is a function of the ego-principle, a mere evolute of *prakṛti.* The unsullied *puruṣa* can be realized only *after* the pure reflection of pure consciousness is apprehended in *asmitā-samādhi.* This realization is at the end of a series of identifications with, and dispassion toward, the grossest to the subtlest evolutes of *prakṛti;* and the series of *samādhi*s (i.e., unifications or *samāpatti*s) explained by Patañjali are such a series.

In Yoga a distinction must be made between two types of knowledge gained by the yogin in *saṃprajñāta.* First there is immediate knowledge *(prajñā)* independent of extraneous influences of the prakṛtic world, the purest level of which is *buddhi,* or in its cosmic aspect *mahat*. This at its highest is *"nirvicāra"* knowledge translated as "I am the whole," the recognition of an organic unity between grasper, grasping, and grasped bringing or "putting back" together, healing *prakṛti*'s formerly fragmented parts as separate realities caused by the divisive and delusive nature of ignorance *(avidyā),* that is, egoic consciousness and extrinsic identity. An epistemological oneness of knower and known, self and world takes place wherein the distinctions of knower, knowing, and known or grasper, grasping, and grasped (*YS* I.41) dissolve and there is no longer the predisposition to separate the perceiver from things perceived or vice versa. Yet there is also the use to which this primary experiential knowledge is put, for the purpose of liberation; that is *vivekakhyāti*.[215] I understand *vivekakhyāti* to mean the discriminative discernment between: (1) the extrinsic nature of consciousness and self-identity located in the mind (in *saṃyoga*)—a reflected, guṇic state of consciousness—and (2) the intrinsic nature of consciousness and self-identity, the authentic "form" of Self *(svarūpa, puruṣa).*

All misidentification with things prakṛtic must eventually dissolve in the process of "cessation" *(nirodha)* in order for emancipation to ensue. There are yogins who become absorbed in the source of all manifestation *(aliṅga)*. Those who attain this state of utter absorption with unmanifest *prakṛti* and consider it to be the final destination are yogins referred to as *prakṛti-laya* (*YS* I.19). They have dissolved their identification with the evolutes and have become identified with undifferentiated, unmanifest *prakṛti* herself. However, they have not yet realized *puruṣa* and so continue in bondage to saṃsāric existence, living a kind of pseudo-liberation.[216] At this point, however, there appears to be nothing further to attain. The yogin does not realize without proper guidance or a *guru* that absorption in unmanifest *prakṛti* is actually not the end of the journey. In this state there are no "objects" except *prakṛti* herself. The yogin must now make efforts to "turn toward" *puruṣa*. However, if this direction does not become clear and the necessary guidance is not available or accepted, the *prakṛti-laya* (yogin) may mistake this point to be the culmination of Yoga, self-awareness becoming identified completely (i.e., misidentified) with *prakṛti.* All other *vṛtti*s of identification have subsided but ignorance has not been completely eradicated. The *prakṛti-laya*'s sense of identity is still rooted in error *(viparyaya),* attachment, and the desire to have control or mastery over *prakṛti*.[217] The identification with *prakṛti* has not been transcended. It is interesting that Vyāsa classifies the "unmanifest" *(aliṅga)* as not being caused by any purpose of *puruṣa:* "No purpose of *puruṣa* brings it about, nor is there any purpose of *puruṣa* in it."[218] It can be concluded that identification with and attachment to unmanifest *prakṛti* merely constitutes a detour on the path of Yoga. From the perspective of the liberated state, *prakṛti-laya* is simply another form of bondage. One could argue that at best *prakṛti-laya* is a "mild" *(mṛdu)* form of practice in comparison to the "moderate" *(madhya)* and "ardent" *(adhimātratva)* forms of practice involving more advanced yogins.[219] Apparently content with this state of identity and "form of practice" where there is as yet an "idea/intention of becoming" *(bhava-pratyaya)*,[220] the yogin must continue to take birth in order to become purified from all misidentification with *prakṛti* and eventually abide in authentic identity as *puruṣa*.

A FURTHER LOOK AT COGNITIVE *SAMĀDHI*

For the purpose of clarifying the analysis given in this chapter on the stages of *saṃprajñāta-samādhi*, it would now seem appropriate to ask the question: How many types of cognitive *samādhi* are there? A critical look at scholarly literature on Yoga reveals that there is a great deal of confusion on this issue. It is of interest to note the following statement by Feuerstein:

> "Joy" and "I-am-ness" . . . must be regarded as accompanying phenomena of every cognitive [ecstasy]. The explanations of the classical commentators on this point appear to be foreign to Patañjali's hierarchy of [ecstatic] states, and it seems unlikely that *ānanda* and *asmitā* should constitute independent levels of *samādhi*.[221]

Our study disagrees with Feuerstein, suggesting that he has misapprehended the specific placement that these ecstatic stages are assigned, at least implicitly so, by Patañjali. I have previously shown how Vyāsa can be read as taking *ānanda-* and *asmitā-samādhi* as later stages of *nirvicāra-samāpatti* and the sorts of experiences these two stages of *samādhi* represent.[222]

Vācaspati Miśra proposes a model of eight types of "unification" *(samāpatti)*. He states: "Thus [with regard] to the 'objects of knowledge' there are four *samāpatti*s, [and there are a further] four [in respect to] the 'grasper' and the 'process of grasping'. Thus there are eight of these."[223] Following from *nirvicāra-samāpatti*—which I have argued is the highest *samāpatti* in Vyāsa's classification, Miśra adds four other stages, in effect doubling Vyāsa's number. These stages, from highest to lowest, may be listed as follows:

(1–2) *Nirasmitā-* and *sāsmitā-samāpatti,* both with "I-am-ness" as the object of support or objective prop.
(3–4) *Nirānanda-* and *sānanda-samāpatti,* both with the sense organs as objects of support or objective props.
(5–6) *Nirvicāra-* and *savicāra-samāpatti,* both with subtle objects as objects of support or objective props.
(7–8) *Nirvitarka-* and *savitarka-samāpatti,* both with gross objects as objects of support or objective props.

Vijñāna Bhikṣu proposes a six-stage model, explicitly rejecting Vācaspati Miśra's view, according to which the mainstay of *vitarka-* and *vicāra-samādhi* is the internalized object *(grāhya),* of *ānanda-samādhi* the instruments of cognition or grasping *(grahaṇa),* and of *asmitā-samādhi* the category of the grasper *(grahītṛ).* Bhikṣu instead regards joy *(ānanda)* as a state that arises when the mind passes beyond the *vicāra* stage; due to an increase in the quality of *sattva* there is a direct experience of a special pleasure termed "joy," which is then made the supportive factor of the ecstasy called *ānanda.*[224] I have already given a critique of both Vācaspati Miśra and Vijñāna Bhikṣu on their views of *ānanda-* and *asmitā-samādhi.* This study agrees, however, with Vijñāna Bhikṣu's adamant denial of a *nirānanda*[225] or a *nirasmitā*[226] form of *samādhi.*

G. Koelman offers a very elaborate analysis of the *samāpatti*s, opting for Vācaspati Miśra's interpretation.[227] Koelman argues that the eight types of *samāpatti*s as delineated in the *Tattva-Vaiśāradī* "are the core of Patañjali's mental discipline" and are indeed "a magnificent piece of psychology."[228] As one scholar suggests, however, "it remains an open question to what degree this [i.e., Koelman's] theoretical model is founded on *bona fide* experiential information."[229] There do not appear to be any sound grounds for justifying a need for a *nirānanda* or a *nirasmitā* stage of *samādhi.* Patañjali's own view seems to be that *nirvicāra-samāpatti* is the highest form of cognitive ecstasy, as this study has attempted to show by using a scheme of classification that adheres to the careful step-by-step process of *samādhi* outlined in both the *Yoga-Sūtra* and the *Yoga-Bhāṣya.*

The *samādhi*s with supportive factors *(sālambana)* are also called *samādhi*s "with seed" *(sabīja).* As Patañjali asserts in *Yoga-Sūtra* I.46: *tā eva sabījaḥ samādhiḥ,* "These *[savitarka, nirvitarka, savicāra, nirvicāra]* are *samādhi* with seed."[230] *Sabīja samādhi* is a technical name for cognitive *samādhi.* In the literature on classical Yoga there appear to be two main interpretations of the term *bīja* as given in *Yoga-Sūtra* I.46. According to Vyāsa, "seed" *(bīja)* refers to the "object" of contemplation or support.[231]

Bhoja Rāja, in his commentary *ad locum,* also explains the term *bīja* by *"ālambana"* or "object of support."[232] The meaning of *Yoga-Sūtra* I.46 in the context of the above interpretation of *bīja* is that the forms of contemplation constituted by the *samāpatti*s do metaphorically have a supporting factor in the object[233] on which the mind has become one-pointed *(ekāgra)*.

Other interpreters maintain for *bīja* its literal meaning of "seed."[234] Rāmānanda Yati and J. W. Hauer follow this interpretation wherein the forms of *samādhi* constituted by the *samāpatti*s have in themselves the seeds or potentialities (i.e., *saṃskāra*s) of new mental processes *(vṛtti*s*),* which necessarily have to actualize themselves and, as a result, create further bondage. Hauer declares that *bīja* stands for the seed of new *vṛtti*s.[235] Rāmānanda Yati understands *bīja* in the sense of "seed of bondage."[236]

Vijñāna Bhikṣu states that the exterior objects (i.e., referring to the prakṛtic realm that is external to *puruṣa*) have qualities not belonging to the *puruṣa*. From these objects arise impressions *(saṃskāra*s*),* characteristics *(dharma*s*),* and so forth, which are the seeds of dissatisfaction and future sorrow (*duḥkha,* see *YS* II.16).[237] Elsewhere Bhikṣu considers that the forms of *samādhi* constituted by the *samāpatti*s are "with seed" both because they have an object of support *(ālambana)* and because they give rise to new mental processes[238] with which the yogin becomes (mis)identified. I comply with Bhikṣu's later interpretation[239] and furthermore suggest that the seed-mechanism of misidentification *(cittavṛtti)* or mistaken identity of the mind *(citta)* with *puruṣa* is the original or "source-seed" that must be uprooted and eradicated. This primal seed of ignorance or *saṃskāra,* as we have seen, takes the form of the *vāsanā*s of erroneous knowledge (*viparyaya-jñāna, YB* II.24).[240]

Most commentators have struggled with *Yoga-Sūtra* I.46, trying to resolve the apparent contradiction in the number of forms of cognitive *samādhi*. Vyāsa's commentary seems to the point:

> Those four unifications have external objects as their seeds; thus, *samādhi* too, is [said to be] with seed. When it is a gross object, the *samādhi* is *savitarka* or *nirvitarka;* when it is a subtle object, it is *savicāra* or *nirvicāra.* Thus is [cognitive] *samādhi* counted to be fourfold.[241]

Apparently ignoring Vyāsa's clear statement, Vācaspati Miśra has asserted that there are eight kinds of cognitive *samādhi.* Vijñāna Bhikṣu understands that there are six kinds. It is not crucial to our study to pursue all of their enumerations, classifications, and differing arguments. However, it is noteworthy that Vyāsa has *not* stated that there are four kinds of cognitive *samadhi,* but rather that cognitive *samadhi* is to be divided "fourfold" *(caturdhā).* As explained earlier, the divisions[242] run as follows:

1. *Savitarka-samāpatti* correlates with *savitarka-samādhi*
2. *Nirvitarka-samāpatti* correlates with *nirvitarka-samādhi*
3. *Savicāra-samāpatti* correlates with *savicāra-samādhi*
4. *Nirvicāra-samāpatti* correlates with *nirvicāra-samādhi, ānanda-samādhi,* and *asmitā-samādhi.*

What is common to the above stages of ecstasy is that what is being known is within the realm of prakṛtic, empirical experience and therefore is exclusive of *puruṣa. Puruṣa,* however, can at no time be made into an object or entity that the yogin takes it upon to realize outwardly or within the mind. Accordingly, all these forms of *samādhi* are labelled *saṃprajñāta,* the *samādhi* of the accurate knowing of objects, including objective and subjective "distinguishables" that pertain to the realm of *prakṛti,* that is, empirical identity. Were I really to know my authentic Self, clearly a manner of "oneness" or identity that is *asaṃprajñāta* is required. It could not be a knowing to which I might give mental shape or form *(vṛtti),* for that would mean it would be of some object, which *puruṣa* cannot be. The insights *(prajñā)* that arise in cognitive *samādhi* cover, comprehend all phenomena, including my empirical persona, and enshrine in its higher stages unabashedly empirical claims that cannot be tested in any "rational" way by argument but can only be fully grasped and understood through direct experience, yogic perception *(yogi-pratyakṣa).*

Patañjali maintains that in cognitive *samādhi* there are still "things of the mind"—mental processes, content, or thought constructs—that get in the way of or hinder our realization of *puruṣa,* intrinsic identity. The mind is likely to sully the purity of *samādhi* in *savitarka* and *savicāra* in the ways explained earlier. The *"nir"* forms are plainly and simply those occasions of attained epistemological oneness when the mind does not interfere as stated. At the moment of the experience of pure knowing or knowingness, the sense of self as normally understood and felt—as an ego-subject that is separate from the object of experience and that misappropriates or lays claim to the experience—no longer veils (or remains an impediment or obstacle to) clear knowledge and understanding. Our misidentification of self—rooted in ignorance *(avidyā)* and given shape through the saṃyogic/saṃsāric processes of *vṛtti* and *saṃskāra* that generate and sustain our notions *(pratyaya)* of egoity *(asmitā)*—is shown to be the product of a profound epistemological distortion that resides deep within the mind yet that can effectively be removed through insight *(prajñā)* or knowledge *(jñāna)* in *samādhi.* However much *puruṣa* is conceived to be concealed or excluded in *saṃyoga,* it must be emphasized that without the presence of *puruṣa* as knower-witness no cognition or knowledge *(vṛtti)* under any circumstances could arise in consciousness or function in the mind. The explanation of the existence of a "path" or "mapping" of Yoga from ordinary experience *(bhoga)* to the liberated "aloneness" *(kaivalya)* is based on the understanding that *puruṣa* is ubiquitous and already present, immanent (though seemingly stained and misidentified as an entrapped entity within *prakṛti*) as the true knower/experiencer of ordinary cognition. Due to *puruṣa*'s immanence, the sequence of "unification" *(samāpatti)*—from *grāhya* to *grahaṇa* to *grahītṛ*—is rendered pertinent and effective for liberation. Through the process of "cessation" *(nirodha),* the yogin succeeds in dissolving or discarding the limitations—in the form of misidentification with *vṛtti*—imposed on self-identity.

Puruṣa is present throughout ordinary states of awareness and indeed the stages of cognitive *samādhi* through an "as if" identification taking the form of a reflected, albeit masquerading consciousness, a pseudo sense-of-self *that in seeking to secure its identity through prakṛti can never truly ground itself because it is itself extrinsic, inauthentic identity, irrevocably conditioned by and contained within the changing guṇic realm.* Patañjali declares that all forms of *saṃprajñāta,* being contemplations on and realizations of supportive factors, are *samādhi*s "with seed" *(sabīja).* Because they are *samādhi*s on the realities perceived within the composite person and are "exterior" to *puruṣa,* they yet contain the seed of ignorance, further bondage, dissatisfaction, and sorrow. Therefore *saṃprajñāta* is to be contrasted with *asaṃprajñāta,* the supracognitive *samādhi* that, at the very highest level of realization, is said to be "seedless" *(nirbīja),*[243] unaffected by ignorance and its *saṃskāra*s and therefore free from all dissatisfaction. Thus the practice and cultivation of *samādhi* continues for the sake of each misidentified being. Even though in *saṃprajñāta* the yogin is established in a one-pointedness *(ekāgratā)* of mind that removes the barriers separating subject from object, the purest and most illuminated or sattvified state of mind *(niruddha, nirodha)*—one in which the yogin is no longer dependent on objects of contemplation for the sake of liberation—is yet to be attained.

We will now go on to complete our study of *samādhi* and the cessation *(nirodha)* of mistaken identity *(cittavṛtti)* in Yoga. Included in this final chapter will be an examination of the enstatic, supra- or transcognitive *(asaṃprajñāta)* state of *samādhi* as well as a consideration of the meaning of the culminating state of liberation called "aloneness" *(kaivalya).*

chapter six

From Knowledge to the "Aloneness" of the Knower

THE SOTERIOLOGICAL ROLE OF *SAṂSKĀRA* IN YOGA

We have seen that one of the practical aims of Yoga is to generate and strengthen the nonafflicted mental processes *(akliṣṭa-vṛtti*s*)* and impressions *(saṃskāra*s*)* that help to eradicate the impurities of the mind rooted in error *(viparyaya)* and its five parts, namely, the afflictions *(kleśa*s*)*.[1] As long as the afflictions are in place, a human being is ineluctably oriented toward experiences in the limited realms of *prakṛti*. The five *kleśa*s are the motivational matrix of the unenlightened mind. The cultivation of discipline in Yoga gives rise to sattvic virtues such as friendliness *(maitrī)* toward other beings, nonviolence *(ahiṃsā)*, compassion *(karuṇā)*, and so forth. As ignorance *(avidyā)* is gradually replaced by knowledge *(vidyā)*, attachment *(rāga)*, aversion *(dveṣa)*, and so on, will also be replaced by their opposites, through their inevitable linking together by the mental impressions *(saṃskāra*s*)*. *Saṃskāra*s of benevolence, dispassion, and the like, in opposition to their corresponding impurities, will, in their turn, counter the influence of ignorance and its web of afflictions (i.e., egoity/I-am-ness, attachment, aversion, desire for continuity/fear of death), contributing in this manner to an increasing light of knowledge,[2] an illumination of consciousness.

Thus, yogic disciplines culminating in *samādhi* are designed to bring about and foster those *saṃskāra*s that can eventually subdue and eliminate the afflictions, gradually assuring an undisturbed "flow of" the mind toward liberation.[3] The more positively impregnated mental activities *(vṛttis)* produce sattvic impressions *(saṃskāras)* and these in turn give rise to a different, positively transformed mental activity that will then produce new impressions, and so on.[4] The yogin's personality likewise becomes transformed—meaning that it becomes morally and cognitively purified of the binding effects of *rajas* and *tamas*. The yogin develops a clarity of knowledge through which *prakṛti* is increasingly appropriated in a nonconflicting and unselfish manner. Purity of the *sattva* implies a mastery over *rajas* and *tamas* and their identity-constricting influences (i.e., attachments, aversions), and consists in a dispassion toward what is perceived and experienced. Purity *(śuddhi)* generally stands for purity of the mental *sattva,*[5] even though the yogin's final "step" is that of becoming free from the influence of the *guṇas* in their entirety and hence also from *sattva*.[6] In this way Yoga seeks to give, in the words of C. Pensa:

> an analytical and "scientific" explanation . . . predominant in Indian religion, according to which true knowledge has such a totally transforming effect on the individual as to release him from the *saṃsāra*. Terms such as knowledge, purification, *samādhi,* liberation, are thus all very closely related and interdependent; but this intimate association and reciprocity could not be had outside the connective tissue represented by the *saṃskāras* and their law.[7]

After considerable journeying on the "path" of Yoga, the yogin seeks to attain an eventual "victory" over *karma* in its form of spiritual ignorance *(avidyā)*. Again, Pensa incisively states:

> Without such a victory there would be no sense in talking about freedom and absolute independence as the final result of the yogic *mārga*. Nevertheless—and here we have a vital point—if this victory-liberation is to be achieved, it must be "sown" continually in accordance with the iron logic of the basic law: liberation may be achieved only on condition that the mind *(citta),* through adequate depuration, be enabled to produce the necessary amount of karmic impulses [*saṃskāras*] endowed with the specific quality of giving rise in their turn to liberation.[8]

In Yoga philosophy *saṃskāra* functions both as a binding influence in the form of ignorance and where *rajas* and *tamas* predominate, or as a liberating force in the form of knowledge *(jñāna)* residing in the *sattva* of the mind. As Pensa implies in the above, in its most sattvic form *saṃskāra* has a profound soteriological significance in Yoga. There are many levels at which the strength of worldly, afflicted *karma* is reduced. For example, there are many expiatory observances of prayer, ritual offerings, and meritorious acts that reduce the power of already existing karmic traits, predispositions, and *saṃskāra*s by adding to the karmic residue *(karmāśaya)* the force of these thoughts and acts.[9] But these efforts do not free one from the entire bondage of *karma* and the inherent dissatisfaction *(duḥkha)* within *saṃsāra* because there is still one's involvement as an egoic identity: the inclination toward dependence on further acts and attachment to the results of those acts (in the form of gainful award engendering happiness/pleasure or loss generating sorrow, pain and aversion) still remains. The true yogic sacrifice—the "interiorized" or "spiritualized" sacrifice *(yajña)*—of egotism itself (as proclaimed, for example, by the early Upaniṣadic sages)[10] must be distinguished in Yoga from "external" or extrinsic forms of sacrifice or ritual that, motivated from a basic misconception of self rooted in a selfish mentality and desirous of material or spiritual gain, are clearly inefficacious for bringing about spiritual emancipation.[11]

The perceptual knowledge attained in *saṃprajñāta* helps to reveal our very identity or being, which due to an epistemological error had seemingly become entangled and dispersed in the prakṛtic realm. At the stage of *nirvicāra-samādhi* (*samādhi* without subtle associations) the knowledge that arises is said to be "truth-bearing" *(ṛtaṃ-bharā)*;[12] the yogin has attained a "knowing-oneness" with the whole of manifest *prakṛti (mahat)*, including the ability to know—through *siddhi*s or "powers" brought about by the application of *saṃyama* or "constraint" (see below)—all of the various manifestations that arise out of *mahat*. At this stage the inner reflective awareness of self has become pure, clear,[13] and capable of contemplating its own true nature or essence. It is, however, only the lucidity and clarity made possible through the reflected presence of *puruṣa* in *asmitā-samādhi* that is intended here. Vijñāna Bhikṣu correctly points out that the word *tatra* ("therein," *YS* I.48) refers to *sabīja-samādhi*,[14] and even there only to the subtlest of the *samādhi*s "with seed," namely *asmitā*-accompanied *samādhi*, the highest form of *nirvicāra* ecstasy. We must bear in mind that *all* forms of cognitive *samādhi* are experiential states that involve objects or mental content and in which misidentification of self is only partially transcended; still contained within the mind is the "seed" of ignorance, further confusion and sorrow that can "sprout" at any time, destabilizing, as it were, the yogin's developed state of one-pointedness. From a different perspective, the forms of cognitive *samādhi* can be regarded as yogic means for obtaining particular knowledge of *prakṛti* and her manifestations or actualizations through the capacity of the mind for epistemic oneness with the object of support and contemplation.[15] At the most subtle awakening in *saṃprajñāta,* the yogin is able through discriminative discernment *(vivekakhyāti)* to distinguish between the finest aspect of *prakṛti*—the *sattva* of the mind—and *puruṣa.* This highly refined discernment gives rise to sovereignty *(adhiṣṭhātṛtva)* over all states of prakṛtic existence and omniscience, that is, "knowingness"/"knowledge of all" *(jñātṛtva).*[16]

Patañjali goes on to state: "The *saṃskāra* born of that [truth-bearing insight] obstructs other *saṃskāras.*"[17] Turning to Vyāsa on this *sūtra* we are informed that:

> Upon the yogin's attainment of insight arising from *samādhi,* a fresh *saṃskāra* made by that insight is produced. The *saṃskāra* generated by the truth-bearing insight obstructs the accumulated residue of the *saṃskāras* of emergence (worldly, afflicted identification). When the *saṃskāras* of emergence are overcome, the ideas and intentions arising from them no longer occur. With the cessation of these ideas, *samādhi* presents itself. Then there is insight arising from the *samādhi;* from that, more *saṃskāras* are generated from the insight. Thus a fresh deposit of such *saṃskāras* is built up. From that again [is generated] insight which in turn produces more *saṃskāras* of insight. Why would this new accumulation of *saṃskāras* not draw the mind into an [afflicted] involvement with it? It is because the *saṃskāras* generated by insight cause the destruction of the afflictions, and so do not constitute anything that would involve an [afflicted state of] mind. In fact, they cause the mind to cease from its [afflicted] activity. Indeed, the mind's [afflicted] endeavor terminates in knowledge.[18]

As the impressions *(saṃskāras)* generated by *samādhi* gather force and are renewed on a regular basis through practice *(abhyāsa),* the impressions of emergence *(vyutthāna)*—which are rooted in and add to an extraverted or extrinsically oriented sense of self—weaken. The "old," former residue *(āśaya)* of the mind constituting the deposits of afflicted, worldly *karma* and *saṃskāras* is gradually replaced with regularly replenished new impressions of *samādhi* generating insight *(prajñā),* that is, yogic perception *(yogi-pratyakṣa),* which again reinforces the impressions or *saṃskāras* of *samādhi.* Thus the past habitual pattern or cycle of egoically appropriated *vṛttis* and afflicted impressions *(saṃskāras)* is broken. Due to the fact that these impressions of insight are of the nonafflicted *(akliṣṭa),*[19] sattvic kind, they do not generate any further afflictions in that they do not add to the rajasic and tamasic components or predispositions of the mind that would perpetuate misidentification as in the situation of *vyutthāna,* the extrinsic mode of human identity.

What *Yoga-Sūtra* I.50 indicates, at least from a soteriological perspective, is the fruit of the "truth-bearing" *(ṛtaṃbharā)* insight *(prajñā).* As the mind becomes purified of affliction—including the *saṃskāras* and personality traits *(vāsanās)* that sustain affliction—it becomes capable of a steady "flow" toward the "good" meaning a "flow" of discernment[20] from which an identity shift can take place, an identity shift involving a transformation of consciousness from a mistaken, saṃsāric identity in *saṃyoga* to authentic or true identity *(svarūpa)* as *puruṣa.* The starting point of this discernment may be, as Vyāsa suggests, a questioning of one's individual identity, pondering on one's state of being by dwelling on questions such as, "Who have I been?" and "What shall we become?"[21] However, one must go beyond this initial inquiry in order to experience the rarefied consciousness of pure *sattva,* which by transcending the individual consciousness, discloses discerning knowledge: "The one who sees the distinction [between extrinsic and intrinsic self-identity] discontinues the cultivation of self-becoming."[22] Having confused true identity for empirical or prakṛtic selfhood by conforming *(sārūpya)* to the changing nature of *vṛtti,* one must then attain the discriminative discernment reflected in the pure, finest *sattva* of the mind *(citta).* In this achievement of knowledge the generation of the false or misidentified sense of self ceases. One no longer has any need to ask questions from the perspective of a confused person who upon seeking liberation remains ensconced in his or her own spiritual dilemma. As Patañjali goes on to inform us, the mind thus inclined toward discernment (i.e., discrimination = *viveka*) has a definite propensity for the liberated state of "aloneness" *(kaivalya).*[23]

Impressions based on the clarity and stability of knowledge in *samādhi* have the power to remold, reshape, and restructure the psychological and epistemological functioning of the mind. As a result of these *saṃskāras* of insight, the new cycle or "wheel" of *saṃskāra-vṛtti-saṃskāra* breaks the former "beginningless" (*YS* IV.10) cycle of saṃsāric identity by impeding, and therefore helping to remove, the worldly, afflicted *saṃskāras* of *vyutthāna.* They prevent their effects (and affects), namely the *vṛttis* of extrinsic identity or worldly identification, rendering them ineffective, obsolete, incapable of functioning. Neither Patañjali nor Vyāsa state exactly why the *saṃskāras* of insight *(prajñā)* annul the appearance of other *saṃskāras.* Bhoja Rāja explains the ability and strength given to this type of *saṃskāra* by the fact that the insight that engenders it is in direct "contact" or alignment with the real nature or "thatness" *(tattva)* of existence,[24] implying an innate "order" or balance in life. This alignment—comprised of knowledge structured in the mind (consciousness) in the form of "truth-bearing" insight *(ṛtaṃbharā-prajñā),* cosmic and individual existence—is something that does not happen with other *saṃskāras* (of a *vyutthāna* nature), being as they are rooted in ignorance and disconnected from the real nature of existence (*atattva,* see n. 24). A preponderance of the latter type of *saṃskāras* forces human identity to contract or "fall" from the natural (intrinsic) order, harmony, and balance of life.

Clarifying Vyāsa, Vijñāna Bhikṣu[25] states that the regular practice and cultivation of *saṃprajñāta* leading to a series of insights *(prajñās)* confirms and strengthens its *saṃskāras* without which the *saṃskāras* of emergence *(vyutthāna)* will continue to arise. A single experience of *prajñā* alone does not thwart the *saṃskāras* of emergence, but the opposing *saṃskāras* built up through sustained practice gradually attenuate[26] them. The mind's power to serve as a vehicle of ignorance and egoity is therefore weakened. Thus a pattern of *samādhi-prajñā-saṃskāra-samādhi* ensues. Through the *vṛttis* of higher perception *(yogi-pratyakṣa)* and their resultant *saṃskāras* of insight, the deluding power of ignorance and its regular pattern of *vyutthāna-saṃskāras* and *vṛttis* that normally exacerbate an afflicted sense of self diminish in power and are eventually expelled altogether.

Why does Patañjali say (*YS* I.50, see n. 17 above) that it is the *saṃskāra* of the *prajñā* that obstructs the production of *vyutthāna-saṃskāras*, and not that it is the *prajñā* itself that does so? One plausible explanation of why Patañjali expresses himself in this way has to do with the importance that the *saṃskāra* is given at this point in the process of "cessation" *(nirodha).* At this stage of *samādhi* the *saṃskāra* helps to generate and sustain insight *(prajñā),* and the existence of the *prajñā* presupposes that all other mental processes must have already subsided; at this moment of yogic praxis there cannot be the production of any afflicted type of *saṃskāras*. Patañjali is saying, according to our understanding, that it is the *saṃskāra* of the insight *(prajñā) as the cause* that checks the appearance of the other *(vyutthāna) saṃskāras*. It is not the *prajñā itself as the effect* that obstructs the effects of the residue of past action. The yogin is operating on the most subtle levels of *prakṛti,* in effect radically reordering the mind by changing the tendency of consciousness to generate identity captivated by the manifest realm as it has normally (and habitually) been understood, or rather misperceived. However, this is not as yet the final awakening in Yoga.

The goal in Patañjali's Yoga as expressed in *Yoga-Sūtra* I.2 (Yoga is *cittavṛttinirodha*), is the utter cessation *(nirodha)* of the afflictions *(kleśas)* in the form of an afflicted, guṇic identity *(cittavṛtti)* of self. It is Patañjali's understanding that insight *(prajñā)* and its *saṃskāra*s are a necessary but not sufficient condition for the complete removal of ignorance and its effects, which include dissatisfaction *(duḥkha)*. Thus *samādhi,* even at this subtle stage of practice, is still "with seed" *(sabīja)*. While *saṃprajñāta* arrests the extrinsic *(vyutthāna-)* mode of selfhood, of egoic, worldly identification and experience *(bhoga)*[27]—experience being one of the purposes of the "seeable" (*dṛśya, YS* II.18), *prakṛti* or the mind *(citta)*—the *saṃskāra*s of insight foster the other purpose or assignment of the mind,[28] which is liberation *(apavarga)*.[29] This involves nothing less than the final eradication or overcoming of *avidyā*'s hold over the mind, a "grip" or monopolizing power that is responsible for the superimposed condition of the "failure-to-see" *(adarśana)* resulting in mistaken identity. Even *prajñā* and its impressions are not capable of overcoming or displacing the latent potential in the mind for epistemological distortion, selfish mentality, and afflicted activity. Insight *(prajñā)* itself is a quality or virtue of the *sattva* of the mind, a special cognition or *vṛtti* of knowledge *(jñāna)* made possible due to the reflected and increasingly intensified presence of *puruṣa.* The locus of identity must, however, shift from the mind to *puruṣa.* The yogin is not satisfied simply with generating purer knowledge-type *saṃskāra*s. As we will soon see, the yogin's goal is to cease to generate any *saṃskāra*s at all, in effect, to transcend the whole saṃskāric-mode of self-identity by terminating the remaining *saṃskāra*s. Yet, we must ask, how can a mind that is being fueled with the *saṃskāra*s of insight in the experience of *samādhi* "with seed," and therefore still under the influence of the afflictions, reach "seedless" *(nirbīja) samādhi?*

ENSTASY *(ASAṂPRAJÑĀTA-SAMĀDHI)*

After *samādhi* in the seeable/knowable and involving objects is attained and perfected, *samādhi* in the "unknowable" or "without the known" *(asaṃprajñāta)* can be cultivated. Ultimately, the stage of "seedless" or "objectless" (nonintentional, contentless) *samādhi* takes place in which all affliction and its effects are "burned away," "scorched," bringing about the total cessation *(nirodha)* of *puruṣa*'s "superimposed condition" (i.e., *cittavṛtti*). Transcending the stages of cognitive *samādhi,* all the potencies *(saṃskāras)* that form the root cause (i.e., *avidyā*) of mistaken identity become purposeless, inactive, and dissolve from consciousness; and the consciousness of the "knower" formerly directed to the objects of experience settles down in the pure knower *(puruṣa)* or experiencer for which there will be nothing then to be "known" or "experienced" soteriologically, that is, for the purpose of liberation. This *samādhi* is the supracognitive *samādhi, samādhi* in the autotransparent knower itself (i.e., the yogin's consciousness "directed toward," "merging in" and identified as *puruṣa*), which can never be an object of knowledge and is, in that sense, unknowable.[30]

Yoga-Sūtra I.18 asserts: "The other [state] is preceded by the practice of the idea of discontinuation and has *saṃskāra* only as residue."[31] Vyāsa refers to "the other" in the above as *"asaṃprajñāta samādhi."*[32] This *sūtra* presupposes two questions: (1) What are the means to attain the supracognitive *samādhi?* (2) What is the nature of this *samādhi?* The phrase *virāma-pratyaya-abhyāsa-pūrvaḥ* ("preceded by the practice of the idea of discontinuation") answers the first question and is explained in different ways by the commentators. Vācaspati Miśra appears to support the notion (which I have argued against in chapter 4) that *virāma* refers to the absence of all *vṛtti*s, implying here the ontological cessation of *vṛtti*s.[33] Vijñāna Bhikṣu, who stresses an epistemological emphasis (*YV* I.18), declares that higher dispassion *(para-vairāgya)* rejects the knowledge or self-identifications (i.e., identification with *vṛtti*s in *saṃprajñāta-samādhi*) as being insufficient. I understand Vijñāna Bhikṣu as saying that the meaning of *virāma-pratyaya* is the awareness of the termination of the misidentification with knowledge *(vṛtti)*.[34] H. Āraṇya explains that the practice of higher dispassion is itself *virāma-pratyaya.*[35] Bhoja Rāja suggests that the abandonment of all concern with *vitarka* and such supports is in itself *virāma-pratyaya.*[36]

Both Vijñāna Bhikṣu and Vācaspati Miśra agree, however, that the practice of *virāma-pratyaya* means to enter repeatedly into a purer awareness than that engaged in cognitive *samādhi.*[37] The process involves, as Bhoja Rāja asserts, establishing this practice again and again, cultivating the mind in this way.[38] Āraṇya seems to imply that the practice is perfected when the identification with the *vṛtti* "I am" from *asmitā* disappears.[39] In the enstatic realization of *asaṃprajñāta* there is no longer misidentification, indeed no longer any soteriological need for identification with objects of support or mental content as in cognitive *samādhi*. This higher *samādhi* is characterized by the presence of residual *saṃskāra*s only *(saṃskāra-śeṣa).* Vyāsa states: "When all [misidentification with] the mental processes and content has subsided and only the *saṃskāra*s remain as residue, such cessation *(nirodha)* is the supracognitive *samādhi*. The means to this *samādhi* is higher dispassion. The practice with supportive factors is ineffective as a means of attaining it."[40] When even the *vṛtti*s of sattvic knowledge revealed in cognitive *samādhi* are mastered and the yogin is detached from them, they are no longer fed or formed into *saṃskāras*. In enstasy *(asaṃprajñāta),* the *saṃskāras* cease to generate *vṛttis* of misidentification or egoity and simply lie as inoperative residue.

Does *asaṃprajñāta* refer to a state of consciousness in which there is no cognition of any kind and therefore is to be rendered as "unconscious" as has been suggested in some translations or interpretations?[41] Taking a more positive approach to the nature of *asaṃprajñāta,* S. Dasgupta comments: "This state, like the other states of the *saṃprajñāta* type, is a positive state of the mind and not a mere state of vacuity of objects or negativity. In this state, all determinate character of the states disappears and their potencies only remain alive."[42] G. Koelman asserts that: "Concentration [sic] without objective consciousness should not be conceived as total absence of knowledge; only knowledge by objectification is absent."[43] Elsewhere, however, Koelman refers to *asaṃprajñāta* as "unconscious absorption"[44] which is somewhat misleading in that the yogin finally attains an awakening of consciousness that reveals intrinsic identity to be *puruṣa.* In this state of *puruṣa*-realization the yogin's consciousness is established in the true form of the seer, the being "who" truly "sees" and is fully conscious *(cetana). Prakṛti* has no capacity to "know" or be conscious of *puruṣa.* Yet this shortcoming on the part of prakṛtic existence including ordinary human consciousness in no way justifies our classifying of *asaṃprajñāta* as an "unconscious" state. Formally speaking, the nonconscious *(acetana)* is reserved for *prakṛti*'s domain and any attempt to portray *puruṣa* as an unconscious state is, from the perspective of Yoga, unwarranted.

Vyāsa's commentary on *Yoga-Sūtra* I.2 specifies that when the last stain of *rajas* is removed, the mind becomes established in the knowledge that *sattva* and *puruṣa* are different. This statement should not be confused with the purpose of *Yoga-Sūtra* I.3. In the final analysis the term *nirodha* as used in *Yoga-Sūtra* I.2 explains the state of the *mind* during *asaṃprajñāta,* whereas *Yoga-Sūtra* I.3 tells us that the seer's identity—the true form of Self *(puruṣa)*—is established in its own authentic nature, and this realization of *puruṣa* takes place in *asaṃprajñāta.* Awareness as restricted to the mind (and which can include illuminating insight or discriminative discernment) is a *vṛtti,* but Self-awareness—the conscious principle *(puruṣa)*—is an immutable constant. Pure consciousness is not at all in the same category as the mental processes. The whole point of *asaṃprajñāta* is to dwell in the true nature of *puruṣa* that, if not Self-aware, would be nonexistent. If *asaṃprajñāta-samādhi* is construed merely as an unconscious state, then what would happen to the unchanging power of consciousness (*citiśakti, YS* IV.34)? The conscious principle—*puruṣa,* the seer—is the power of seeing (*YS* II.20), pure consciousness itself, and it is a mistake to proclaim this principle as unconscious in *asaṃprajñāta-samādhi*. *Yoga-Sūtra* I.18 only seems to contrast *enstasy—puruṣa* abiding in its true nature—with the ecstatic states outlined in *Yoga-Sūtra* I.17, not by indicating the true nature of *puruṣa* (as realized in *asaṃprajñāta*), but rather by explaining what happens to the mind after *asaṃprajñāta* takes place: simply that, according to Vyāsa, it receives *nirodha-saṃskāra*s (see below for explanation). While it may be said that in enstasy *(asaṃprajñāta)* there is a temporary suspension of the mental processes as well as any identification with objects (i.e., the functioning of *vṛtti*), it would be misleading to conclude that higher *samādhi* results in a definitive cessation of the *vṛtti*s in total (see chapter 4), predisposing the yogin to exist in an incapacitated, isolated or mindless state and therefore incapable of living a balanced, useful, and productive life in the world.

In *Yoga-Sūtra* I.51 the final stage in the process of *nirodha* is enumerated as follows: "With the cessation of even that *[saṃskāra* of *prajñā]*, the cessation of everything else [i.e., all misidentification] ensues and that is seedless *samādhi*."[45] Vyāsa explains:

> This (higher *samādhi*) not only opposes the (identification with) insight (attained in cognitive) *samādhi* but impedes even the *saṃskāra*s generated by that insight. Why? Because the *saṃskāra* brought about by cessation *(nirodha)* counteracts the *saṃskāra*s generated by (cognitive) *samādhi*. The existence of *saṃskāra*s being formed in the mind as a result of this cessation is inferred from the experience that the cessation remains steady for progressively longer periods of time. The mind [as a vehicle for ignorance], along with the *saṃskāra*s of *samādhi* on external objects (i.e., emergence or externalization = *vyutthāna*) and the *saṃskāra*s of cessation which lead one to liberation, are dissolved into their own original basis. Thus, the *saṃskāra*s [of *nirodha*] do not cause the mind [in its previous state of ignorance] to continue to exist but prevent its involvement. Since that mind, no longer empowered, withdraws together with the *saṃskāra*s (which lead to liberation), the *puruṣa* is established in its own true nature and is therefore called pure, alone, and free or liberated.[46]

In the above it has been understood that by the use of the term *vyutthāna*—referring to the extrinsic or attached modes of self—Vyāsa is including *saṃprajñāta-samādhi,* which in contrast to enstasy *(asaṃprajñāta)*—the topic of *Yoga-Sūtra* I.51—involves ecstatic experiences of identification that are yet "external" to authentic identity *(puruṣa)*. There still remain dependency factors of support that by lying "outside" the domain of true selfhood, in *prakṛti*'s realm, prolong the yogin's susceptibility to the deeply embedded "seeds" of ignorance *(avidyā)* that can germinate into further dissatisfaction *(duḥkha)*. Up to the level of insight and self-mastery attained in *saṃprajñāta*, the term *"vyutthāna"* served as an antonym to *samādhi* (and *nirodha*) and denoted a "movement" of the mind "away" from *puruṣa* toward objects of perception, thereby generating an extrinsic identity of self, compulsive attachment to objects, and afflicted, worldly involvement. However, in contrast to enstasy ("standing or abiding in the Self"), it can be said that the ecstatic states of cognitive *samādhi* are also extrinsic modes of self-identity *(vyutthāna)*, that is, they arise within the context of prakṛtic experience and are based on an "externalized" or extrinsic nature and awareness of selfhood. The innermost core of Patañjali's Yoga constituting the climax of yogic purification is said to be *nirbīja* ("without seed"), in comparison with cognitive *samādhi*, which being classified as *sabīja* ("with seed"), is considered an exterior part (*bahiraṅga, YS* III.8)[47] of Yoga.

Enstasy *(asaṃprajñāta)* not only eliminates any dependency on insight *(prajñā)* as a basis for self-identity but also overcomes the *saṃskāra*s of *prajñā*. All prakṛtic (guṇic) self-understanding persisting within the core of the mind *(citta)*—whether informed through corporeal or bodily identifications, whether in the form of affective, emotional, moral, cognitive, or egoistic identities, memories or *saṃskāra*s of former attachments *(rāga)*, aversions *(dveṣa)* or fear of death and desire for continuity *(abhiniveśa)*—must all be transcended. The *Yoga-Sūtra* attests to contemplative experiences that cross the boundaries of ordinary human perception and initiate an exploration into an ontologically different mode of consciousness. In *asaṃprajñāta-samādhi* the yogin's quest for authentic identity deepens and is now focused directly on the "extricated" and undefiled presence of *puruṣa*, a liberating realization resulting in the discovery of a trans-empirical and indestructible foundation of being; it is the recognition of a previously concealed, yet unchanging identity that is eternally pure *(śuddha)*, "alone" *(kevala)*, and free *(mukta)*.[48]

Vyāsa tells us that while "cessation" *(nirodha)* overcomes any attachment to insight *(prajñā)*, the *saṃskāra*s of *nirodha* thus generated counteract the *saṃskāra*s of insight. A single "experience" or realization of *puruṣa* in *asaṃprajñāta*, however, is unlikely to accomplish this task all at once. When regular practice undertaken with proper attention and reverence is cultivated and strengthened over time,[49] it causes an unbroken flow of calm or serenity in the mind and the final results accrue.[50] Vyāsa suggests that a calm flow of the mind arises only through sustained practice, which brings about the *saṃskāra*s of *nirodha*, for initially the state of peacefulness in the mind can easily be unsteadied and overwhelmed by the *saṃskāra*s of "extroversion" or "emergence" *(vyutthāna).*[51] Only after the initial enstatic realizations in *asaṃprajñāta* and through its transformative or "maturing" effects on the mind can the transcendence of the identifications in the ecstatic levels of *saṃprajñāta* occur.[52]

Asaṃprajñāta-samādhi, which initially coincides with a temporary stage of *puruṣa*-realization, presupposes a total turnabout or *metanoia* of consciousness, a complete shift in identity and transformation of understanding. Contrary to what C. Pensa[53] writes, the supraconscious *samādhi* is ultimately the *only* avenue to recover an awareness of our transcendent identity and autonomous freedom as *puruṣa*. For only this transphenomenal state of *samādhi* can fully kindle a fire of enstatic transcendence that does not involve the once powerful habit pattern or trait *(vāsanā)* of egoity *(asmitā).* In *asaṃprajñāta,* counter-*saṃskāra*s are generated based on *puruṣa*-realization that gradually render obsolete all of the remaining types of *saṃskāra*s. The yogin develops the "habit" of entering into the state of pure identity as *puruṣa* by regularly ascending into supraconscious *samādhi*. The former "habit" of egoic or saṃsāric identity is weakened when the yogin returns from the enstatic consciousness *(asaṃprajñāta)* to the normal waking state of the mind. The "eight-limbs" of Yoga *(aṣṭāṅga)* outlined by Patañjali in the *Sādhana-Pāda* (*YS* II.29)[54] can be seen as aids in this progressive shift from egoity to *puruṣa*. Yet, in the final analysis, the afflictions *(kleśa*s*)* are terminated not through any specific exercise, technique, attitude, behavior, or intention but solely by the dispassionate "act" of de-identifying completely with any notion of our psychophysical being as constituting authentic identity, *puruṣa.*

The direct means to enstasy *(asaṃprajñāta),* as stated by Vyāsa,[55] is higher dispassion *(para-vairāgya).* The yogin must take the step of becoming utterly dispassionate toward[56] (detached from) the much esteemed yogic state of discernment *(khyāti)* (between the finest aspect of *prakṛti*—the *sattva*—and *puruṣa*) and the supreme knowledge and power that proceed from it.[57] Higher dispassion, according to Vyāsa, is the finest, most subtle limit of knowledge;[58] the yogin's thirst for liberating knowledge is quenched through knowledge of *puruṣa* as revealed in the last stage of insight *(prajñā),* which is said to be sevenfold (*YS* II.27).[59] Vyāsa specifies that knowledge of *puruṣa* (*puruṣa-jñāna, YS* III.35) is attained by performing *saṃyama* ("constraint") on the idea of *puruṣa* being, by nature, pure consciousness.[60] Vijñāna Bhikṣu notes that outside this particular *saṃyama* there is no other means given for direct perception of *puruṣa.*[61] Clarifying the nature of this high-level perception, Vyāsa discloses that it is *puruṣa* that sees this knowledge of itself (as the knower) when no other processes of apprehension or ideas arise in the mind.[62] It is the purest reflection of *puruṣa,* whereby the yogin realizes that there is no further need to look or seek "outside" *puruṣa*—within *prakṛti*'s domain—in order to gain liberation. The mind has temporarily attained fulfillment of what it had to do: to act as a vehicle for the liberating knowledge of *puruṣa.*[63] However, it is still subject to the "seed" of *avidyā* and needs further purification. All *prajñā,* thus, is but a temporary state; it is not the purest state of knowing/seeing, that being a permanent power belonging to the knower/seer, *puruṣa* alone.

The higher dispassion, as Vyāsa suggests, grows in stages. Upon returning from *asaṃprajñāta* to the waking state, the yogin observes the time that has elapsed and thereby infers that the state of *nirodha (niruddha)* has indeed occurred. It is important to note that the state of mind being referred to here as *nirodha (niruddha)* is, formally speaking (*YB* I.1), the purest state of the mind that follows from the one-pointed state of mind *(ekāgra)* in cognitive *samādhi.* It is the accumulated force of the experiences of *nirodha* that creates impressions until dispassion develops to the utmost degree. If this were not so, the increased intensity and length of the enstatic "experience" would not result. Thus, the yogin infers that both *nirodha* and its impressions do take place.[64] Having transcended all *vṛtti*-knowledge and mental content through higher dispassion, the *guṇa*s no longer hold any epistemological power over the yogin. There is no memory *(smṛti)* carried over from the "experience" in *asaṃprajñāta.*

Yet a question ensues: Since the *nirodha*-state of the mind (generated from *asaṃprajñāta*), not being a *vṛtti,* does not produce a corresponding idea, cognition, or insight, how is it possible for a *saṃskāra* of *nirodha* to form? One response to this query, given by H. Āraṇya, is that the flow of ideas and apprehensions exists before the experience of *nirodha* and continues after it. The break in that flow is recognized by the mind and this recognition constitutes the *nirodha-saṃskāra.* As these breaks occur more frequently and are prolonged through practice, the tendency to enter into the state of *nirodha* increases.[65] Finally, misidentification with the flow of ideas *(pratyaya)* and mental processes *(vṛtti)* permanently ceases and the yogin forever abides in the true enstatic nature of *puruṣa,* the seer (*YS* I.3). This supracognitive awareness must be cultivated under all conditions including during: (1) the "formal" practice *(sādhana)* of *samādhi* in the meditative posture, and (2) ordinary involvement in the world. While performing all the necessary duties of the world—personal or otherwise—the yogin continues to reflect upon all knowledge *(vṛtti)* as it arises in the mind. The yogin then traces this "flow" of knowledge back to the pure knower *(puruṣa)* of knowledge until the *saṃskāras* that formerly corrupted the attention needed for this purpose become so weakened that enstasy becomes increasingly integrated with the wakeful state. Up to this time the yogin's attention had been interrupted constantly by the prakṛtic identifications. But now after a profound journey of purification and illumination of understanding, the yogin, remaining alert, aware and open to the everyday world, finds repose in an uninterrupted, "seedless" *samādhi* where identification with *vṛtti*s, thoughts, emotions, relationships, and so forth, is recognized as a nonenslaving association. Prior to *nirbīja-samādhi,* this trans-empirical awareness must be diligently cultivated by overcoming the *saṃskāra*s of mistaken identity, attachment, and so on, including the objects and mental content that left their imprints in *saṃprajñāta-samādhi.* Bhoja Rāja describes it thus: As the yogin progresses through the stages of cognitive *samādhi,* the knowledge-*vṛtti* at each stage is dissolved into its own saṃskāric cause; as each *vṛtti* arises from a *saṃskāra,* the yogin discerns "not this, not this" *(neti neti).* Denying *vṛtti*s any intrinsic worth, pure consciousness is pursued with greater intensity until the culminating state of "seedless" *samādhi* is reached.[66] This view as articulated by Bhoja Rāja echoes an important teaching of the Upaniṣads.[67]

The process of cessation *(nirodha)* results in an expansion of insight, self-understanding, and identity in *samādhi,* followed by a creative potency. *Nirodha* does not mean the destruction, suppression, or negation[68] of the mental processes or the realm of the *guṇa*s in total, as we have argued earlier.[69] It is not a deadening of the mind but entails a form of mental initiative that allows for a sattvification (i.e., purification and illumination) of consciousness (the mind). The final cessation of mistaken identity thus can be viewed as a positive process disclosing a finer attunement between *puruṣa* and *prakṛti* and producing *saṃskāra*s in no less fashion than is the case with the *vṛtti*s.[70] However, as the *saṃskāra*s of *nirodha* grow progressively more intense, they end up turning, paradoxically, against any form of mental activity based on egoity, misidentification, and ignorance, including their own existence. The consequence of all this can be none other than *kaivalya: puruṣa* entirely free shines with its own power of consciousness *(citiśakti).*[71] The process of final cessation *(nirodha)* epitomizes well the bipolarity of the yogic "path" where both *abhyāsa* (i.e., the "practice of the idea of discontinuation"—*virāma-pratyaya-abhyāsa*—of misidentification with *vṛtti, YS* I.18) and *para-vairāgya* (i.e., the higher dispassion that serves as the final means to enstasy) are the primary methods that the yogin must utilize in order to be properly prepared for the "event" of liberation.

A brief summary of the process of *nirodha* as it passes through the various states of mind can now be formulated. In the following order of development, *nirodha* involves: (1) turning the mind away from external, grosser identifications resulting in restless, agitated, or rajasic *(kṣipta)* and dull, somnolent, or tamasic *(mūḍha)* states of mind, allowing for (2) the beginnings of *samādhi* as in the distracted *(vikṣipta)* state of mind when, for a short period *sattva* gains ascendency; the *saṃskāras* of *vikṣipta* are gradually supplanted by those of (3) one-pointedness *(ekāgratā)* and the "truth-bearing" insight where the binding power of the rajasic and tamasic or afflicted modifications *(kliṣṭa-vṛtti*s*)* and their *saṃskāra*s is discarded so that the "tide" or current of the *saṃskāra*s of a *vyutthāna*-nature no longer waxes or wanes giving a wavering, unsteady nature to the mind. Consequently, (4) the discriminative discernment of the distinction between *puruṣa* and the finest aspect of *prakṛti—sattva*—can take place. All attachment even to the purely sattvic, nonafflicted *(akliṣṭa) vṛtti*s of insight *(prajñā)* along with their *saṃskāra*s dissolves when the state of *nirodha/niruddha* gains considerable strength and momentum. In *asaṃprajñāta, puruṣa* dwells by itself and this enstatic "experience" generates a *nirodha-saṃskāra*. Moreover, as Bhoja Rāja affirms, "the *saṃskāra*s born of *nirodha* burn the *saṃskāra*s born of 'one-pointedness' *(ekāgratā)* and also burn themselves."[72] There being no stage of saṃsāric involvement after this, no other *saṃskāra*s can replace the *nirodha-saṃskāra*s that have "burnt" or "consumed" themselves.

The higher dispassion arising from the discernment of *puruṣa* (*YS* I.16) is the crucial means that prevents the mind from being overtaken by the *vyutthāna*-mode of identification; it is an advanced stage of mastery *(vaśīkāra)*—following from the lower form of dispassion *(vairāgya)* defined in *YS* I.15[73]—where the yogin is no longer under the binding influence of the *avidyā*-dominated play of the *guṇa*s (i.e., *saṃyoga*). Soteriologically, the *guṇa*s have become "void of purpose" (*artha-śūnya, YB* I.18). Epistemologically, the yogin is freed from the limited forms of perception and self-understanding based on *saṃprajñāta*-identifications. This state is also referred to as "having *saṃskāra* only as residue" (*saṃskāra-śeṣa,* see n. 31). If this state is in its initial stages and is not sufficiently established in the mind, further misidentification with objects (and therefore of selfhood) can arise.[74] Eventually this subtle residue of *saṃskāra*s dissolves in a last purificatory stage of the mind and the yogin permanently lives in "a state, as it were, of the absence of objects [of support] . . . the seedless *samādhi* which is supra-cognitive."[75]

It appears to be the case that both Patañjali and Vyāsa use the term *saṃskāra* to refer to mental impressions that are structured and function within the overall context of spiritual ignorance *(avidyā)*—a misapprehension of authentic identity, of the true nature of *puruṣa—and* within the context of liberating knowledge *(jñāna, prajñā)* that frees the yogin from ignorance and its effects (and affects). *Saṃskāra* means a mental impression based on some degree of ignorance of *puruṣa* and can include knowledge *(jñāna)* or insight *(prajñā)* as it continues to function within the broader epistemological framework of the "failure-to-see" *(adarśana),* that is, the failure to identify as *puruṣa* and "see" clearly from the perspective of *puruṣa. Saṃskāras* arise within the context of our primary analogue of empirical discourse—*cittavṛtti*—wherein there lies any potential for, including any present manifestation of, mistaken identity. This is obviously the case for impressions *(saṃskāras)* of an afflicted, extrinsic *(vyutthāna)* nature. Yet it is not so apparent for impressions generated by insight *(prajñā)* and the final state of cessation *(nirodha). Saṃskāras*, therefore, paradoxically refer to one of the principal building blocks or forms of ignorance in the process of *saṃyoga* and misidentification *as well as referring to one of the principal removers or eliminators of ignorance and the situation of saṃyoga or misidentification. Vṛttis*, as we have seen,[76] also perform a similar paradoxical role in Yoga. However, even though the *saṃskāras* of *prajñā* counteract and annul the rajasic and tamasic *saṃskāras* in the *vyutthāna*-mode of empirical identity, and the *nirodha-saṃskāras* in turn obstruct and supersede the sattvic *saṃskāras* of insight in cognitive *samādhi,* both of these types of *saṃskāras (prajñā* and *nirodha)* remain only until the seed-mechanism *(cittavṛtti)* of our mistaken identity with the "seeable" is completely eradicated and their purpose—to bring about experience and liberation—has been fulfilled.[77] The use of the *saṃskāras* of *prajñā* and *nirodha* are similar to the act of using a thorn to remove another thorn and then discarding both when the job is done. The mind thus ceases to generate further *saṃskāras* and has become utterly pure, *saṃskāra*-free, transparent to all modes of misidentification. When Vyāsa tells us that the *saṃskāras* of the yogin have become "burned," their seeds "scorched" (*YB* IV.28), it is meant that *avidyā*—the cause of *saṃyoga* and all the *saṃskāras* that take the form of habit patterns of misconception or error (*viparyaya-vāsanās*, *YB* II.24)—has been burned, and not that the mind or "consciousness-of" (the power of identification) or the functioning of mental impressions and memory in total have been destroyed.[78] The yogin's understanding and the functioning *(vṛtti)* of the mind have been transformed, not negated.

In short, only ignorance *(avidyā)* and its concomitant—misidentification (the superimposition of identity in *saṃyoga*)—are eliminated in Yoga. It is, in a sense (and a very specialized sense at that), correct to say that in Yoga "*prakṛti* dissolves"; but we must be very careful to pinpoint exactly what we mean when we say this. After all, the nature of manifest *prakṛti* is to be engaged in a process of constant change and transformation involving the three *guṇa*s, a process that incorporates periods of manifestation ("creation"), stabilization (sustenance, maintenance), and dissolution of formed reality. "Dissolution," "a returning to the source" (i.e., of unmanifest *prakṛti*) is an intrinsic dynamic of the conditional realm of the *guṇa*s. This study submits that it is *prakṛti* in her mental/psychological formation of *saṃskāra*s and *vṛtti*s of misidentification (mistaken identity) that dissolves in Yoga.[79] The former and habitually impure mind or selfish mentality rooted in misperception/misconception *(viparyaya)* and its *saṃskāra*s (and habit patterns or *vāsanā*s) is transformed into a purified mind rooted in knowledge. The psychology of limited counterproductive states of mind is transformed through direct insight into the true nature and states of *prakṛti,* thereby undoing an afflictive process *(kliṣṭa, kleśa)* of egoity built on the "failure-to-see" *(adarśana, avidyā).* Clearly Yoga philosophy, far from negating human nature, has profound ramifications for psychological improvement. The superimposed condition of *puruṣa* or state of *saṃyoga* that is the cause (*YS* II.17) of impending dissatisfaction or sorrow (*duḥkha, YS* II.16) is discontinued or discarded and there is no purpose for the further production of *saṃskāra*s. This finality to the process of "cessation" *(nirodha)* is called "seedless" *(nirbīja-) samādhi,* meaning that the "seed" of all ignorance has been eliminated. Thus Yoga as a spiritually emancipating process takes place within the framework of misidentification/superimposition and its annihilation. Through a series of de-identifications of selfhood with phenomenal existence involving a sustained discipline of practice coupled with a dispassionate awareness, Yoga yields greater insight into the nature of the mind, thus opening the way for clearer knowledge of *puruṣa* until there arises an unmistakable identity as *puruṣa.*

"ALONENESS" *(KAIVALYA):* IMPLICATIONS FOR AN EMBODIED FREEDOM—A FINAL ANALYSIS AND ASSESSMENT OF THE *YOGA-SŪTRA*

The term *kaivalya,* meaning "aloneness,"[80] has elsewhere been translated as "absolute freedom,"[81] "total separation,"[82] "transcendental aloneness,"[83] "independence,"[84] "absolute isolation,"[85] and "isolation."[86] In the classical traditions of Sāṃkhya and Yoga, *kaivalya* is generally understood to be the state of the unconditional existence of *puruṣa*. In the *Yoga-Sūtra, kaivalya* can refer more precisely to the "aloneness of seeing" *(dṛśeḥ kaivalyam)* that, as Patañjali states, follows from the disappearance of ignorance *(avidyā)* and its creation of *saṃyoga*[87]—the conjunction of the seer *(puruṣa)* and the seeable (i.e., *citta, guṇas*)—explained by Vyāsa as a mental superimposition. "Aloneness" thus can be construed as *puruṣa*'s innate capacity for pure, unbroken, nonattached seeing/perceiving, observing or "knowing" of the content of the mind *(citta)*.[88]

In an alternative definition, Patañjali explains *kaivalya* as the "return to the origin" *(pratiprasava)* of the *guṇa*s that have lost all soteriological purpose for the *puruṣa* that has, as it were, recovered its transcendent autonomy.[89] This *sūtra* (*YS* IV.34) also classifies *kaivalya* as the establishment in "own form/nature" *(svarūpa),* and the power of higher awareness *(citiśakti)*.[90] Although the seer's *(puruṣa)* capacity for "seeing" is an unchanging yet dynamic power of consciousness that should not be truncated in any way, nevertheless our karmically distorted or skewed perceptions vitiate against the natural fullness of "seeing." Having removed the "failure-to-see" *(adarśana),* the soteriological purpose of the *guṇa*s in the saṃsāric condition of the mind is fulfilled; the mind is relieved of its former role of being a vehicle for *avidyā*, the locus of selfhood (egoity), and misidentification, and the realization of pure seeing—the nature of the seer alone—takes place. *Yoga-Sūtra* IV.34 completes the definition of Yoga as *cittavṛttinirodha,* whereupon the seer abides in its own form or pure identity (*YS* I.3).

According to yet another *sūtra* (*YS* III.55), we are told that *kaivalya* ensues when the *sattva* of consciousness has reached a state of purity analogous to that of the *puruṣa*.[91] Through the process of sattvification—the subtilization or "return to the origin" *(pratiprasava)* in the *sattva*—the transformation *(pariṇāma)* of the mind *(citta)* takes place at the deepest level, bringing about a radical change in perspective: the former impure, fabricated states constituting a fractured identity of self are dissolved or discarded, resulting in the complete purification of mind. The mind thus purified probably refers to the "one mind" (*cittaṃ ekaṃ, YS* IV.5)[92] in its most refined and subtle form of *sattva* (or *buddhi*), which being pure *like puruṣa* is associated with "aloneness."[93] For Patañjali goes on to say: "There [in that one mind], what is born of meditation is without [karmic] residue."[94] When the *guṇa*s have fulfilled their purpose for providing experience and liberation, their afflicted condition dissolves forever and *puruṣa,* absolutely disjoined from them in their form of ignorance, is no longer incorrectly associated with sorrow and dissatisfaction *(duḥkha)*.[95] Through knowledge and its transcendence, self-identity overcomes its lack of intrinsic grounding, a lack sustained and exacerbated by the web of afflictions in the form of attachment, aversion, and the compulsive clinging to life based on the fear of extinction. The yogin is no longer dependent on liberating knowledge (mind-*sattva*),[96] is no longer attached to *vṛtti* as a basis for self-identity. The beginningless succession of changes of the *guṇa*s (or empirical characteristics) that was incorrectly assumed to be related to authentic identity *(puruṣa),* and that was itself the first notion of bondage, comes to an end. This ending, it must be emphasized, does not mark a definitive disappearance of the *guṇa*s from *puruṣa*'s view.[97] For the liberated yogin, the *guṇa*s cease to exist in the form of *avidyā*, its *saṃskāra*s, *vṛtti*s, and false cognitions, notions or fixed ideas *(pratyaya)* of selfhood that formerly veiled true identity. The changing guṇic modes cannot alter the yogin's now purified and firmly established consciousness. The mind has been liberated from the *egocentric world of attachment to things prakṛtic.* Now the yogin's identity (as *puruṣa*), disassociated from ignorance, is untouched, unaffected by qualities of mind,[98] uninfluenced by the *vṛtti*s constituted of the three *guṇa*s. The mind and *puruṣa* attain to a sameness of purity (*YS* III.55), of harmony, balance, evenness, and a workability together: the mind appearing in the nature of *puruṣa.*[99]

According to J. Gonda, the various methods and limbs of Yoga have but one purpose, the isolation *(kaivalya)* of the spirit. Gonda sees *kaivalya* as incorporating the perfect simplicity and uniformity of the nucleus of personality.[100] As an addendum to Gonda's position it can be stated that *kaivalya* in no way presupposes the destruction or negation of the personality of the yogin, but is an unconditional state in which all the obstacles or distractions preventing an immanent and purified relationship or engagement of person with nature and spirit *(puruṣa)* have been removed. The deep-rooted "knots" *(granthi)* of the mind[101] in the form of habit patterns *(vāsanās)* of misconceived knowledge *(viparyaya-jñāna)*[102] have been undone ("untied"). The mind, which previously functioned under the sway of ignorance coloring and blocking our awareness of authentic identity, has now become purified and no longer operates as a locus of misidentification, confusion, and dissatisfaction *(duḥkha)*. *Sattva,* the finest quality *(guṇa)* of the mind, has the capacity to be perfectly lucid/transparent, like a dust-free mirror in which the light of *puruṣa* is clearly reflected and the discriminative discernment *(vivekakhyāti)*[103] between *puruṣa* and the *sattva* of the mind (as the nature of the "seeable") can take place.[104] The crucial (ontological) point to be made here is that *prakṛti* ceases to perform an obstructing role in *kaivalya*. In effect, *prakṛti* herself has become liberated[105] from *avidyā*'s grip including the misconceptions, misappropriations, and misguided relations implicit within a world of afflicted selfhood. The mind has been transformed, liberated from the egocentric world of attachment, its former afflicted nature abolished; and self-identity left alone in its "own form" or true nature as *puruṣa* is never again confused with all the relational acts, intentions, and volitions of empirical existence. Vyāsa explicitly states that emancipation happens in the mind and does not literally apply to *puruṣa,* which is by definition already free and therefore has no intrinsic need to be released from the fetters of saṃsāric existence.[106] While this is true from the enlightened perspective, it would not be inappropriate to suggest that, figuratively speaking, in the state of "aloneness" *(kaivalya) puruṣa* and *prakṛti* are simultaneously liberated in that, all ignorance having been removed, *they are both "known," included, and are therefore free to be what they are.* There being no power of misidentification remaining in *nirbīja-samādhi,*[107] the mind ceases to operate within the context of the afflictions, karmic accumulations, and consequent cycles of *saṃsāra* implying a mistaken identity of selfhood subject to birth and death.

The *Yoga-Sūtra* has often been regarded as calling for the severance of *puruṣa* from *prakṛti;* concepts such as liberation, cessation, dispassion, and so on, have been interpreted in an explicitly negative light. Max Müller, citing Bhoja Rāja's commentary[108] (eleventh century CE), refers to Yoga as "separation" *(viyoga).*[109] More recently, numerous other scholars[110] have endorsed this interpretation, that is, the absolute separateness of *puruṣa* and *prakṛti.* In asserting the absolute separation of *puruṣa* and *prakṛti,* scholars and nonscholars alike have tended to disregard the possibility for other (fresh) hermeneutical options, and this radical, dualistic metaphysical closure of sorts surrounding the nature and meaning of Patañjali's Yoga has surely proved detrimental to a fuller understanding of the Yoga *darśana* by continuing a tradition based on an isolationistic (and therefore one-sided) reading or perhaps misreading of the *Yoga-Sūtra* and Vyāsa's commentary. Accordingly, the absolute separation of *puruṣa* and *prakṛti* can only be interpreted as a disembodied state implying death to the physical body. However, Patañjali observes that the "desire for continuity" *(abhiniveśa)* in life arises even in the sage,[111] although it would be accurate to say that the sage, having developed dispassion toward all things, is no longer enslaved by this basic "thirst" or "clinging to life" or by any fear of extinction. To dislodge the sage from bodily existence is to undermine the integrity of the pedagogical context that lends so much credibility or "weight" to the Yoga system. Thus it need not be assumed that in Yoga liberation coincides with physical death.[112] This would only allow for a soteriological end state of "disembodied liberation" *(videhamukti)*. What *is* involved in Yoga is the death of the atomistic, egoic identity, the dissolution of the karmic web of *saṃsāra* that generates notions, specifically misconceptions, that we are merely "subjects," each one of us trapped in the prakṛtic constitution of a particular body-mind.

The transformation from ignorance into the enlightened perspective requires a fundamental restructuring of ideas of self that takes place through a process that we have termed the "sattvification" of the mind or consciousness. In the ordinary consensus reality of empirical existence the sense of self misidentified with any aspect of *prakṛti* thinks that it is the seer. Upon meditative reflection it is disclosed that the empirical I-sense is not the seer,[113] but merely masquerades as the seer. A high-level power of discernment ascertaining the difference between the seer and the seeable (which includes our empirical I-sense) arises and aids in the dissolution of any remaining fixed or reified notions of self and world that maintain egoity and its compulsive attachment to the "things" of the world. The separate, empirical, and prakṛtic I-sense in *saṃyoga* (often equated with the principle of *ahaṃkāra*) is then understood to be a function within *prakṛti* catalyzed by the affliction of *asmitā*. But due to the purification attained in *samādhi*, the sense of self no longer interferes in the act of perception thus resulting in a state of "unification" *(samāpatti)* or nonseparation between seer, seeing, and the seeable. As *YS* III.55 implies, *kaivalya* requires the presence of both *puruṣa* and *prakṛti* in the act of pure "seeing," *puruṣa* "providing" the consciousness of the seer who actually "sees," and *prakṛti* supplying the arena of the seeable, the existence of the seen.[114]

Not being content with mere theoretical knowledge, Yoga is committed to a practical way of life implying "physical training, exertion of will power and acts of decision, because it wants to deal with the complete human situation and provide real freedom, not just a theory of liberation."[115] To this end, Patañjali included in his presentation of Yoga an outline of the "eight-limbed" path *(aṣṭāṅga-yoga)*[116] dealing with the physical, moral, psychological, and spiritual dimensions of the yogin, an integral path that emphasizes organic continuity, balance, and integration in contrast to the discontinuity, imbalance, and disintegration inherent in the condition of *saṃyoga*. The idea of cosmic balance and of the mutual support and upholding of the various parts of nature and society is not foreign to Yoga thought. Vyāsa deals with the theory of "nine causes" *(nava kāraṇāni)* or types of causation according to tradition.[117] The ninth type of cause is termed *dhṛti*—meaning "support," "sustenance"—and is explained by Vyāsa as follows: "The cause of sustenance for the sense organs is the body; and that [body] is supported by these [sense organs]. The elements sustain the bodies and the bodies support each other; and because there has to be mutual support, animal, human, and divine bodies support all entities."[118] On the basis of Vyāsa's explanation of *dhṛti,* we can see how mutuality and sustenance are understood as essential conditions for the maintenance of the natural and social world. There is an organic interdependence of all living entities wherein all (i.e., the elements, animals, humans, and divine bodies) work together for the "good" of the whole and for each other.

At this point I would like to emphasize a much overlooked aspect of Yoga thought. Far from being exclusively a subjectively oriented and introverted path of withdrawal from life, classical Yoga acknowledges the intrinsic value of "support" and "sustenance" and the interdependence of all living (embodied) entities, thus upholding organic continuity, balance, and integration within the natural and social world. Having achieved that level of insight *(prajñā)* that is "truth-bearing" *(ṛtaṃbharā),*[119] the yogin perceives the natural order *(ṛta)* of cosmic existence, "unites" with and embodies that order. To fail to see clearly *(adarśana)* is to fall into disorder, disharmony, and conflict within oneself and with the world. In effect, to be ensconced in ignorance implies a disunion with the natural order of life and inextricably results in a failure to embody that order. Through Yoga one gains proper access to the world and is therefore established in right relationship to the world. Far from being denied or renounced, the world, for the yogin, has become transformed, properly engaged. The term 'Yoga,' which can mean "addition,"[120] carries with it the philosophical connotations of an inclusiveness in that Yoga ultimately *adds or includes the power of consciousness that is puruṣa but not to the exclusion of prakṛti.* Seen here, *saṃyoga* amounts to no more than a misperceived union resulting in a misalignment of *puruṣa* and *prakṛti.* Yoga, understood as a disengagement with the world of *saṃyoga*[121] (i.e., ignorance, misidentification, dissatisfaction, sorrow), corrects this misalignment, allowing for a proper alignment in consciousness between these two principles.

Yoga is the "skill in action" (cf. *BG* II.50) that enables the yogin to disengage or unfocus the *attention* away from the distracted mind caught within the changing world of prakṛtic identity dependent on the "consciousness-of-objects" *(citta, vṛtti).* The yogin then develops the capacity for (re)focusing on and "retrieving" the unchanging pure consciousness *(puruṣa).* The process of *nirodha* is an effort at breaking away, letting go of the ordinary focus of consciousness that generates the notion of an empirical/conceptual self standing apart from the objective world. Thus, for the skillful yogin *saṃyoga* ceases, but not for the empirical selves since the world based on *saṃyoga* (saṃsāric/extrinsic identity) is their common experience.[122] By our conforming *(sārūpya)* to the modifications *(vṛtti)* of the mind *(citta), puruṣa* (the seer) appears to take on the nature of the realm of the seeable *(dṛśya)* in the state of *saṃyoga,* giving rise to mistaken identity. The world of *saṃyoga* and mistaken identity, not *prakṛti* in total (i.e., the everyday world of nature, forms and phenomena as well as their unmanifest source) constitutes the "nature/essence of the seeable" (*dṛśyasya-ātmā, YS* II.21) that eventually disappears for the liberated yogin (see above).

The status of *saṃyoga* and its saṃsāric identifications are being emphasized here as an epistemological error rather than an ontological realm (i.e., *prakṛti*). Yet such an afflicted state of affairs in *saṃyoga* remains for those who have not attained liberating insight. By focusing on the true nature of the seer *(puruṣa),* Yoga does not mean to negate *prakṛti* or suggest a radical withdrawal from the seeable, thereby removing *prakṛti* (formed reality, relative states of existence) completely from the yogin's view. The yogin does not become a "mind-less" (or "body-less") being. Rather, the yogin is left with a transformed, fully sattvified mind, that, due to its transparent nature, can function in the form of nonbinding *vṛtti*s—whether of a cognitive or affective/emotive nature—thoughts, ideas, intentions, and so forth. Āraṇya argues that liberated yogins who embark on their role as a teacher *(guru)* "for the benefit of all" do so through their ability to create or construct a new (individualized) mind (*nirmāṇa-citta, YS* IV.4) "which can be dissolved at will" and does not collect *saṃskāra*s of ignorance. Such a mind, Āraṇya continues, cannot "give rise to bondage,"[123] can no longer veil the yogin's true identity as *puruṣa.*

In contradistinction to the interpretation mentioned above, which views Yoga as a radical "separation" between spirit and matter/psychophysical being, I am suggesting that far from being incompatible principles, *puruṣa* and *prakṛti* can engage or participate in harmony, having attained a balance or equilibrium together. The enstatic consciousness of *puruṣa* can coexist with the mind and indeed all of *prakṛti.*[124] The yogin fully reconciles the eternally unchanging seer with the eternally changing realm of relative states of consciousness only by allowing the mind, in the experience of *samādhi,* to dwell in its pure sattvic nature in the "image of *puruṣa,*" and then to be engaged once again in the field of relative existence. The process of "cessation" *(nirodha)* deepens from cognitive (*saṃprajñāta, YS* I.17) *samādhi* into supracognitive *(asaṃprajñāta) samādhi,*[125] where it can be said that the seer abides in its own form/intrinsic identity *(tadā draṣṭuḥ svarūpe'vastānam).*[126]

According to Vyāsa, the repeated practice of the "experiences" of enstasy gradually matures the yogin's consciousness into *kaivalya,* "aloneness" or permanent liberation. The steadfastness of the consciousness in *kaivalya* should not be misconstrued as either being or leading to sheer inactivity, pacifism, or lethargy; rather, stability in *nirbīja-samādhi* allows for a harmony in activity in which the *guṇa*s, no longer struggling for predominance, do not conflict with each other and are attuned to *puruṣa.* We need not read Patañjali as saying that the culmination of all yogic endeavor—*kaivalya*—is a static finality or inactive, isolated, solipsistic state of being. In fact, *Yoga-Sūtra* IV.34 tells us that *kaivalya* has as its foundation the very heart of the unlimited dynamism or power of consciousness *(citiśakti)* that *is puruṣa;*[127] like an incandescent flame *puruṣa* is utterly white hot in contrast to the sputtering, affected "flame" of the mind and self-identity in *saṃyoga.* In terms of our primary analogue of empirical existence *(citta-vṛtti), puruṣa is not "active,"* or better still *puruṣa is not seen to be "active."* In terms of *puruṣa*'s inexhaustibility, *puruṣa constitutes a supremely dynamic presence* that allows for a state of nonafflicted activity (*YS* IV.30 and *YB* IV.30). To conclude that in the liberated state the yogin is incapable of any activity whatsoever simply amounts to a tautalogical statement, indeed implies a circular argument addressed from a prakṛtic or guṇic rather than enlightened perspective.[128]

In the liberated state of "aloneness" it can be said that *prakṛti* is so integrated in the yogin's consciousness that it has become "one" with the yogin. *Kaivalya* can be seen to incorporate an integrated, psychological consciousness along with the autonomy of pure consciousness, yet pure consciousness to which the realm of the *guṇa*s (e.g., psychophysical being) is completely attuned and integrated. On the level of individuality, the yogin has found his (her) place in the world at large, "fitting into the whole";[129] no longer struggling to maintain or seek an identity rooted in *prakṛti*'s domain, the yogin is established in a lasting contentment/peace that transcends the changing nature and conditions of empirical reality. This epistemic transformation and reassessment of experience involves the recognition and inclusion of a formerly concealed, nonappreciated, and obscured mode of being and constitutes Yoga's understanding of immortality, a spiritual recovery wherein authentic identity is uncovered, disclosed.

In the last chapter of the *Yoga-Sūtra (Kaivalya-Pāda),* "aloneness" *(kaivalya)* is said to ensue upon the attainment of *dharmamegha-samādhi,* the "cloud of *dharma*" *samādhi.* This *samādhi* follows from the discriminative discernment *(vivekakhyāti)* and is the precursor to "aloneness."[130] The high-level discriminative vision (also called *prasaṃkhyāna* in the texts) is the fruit of *saṃprajñāta-samādhi* but is not itself *dharmamegha-samādhi.*[131] The yogin must be disinterested in and detached from *vivekakhyāti* and the resulting sovereign power and omniscience.[132] Having relinquished all thirst for the "seen" and the "heard," indeed for the *guṇa*s themselves,[133] the yogin discards all involvement with the saṃsāric realm of attachment and pride because of the awareness of the undesirable (sorrowful) consequences of such re-entrance.[134] The inclination toward misidentification with *vṛtti* has ceased. The yogin has abandoned any search for (or attachment to) reward or "profit" from his or her meditational practice. A perpetual state of discerning insight follows[135] through which the yogin is always aware of the fundamental distinction between: extrinsic identity/the world of change, and intrinsic identity/pure unchanging consciousness. *Yoga-Sūtra* IV.29 states: "Indeed, following from [that elevated state of] meditative reflection, for the one who has discriminative discernment and is at all times nonacquisitive, there arises the 'cloud of *dharma*' *samādhi.*"[136] Vyāsa asserts that because the seed-*saṃskāra* of taint is destroyed, no further ideas rooted in ignorance and based on an afflicted identity of self can arise.[137]

Dharmamegha-samādhi, so it appears, presupposes that the yogin has cultivated higher dispassion *(para-vairāgya)*—the means to the enstatic consciousness realized in *asaṃprajñāta-samādhi* (*YB* I.18).[138] Thus, *dharmamegha-samādhi* is more or less a synonym of *asaṃprajñāta-samādhi* and can even be understood as the consummate phase of supracognitive *samādhi* or enstasy, the final step on the long and arduous yogic journey to authentic identity and "aloneness."[139] A permanent identity shift—from the perspective of the human personality to *puruṣa*—takes place. Now free from any dependence on or subordination to knowledge or *vṛtti,* and detached from the world of misidentification *(saṃyoga),* the yogin yet retains the purified guṇic powers of virtue including illuminating "knowledge of all"[140] (due to purified *sattva*), nonafflicted activity[141] (due to purified *rajas*), and a healthy, stable body-form (due to purified *tamas*). Fully awakened into the self-effulgent nature of *puruṣa,* the yogin witnesses, observes, perceives *prakṛti,* yet ceases to be ensnared and consumed by the drama or play of the *guṇa*s whether in the form of ignorance or knowledge, cause or effect, personal identity or sense of otherness. The auto-transparent knower, knowledge, and action coexist in a state of mutual attunement.

One problem that easily arises in Yoga hermeneutics is when the knower and knowledge are completely sundered and the doctrine of "aloneness" *(kaivalya)* becomes reified into a radically dualistic, orthodox perspective that paralyzes the possibility of developing fresh ways to understand the relation between the knower and knowledge. Initially there must be some relation, some continuum (i.e., consciousness and its modes: reflected or pure), or liberation would not be possible because one could never make the transition from delusion to enlightenment. The point of their distinction is that one must not try to attempt to understand or grasp the transcendent knower from a relative, empirical, and therefore inept perspective.

Yoga-Sūtra IV.30 declares: "From that *[dharmamegha-samādhi]* there is the cessation of afflicted action."[142] Hence the binding influence of the *guṇa*s in the form of the afflictions, past actions, and misguided relationships is overcome; what remains is a "cloud of *dharma*" that includes an "eternality of knowledge" free from all impure covering (*āvaraṇa-mala, YS* IV.31) or veiling affliction and where "little (remains) to be known."[143] The eternality or endlessness of knowledge is better understood metaphorically rather than literally: it is not knowledge expanded to infinity but implies *puruṣa*-realization that transcends the limitations and particulars of knowledge *(vṛtti)*.

The culmination of the Yoga system is found when, following from *dharmamegha-samādhi,* the mind and actions are freed from misidentification and affliction and one is no longer deluded/confused with regard to one's true nature and identity *(svarūpa)*. At this stage of practice the yogin is disconnected *(viyoga)* from all patterns of egoically motivated action. Vijñāna Bhikṣu argues that while cognitive *samādhi* abolishes all the *karma* except the *prārabdha karma*—the *karma* that is already ripening in the present—the enstatic realization in *asaṃprajñāta-samādhi* has the potency to destroy even the *prārabdha karma,*[144] including all the previous *saṃskāra*s.[145] The *karma* of such a yogin is said to be neither "white" *(aśukla),* nor "black" *(akṛṣṇa),* nor "mixed."[146] There is a complete exhaustion or "burning up" of the afflictions *(kleśa*s*)* and latent impressions *(saṃskāra*s*)*. According to both Vyāsa[147] and Vijñāna Bhikṣu,[148] one to whom this high state of purification takes place is designated as a *jīvanmukta:* one who is liberated while still alive (i.e., embodied). The modern commentator, H. Āraṇya, also asserts that through freedom from affliction in the form of *saṃskāra* the yogin attains to the status of a *jīvanmukta.*[149]

By transcending the normative conventions and obligations of karmic behavior, the yogin acts morally not as an extrinsic response and out of obedience to an external moral code of conduct, but as an intrinsic response and as a matter of natural, purified inclination. The stainless luminosity of pure consciousness is revealed as one's fundamental nature. The yogin does not act *saṃsārically,* that is, ceases to act from the perspective of a delusive sense of self confined within *prakṛti*'s domain. Relinquishing all obsessive or selfish concern with the results of activity, the yogin remains wholly detached from the egoic fruits of action.[150] The yogin does not, for example, indulge in the fruits of ritual action, in the merit *(puṇya)* and the demerit *(apuṇya)* generated by good and bad observance of traditional ritualistic religion. By the practice of a detached ethic, the yogin must transcend this ritualistic, self-centered mentality. This does not imply that the yogin loses all orientation for action. Dispassion (detachment) in its highest form (*para-vairāgya, YS* I.16) is defined by Vyāsa as a "clarity of knowledge" *(jñāna-prasāda).*[151] It is attachment (and compulsive desire), not action itself, that sets in motion the law of moral causation *(karma)* by which a person is implicated in *saṃsāra.* The yogin is said to be attached to neither virtue nor nonvirtue, and is no longer oriented within the egological patterns of thought as in the epistemically distorted condition of *saṃyoga.* This does not mean, as some scholars have misleadingly concluded, that the spiritual adept or yogin is free to commit immoral acts,[152] or that the yogin is motivated by selfish concerns.[153]

Actions must not only be executed in the spirit of unselfishness (i.e., sacrifice) or detachment, they must also be ethically sound, reasonable, and justifiable. If action were wholly contingent upon one's mood or frame of mind, it would constitute a legitimate pretext for immoral conduct. Moreover, the yogin's spiritual journey—far from being an "*a-moral* process"[154]—is a highly moral process! The yogin's commitment to the sattvification of consciousness, including the cultivation of moral virtues such as compassion *(karuṇā)*[155] and nonviolence *(ahiṃsā),*[156] is not an "a-moral" enterprise, nor is it an expression of indifference, aloofness, or an uncaring attitude to others. Moral disciplines are engaged as a natural outgrowth of intelligent (sattvic) self-understanding, insight, and commitment to self-transcendence that takes consciousness out of *(ec-stasis)* its identification with the rigid structure of the monadic ego, thereby reversing the inveterate tendency of this ego to inflate itself at the expense of its responsibility in relation to others.

Having defined the "goal" of Yoga as "aloneness" *(kaivalya),* the question must now be asked: what kind of "aloneness" was Patañjali talking about? "Aloneness," I submit, is not the isolation of the seer *(draṣṭṛ, puruṣa)* separate from the seeable *(dṛśya, prakṛti),* as is unfortunately far too often maintained as the goal of Yoga, but refers to the "aloneness" of the power of "seeing" (*YS* II.20, 25) in its innate purity and clarity without any epistemological distortion and moral defilement. The cultivation of *nirodha* uproots the compulsive tendency to reify the world and oneself (i.e., that pervading sense of separate ego irrevocably divided from the encompassing world) with an awareness that reveals the transcendent, yet immanent seer *(puruṣa)*. Through clear "seeing" *(dṛśi)* the purpose of Yoga is fulfilled, and the yogin, free from all misidentification and impure karmic residue (as in the former contextual sphere of *cittavṛtti*), gains full, immediate access to the world. By accessing the world in such an open and direct manner, in effect "uniting" (epistemologically) with the world, the yogin ceases to be encumbered by egoism (i.e., *asmitā* and its egoic attitudes and identity patterns), which, enmeshed in conflict and confusion and holding itself as separate from the world, misappropriates the world. While such a selfish appropriation of the "things" of the world may achieve a temporary or extrinsic sense of satisfaction, it also contains the seed of its own dissatisfaction *(duḥkha)* because the *only* avenue to intrinsic well-being or happiness[157] according to Yoga is to live not as a mistaken identity ineluctably making efforts at trying to fill up its own inner "lack" of permanency, but to abide as the permanent seer *(draṣṭṛ, puruṣa)* or experiencer *(bhoktṛ)*[158] that "sees" and "experiences" the world without any selfish seed of desire or lack.

In enstasy *(asaṃprajñāta-samādhi),* unlike cognitive *(saṃprajñāta-) samādhi,* there is no objective prop bolstering a reflected self-identity; there is no separated object or subject but the *puruṣa,* nor is there any power of knowing except that of *puruṣa*. This is the basis of *kaivalya,* "aloneness," not because there is an opposition, separation or conflicting modes of identity, but because there is no mistaking of *prakṛti* for *puruṣa* (that is, no misconception of *puruṣa*'s identity). Authentic identity is no longer misperceived as existing "outside" of itself. Clearly then, Yoga is not a Cartesian-like dichotomy (of thinker and thing).[159] Nor can Yoga be described as a metaphysical union of an individuated self with the objective world of nature or the more subtle realms of *prakṛti*. Rather, Yoga can be seen to unfold—in *samādhi*—states of epistemic oneness that reveal the non-separation of knower, knowing, and the known (*YS* I.41), grounding our identity in a nonafflicted mode of action. *Kaivalya* implies a power of "seeing" in which the dualisms rooted in our egocentric patterns of attachment, aversion, fear, and so on, have been transformed into unselfish ways of being with others.[160]

The psychological, ethical, and social implications of this kind of identity-transformation are, needless to say, immense. I am suggesting that Yoga does not destroy or anesthetize our feelings and emotions thereby encouraging neglect and indifference toward others. On the contrary, the process of "cessation" *(nirodha)* steadies one for a life of compassion, discernment and service informed by a "seeing" that is able to understand (literally meaning "to stand among, hence observe")—and is in touch with—the needs of others. What seems especially relevant for our understanding of Yoga ethics is the enhanced capacity generated in Yoga for empathic identification with the object one seeks to understand. This is a far cry from the portrayal of the yogin as a disengaged figure, psychologically and physically removed from the human relational sphere, and who in an obstinate and obtrusive fashion severs all ties with the world and nature. Such an image of a wise yogin merely serves to circumscribe our vision of humanity and, if anything else, stifle the spirit by prejudicing the spiritual, abstract (and disembodied) realm over and against nature and our human embodiment. Throughout our study we have been consistently arguing that in Yoga philosophy "seeing" is not only a cognitive term but implies purity of mind (and physical discipline), that is, it has moral content and value. Nor is "knowledge" *(jñāna, vidyā)* in the Yoga tradition to be misconstrued as a "bloodless" or "heartless" gnosis.

Yoga involves the sacrifice of attachment to the limiting power of the "owned" (*sva, YS* II.23), which includes the mind *(citta),* for the unlimited power of the "owner" (*svāmin, YS* II.23) or power of "seeing," a sacrifice of one's separated, fragmented self—with all of its hopes and fears, likes and dislikes, pleasures and sorrows, ambitions/successes and failures—for the purpose of the unfractured consciousness of the seer—the "one" who truly "sees." This entails a sacrifice of all mistaken identity or misidentification with the seeable *(dṛśya)* in *saṃyoga* for the purpose of authentic identity as *puruṣa.* The perspective referred to as *Pātañjala Yoga Darśana* culminates in a permanent state of clear "seeing" brought about through the discipline of Yoga. Yoga thus incorporates both an end state or "goal" and a process, that is, being and becoming.[161]

On the "path" of Yoga one places one's faith (*śraddhā, YS* I.20) in the presence or awareness of *puruṣa,* which is without qualities *(nirguṇa)* or properties and yet is the authentic foundation of one's existence. Yoga does not call for mere blind faith but stresses the need for clarity of mind—initially grounded in the direct experience of *sattva*—which, as Vyāsa asserts: "like a good mother protects a yogin."[162] When *puruṣa* is perceived as being distinct (*YS* III.49) from the extrinsic (guṇic) identity of self—however sattvic—which lays claim to the experience in the form of "my knowledge," "my reward," "my experience," the yogin then loses interest in any attachment to the things of the mind; the personality is purified and relinquishes all claim to authentic identity. With this shift in identity from egoity and its limited knowledge-component (both of which are a part of the seeable) to the knower of all knowledge, from misidentification with *citta* to identity as *puruṣa,* the obfuscations of past conditioning *(saṃskāras, vāsanās)* are removed and the yogin finds his/her right place in the world "fitting in" to the world (the cosmos) at large. A clarity of the inner self (*adhyātma-prasāda, YS* I.47) or right "internal" order *(ṛta)* is revealed in which "truth-bearing insight" (*ṛtaṃbharā-prajñā, YS* I.48), free from any trace of erroneous knowledge, arises in the yogin's consciousness.[163]

We must bear in mind that in Yoga there is no bifurcation or dichotomization between the cosmological and the psychological, the macrocosmic universe and the microcosmic human being.[164] The superimposition (*adhyāropa, YB* II.18)—a projection of changing, impure, sorrowful states as real existences "in" *puruṣa*—caused by ignorance provides the fundamental structure of our cosmological/objective world and psychological/subjective world in *saṃyoga;* the "inner" world of self and "outer" world of the universe are both normally experienced as a bifurcation within *prakṛti,* a subject-object duality implying a given, reified world as referenced to a separate sense of self. In Yoga, the structures of the world *(prakṛti),* as experienced directly in *samādhi,* function heuristically as contemplative directives for the purpose of subtilizing and sattvifying the yogin's consciousness: *prakṛti* is utilized for the liberating of identity from "within" the microcosmic, psychophysical organism.

Clearly seen, the body-mind and *prakṛti* in general are no more impediments to *puruṣa*-realization. Nor, from the perspective of Yoga philosophy, is *prakṛti* designated as being either ontologically unreal or a mere projection of the mind. The process of "cessation" *(nirodha),* which may be considered an ongoing sacrifice of egoity in Yoga, involves a continual surrender of perspectives or fixed notions/ideas/cognitions *(pratyaya)* of self to the point where the fragmented, dis-eased world of *saṃyoga* ends and a healing vision of self and world, now both properly harnessed and "put back together," issues forth. Cognition and attention, no longer separated from the known and the attended, cease to function as binding patterns of misidentification and attachment as in the network or mental-complex of *cittavṛtti.* The sacrifice (Latin *sacer facere,* "to make sacred") of egoic identity for the purpose of identifying as *puruṣa* (that is, spiritual emancipation) is precisely what renders *prakṛti* sacred and ultimately reveals her intrinsic significance and value. By implication, in "aloneness" *(kaivalya)* sacrifice becomes an effortless, automatic (spontaneous) sanctification of the totality of life.

Yoga, in its program of purification, goes beyond the position of classical Sāṃkhya (see n. 112), which seems to rest content with a discriminating knowledge *(viveka)* leading to a final isolation of *puruṣa* or absolute separation between *puruṣa* and *prakṛti.* At the end of the day, *prakṛti*'s attunement to, or alignment with the purpose of *puruṣa* appears to be all for nought. Yet, if *puruṣa*—the conscious principle—were free to start with, why would consciousness get "involved" with *prakṛti? Puruṣa*'s seeming "entanglement" does intelligize *prakṛti,*[165] which on her own is said to be devoid of consciousness (*YS* IV.19).[166] The end result of *puruṣa*'s apparent "involvement" with *prakṛti,* the state of liberated knowingness or omniscience, is enriching and allows for a verifying and enlivening of human nature, identity, and consciousness. From an integral perspective, one can argue that *prakṛti* performs her task of providing experience and liberation so that consciousness—in its reflective mode or capacity as the mind—may have content and function in various intentional, relational, and practical modes. *Puruṣa* is perceived to shine only through an experiential journey into subtler realms of *prakṛti,* thereby disclosing finer insights into the nature of consciousness.

Interpretations of Yoga that adhere to an absolute separation, implying a final unworkable duality between spirit and matter, amount to an impoverishment of ideas. Simply to foist, as many have done, this radical dualistic perspective—often inherited from interpretations of classical Sāṃkhya—onto Patañjali's system results in a parochialization and trivialization of classical Yoga, marginalizing its importance and reducing its overall integrity as one of the six major orthodox Hindu *darśana*s.[167] In Yoga, however, knowledge can be utilized in the integrity of being and action. Thus, Vyāsa states that "the knower is liberated while yet living."[168] The *puruṣa* is "alone" not because it is "at home" in a purely atomistic or monadic state[169] bereft of any accessibility—any open "door" or "window"—to an external realm of existence and therefore having no connection whatsoever to *prakṛti.* Rather, the *puruṣa* is "alone" because it transcends the faulty mechanism of *saṃyoga,* which, like a broken wheel on a cart, brings about frustration and, if not properly attended to, unending dissatisfaction.[170]

Seen here, our sense of self is "tossed" or "whirled about" within the confining boundaries of identity implicit in the scheme or saṃsāric wheel of *cittavṛtti*. Free of such confinement, including all forms of obsession and all ideas of "acquiring" and "possessing," *puruṣa* is never a product of, nor is it affected or influenced by, the *guṇa*s and *karma*. *Puruṣa* shines in its own nature and glory only after one has overcome all misconceptions about reality. Having discarded all forms of misconception or "afflicted space" within the mind, the "wheel" of life through which consciousness and self-identity function can move smoothly, unimpaired.

Can *puruṣa*'s existence embrace states of action and knowledge, person and personality? The tradition of Yoga answers in the affirmative. Vyāsa asserts that having gone beyond sorrow, "the omniscient yogin, whose afflictions and bondage have been destroyed, disports himself [herself] as a master."[171] Established in the true nature of *puruṣa,* the yogin is now truly empowered to radiate the light of *puruṣa.* In *kaivalya*[172] the enstatic consciousness and *sattva* of the mind "merge," as it were, in a "sameness" of purity resulting in a perfect attunement of mind and body in relation to *puruṣa.* The karmic power of *avidyā* functioning within *prakṛti* ceases to have a hold over the yogin, the karmic ego having been exploded, its barriers dissolved. The yogin's attention is no longer sucked into the vortex of the conflicting opposites *(dvandvas)* in *saṃsāra,* is no longer embroiled in the polarizing intentionalities of desire: the vectors of attraction (i.e., attachment or *rāga*) and revulsion (i.e., aversion or *dveṣa*). Yogic emancipation does not imply a state of apathy or passivity but rather suggests a mode of comportment different from that which takes place according to the tensions in the opposition between activity and passivity. Free from the egoic intrusions of worldly existence, the yogin is said to be left "alone."

The *puruṣa* can be said to express itself in the time-space continuum in a particular body and with a particular personality and mind. Yoga does not deny the existence of individuality; it allows for a trans-egoic development that is not the dissolution of the individual person and his/her personality, but, rather, that includes their extension into the recognition, moral integrity, and celebration of the interconnectedness (because of the nonseparation, i.e., *prakṛti* is "one") of all embodied beings and life as a whole. Enstasy is lived simultaneously with our psychophysical being. The link between the enstatic consciousness *(puruṣa)* and the world is the purified *sattva* of the mind.

We must question assertions to the effect that having attained liberation the psychical apparatus of the yogin is destroyed,[173] or that in the enlightened state the yogin's body lives on in a state of catalepsy until death.[174] What disappears for the yogin is the "failure-to-see" *(adarśana)*[175]—the worldview born of *avidyā* that generates the parasitic consciousness of self in *saṃyoga*—not *prakṛti* herself. The purified mind and evolutes of *prakṛti* (e.g., intellect, ego) can now be used as vehicles for an enlightened life of interrelationship, interaction, and service, such as imparting knowledge to others: the purity and cognitive power impersonated in the *guru* or spiritual adept is transformed from an end into an available means. When one who is accomplished in Yoga (i.e., has reached the state of *nirbīja-samādhi*) opens one's eyes to the world of experience, the knower or experiencer *(puruṣa)* will be one's true center of experience. The *guṇas* (i.e., *vṛttis*) will be subordinate to the knower[176]/experiencer,[177] the "owner" of the field of the seeable.[178] Once the final stage of emancipation is reached, the lower levels of insight previously gained are not destroyed but are included by means of a nonbinding appropriation and incorporation of those insights in the light of freedom.

This study therefore suggests that through the necessary transformation of consciousness brought about in *samādhi,* an authentic and fruitful coherence of self-identity, perception, and activity emerges out of the former fragmented consciousness in *saṃyoga.* In Yoga the state of freedom does not necessitate being without thoughts or *vṛtti*s. Freedom means to identify as the very knower *(puruṣa),* which, while present to the mind and its modifications *(vṛtti*s*),* remains eternally unattached, never enslaved, subsumed, or consumed by the realm of the seeable. This realization includes a "knowledge born of discrimination" that is liberating, inclusive of all objects (and conditions) and all times, and is nonsequential.[179] The experience of transparency in *kaivalya* reveals the simultaneity and interconnectedness of all beings, conditions, and things without abandoning, distorting, or displacing the sattvic realizations—cognitive and ethical—characteristic of the former states of clarity, insight, and understanding. What is discarded in Yoga is not the mind in total, but ignorance and its creation of misidentification with phenomena or mistaken identity. When it is said that one has realized *puruṣa* through "cessation" *(nirodha),* it is meant that there is no further level to experience for one's liberation. *Nirodha* does not indicate the denial of formed reality or the negation of relative states of consciousness. Nor need *nirodha* imply being rooted in a conception of oneself that abstracts from one's identity as a social, historical, and embodied being. *Nirodha* refers to the expansion of understanding necessary to perceive every dimension of reality from the perspective of pure, untainted consciousness.

If Patañjali's perception of the world of forms and differences had been destroyed or discarded, how could he have had such insight into Yoga and the intricacies and subtle nuances of the unenlightened state?[180] If through *nirodha,* the individual form and the whole world had been cancelled for Patañjali, he would more likely have spent the rest of his days in the inactivity and isolation of transcendent oblivion rather than presenting Yoga philosophy to others! Rather than being handicapped by the exclusion of thinking, perceiving, experiencing, or activity, the liberated yogin actualizes the potential to live a fully integrated life in the world having overcome all enslavement to *avidyā.* The yogin simultaneously lives as it were in two worlds: the dimension of the unqualified *(nirguṇa)* existence of *puruṣa,* and the relative dimension *(saguṇa),* yet two worlds that work together as one.

There is then no reason why *kaivalya* cannot be seen as a "bridge" concept, bridging together or harnessing two formerly undisclosed principles or powers by correcting a misalignment between them based on a misconception or misperception of authentic identity. In this context *kaivalya* is an analogical term and can be understood with an epistemological emphasis. In Yoga, the *guru* is not physically isolated or alone but remains free even in the midst of relationships and commitments. The liberated yogin can exist in relation to the world not being morally or epistemologically enslaved by worldly relationship. The yogin is *in* the world but is not defined by worldly existence. The yogin's identity is not *of the world,* that is, is not *of a worldly afflicted nature*. Having himself/herself passed through innumerable lifetimes as a human being experiencing various joys and sorrows, the *guru* understands ordinary human life as well as the plight of the aspiring yogin. To be sure, the *guru* does not "experience" thoughts and emotions in the same way that an ordinary person does. The adept's consciousness transcends all mental activity including the affects of good (merit) and evil (demerit). However, it is said the adept "cannot but do what is perfectly consonant with his own nature, cannot but do the right thing"[181] because the adept is perceived to act not for self-gratification alone but for the spiritual benefit of others.

The purified body-mind of the yogin is used as an instrument for benevolent action in the world, while at the same time, the ego-personality is continually transcended through dispassionate acts of conscious self-surrender. Identity thus is not a mental, subjective state that can indulge and enjoy according to its own whims, but refers to an ontological category. Transcending the affective dimension in Yoga does not signal the end of the yogin's feeling-emotional nature; feelings, desires, and emotions, like cognition, are not simply reducible to the category of affliction, nor are either they or their objects to be obliterated or suppressed in Yoga.[182] As a fully liberated being the yogin is now able to engage life spontaneously and innocently yet animate freely a full range of feelings, emotions, and passions without being overtaken by them and without causing harm to others. Pedagogically this would have important implications in that the entire spectrum of human emotion could be used by the adept for the purpose of instruction.

Like the Buddha, Patañjali regards *duḥkha* as the fundamental emotion or affect in response to the contingency of saṃsāric identity and existence. Overcoming dissatisfaction *(duḥkha)* yet-to-come (*YS* II.16) is one of the principal aims of Yoga and for this to take place dispassion is essential. But dispassion *(vairāgya)* is not a severing, narrowing, or flattening out of our affective lives. The relationship between subject and object in Yoga is freed to transcend mundane intention and expectation. Moreover, the advanced yogin can experience ordinary pleasure and sorrow without wavering—feeling more satisfied or diminished—in his or her identity, for all is experienced in the light of *puruṣa*. For example, the *guru*'s participation in the field of action and simultaneous nonattachment to the fruits of action[183] are grounded in an identity that transcends the three *guṇa*s. The freedom granted to the yogin is not merely a "negative" freedom or "freedom from" the fetters of worldly turbulence, misidentification, and sorrow, but can be more positively construed to incorporate a "freedom to," meaning that the yogin can embody a highly developed, virtuous state in a manner that does not distort the yogin's understanding and identity.

I conclude here that there is no reason why the liberated yogin cannot be portrayed as a vital, creative, thoughtful, empathetic, balanced, happy, and wise person. Having adopted an integrative orientation to life, the enlightened being can endeavor to transform, enrich, and ennoble the world. I am therefore suggesting that there is a rich affective, moral, and cognitive as well as spiritual potential inherent in the realization of *puruṣa,* the "aloneness" of the power of consciousness/seeing.

The Sanskrit commentators on the *Yoga-Sūtra* and the *Yoga-Bhāṣya,* including Vācaspati Miśra and Vijñāna Bhikṣu, tend to favor the ideal of "liberation in life" or "embodied liberation" *(jīvanmukti).* The tradition clearly acknowledges an "altruistic" motive in the pursuit of enlightenment[184] that can be considered an integral part of classical Yoga, since the *guru* is recognized as a major catalyst for spiritual (and social) transformation in India and elsewhere. The *Yoga-Sūtra* functions as a text that from its very incipience (*YS* I.1-4) serves to direct the attention of the aspirant to the "goal" of *puruṣa*-realization; along the way it strongly encourages aspiration (e.g., *YS* I.21) by inculcating the yogin toward liberating insight and awareness instilled by practice and dispassion. But, as we have seen, the yogin must eventually surrender all attachment to the idea of acquiring or obtaining pure identity *(puruṣa).* Traditionally in Yoga it is often held that yogic technique ultimately succeeds only through the grace and compassion of the realized or fully awakened *guru.* That is to say, spiritual emancipation is made accessible to one who receives guidance from a liberated being *(jīvanmukta)* and who in turn is committed to yogic discipline.

While still functioning within the prakṛtic constitution of a body and mind, the yogin-adept is thus never deluded into any association with affliction implying a desire for continuity (*abhiniveśa, YS* II.9) based on a misidentification with mortal states and the consequent fear of death. Even though the prakṛtic apparatus will eventually perish, the yogin remains established in immortal consciousness, the true nature of *puruṣa*. Yoga does account for transformation into other births due to the outflowing nature of *prakṛti* (*YS* IV.2, *YB* IV.2; see discussion in chapter 2). But that Patañjali has not made an objective investigation into how the yogin is going to continue in existence after death to the physical body is not surprising. For one, classical Yoga does not admit of any need for a migratory subtle body *(sūkṣma-śarīra)*.[185] As a disembodied state (i.e., conceived as such after physical death), *kaivalya* need not be interpreted as an isolated, self-contained, relationless realm. If we are to assume that there exist a plurality of *puruṣa*s, *prakṛti* can be seen as a stepping stone for the eventual exit of liberated *puruṣa*s from "this world" into a state of mutual interrelatedness and intersubjectivity, thereby giving a different perspective to the meaning of the "flight of the alone to the alone." Or again, from this pluralistic perspective, all *puruṣa*s (and *īśvara*?) could be seen to intersect resulting in an interfusion or ontological merging of sorts, all being omnipresent and of one nature—pure consciousness—with no prakṛtic barriers and therefore without the distorting power of ignorance *(avidyā)* that generates such barriers or impediments to *puruṣa*-realization.

Patañjali's real concern, however, is with the transformation of human nature, consciousness, and identity in this very world—a world that includes our body, personhood, nature, and innumerable conditions and objects of experience. To repeat, "Patañjali's practical and pragmatic orientation emphasizes that spiritual emancipation can take place in this very lifetime and can be understood as an embodied state of freedom."[186] Are there an apparently innumerable number of omnipresent yet discrete *puruṣa*s? Nowhere in the *Yoga-Sūtra* does Patañjali make a direct case for multiple *puruṣa*s.[187] Indeed, if the culminating realization in Yoga incorporates all objects (space) and time and is simultaneous (*YS* III.54)—*puruṣa*'s nature being ubiquitous—then how can there be a large number of omnipresent, distinct, and different *puruṣa*s occupying the same space (as it were) and yet in principle purporting to have no distinguishing characteristics (for all are pure consciousness and "attributeless" by nature)? One way of resolving this problem (as has been suggested in chapter 2) is to argue that the issue of innumerable *puruṣa*s is largely an epistemological one having to do with a plurality of individualized minds through which pure consciousness discloses itself. To be sure, one of the major implications of multiple *puruṣa*s for Patañjali's system would be to underline the uniqueness of each individual's perspective or consciousness.[188]

Whether or not Patañjali actually adhered to the notion of a plurality of *puruṣa*s remains an open question. In fact, Patañjali's psychological and epistemological orientation does not lend itself easily to metaphysical speculation. Merely labelling Patañjali's philosophy as being dualistic or otherwise does not satisfy the practical concerns of Yoga per se. I have suggested, however, in chapter 2 that Patañjali can be understood as having adopted a provisional, practical dualistic metaphysics but that there is no proof that his system culminates in a metaphysical duality. Building upon our previous argument that views Yoga from an integral perspective, I am suggesting that in *kaivalya* the liberated identity of *puruṣa* can incorporate an integration of spirit and matter—including our psychophysical being and nature—such that *puruṣa* may be seen to contain every potential experience, in fact everything within itself. Or, one could say that following from the complete purification or sattvification of the mind, *puruṣa* knows itself to be everything. At this level of realization, one is no longer held captive to any sense of duality. One beholds *puruṣa*—one's true identity or Self—in the entire cosmos, and the entire cosmos, which is also one's Self, in *puruṣa*.

The practical and soteriological orientation in the *Yoga-Sūtra* can in no way be separated from the pedagogical dimension of Yoga. The diversity and flexibility of methods and the actual process of purification and illumination of consciousness is of much greater importance to Patañjali than a metaphysical systemization of reality. Patañjali, a Yoga master and wise pedagogue, emphasizes the processes leading up to *puruṣa*-realization and he clearly prefers a schema that attempts to establish the identity and distinctness of the seer *(draṣṭṛ, puruṣa)* or pure consciousness against all that is of the nature of the seeable *(dṛśya)* including the objectifiable processes of the mind *(citta)*, that is, the modifications *(vṛtti)* and objective content or constructs *(pratyaya)* of awareness. Moreover, *realizing* the distinctness and pure, nonfractured identity of the *puruṣa* is of greater concern than any grand explanation of ultimate reality whether that reality be dualistically or nondualistically understood. This study suggests that the duality of the seer and the seeable in the *Yoga-Sūtra* is best conceived, at least initially, as a provisional, relative one that is meant to serve the practical and pedagogical purpose of allowing the yogin to distinguish, in his or her understanding, reality as "seen" by *puruṣa*—from the perspective of intrinsic identity—and reality as "seen" by the mind and its influences and from the perspective of egoity or extrinsic identity.

Patañjali does not view the "discriminative discernment" *(vivekakhyāti)* between *puruṣa* and *prakṛti* merely in inferred or abstract, metaphysical terms of principles. In classical Yoga discriminative discernment necessitates a consciousness of mastery over the forces of *rajas* and *tamas* whereby the mind is fully sattvified, transformed, purified through the recognition that mind-*sattva* and *puruṣa* are distinct.[189] *Vivekakhyāti* incorporates moral value and content as well as cognitive clarity. As Vyāsa asserts (*YB* I.12), the "stream of the mind" that commences with "discrimination" *(viveka)* and terminates in "aloneness" flows to the "good," while the failure to discriminate properly leads to "evil."[190] Experiences of identity in the situation of *saṃyoga* are based on the failure to distinguish between the absolutely unmixed *puruṣa* and the mind *(sattva),*[191] between the "seer-consciousness" that truly "sees" objects (including the subtlest content of the mind) and the self-consciousness that has conformed to the changing nature of the mind. Ordinary human consciousness is of the nature of the "seeable" and assuming itself to be the seer misperceives the reality of *puruṣa* as well as *prakṛti.* This study is suggesting that an epistemologically nuanced emphasis be given to the nature of discriminative discernment *(vivekakhyāti)* in Yoga. What is being emphasized is for the yogin to distinguish between levels of perception, understanding, and knowledge (i.e., states of consciousness) rather than ontological categories alone.

It would not be true to the style or spirit of Patañjali's thought to end up reifying *kaivalya* into an ultimate principle of existence, "all else" falling under the category of "illusion," for such an interpretation can easily lead to a form of idealism that accentuates a sense of aversion *(dveṣa)* toward and emotional alienation from the world. But to withdraw from the world and merely renounce one's responsibilities while remaining in an afflicted condition oneself (e.g., self-pity, envy, hypocritical or self-righteous behavior, pride, or a plain lack of energy and confidence) can only generate egoity, forms of spiritual mediocrity, a misappropriation of yogic technique/methods, and pseudo-liberation—all of which are not to be equated with Yoga. The dualistic framework that Patañjali adopts reflects the condition of the aspiring yogin. It instills a pragmatic and practical orientation that engages the yogin-practitioner in the cultivation of a spiritual discipline capable of leading the yogin from states of ignorance/impurity/mistaken identity to knowledge/purity/authentic identity. The reality of the body, mind, nature, and materiality in general—so real to one on the "path" of Yoga—is not denied. Idealistic interpretations of reality are, in fact, refuted in Yoga.[192]

Kaivalya can be said to represent the culminating fruit of the yogin's commitment to the realization of an underlying identity or reality that engages *puruṣa* and *prakṛti* both, thereby transcending all conceptual understanding, including all dualistic or nondualistic notions, regarding that identity or reality. Koelman argues that Patañjali's Yoga can adapt itself to different philosophical backgrounds: whether there is a distinct *puruṣa* for each human personality as classical Sāṃkhya teaches, or whether there is ultimately one supreme Self *(paramātman)* as Śaṅkara's Advaita Vedānta maintains is, according to Koelman, indifferent to Yoga technique as such.[193]

The process of "cessation" *(nirodha)* seeks to disclose the experiencer, the unseen seer also referred to in the *Upaniṣad*s.[194] The purpose of yogic meditative discipline is to reveal the object of perception as it is "in itself" (i.e., in *samādhi*) and break through to the point where there can be no epistemological distortion between the seer and the seeable. The yogin sacrifices the characteristic feature of ordinary human identity, which is its bipolar nature, its tension between subject and object. *Puruṣa* is transcendent, yet is also an immanent (ineffable) presence that can only be expressed metaphorically. Patañjali does not espouse negative descriptions of the nature of *puruṣa* but prefers metaphors in the context of "seeing" *(draṣṭṛ, dṛś, dṛśi, dṛśi-mātra),* "cognizing" *(citi, citi-śakti),* and "owning" (i.e., referring here to the "owner" or *svāmin*) that comply with his epistemological and psychological rather than a metaphysical approach.

What contribution does Patañjali make to the rich, historical, and philosophical "tradition" of Hinduism? We shall confine our comments here within the context of the *ṣaḍ-darśana*s—the so-called six orthodox Brāhmaṇic perspectives of life. Sāṃkhya, with its emphasis on ontology, is concerned with enumerating and describing the principal categories of existence. All experience—succinctly fitted into an ontologically oriented framework—culminates in a complete severance of *puruṣa* and *prakṛti,* a radical metaphysical duality. The stress in the Nyāya school is on principles of logic and reasoning and deals largely with epistemological issues and procedures. The Vaiśeṣika system (Vaiśeṣika means "pertaining to individuality or particularity") is concerned with differences between material states, with the physical properties of matter, and, by experimentation, how the self and mind use those properties. Vaiśeṣika stresses ontological questions and distinctions about the nature of reality. Both Nyāya and Vaiśeṣika are highly analytical in their approaches. The tradition of Pūrva Mīmāṃsā, in keeping with the exegetical tradition of Vedic ritualism, is mainly concerned with the meaning and implementation of *dharma,* understood here as "right action" as in the Vedic solemn ritual and *karma* in its strictest sense. Uttara Mīmāṃsā (i.e., Vedānta) insists on the crucial, authoritative role given to scripture for validating metaphysical and soteriological matters; and, in the case of Advaita Vedānta, the need for knowledge *(vidyā,* *jñāna)* as the means for attaining *brahman,* the ultimate Reality of the Upaniṣads, is clearly emphasized.

Granting validity to above schemes, Patañjali's overriding concern is with the practical implications of all the enumerating, reasoning, experimenting, ritual action and scriptural authority. How may we finally experience and know that our true identity is immortal, eternally pure, wise, and free? One of Patañjali's main contributions lies in showing how and by what methods, consciousness, misidentified with *prakṛti* (matter, psychophysical being, nature), can be purified, illuminated, and restored to its original authentic identity as *puruṣa,* a state of freedom termed the "aloneness of seeing" *(dṛśeḥ kaivalyam).* Despite the opinion of some—that Patañjali has made little if any contribution to Yoga philosophy—this study suggests that Patañjali's presentation of Yoga makes a significant philosophical contribution to our understanding of Yoga.[195]

More specifically, Patañjali's unique contribution (and one might say his real "genius") lies in his ability to overcode previous teachings on Yoga adding a profoundly articulate and integral understanding of Yoga as defined in *Yoga-Sūtra* I.2. The definition of Yoga as *cittavṛttinirodha* masterfully incorporates a sophisticated philosophical theory of Yoga along with a rich diversity of yogic practices. This central definition of Yoga can be seen as "threading together" the *Yoga-Sūtra* as a whole as well as skillfully communicating the meaning and essence of Yoga as being: (1) process and transformation implying spiritual growth and development, and (2) a culminating state of freedom, of enlightened identity (i.e., consciousness and being). Classical Yoga reveals how *puruṣa* and *prakṛti*—the two components (spiritual and material) of our human nature and identity—can work together in harmony and attain the highest "good" as well as the highest cognitive realization in the liberated state of "aloneness" *(kaivalya).* The reality of nature, the mind, and our human embodiment need not be ultimately denied, disposed of, or rendered inherently problematic.

Patañjali wrote (spoke?) not from the standpoint of revealed scripture or theoretical clarification, but from the perspective of concrete experience. The aphoristic method of the *Yoga-Sūtra* leaves much unsaid, throwing aspirants back upon themselves with a powerful stimulus to self-inquiry, self-testing, and self-discovery but within the established tradition (i.e., already discovered "truths") of Yoga. To practice Yoga does not give one a platform to engage licentiously in an "independent consciousness research"[196] project or an open-ended experimentation or inquiry into the nature of consciousness. For nothing can really be added to the knowledge contained in Yoga. Moreover, Yoga is rooted in a pedagogical dynamic—

the *guru-śiṣya* relation—which functions as a vital building block and catalyst for self-transformation and direct experience of pure identity. While recognizing the practical and heuristic (albeit provisional) value of forms of belief, creeds, theories, models of reality, debate, questions and answers, and points of view, the purpose in Yoga is to move beyond their limited, conceptual, and subjective dimensions and engage Yoga directly. Thus, after declaring that Yoga alone is the teacher, Vyāsa cites an ancient expression: "By Yoga Yoga is to be known; Yoga progresses from Yoga. He who cares for Yoga, forever remains in Yoga."[197]

Yoga presupposes the integration of knowledge and activity; there can be no scission between *theoria* and *praxis*. The *Yoga-Sūtra* is a philosophical text where *praxis* is deemed to be essential. Without actual practice the theory that informs Yoga would have no authentic meaning. Yet without examination and reflection there would be no meaningful striving for liberation, no "goal" as it were to set one's sight on. In an original, inspiring, and penetrating style, Patañjali bridges metaphysics and ethics, transcendence and immanence, and contributes to the Hindu fold a form of philosophical investigation that, to borrow J. Taber's descriptive phrase for another context, can properly be called a "transformative philosophy." That is to say, it is a philosophical perspective that "does not stand as an edifice isolated from experience; it exists only insofar as it is realized in experience."[198]

Yoga philosophy is primarily a means for transforming our understanding and perception of reality; it is not overly concerned with a metaphysical categorization, enumeration, objectification, or systemization of reality, that all too easily can be misappropriated and lead to reified notions of self and world. Grounded in a pedagogical context, Yoga ontology (*YS* II.19) is initially abstracted from direct experience and acts as a contemplative directive for the realization of the underlying, transconceptual realities; a "realized" ontology follows from Yoga epistemology. Patañjali's soteriological, practical, and transformative approach does not mean that his system fails to consider the ontological implications of Yoga. Rather, Yoga philosophy, like other systems of Indian thought (e.g., within Buddhism and nondualistic Vedānta), is representative of a form of "thought about being that is rooted in and motivated by a desire for absolute liberation, a kind of 'soteriontology'."[199] Moreover, this study suggests that Patañjali's Yoga has profound implications for an embodied state of liberation.

Having expounded a central, foundational definition of Yoga (*YS* I.2), Patañjali pragmatically lays out various means to liberation through which the pure power of "seeing"—the nonseparation of knower, knowing, and known—is revealed. In what state, being, or consciousness may *puruṣa* be said to dwell in *kaivalya?* Perhaps *kaivalya* is a transition to a nondualistic state: the unmodifiable, immutable *brahman* or one indivisible reality acknowledged in schools of Vedānta. The *Yoga-Sūtra,* having done the work of providing practical guidance that leads to *kaivalya,* remains silent[200] and lets the experience or realization itself answer. In enstasy *(asaṃprajñāta-samādhi)* the yogin moves beyond the "seeable," beyond all prakṛtic limitations of consciousness and identity, and directly "experiences," or rather *identifies as puruṣa*. Yoga brings about a trans-empirical or transworldly dimension that, being both world-transcending and world-transforming, does not negate self and world but properly bridges or aligns them. As *puruṣa* is self-luminous,[201] in *kaivalya*—the *telos* of all knowledge—"*puruṣa* stands alone in its true nature as pure light."[202]

Puruṣa "knows" itself and the realm of the seeable by its own light of consciousness. Thus *puruṣa* is "known" only by *puruṣa* and not by the mind.[203] In knowing itself, *puruṣa* is free to be itself, to abide in its inviolable identity, nature, and glory. Through praxis a transformation of consciousness takes place involving a transformed perception of self-identity and the world. Even "knowing *puruṣa*" is a metaphor for an experience or state that is better described as a coming-to-dwell *as* the formless knower in pure knowingness/pure seeing. Self-identity no longer needs to know itself reflexively, but is peaceful and immutable because it needs or lacks nothing. In *kaivalya* the rupture from authentic identity is healed and a fullness of being emerges.

Conclusion

Although several valuable, contemporary scholarly writings have helped to present Patañjali's philosophy to a wider academic and popular audience, our study suggests that Patañjali has far too often been misinterpreted or misrepresented due to the use of inappropriate methodology: partial and misleading definitions of Sanskrit yogic terms and reductionistic hermeneutics leading to an imposed radical, dualistic finality or closure to Patañjali's perspective of Yoga. Many scholars have repeatedly given ontological definitions and explanations for terms that, this study maintains, are more appropriately understood with an epistemological emphasis. Consequently, the specialized sense inherent in Yoga soteriology is diminished. The soteriological intent of Yoga need not preclude the possibility for an integrated, embodied state of liberated identity. A bias is invariably created within the language encountered in the translations and interpretations of the *Yoga-Sūtra* resulting in an overemphasis on content, due consideration not having been given to form, structure, and function.

It is crucial to view Yoga contextually—as it is understood, experienced, and embodied by the yogin—and not simply to impute a content-system to the whole process of Yoga. The bias extends to the ontological priorities of *puruṣa* over *prakṛti* and by consequence the priority of axiology over epistemology. *Puruṣa* is generally explained or understood as the enlightened and ultimately hegemonic principle of pure consciousness, our true identity that alone has intrinsic spiritual value. *Prakṛti,* we are often told, is the nonspiritual cosmogonic principle comprised of the three *guṇa*s (*sattva, rajas,* and *tamas*), has a deluding, binding, yet paradoxically subservient nature (for the purpose of *puruṣa*), and eventually disappears from the yogin's (i.e., the "seer's") purview, having been granted no real value or place in the liberated state. It is not clear that the language of the *Yoga-Sūtra* is explanatory. It could equally be descriptive, in which case the axiological and ontological priorities would collapse thereby challenging the widely held scholarly view that the relationship between *puruṣa* and *prakṛti,* the seer *(draṣṭṛ)* and the seeable *(dṛśya),* is exclusively or definitively an asymmetrical relation, that is, *prakṛti* exists for the purpose of *puruṣa* and her value is seen merely in instrumental terms and within the context of a soteriological end state that excludes her.

In Patañjali's central definition of Yoga (*YS* I.2)—the focus of this study—*nirodha* has frequently been understood as an ontological cessation, suppression, or "deadening" of the mind *(citta)* and its modifications *(vṛtti),* and this misunderstanding has led, I suggest, to some major interpretive errors. First, one can witness a reductionistic application of positivistic presuppositions to a trans-empirical, transconceptual, mystical system: scholars have often concluded that when liberation *(apavarga)* or "aloneness" *(kaivalya)* has been attained, the yogin will no longer be capable of experiencing or engaging the world since the body and mind will have ceased to function (at least effectively so). Second, the pedagogical context of Yoga involving the oral/historical teaching tradition has either been ignored or else this important foundational dynamic within Yoga has not been sufficiently taken into consideration and incorporated into the philosophy. Our hermeneutic must include a way of reading the tradition of Yoga within its cultural/religious context.

Third, by explaining *nirodha* as an ontological cessation or negation of *vṛtti*s, many scholars have given a negative, one-sided, and spurious definition of Yoga. The result is a volatile concept of *nirodha,* one that emphasizes Yoga as being a form of world-denial and psychophysical negation or suppression. Seen here, phenomenal reality for the liberated yogin (including the mind-body complex) is rendered as a meaningless or purposeless existence and "dissolves" into or returns to its "preformed" state, the unmanifest, nonconscious, undifferentiated (disembodied) realm of the *guṇa*s that has lost all connection with consciousness. Consequently, Patañjali's philosophy *as a whole* becomes parochialized, even trivialized, and can be viewed as unapproachable, unintelligible, unattractive, and impractical.

Puruṣa indeed has precedence over *prakṛti* in Patañjali's system, for *puruṣa* is what is ordinarily "missing" in human life and is ultimately the state of consciousness one must awaken to in Yoga. According to this study, the liberated state of "aloneness" *(kaivalya)* need not denote an ontological superiority of *puruṣa,* or an exclusion of *prakṛti. Kaivalya* can be positively construed as an integration of both principles—an integration that, I have argued, is what is most important for Yoga. The sheer questioning of why *puruṣa*—being by nature ever-pure, wise, and free—would care or even bother to be involved or integrated with "insentient" *prakṛti* is itself laced with a radical dualistic assumption about Yoga that is perhaps more indicative of a spiritually elitist understanding of Patañjali's thought: *prakṛti,* conceived to be the "inferior," less worthy, and therefore undesirable reality of the two, is left behind for good in the enlightened state. Moreover, the calling into question of *puruṣa*'s association with matter presupposes that the nature of *puruṣa* and *prakṛti*'s "togetherness" or "union" is intrinsically rooted in ignorance and can therefore only generate mistaken identity, suffering, frustration, and dissatisfaction *(duḥkha).*

But what if the nature of the relationship *itself* (between *puruṣa* and *prakṛti*) is transformed from the binding, obfuscated involvements inherent in the situation of *saṃyoga* to the liberating mode of activity and "seeing" inherent in Yoga? Yoga can be understood then as having corrected a basic "misalignment"—rooted in "misconception"—between *puruṣa* and *prakṛti,* implying therefore the disclosure of a clearly established "union" or "alignment" between these two principles. The problem of "self" and "identity" in Yoga lies not in ontology—the existence of *puruṣa* and *prakṛti* are not in doubt—but in perception, self-understanding, and the activity of decision making. How and what we perceive and how we choose to act are crucial considerations in Yoga.

Admittedly, the more integrative approach to Patañjali's Yoga *darśana* suggested in this study does raise some rather provocative questions that I feel need to be raised in order to reflect adequately on the profundity and practical emphasis of this foundational scripture of Yoga, the *Yoga-Sūtra.* Instead of assuming an absolute incommensurability between *puruṣa* and *prakṛti,* we can ask: Have these two principles—usually conceived as eternally existent—ever *been* separate (i.e., absolutely disjoined)? Could they ever *be* separate? Does pure consciousness *in itself,* as a purely isolated, relationless state—a formless, all-pervading consciousness or reality eternally separate from all matter or form—actually exist? Or, not unlike the term *citta,* could it (i.e., pure consciousness) be understood as a heuristic notion, perhaps even a stage along the way ("experienced" in *asaṃprajñāta-*

samādhi), that skillfully serves to lead to the fullness of our identity as revealed in *kaivalya?* There is no ultimate evidence given in the *Yoga-Sūtra* to conclude, on a definitive basis, that the unbound identity of the seer *(draṣṭṛ, puruṣa)* does not or cannot engage with or even include the realm of the seeable *(dṛśya, prakṛti)*.

To break *puruṣa* and *prakṛti* apart, to keep one and try to discard the other, is an enterprise that creates disequilibrium or imbalance involving confused notions of identity or "self" that, I submit, are clearly inimical to Yoga. Such notions may have a compulsive attachment-orientation (*rāga, YS* II.7) whereby we succumb to the world and can become easily enmeshed in forms of narcissism and egocentrism by aggressively objectifying and exploiting the world and others. Or such notions may be stringently rooted in an aversion-orientation (*dveṣa, YS* II.8) involving an exaggerated and impoverished sense of "isolation" from the world, a form of escape or flight of self with an impulse toward self-negation. Both of these extremes: worldly entrapment and escape from the world, must be transcended in Yoga.

Patañjali's definition of Yoga (*YS* I.2) can be seen as an effective prescription for correcting the deluded or confused state of affairs in *saṃyoga*. Epistemologically, the mind *(citta)* has two basic opposing tendencies or qualities: ignorance *(avidyā)* of reality, and knowledge *(jñāna)* of reality. The degree or level of knowledge that exists depends to what extend our psychophysical being has undergone the purifying and illuminating process of sattvification—sattvification implying a process through which ignorance is gradually discarded and knowledge predominates. Paradoxically, the mind that under the grip of ignorance formerly acted as a locus for misidentication in *saṃyoga* and was burdened and restricted in its power of perception, becomes—through a transformative process in Yoga—an instrument of liberating knowledge or insight *(prajñā)*. This knowledge, it has been argued, is then incorporated and integrated in the state of "aloneness" *(kaivalya)*.

Viewed from another angle, under the influence of *avidyā* the reflected consciousness of *puruṣa* in the mind makes *puruṣa* appear embroiled in *saṃsāra,* selfhood being conceived within prakṛtic existence as a mere product or creation of the three *guṇa*s *(triguṇa)*. Thus, one's identity is confined within the *cittavṛtti* schematic, resulting in a misidentification with and misappropriation of *prakṛti*. Through the process of the "cessation" *(nirodha)* of the misidentification with *vṛtti,* ignorance—in the form of the *saṃskāra*-complex of personality traits or habit patterns *(vāsanā*s*)* entrenched in erroneous knowledge *(viparyaya-jñāna)* or misperception—is sifted out from the yogin's view. Impurity *(aśuddhi)* dissolves, leading to an increasing light of knowledge (*jñāna-dīpti, YS* II.28), and the mind, inclined toward discriminative discernment *(viveka-khyāti),* then has a propensity for *kaivalya* (*YS* IV.26). The result of this transformed state of identity is nothing less than the "aloneness of seeing" unencumbered in its fullness. I have proposed that the *Yoga-Sūtra* does not uphold a "path" of liberation that ultimately renders *puruṣa* and *prakṛti* incapable of "cooperating" together. Rather, the *Yoga-Sūtra* seeks to "unite" these two principles without the presence of any defiled understanding, to bring them "together," properly aligning them in a state of balance, harmony, and a clarity of knowledge in the integrity of being and action.

By viewing the *Yoga-Sūtra* as having given a legitimate voice to the quest for an absolute separation of *puruṣa* and *prakṛti,* scholars and other writers on Yoga may well have misread Patañjali, portraying the great master as having taught a form of radical dualism—a dualism that has often been at the center of controversy and may even be considered an anomaly within Hinduism. A dominant philosophical position within Hinduism that is prior to the *Yoga-Sūtra,* and that includes Upaniṣadic writings and the *Mahābhārata,* has been nondualistic or panentheistic. Thus, most Yoga thought or schools that preceded Patañjali, or that subsequently developed after the *Yoga-Sūtra,* have advocated some form of nondualism or theism. Indeed, yogic (Hindu) teachings that arose after Patañjali—as recorded, for example, in the *Yoga Upaniṣads, Yogavāsiṣṭha,* Hindu tantric works (e.g., the *Mahānirvāṇa-Tantra*), works in Kashmiri Śaivism, and *haṭha-yoga*—can be seen as reaffirmations of a nondual understanding of reality and are informed more by the metaphysics of, for example, (Advaita) Vedānta than by the Sāṃkhyan dualistic framework. Are we to understand Patañjali's Yoga as a system that "can almost be regarded as an interlude in a tradition that was from the outset nondualistic"?[1]

Notwithstanding the long-lasting success and primarily practical influence of the *Yoga-Sūtra* as well as the overall status granted to classical Yoga as one of the six orthodox philosophical schools *(darśana*s*)* of Brāhmaṇical Hinduism, we suggest that the inappropriate label of "radical dualism" inflicted upon Patañjali's philosophy, combined with a somewhat attenuated or elusive concept of "God" *(īśvara),* has disparaged its integrity and prevented the Yoga *darśana* from assuming greater religious, philosophical, and cultural significance than it truly deserves. This study has argued for a more open-ended approach to Patañjali's thought, an approach that, it has been suggested, orients us toward or more closely aligns us with the intent or purpose of Yoga itself.[2]

Thus, Patañjali's Yoga, defined as *cittavṛttinirodha,* need not imply the extinction or evaporation of our "personhood" along with the objective, material world. Rather, it seems more accurate to assert that Yoga culminates in the eradication of spiritual ignorance *(avidyā)*—the root cause of our misidentification with, and attachment to, worldly (or otherworldly!) existence. In this way, Yoga removes our selfishness, suffering, and dissatisfaction *(duḥkha)* rooted in an afflicted and mistaken self-identity *(asmitā)*. I have emphasized how Yoga as "the cessation of [the misidentification with] the modifications of the mind" can be seen as a bipolar process of practice *(abhyāsa)* and dispassion *(vairāgya),* a process that has been articulated through a detailed analysis of Patañjali's stages of cognitive *samādhi (saṃprajñāta)* and the state of supracognitive *samādhi (asaṃprajñāta)*. In our exposition of the multileveled process of *samādhi* an attempt has been made to show how the expansion of consciousness and burgeoning of knowledge and ethical virtues attained through the rarified *sattva* of the mind contribute to the cessation of *puruṣa*'s superimposed, object-oriented condition of externalization/emergence *(vyutthāna)* and extrinsic identity, thus leading to the objectless enstasy *(asaṃprajñāta)*.

In the process of *nirodha* two seemingly antithetical impulses can be discerned: One presses for a deconstruction and unmasking of a prakṛtic identity of self—its cognitions, emotive dispositions, beliefs, worldview, and so forth—and the other for an integration and reconciliation of individuality/personhood/embodiment and its place in the world. Yoga allows for a dynamic interplay and creative tension between identification and association within the empirical world *(prakṛti)* and a trans-empirical or transworldly identity *(puruṣa)*. Through the summation and transmutation of all past experience, achieved in *asaṃprajñāta,* Yoga can thus be recognized as a highly developed and integrated state of mystical illumination that extends and enhances our self-identity. Liberated from the pain of self-limitation and all destructive personality traits or habit patterns *(vāsanā*s*),* and having incorporated an expanded and enriched sense of personal/empirical identity embodying virtues such as nonviolence *(ahiṃsā),* compassion *(karuṇā),* and yogic insight *(prajñā),* the yogin can dwell in a state of balance and fulfillment serving others while feeling/being truly at home in the world. The yogin can function in relation to the world not being morally or epistemologically enslaved by worldly relationship. Freedom therefore is not to be equated with living in an everyday world conditioned by attachment; it is living and acting in the everyday world with *puruṣa*-realization. Nor is freedom to be confused with escape from the world. Freedom denotes a transformation of our entire way of being or mode of action as embodied within the lived world itself.

Both morality and perception (cognition) are essential channels through which human consciousness, far from being negated or suppressed, is transformed and illuminated. Yoga combines discerning knowledge with an emotional, affective, and moral sensibility, allowing for a participatory epistemology that incorporates the moral amplitude for empathic identification with the objects or persons one seeks to understand. The enhanced perception gained through Yoga must be interwoven with Yoga's rich affective and moral dimensions to form a spirituality that does not become entangled in a web of antinomianism, but that retains the integrity and vitality to transform our lives and the lives of others in an effective manner. By upholding an integration of the moral and the mystical, Yoga supports a reconciliation of the prevalent tension within Hinduism between: (1) spiritual engagement and self-identity within the world *(pravṛtti)*, and (2) spiritual disengagement from worldliness, and self-identity that transcends the world *(nivṛtti)*. Yoga discerns and teaches a balance between these two apparently conflicting orientations.

This study has attempted to counter the radically dualistic, isolationistic, and ontologically oriented interpretations of Yoga presented by many scholars—where the full potentialities of our human embodiment are constrained within a radical, rigid, dualistic metaphysical structure—and propose instead an open-ended, morally and epistemologically oriented hermeneutic that frees Yoga of the long-standing conception of spiritual isolation, disembodiment, self-denial, and world-negation and thus from its pessimistic image. Our interpretation does not impute that *kaivalya* denotes a final incommensurability between spirit and matter. It was suggested that while Patañjali can be understood as having adopted a provisional, practical, dualistic metaphysics, there is no proof that his system ends in duality.

Throughout our study I have endeavored to show where writings on Patañjali—ranging from traditional Yoga scholiasts to modern academics—have often explained the meanings of key yogic terms such as *nirodha* and *kaivalya* in an unclear, confused, or misleading manner. I have undertaken to clarify the meanings of central terms in Yoga and add new meanings, showing how the latter relate to the literal or conventional meanings generally used. Thus, I have suggested improvements over past translations and interpretations of the *Yoga-Sūtra*, and have consulted (for analytical and critical purposes) the works by Vācaspati Miśra, Bhoja Rāja, Vijñāna Bhikṣu, H. Āraṇya, and others who have contributed to the exegetical tradition of classical Yoga. This study has taken the view that Vyāsa's commentary, the *Yoga-Bhāṣya*, provides the key to unlocking the profundity of meaning contained within the *Yoga-Sūtra,* thus illuminating our understanding of Patañjali.

As well as being one of *the* seminal texts on yogic technique and transformative/liberative approaches within Indian philosophy, Patañjali's *Yoga-Sūtra* has to this day remained one of the most influential spiritual guides in Hinduism. In addition to a large number of people within India, millions of Westerners are actively practicing some form of Yoga influenced by Patañjali's thought, clearly demonstrating Yoga's relevance for today as a discipline that can transcend cultural, religious, and philosophical barriers. The universal and universalizing potential of Yoga makes it one of India's finest contributions to our modern/postmodern struggle for self-definition, moral integrity, and spiritual renewal. The main purpose of this present study has been to consider a fresh approach in which to reexamine and assess classical Yoga philosophy, one that helps to disclose the integrity of the Yoga *darśana*. There is, I submit, nothing in what I argued that can be proven to be incompatible with Patañjali's thought. Thus, it is my hope that some of the suggestions presented in this study can function as a catalyst for bringing Patañjali's Yoga *darśana* into a more fruitful dialogue and encounter with other religious and philosophical traditions both within and outside of India.

NOTES

CHAPTER 1. SELECTED BACKGROUND MATERIAL

1. G. Feuerstein (1979a), *The Yoga-Sūtra of Patañjali: A New Translation and Commentary,* p. 26.

2. M. Eliade (1969), *Yoga: Immortality and Freedom,* p. 4.

3. G. Larson (1978), Review: Gaspar M. Koelman (1970), *Pātañjala Yoga: From Related Ego to Absolute Self,* in *PEW,* 28.2: 236–239.

4. G. Feuerstein (1989), *Yoga: The Technology of Ecstacy,* p. 15. The best historical and thematic reference on Yoga, to which this chapter is indebted, is the above-mentioned work by Feuerstein.

5. See ibid., pp. 40–62, for a discussion on most of these forms of Yoga.

6. M. Monier-Williams (1899), *A Sanskrit-English Dictionary,* p. 853.

7. G. Feuerstein (1989: 16) and (1975), *Textbook of Yoga,* p. 3.

8. The word Yoga, as Feuerstein mentions (1989: 16), is also related to German *joch,* Swedish *ok,* Latin *iugum,* Greek *zugos,* French *joug,* and Russian *igo,* which all have similar meanings.

9. Monier-Williams, (1899: 853).

10. See Eliade (1969: 361).

11. *BG* IV.3.

12. See Hauer's (1958), *Der Yoga,* and M. Falk's (1941), *The Unknown Early Yoga and the Birth of Indian Philosophy;* see also K. Werner (1977), *Yoga and Indian Philosophy.*

13. Contemporary scholarship tends to agree on this point. Feuerstein (1989: 97) writes: "traces of an early form of Yoga can even be detected in the Indus civilization that flourished in the second and third millennia BCE). According to this view, Yoga thus antedates the invasion of the Sanskrit-speaking tribes from the steppes of Southern Russia, who called themselves Aryans ("noble folk") and who had long been thought to have given birth to the tradition of Yoga." There are some major problems in trying to discern the religious life of the people of the Indus Valley Civilization. However, there are some examples available of their writing, in a pictographic script, mainly upon small seals that may have been used to seal bags of grain. Scholars have looked for materials that prefigure religious phenomena in the later development of Indian culture. One of the seals discovered portrays a male, ithyphallic, horned person, perhaps a human being, perhaps a deity, sitting in what appears to be a yogic posture—a variant of the lotus position—with animals around him. This figure has been associated with the important god of Hinduism, Śiva, who is considered to be a great yogin, and who

is often referred to as Paśupati—the "lord of the animals." This suggests that the practice of Yoga and the worship of the god Śiva are derived from this pre-Aryan Indus Valley Civilization. For more on the Indus Valley Civilization and Yoga, see Feuerstein (1989: 97–101); see also J. Marshall (1931), *Mohenjo Daro and the Indus Civilization;* M. Wheeler (1968), *The Indus Civilisation;* and B. Allchin and R. Allchin (1982), *The Rise of Civilisation in India and Pakistan.*

14. See Joshi (1965), "On the Meaning of Yoga." *PEW,* 15.1: 53.

15. See Dasgupta (1922), *History of Indian Philosophy,* vol. 1, p. 226.

16. References from the *ṚV* are taken from Swami S. P. Sarasvati, trans. (1977, 1987), *Ṛg-Veda Saṃhitā*, vols. 2, 5, 6, and 13. Unless otherwise noted, translations from Sanskrit sources used in this study are mine. *ṚV* X.114.9 in (1987), vol. 13, p. 4592: *kaś chandasāṃ yogaṃ ā veda dhīraḥ ko dhiṣṇyāṃ prati vācaṃ papāda.*

17. Joshi (1965: 54).

18. The Sanskrit text of the Upaniṣads can be located in S. Radhakrishnan (1953), *The Principal Upaniṣads;* page numbers following references to passages from the *Upaniṣads* are taken from Radhakrishnan's book. See p. 257 for text of *BĀ Up* IV.3.10: *na tatra rathāḥ, na rathayogāḥ, napanthāno bhavanti; atha rathān, rathayogān, pathaḥ sṛjate*. "There are neither chariots nor animals for yoking to chariots, nor paths; then he produces chariots, animals for yoking to chariots and paths."

19. E.g. *ṚV* III.42 and *Śatapatha Brāhmaṇa* III.5.1.24.

20. See *Kaṭha Up* I.3; *Mait Up* II.6; *Mahābhārata, Vanaparva,* 211.23.

21. Dasgupta (1922: 226).

22. S. Dasgupta (1930), *Yoga Philosophy in Relation to Other Systems of Indian Thought,* pp. 39, 44.

23. S. Dasgupta (1922: 226).

24. Cf. *Atharva Veda* XIX.43.1; *ṚV* IV.1.1; and *Yajur Veda* II.2.

25. Joshi (1965: 55).

26. The term Veda ("knowledge") refers to the oldest section of the sacred canon of Hinduism comprising the *Ṛg Veda, Yajur Veda, Sāma Veda* and *Atharva Veda.* The hymns *(sūkta, mantra)* of these ancient collections composed as early as 1200 BCE (i.e., the *Ṛg Veda),* are traditionally acknowledged to have been "heard" or "perceived" by seers *(ṛṣis)* and are regarded as part of revealed scripture *(śruti).*

27. See *ṚV* X.90.12–13; cf. Eggeling, *The Sacred Books of the East,* vol. 43, p. xv.

28. *ṚV* X.90.16ab.

29. *ṚV* V.81.1 in (1977), vol. 5, p. 1802: *yuñjate mana uta yuñjate dhiyo viprāḥ.*

30. See R. Panikkar (1977), *The Vedic Experience: Mantra-mañjarī*, pp. 350–351 for a discussion of the term *ṛta.*

31. Ibid., p. 354.

32. See *Atharva Veda* XI.8.6.

33. See Uma Vesci (1985), *Heat and Sacrifice in the Vedas.*

34. See, for example, *ṚV* I.23.5 and V.68.4.

35. J. Miller (1974), *The Vedas: Harmony, Meditation and Fulfilment,* p. 45. I am grateful to G. Feuerstein (1989, p. 103) for having introduced me to Miller's stimulating work. See also Antonio de Nicholas's (1976), *Meditations Through the Ṛg Veda* (New York: Nicolas Hayes) for insights on issues raised in this section of our study.

36. J. Gonda (1963: 68–69). Concerning *dhītiḥ*, Gonda writes (p. 171): the "suffix *(ti)* helps to form words expressing that the idea conveyed by the root manifests itself and is realized as an actuality."

37. The *dhītayaḥ* (plural of *dhītiḥ*) refer to materialized visions, often inspired hymns. The term *dhīta* denotes "an object of visionary sight"; the adjective *dhīra* means "gifted with vision" and hence "able on account of the possession of a vision." The quality expressed by *dhīra* may enable a sage or wise person to overcome practical difficulties of various kinds. Thus there are a whole family of concepts that originate in the *Ṛg Veda* and that precede the related term *dhyāna* of classical times.

38. See Miller (1974: 61).

39. Ibid., p. 354.

40. *ṚV* V.40.6 in (1977), vol. 5, p. 1672: *gūḷhaṃ sūryaṃ tamasāpavratena turīyeṇa brahmaṇāvindad atriḥ.*

41. See Miller (1974: 97). This is in reference to the fourth *brahman*. Vedic Sanskrit employed two words for prayerful or meditative contemplation: *brahman* and *dhī.* Both have different meanings yet are closely linked together. The term *dhī* refers to visionary insight, intense thought, and reflection; and *brahman* is derived from the verbal root *bṛh,* meaning "to grow, expand."

42. Ibid., p. 100. This is evidenced in the text quoted in n. 40 (above); cf. also *ṚV* I.50.10 and I.164.21.

43. See ibid., on *ṚV* VIII.48.3: "we have become immortal; we have gone to the light; we have found the gods." See also ibid., p. 92, where Miller writes:

> In the state of heightened awareness as was familiar to Vedic sages they beheld the "golden one" (*apaśyāma hiraṇyayam ṚV* I.139.2) not with visionary thoughts or mental insight *(dibhiś cana manasā)* but "with the very eyes of Soma [our] very eyes" *(svebhir akṣ abhiḥ somasya svebhir akṣabhiḥ)* or as the verse could also be translated "with the very eyes of Soma, indeed its very eyes," the meaning being the same, as "its very eyes" become the eyes of the seers. These "eyes" may mean the perception granted through ecstasy, since after drinking Soma the bards could exclaim "we have become immortal, we have come to the light, we have found the gods" (VIII.48.3), the juxtaposition of gods (i.e., divinity), of light (i.e., enlightenment) and immortality (i.e., the abolition of limitation) expressing the gradation of the rapture experienced. The direct mention that there is no mental visioning but an actual realization through the eyes granted by Soma, the insight of the god-intoxicated spirit, lifts up the vision to a higher level than that so far considered. It is also remarkable that the eyes of Soma are equated with "very eyes" as it can be taken that the essence of the seer's perception or "eyes" is one with Soma. From this it may be easily inferred that the eyes of the immortal spirit which are the real eyes, are referred to here.

Such a declaration as outlined by Miller constitutes one of the nearest of Ṛg-Vedic approaches to *YS* III.3 on *samādhi.*

44. See, for example, A. B. Keith (1925), *Religion and Philosophy of the Veda and Upaniṣads,* p. 311, who takes this position.

45. See Miller (1974: 191). In the *Nāsadīya Sūkta* or hymn of creation (*ṚV* X.129), the manifest worlds are said to have been produced by virtue of the excessive self-heating *(tapas)* of the primordial Being. For a translation and commentary on *ṚV* X.129, see J. Miller, "The Hymn of Creation: A Philosophical Interpretation," in G. Feuerstein and J. Miller (1971), *A Reappraisal of Yoga: Essays in Indian Philosophy,* pp. 64–85.

46. See the *puruṣayajña* in *ŚB* I.3.2.1 and Panikkar (1977: 392–393).

47. See *ŚB* II.3.1–39 and the *Prāṇāgnihotra Up.* Interestingly, the *ŚB* does contain clear references dealing with speculation on the nature of the source of manifest existence, the life-force or breath *(prāṇa)* and rebirth, all within the context of Vedic sacrificial mysticism.

48. *Svarga* ("heaven") or *svarga-loka* ("heavenly realm") is the domain of the deities and, as the *Bhagavadgītā* (see IX.20–21) states, of virtuous people who devote themselves to the Divine through forms of sacrifice *(yajña),* but who will nonetheless be reborn as soon as their merit *(puṇya)* is exhausted. One cannot rely on a heavenly state for attaining everlasting security free from the pain *(duḥkha)* of the saṃsāric world of change. "Heaven" should not be made equivalent to liberation itself. From the enlightened perspective, heaven is still implicated in saṃsāric existence.

49. See Radhakrishnan (1953), *The Principal Upaniṣads,* p. 764.

50. See *BĀ Up* III.4.1.

51. *BĀ Up* III.4.2 (p. 220).

52. See *BĀ Up* I.4.10 (p. 168): *aham brahmāsmi.*

53. See *YS* II.12–16.

54. See *BĀ Up* IV.4.22 (p. 279).

55. *BĀ Up* IV.4.13 (p. 276).

56. *BĀ Up* IV.4.20 (p. 278).

57. See *BĀ Up* II.4.12 (p. 200).

58. See, for example, *BĀ Up* II.3.6; III.9.26; IV.2.4; IV.4.2.

59. This method is used, for example, in *tāraka-yoga* dealt with in the *Advaya-Tāraka* ("Nondual Deliverer") *Up,* one of *the Yoga Upaniṣads.* This approach is also illustrated in the *Nirvāṇa-Ṣaṭka,* a well-known didactic poem ascribed to Śaṅkara, the great eighth–ninth century CE exponent of nondual (Advaita) Vedānta.

60. See *BĀ Up* III.8.9–11 (pp. 232–233).

61. *Chānd Up* III.17.4 (p. 396).

62. *Chānd Up* III.16.1 (p. 394): *puruṣo vāva yajñaḥ.*

63. R. E. Hume, trans. (1921), *The Thirteen Principal Upaniṣads,* pp. 272–273.

64. *Tait Up* II.4.1 (p. 545): *yoga ātmā.* Elsewhere, in another section of the *Tait Up* (III.10.2), the compound *yoga-kṣema* is used, meaning, according to Radhakrishnan, "acquisition" and "preservation" respectively. This suggests that the technical designation of the term Yoga had not yet attained preeminent status.

65. Alongside Hinduism and the philosophical and mystical insights of the Upaniṣadic sages, Jainism and Buddhism become major socioreligious movements in India. Founded by Vardhamāna Mahāvīra (sixth century BCE), an older contemporary of Gautama the Buddha, Jainism is a non-Vedic, dualistic system and shares common features with Yoga. Jainism excels in its rigorous observance of moral precepts, especially "nonharming"/"nonviolence" *(ahiṃsā).* This foundational ethical ideal, together with an extensive teaching about the moral force/intention *(karma)* inherent in human

behavior, has exerted a lasting influence on the tradition of Yoga. Also noteworthy is the Jaina soteriological doctrine termed *kevala* and the doctrine of the individual self or *jīva*. The liberated or released self is called *kevalin*. Later Jaina writers have articulated ideas and practices that are similar to Hindu forms of Yoga. For example, the esteemed scholar Haribhadra (eighth century CE) has utilized some of the codifications of Patañjali. Haribhadra's *Yogadṛṣṭisamuccaya* outlines four systems of eightfold Yoga where he lists Patañjali's *aṣṭāṅga-yoga* and goes on to align it with his own eightfold system. His "seed of Yoga" (*Yoga-Bindu* 367) states that the code of more advanced Yoga discipline is meditative practice. For more on Jaina Yoga, see G. Feuerstein (1975: 63-69) and (1989: 129-138). For a recent study that focuses on the doctrine of "nonviolence" *(ahiṃsā)* within an Indic (including a Jaina) context, see C. Chapple (1993), *Nonviolence to Animals, Earth, and Self in Asian Traditions*. For studies on Jainism see W. Schubring (1962), *The Doctrine of the Jainas;* and P. S. Jaini (1979), *The Jaina Path of Purification*. Gautama the Buddha (sixth century BCE), the founder of Buddhism, is referred to in the Pali canon as being devoted to meditation, and the later Sanskrit scriptures of Mahāyāna Buddhism often refer to him as a yogin. Sometimes understood as a pragmatic version of Yoga, his teaching is founded in a rejection of (Brāhmaṇic) metaphysical speculation, especially regarding the notion of an eternal Self *(ātman)*. The Buddha's noble eightfold path to liberation from suffering *(duḥkha)* emphasized practical discipline and direct experience to countermand the human tendency to theorize about spiritual life and reify it rather than to encounter it directly. For example, the eighth member of the noble eightfold path, termed *samyak-samādhi* ("right concentration"), consists of eight stages of meditative practices (known as *jhāna* in Pali and *dhyāna* in Sanskrit) for the purpose of transcending individuated consciousness and leading to enlightenment, or *nirvāṇa*. The contribution of Buddhism to the development of the tradition of Yoga has been considerable, just as the preceptors of Yoga have contributed over time to the unfolding of Buddhist teachings. There has been a long historical interplay between Buddhism and Hinduism that culminated in the movements of Tantrism, some schools of which are not easily identifiable as being either Buddhist or Hindu. The *Yoga-Sūtra* of Patañjali adopts a terminology at times close to Mahāyāna Buddhism. The important connections between classical Yoga and Buddhism have been noted by scholars though no rigorous detailed studies to my knowledge have hitherto been undertaken. Particularly the parallels between the *YS* and the *Abhisamayālaṅkāra* deserve closer examination; and the parallel use of some key terms in the *YS* and texts such as the *Laṅkāvatāra-Sūtra* and the *Madhyāntavibhāgabhāṣya*—both of the later texts associated with the Yogācāra Buddhist tradition—are worthy of more serious scrutiny. For more specialized studies related to the above, see: L. de la Vallée Poussin (1936-37), "Le Bouddhisme et le Yoga de Patañjali," *Mélanges chinois et bouddhiques,* pp. 223-242; and É Senart (1900), "Bouddhisme et Yoga," *Revue de l'Histoire des Religions,* vol. 42, Nov., pp. 345-364. For other studies on Yoga and Buddhism, see: M. Eliade (1969: 162-199); and G. Feuerstein (1975: 54-62) and (1989: 139-146). For other studies on Buddhism, see: T. Stcherbatsky (1923), *The Central Conception of Buddhism;* B. Sangharakshita (1980), *A Survey of Buddhism;* and Paul Williams (1989), *Mahāyāna Buddhism: The Doctrinal Foundations*. As stated in the Introduction, this study does not examine yogic paths and techniques within Jainism and Buddhism, nor is it concerned with an investigation into the influences of Jainism and Buddhism on Hindu Yoga and, in particular, the *YS* of Patañjali. A study along these lines would necessarily involve an analysis of material that, for lack of space, lies outside the scope of this present study. For a brief added look at a few of the parallels between Jainism and Buddhism in relation to Patañjali's Yoga, see n. 40 in chapter 2 of this study.

66. *Kaṭha Up* I.2.12 (p. 613).
67. *Kaṭha Up* I.2.23 (p. 619).
68. *Kaṭha Up* I.3.3-4 (pp. 623-624).
69. *Kaṭha Up* I.3.10-11 (p. 625).
70. *Kaṭha Up* II.3.11 (p. 645).
71. *Śvet Up* I.3 (p. 710).
72. *Śvet Up* I.11 (p. 716).
73. *Śvet Up* I.13-14 (p. 717).
74. *Śvet Up* III.8 (p. 727); cf. *ṚV* V.40.6 in n. 40 above and *BG* VIII.9.
75. See *Śvet Up* VI.21 (p. 749).
76. Although the *Mait Up* most likely belongs to the second century BCE, it undoubtedly contains passages that are considerably older.
77. *Mait Up* III.2 (p. 805).
78. *Mait Up* II.7 (p. 804).
79. *Mait Up* IV.4 (p. 811).
80. *Mait Up* IV.1 (p. 809).
81. *Mait Up* VI.18 (p. 830).
82. We note here the switching of concentration and meditation in this sequence and the citing of *tarka* (which is not a part of the eight-limbed scheme outlined by Patañjali). There is also the absence of any acknowledgment of ethical restraints *(yama)* and self-discipline/observances *(niyama),* which constitute the foundation of the eight-limbed Yoga *(aṣṭāṅga-yoga)* of Patañjali. However, this does not mean that moral guidelines were entirely neglected in the *Mait Up;* they were simply not formalized.
83. See Eliade (1969: 125) and Hauer (1958: 95-117).
84. Dasgupta (1922: 227).
85. *BG* III.4 (p. 133); see G. Feuerstein (1990), *Encyclopedic Dictionary of Yoga,* p. 232. For Sanskrit text of the *BG* consult page numbers given in S. Radhakrishnan (1948), *The Bhagavadgītā*; translations are mine.
86. *BG* II.48 (p. 120).
87. *BG* III.4 (p. 133).
88. *BG* III.6-7 (p. 134).
89. *BG* III.22 (p.140).
90. See, for example, *BG* III.25 and VI.18.
91. *BG* VI.29 (p. 203).
92. G. Feuerstein (1989: 160).
93. *BG* IV.17-18 (pp. 162-163).
94. *BG* IV.20 (p. 164).
95. *BG* IV.33 (p. 168).
96. In fact, all eighteen chapters of the *BG* can each be called a "different" Yoga. Although Yoga is not systematically outlined in the *BG,* it can be argued that the text aims for an integral philosophical approach.
97. *BG* IX.4-5 (pp. 238-239).
98. See *BG* XVIII.57-58 (p. 372).

99. *BG* XIII.34 (p. 313).
100. See *BG* II.71–72 (p. 129).
101. *BG* VI.15 (p. 198).
102. *BG* XVIII.54–55 (p. 371).
103. *BG* XV.18 (p. 332).
104. *BG* VI.31 (p. 204).
105. *BG* VI.47 (p. 211).

106. For example, the *Bhāgavata-Purāṇa* (ca. ninth to eleventh century CE) is the most important scripture of the *Bhāgavata* sect. Its philosophical foundations are by and large those of nondual Vedānta tempered by the conception and worship of the personal form of the Lord, as *Kṛṣṇa*. The *Bhāgavata-Purāṇa* is imbued with Yoga and Sāṃkhya teachings. All the elements of Patañjali's *aṣṭāṅga-yoga* ("eight-limbed Yoga") are present, yet the overall focus is on service and devotion to the personal God. Thus the main path advanced in this Purāṇa is clearly *bhakti-yoga*. This is contrasted with "Yoga," which likely refers to the "dualistic" approach usually assigned to classical Yoga. Of particular interest is the section in the *Bhāgavata-Purāṇa* known as the *Uddhāva-Gītā* (XI.6–29) where Kṛṣṇa expounds the Yoga of devotion *(bhakti)* to the sage Uddhāva. This section includes a discourse (XI.20.6–9) where the three approaches of *jñāna-yoga, karma-yoga,* and *bhakti-yoga* are distinguished. See J. M. Sanyal (1973). Also, a noteworthy exponent of Hindu *bhakti* is Rāmānuja (eleventh century CE), the founder of the Viśiṣṭādvaita school of Vedānta and the leading theologian and philosopher of the medieval *bhakti* movement. An enthusiastic proponent of Vaiṣṇavism, his gifted intellect and zeal made him the chief opponent of Śaṅkara's philosophy. For Rāmānuja, *bhakti* is not a state of profuse emotionalism but is one firmly rooted in wisdom *(jñāna)*. The highest devotee is a knower *(jñānin)* of the Lord. In his approach he sought to integrate *karma-yoga, jñāna-yoga,* and *bhakti-yoga,* but emphasizing union with the Lord ultimately through *bhakti;* see J. Lipner (1986), *The Face of Truth: A Study of Meaning and Metaphysics in the Vedāntic Theology of Rāmānuja;* and R. C. Lester (1976), *Rāmānuja on the Yoga.* The pure nondualist, Vallabha, and the ecstatic Kṛṣṇa Caitanya, both of roughly the fifteenth century CE, recommend *bhakti* as the principal means of liberation. Both were Vaiṣṇava preceptors and great *bhakti* yogins.

107. Franklin Edgerton, trans. (1965), *The Beginnings of Indian Philosophy,* p. 261.

108. Ibid., p. 262.

109. *MBh* XII.188.15 (p. 1058): *vicāraś ca vitarkaś ca vivekaś copajayate*. Sanskrit text is from S. K. Belvalkar, et al., eds., (1958), *The Mahābhārata,* Śāntiparvan 2 and 3, vol. 16. In Patañjali's terminology, the terms *vitarka* and *vicāra* can refer to stages of cognitive *samādhi* (i.e., *saṃprajñāta, YS* I.17), and *viveka* is discriminative knowledge that distinguishes between *puruṣa* (the seer) and *prakṛti* (the seeable). In a later section of the *MD* (XII.294.7–8) Vasiṣṭha instructs Janaka on the method of Yoga using key yogic terms such as *prāṇāyāma* (breath-control), *dhāraṇā* (concentration), and *ekāgratā* (one-pointedness of mind), all which are given more technically precise explanations in the *YS*. See Belvalkar (1951: 1631), and Edgerton (1965: 326 n. 1).

110. *MBh* XII.188.22; see Edgerton, trans. (1965: 262). An in-depth look at Yoga in the *MD* would necessarily involve a thorough and independent study in its own right.

111. Feuerstein (1974: 69).

112. This Yājñavalkya is not to be confused with the revered adept of the *BĀ Up* (eighth century BCE).

113. *YYS* I.43: *saṃyogo yoga ity ukto jīvātmāparamātmanoḥ*. Text from K. S. Śāstri, ed. (1938), *The Yogayājñavalkya,* p. 5. Probably a different Yājñavalkya authored the *Yājñavalkya-Smṛti,* a work on law and ethics *(dharma)* written around the first to third century CE. In one verse (I.8) this text notes that the highest teaching *(dharma)* is that which leads to the vision of the Self *(ātma-darśana)* by means of Yoga. This Yājñavalkya has also been credited with the authorship of the *YYS*. P. C. Divanji (1953, 1954), "The Yogayājñavalkya," mentions the period of 200–400 CE as a possible date for the *Yoga-Yājñavalkya*. Feuerstein (1989: 300) argues it is a later work, perhaps belonging to the twelfth century CE, or even later.

114. From *Tantric Texts,* A. Avalon, ed. (1929), *Mahānirvāṇa Tantra,* XIV.123 (p. 463): *yogo jīvātmanor aikyam*. The eleventh-century CE dating is given by Feuerstein (1989: 309).

115. Text from Feuerstein (1974: 70) *śivaśaktisamāyogaḥ yogaiva na samśayaḥ*; see also *Tantrasāra* by Abhinavagupta, Kashmir Series of Texts and Studies, no. 17, (1918), edited by M. S. Kaul.

116. See H. H. Wilson, trans. (1870), *The Vishnu Purana,* vol. 5, pp. 227–228. The *Viṣṇu-Purāṇa,* which deals with Yoga in its short sixth book, understands Yoga as the path of meditation *(dhyāna)*.

117. According to the *BG* (II.49), *buddhi-yoga* consists in one's taking refuge in the faculty of intelligence *(buddhi)* in order not to be impelled by the fruit of one's deeds. Later on in the *BG* (X.10) *buddhi-yoga* is said to be given by Lord Kṛṣṇa to those who worship Him with love. See also *BG* XVIII.57.

118. See *BG* IX.28 and *Muṇḍaka Up* III.2.6.

119. See *MBh* XII.188.1ff. where a fourfold meditation is taught, the goal of which is "extinction" *(nirvāṇa)*. The *BG* (XVIII.52) emphasizes that *dhyāna-yoga* must be cultivated in conjunction with dispassion *(vairāgya)*. See also chapter VI in the *BG,* entitled "Dhyāna-Yoga."

120. See the *Tri-Śikhi-Brāhmaṇa Up* (II.23), one of the *Yoga-Upaniṣads*, where *kriyā-yoga* is contrasted with *jñāna-yoga* and equated with *karma-yoga*. According to the *Bhāgavata-Purāṇa* (XI.27.49), *kriyā-yoga* can be either Vedic or tantric ritual practice. Both approaches lead to union with the Divine. In *YS* II.1 *kriyā-yoga* is said to be comprised of asceticism *(tapas),* study/personal recitation *(svādhyāya),* and devotion to *īśvara (īśvara-praṇidhāna)*. In modern times (twentieth century) *kriyā-yoga* was taught by Paramahansa Yogananda as a form of *rāja-yoga*.

121. *Nāda-yoga* is a prominent teaching in the *Yoga-Upaniṣads*. It is indirectly referred to earlier in the *Maitrāyaṇīya Up* (VI.22), where we are told of those who listen to the sound *(śabda)* inside the heart by placing the thumb against the ears. According to Bhartṛhari (ca. sixth century CE), the highest form of being is the soundless Word *(vāc),* which is imbued with the power *(śakti)* to burst forth *(sphuṭ)* into creative expression. The "bursting forth" of the Word *(sphoṭa),* also called *Śabda-Brahman* or Word-*Brahman,* is the immanent ground of all manifestation, including all things and all meaning, down to the grossest forms and is an idea which may be derived from the Upaniṣads (see *BĀ Up* IV.1.2 and *Mait Up* VI.22—see above).

122. *YB* I.1 (p. 1): *yogaḥ samādhiḥ*. The Sanskrit text of the *YS,* the *YB* of Vyāsa, the *Tattva-Vaiśāradī* of Vācaspati Miśra, and the *Rāja-Mārtaṇḍa* of Bhoja Rāja is from *The Yoga-Sūtra of Patañjali* (1904), K. S. Āgāśe ed.

123. An in-depth analysis of the term *samādhi* in classical Yoga is given later in chapters 4–6.

124. Eliade (1969: 77); cf. Feuerstein (1989: 11).
125. Feuerstein (1979a: 26).
126. M. Müller (1899: 309).
127. *RM* I.1 (p. 1): *puṃ prakṛtyor viyogo'pi yoga.*
128. See P. T. Raju (1985), *Structural Depths of Indian Thought,* p. 344.
129. *BG* II.50 (p. 120): *yogaḥ karmasu kauśalam.*
130. *BG* II.53 (p. 122): *śrutivipratipannā te, yadā sthāsyati niścalā; samādhāv acalā buddhis, tadā yogam avāpsyasi.*
131. *TV* I.1 (p. 2): *"yuja samādhau" ity asmād vyutpannaḥ samādhy artho na tu "yujir yoge" ity asmāt saṃyogārtha ity arthaḥ.*
132. See n. 29 above.
133. Examples of this usage include: *ṚV* I.82.6; *Kauṣītaki Up* II.6; *Kena Up* I.1; *BĀ Up* V.13.2.
134. It is unlikely, as I go on to state in chapter 2, that the Patañjali who authored the *Mahābhāṣya* is the same Patañjali who is credited for writing the *YS*. It remains, however, an unresolved issue.
135. As this study attempts to do in later chapters (esp. 4–6).
136. See Mādhavācārya (1882), *The Sarva-Darśana Saṃgraha,* pp. 242–243.
137. Ibid., p. 243.
138. U. Arya (1986: 75). In his study (1979b) entitled, *The Yoga-Sūtra of Patañjali: An Exercise in the Methodology of Textual Analysis,* Feuerstein (p. 28) mentions the interesting hypothesis, initially put forward by K. B. R. Rao (1966: 375), that Vyāsa (cf. *YB* II.19) subscribed to the so-called *eka-uttara* ("increasing by one") theory. He writes (ibid.), "This is an ontogenetic model operating on the principle of progressive inclusion."
139. Mādhavācārya (1882: 243).
140. See Sanskrit text of *YSS* in G. Jha, trans. (1894), *The Yogasāra-Saṃgraha of Vijñāna Bhikṣu,* p. 22 reads: *ārurukṣuyuñjamānayogārūḍhapāḥ.*
141. *BG* VI.3 (p. 188).
142. *BG* VI.4 (p. 188).
143. *BG* VI.18 (p. 199).
144. *BG* II.56 (p. 123).
145. *YB* III.51 (p. 169): *catvāraḥ khalvamī yoginaḥ prāthamakalpiko madhubhūmikaḥ, prajñājyotir, atikrāntabhāvanīyaś ceti.*
146. See *YS* II.27 (p. 97): *tasya saptadhā prāntabhūmiḥ prajñā.*
147. *YB* III.51 (p. 169): *tatrābhyāsī pravṛttam ātrajyotiḥ prathamaḥ. ṛtaṃbharāprajño dvitīyaḥ. bhūtendriyajayī tṛtīyaḥ sarveṣu bhāviteṣu bhāvanīyeṣu kṛtarakṣābandhaḥ kartavya sādhanādimān. caturtho yas tv atikrāntabhāvanīyastasya cittapratisarga eko'rthaḥ, sapta vidhāsya prāntabhūmiprajñā.* Also worthy of mention is the later (ca. 1800 CE) *Śiva-Saṃhitā* (V.10–14), one of the principal manuals of *haṭha-yoga,* which distinguishes four types of students depending on the practitioner's commitment to spiritual life:

1. The weak or mild *(mṛdu)* practitioner, who is unenthusiastic, fickle, timid, unenergetic, etc., and is fit for *mantra-yoga;*
2. The moderate *(madhya)* practitioner, who is endowed with evenmindedness, patience, a desire for virtue, kind speech, etc., and is fit for *laya-yoga;*
3. The exceptional *(adhimātra)* practitioner, who demonstrates firm understanding, self-reliance, bravery, vigor, faithfulness, delight in Yoga practice, etc., and is capable of practicing *haṭha-yoga;*

4. The extraordinary (*adhimātratama*) yogin, who displays energy, enthusiasm, charm, heroism, fearlessness, purity, skilfulness, surrender to the teacher, control over the senses, etc., and is fit to practice all types of Yoga—referring here to *rāja-yoga* (V.9).

See B. D. Basu, ed. (1914), *The Yoga Śāstra: Śiva Saṃhitā*, in *The Sacred Books of the Hindus,* vol. 15, pp. 54-56.

148. *YB* I.20 (p. 24): *te khalu nava yogino mṛdumadhyādhimātropāyā bhavanti, tad yathā mṛdūpāyo, madhyopāyo'dhimātropāya iti. tatra mṛdūpāyas trividhaḥ mṛdusaṃvego, madhyasaṃ vegas tīvrasaṃvega iti. tathā madhyopāyas tathādhimātropāyā iti.* "Yogins are of nine kinds, according to the methods which they follow, either mild or moderate or ardent, and then sub-divided according to the energy—mild, moderate or ardent—with which they practise their respective methods. A mild method may be practiced with mild or moderate or ardent energy and likewise with the moderate method and likewise with the intense." Thus the nine kinds of yogins are those of: (i) mild method with mild energy or intensity; (ii) mild method with moderate energy or intensity; (iii) mild method with ardent energy or intensity; (iv) moderate method with mild energy or intensity; (v) moderate method with moderate energy or intensity; (vi) moderate method with ardent energy or intensity; (vii) ardent method with mild energy or intensity; (viii) ardent method with moderate energy or intensity; (ix) ardent method with ardent energy and intensity.

149. *TV* I.21 (p. 24): *mṛdumadhyādhimātrāḥ prāgbhavīya saṃskārādṛṣṭa vaśādy eṣāṃ te tathoktāḥ.*

150. As will be discussed in chapter 3; cf. *YS* II.12-13 and IV.8.

151. *YS* I.21 (p. 24): *tīvrasaṃvegānām āsannaḥ.*

152. *YB* I.21 (p. 24): *samādhilābhaḥ samādhiphalaṃ ca bhavati.*

153. *TV* I.21 (p. 24): *samādheḥ saṃprajñātasya phalam asaṃprajñātatas tasyāpi kaivalyam.*

154. *YS* I.22 (p. 25): *mṛdumadhyādhimātratvāt tato'pi viśeṣaḥ.* It appears that the *YS* can be seen to yield, at the most, a ninefold classification of yogins.

155. Cf. Feuerstein (1979a: 41).

156. M. Eliade (1969: 5).

157. *Śiva Purāṇa* VII.2.15, 38.

158. Eliade (1969: 5). See also Feuerstein (1989: 20).

159. *BG* IV.34 (p. 169).

160. Joel D. Mlecko (1982), "The Guru in Hindu Tradition," in *NUMEN,* vol. 29, fasc. 1, July, p. 34.

161. See *Śiva-Saṃhitā* (1914) p. 25: *bhavedvīr yavatī vidyā guruvaktra samud bhavā, anyathā phalahīnā syānnir viryāpyati duḥkhadā.*

162. The word *dīkṣā* and its underlying concept goes back to the *Atharva Veda* II.5.3.

163. R. K. Mookerji, ed. (1951), *Ancient Indian Education,* pp. 214-215.

164. Lama A. Govinda (1972), *The Way of the White Clouds,* p. 3.

165. G. Feuerstein (1984), "Worshipping the Guru's Feet," *The Laughing Man,* vol. 4, no. 4, p. 11.

166. See Feuerstein (1989: 27). On *dīkṣā*, see the important medieval Hindu tantric work, the *Kulārṇava Tantra* (X.1 and XIV.39).

167. *ṚV* IV.7.6.

168. *Yajur Veda* VII.27.
169. Mookerji (1951: xxvi).
170. *Tait Up* I.3.3 (p. 529).
171. *Chānd Up* IV.4.3.
172. *Kaṭha Up* I.2.8 (p. 610). The teacher-disciple context in India as well as elsewhere can have its negative or perverted side: see the *Maitrāyaṇīya Up* VII.8 ff. (pp. 854–855), which warns against false teachers who merely deceive the naïve.
173. See Monier-Williams (1899: 201).
174. See, for example, *BĀ Up* IV.5.15 (p. 286); see also n. 58 above.
175. See *Tait Up* III.1–6 (pp. 553–558).
176. See *Chānd Up* VI.12.3 and VI.13.3 (p. 463). In VI.12, it is stated that the invisible essence that maintains the life of the Nyagrodha tree, indeed the whole world, is the same as the essence of our human identity. The one who *knows* this essence, *is* this essence. The discussion that then ensues (VI.14.1–2) elaborates on the spiritual aspirant's need for a teacher in order to reach the perfected state of liberation.
177. Mookerji (1951: 114).
178. Shashibhusan Dasgupta (1962), *Obscure Religious Cults,* p. 88.
179. See M. P. Pandit (1965), *The Kulārṇava Tantra,* pp. 98–99.
180. See Mlecko (1982: 45).
181. Dasgupta (1962: 88).
182. The *Advaya-Tāraka Up* (16) gives an esoteric explanation of the word *guru,* deriving it from the syllable *gu,* indicating "darkness," and *ru,* indicating "dispeller." Thus, the *guru* is one who dispels the disciple's spiritual ignorance. See A. Mahadeva Sastri, ed. (1920), *The Yoga Upaniṣads, with the Commentary of Sri Brahma-Yogin,* p. 9. The *Advaya-Tāraka Up* (16 and 17) states: *guśabdas tv andhakāraḥ syāt ruśabdas tannirodhakaḥ, andhakāranirodhitvāt gurur ity abhidhīyate. gurur eva paraṃ brahma gurur eva parā gatiḥ, gurur eva parā vidyā gurur eva parāyaṇam.* "The syllable *gu* [signifies] darkness; the syllable *ru* [signifies] the destroyer of that [darkness]. By reason of [the power] to destroy darkness, one is called *guru.* The *guru* alone is the supreme God. The *guru* alone is the supreme path. The *guru* alone is the supreme knowledge. The *guru* alone is the supreme resort."
183. See n. 65 above.
184. Feuerstein (1989: 38). Feuerstein's book (ibid.) entitled, *Yoga: The Technology of Ecstasy,* has already attempted this kind of in-depth survey of the history, literature, and branches of Yoga with varying degrees of success. To illustrate his point of yogic paths occasionally having incompatible goals, Feuerstein contrasts the ideal of *rāja-yoga,* which he states (p. 38) "is to recover one's true Identity as the transcendental Self standing eternally apart from the realm of Nature," with the ideal of *haṭha-yoga,* which he adds (ibid.) "is to create an immortal body." *Rāja-yoga* most commonly refers to Patañjali's Yoga system. As I go on to suggest, the radically dualistic understanding of the *YS* does not do justice to the integrity of Patañjali's Yoga.

CHAPTER 2. THE *YOGA-SŪTRA*

1. Francis Humphreys (1981), Review: Georg Feuerstein (1980), *The Philosophy of Classical Yoga,* in *BSOAS,* vol. 44, part 2, pp. 393–394.

2. K. S. Joshi (1965: 53).

3. The *YS* belongs to the authoritative traditional or "remembered" *(smṛti)* literature within Hinduism and thus is not considered to be a "revealed" *(śruti)* or primary scripture. Yoga is mentioned in the writings of other Brāhmaṇic schools, for example, in the *Vaiśeṣika-Sūtra*s of Kaṇāda (V.2.17) and the *Nyāya-Sūtra*s of Akṣapāda (IV.2.46). Bādarāyaṇa's refutation of Yoga in the *Brahma-Sūtra*s (II.1.3) may have been intended for Patañjali's Yoga although this is uncertain. There are evaluations and critiques of Yoga thought and practice in different schools within Vedānta such as in the writings of Śaṅkara (ca. 800 CE), the great Advaita Vedāntin (see also below), as well as in the writings of Rāmānuja (eleventh century CE), the founder of Viśiṣṭhādvaita Vedānta. The oldest available commentary on the *YS* is the *Yoga-Bhāṣya* ("Discussion on Yoga") or *Vyāsa-Bhāṣya* by Vyāsa. It was composed around the fifth–sixth centuries CE and is the basis for all subsequent exegetical efforts in classical Yoga. Vyāsa is often alleged to be the same person who compiled the *MBh,* together with the *BG,* the vast Purāṇa literature as well as other works. This idea, however, does not appear to have any basis in reality given the development of ideas and *śāstra* expressions found in the *YB*. Both Frauwallner (1953: 482) and Chakravarti (1951: 138ff.) suggest that the author of the *YB* is indebted to the work of the Sāṃkhyan revisor, Vindhyavāsin (see n. 73 below). In an unpublished paper (1995) entitled "Yoga, Vyākaraṇa and the Chronology and Works of Some Early Authors" (cited with permission), A. Aklujkar has outlined several arguments that tend to attribute the authorship of the *YB* to Vindhyavāsin himself. The name Vyāsa means "collector" and here may refer more generically to a title rather than to a personal name. Unfortunately, as is the case with Patañjali, we know very little about Vyāsa. Vyāsa, the commentator on the *YS,* was in all likelihood a highly advanced yogin (cf. J. W. Hauer, 1958) since he wrote with great authority on esoteric matters pertaining to yogic discipline. Vyāsa's *Bhāṣya (YB)* plays a crucial part in our interpretation of Patañjali's thought and enlightens our understanding of the *YS.* Vācaspati Miśra's *Tattva-Vaiśāradī* ("Clarity on the Categories [of Existence]"), a *ṭīkā* (a gloss or commentary on a commentary) on the *YB,* is considered by some to be the most important work after Vyāsa. In addition to the *TV,* Vācaspati (ninth century CE) wrote outstanding commentaries on, for example, Sāṃkhya, Nyāya, and the Vedānta systems. He did not attempt to establish a philosophical system of his own (although he was a Vedāntin) and was content to attempt a lucid explanation of whichever text or philosophical system he was writing on. His knowledge often appears theoretical rather than practical and in the *TV* he tends to expand on philological and epistemological issues at the expense of more practical deliberation. His commentary on Vyāsa is arguably the most helpful one. *Rāja-Mārtaṇḍa* ("The Royal Sun"), also known as *Bhoja-Vṛtti,* is by the eleventh century CE king, Bhoja Rāja. He was an accomplished poet as well as being a patron of the arts, sciences, and spiritual traditions. Bhoja's commentary is on Patañjali and is almost totally independent, although it incorporates some of the *YB*. It is a work, as a *vṛtti* is intended to be (note here that the term *vṛtti* is being used in a different sense from its technical usage in the *YS*), with only brief argumentation here and there. From the fourteenth century CE there exists an admirable systematic account of classical Yoga in Mādhavācārya's *Sarva-Darśana Saṃgraha.* In the sixteenth or seventeenth century CE Rāmānanda Yati wrote *Maṇi-Prabhā* ("Jewel Lustre"), a brief *ṭīkā* on Vyāsa. Also in the sixteenth century Vijñāna Bhikṣu authored an elaborate commentary called *Yoga-Vārttika* ("Exposition on

Yoga"), considered by some to be the second most important commentary on Vyāsa. Bhikṣu also wrote the *Yogasāra-Saṃgraha* summarizing his interpretation of Patañjali's philosophy. Vijñāna Bhikṣu was a renowned scholar and yogin who interpreted Yoga from a Vedāntic point of view. One of his main contributions is his attempt to establish points of unity between the dualistic perspective of Sāṃkhya and theistic/nondualistic thought in Vedānta, and some of his comments also provide valuable insights into the experiential dimension of Yoga itself. We can also mention *Pradīpikā* ("That Which Sheds Light")—the work (i.e., *vṛtti*) by Vijñāna Bhikṣu's disciple Bhāvāgaṇeśa, and Nāgojī Bhaṭṭa's works *(vṛttis): Laghvī* and *Bṛhatī.* Both of the above authors (sixteenth and eighteenth centuries respectively), for the most part, echo Vijñāna Bhikṣu. Nārāyaṇa Tīrtha's seventeenth or eighteenth century *Bhāṣya* entitled, *Yoga-Siddhānta-Candrikā* ("Moonlight on the Tenets of Yoga"), and *Sūtrārtha-Bodhinī* ("Illumination of the Meaning of the *Sūtras*")—a *vṛtti*—are two works not dependent on Vyāsa. Nārāyaṇa Tīrtha writes from a Vedāntic point of view and especially draws upon the discipline of devotion *(bhakti)* in his interpretation. Other writings that can be noted are Rāghavānanda Sarasvatī's *Pātañjala-Rahasya* ("The Secret of Patañjali's System"), a subcommentary *(upa-ṭīkā)* of uncertain but recent date on Vācaspati's work, and Sadāśivendra Sarasvatī's (eighteenth century) *Yoga-Sudhā-Ākāra* ("Mine of Ambrosia"). Ananta-deva Pandit's (nineteenth century) *Padacandrikā* ("Moonlight on Words"), for the most part, scans the *RM* of Bhoja Rāja. Baladeva Miśra's *Yoga-Pradīpikā* is a twentieth-century work summarizing Vācaspati's work. Also from the twentieth century is Hariharānanda Āraṇya's *Bhāsvatī* ("Elucidation") as well as his (1963) *Yoga Philosophy of Patañjali.* Āraṇya was a Sanskrit scholar and a practitioner of Sāṃkhya-Yoga. It is probable that many ancient commentaries have been lost to arson by Muslim conquerors as well as having disappeared due to the discontinuity of a line of teachers and neglect by owners. One example of a lost commentary is that of a versified version (eleventh century) from which al-Bīrūnī, the famous Persian traveler, translated into Arabic; on this see S. Pines and T. Gelblum (1966, 1977). There are a number of other, lesser-known works, known by name only. On the whole, these secondary commentaries do not excel in originality, relying largely on Vyāsa. With some exceptions, the secondary literature on classical Yoga can tend to be dry and repetitive, which underlines the notion that Yoga, in its authentic context, has always been an esoteric discipline taught mainly through oral instruction. It is not a tradition of bookish speculation or mere "book learning" (Feuerstein, 1989: 176). Throughout this study I have incorporated an analysis, sometimes critical, of the most important Sanskrit literature on Patañjali and Vyāsa including works by Vācaspati Miśra, Vijñāna Bhikṣu, Bhoja Rāja, H. Āraṇya, and others who have contributed to the exegetical tradition of classical Yoga. Many of the secondary works do not appear to have come out of Patañjali's school itself, and therefore their expositions need to be examined with a good measure of discernment. There is also the very detailed commentary attributed to Śaṅkara (ca. 800 CE), the great exponent of Advaita Vedānta. The *Yogasūtrabhāṣyavivaraṇa* (= *YSBhV*) ("An Exposition on the Commentary [of Vyāsa] on the *Yoga-Sūtra*"), which is more properly called *Pātañjalayogaśāstravivaraṇa,* is a work explaining the *YB* and is not so overly Vedāntic as to obscure the Sāṃkhyan tenets. Trevor Leggett (1990), in the "Technical Introduction" to his useful translation of the *Vivaraṇa* entitled, *The Complete Commentary by Śaṅkara on the Yoga Sūtra-s,* pp. 17–18, supports the view that the *Vivaraṇa* is a genuine work of Śaṅkara as do P. S. Rama Sastri and S. R. Krishnamurti Sastri, the editors of the *YSBhV* which was published in 1952 as volume 94 of the Madras Government Oriental Series. Leggett subscribes to the text's authenticity, although he admits that the matter is still open. Studies/comments by P. Hacker, H. Nakamura, S. Mayeda, and T. Vetter represent part of a growing consensus among scholars that tends to accept the *YSBhV* as Śaṅkara's own work. However, any efforts to prove that it is a work of the first Śaṅkarācārya are on the whole unconvincing, especially regarding matters of style and ideology (on this see, for example, see G. Larson's comments in 1987: 626). There is presently nothing in the evidence that would prevent one from arguing that the author of the *Vivaraṇa* was one of Śaṅkara's later followers thereby implying that the text may be somewhat later than the time of Śaṅkara. Gopinath Kaviraj has argued (see [as cited by Larson, ibid.] "Literary Gleanings, Jayamaṅgalā," *Quarterly Journal of the Andhra Historical Research,* Oct. 1927, pp. 133-136) that the *Vivaraṇa* is a fourteenth-century work by a certain Śaṅkarācārya. In his article entitled, "Philological Observations on the So-Called Pātañjalayogasūtrabhāṣyavivaraṇa" (*Indo-Iranian Journal* 25 [1983]: 17-40), A. Wezler stipulates that the question of authorship of the *Vivaraṇa* remains unanswered for the time being. W. Halbfass (1991: 205-242) offers a scholarly analysis and critical assessment dealing with the unsettled issue of the *Vivaraṇa*'s authorship, including its philological status, historical role, and philosophical position. In a recent article (1992), T. S. Rukmani (see "The Problem of the Authorship of the *Yogasūtrabhāṣyavivaraṇa,*" *JIP* 20: 419-423) outlines several noteworthy reasons to question Śaṅkarācārya's authorship of the *YSBhV*. Doubts about the text's provenance and its heavy reliance on (i.e., it is a subcommentary to the exposition of Patañjali by Vyāsa), yet uncommon exegetical independence from the classical Yoga school have, for the purpose of this study, precluded my taking further notice of it. In this study, as the reader will see, I have been directly guided by Vyāsa's own work.

4. See R. Garbe (1894), *Sāṃkhya and Yoga;* see also R. Garbe (1922), "Yoga," in *Encyclopedia of Religion and Ethics,* vol. 12, pp. 831-833.

5. See Dasgupta (1922), *A History of Indian Philosophy,* vol. 1, pp. 231-233.

6. See *RM* (p. 1) in "Introduction" (stanza 5).

7. T. S. Rukmani (1981), *Yogavārttika of Vijñāna Bhikṣu, Samādhipāda,* p. 3.

8. As Eliade mentions (1969: 9).

9. Jacobi (1929), "Über das ursprüngliche Yoga-System," pp. 583-584; see also H. Jacobi (1911), "The Dates of the Philosophical Sūtras of the Brahmans," *JAOS* 31: 26; and J. Prasad (1930), "The Date of the *Yoga-sūtras,*" *JRAS* 84: 365-375.

10. Keith (1949), *Sāṃkhya System,* pp. 69-70.

11. See J. H. Woods, trans. (1914), *The Yoga-System of Patañjali,* pp. xvii-xx. The evidence so painstakingly collected by Woods and the arguments advanced by him fix the date of the *YS* somewhere between 300 and 500 CE. All the evidence Woods has collected, and various arguments he uses to narrow down the date of the *YS* to somewhere between 400 and 500 CE, seem more relevant for fixing the date of the *Bhāṣya* of Vyāsa. Both Jacobi and Woods dispute the common authorship of the *Mahābhāṣya* and the *YS* mainly on the basis of internal evidence. Jacobi (1911: 26) points out that there is no corresponding tradition among the grammarians regarding this common authorship. Woods (1914: xv-xvii) argues that in regard to philosophical terms and concepts there is no real accord between the two to support their common authorship. There are very wide differences of terminology that cannot be accounted for as being

merely due to differences in subject matter. For a summary of some of the above as well as other views, see M. Eliade (1969: 370–372).

12. See Hauer (1958), *Der Yoga,* p. 233.

13. See E. Frauwallner (1953), *Geschichte der indischen Philosophie,* 1, p. 285.

14. See H. von Glassenapp (1958), *Die Philosophie der Inder,* pp. 221–222.

15. See M. Winternitz (1967), *History of Indian Literature,* vol. 3, part 2, p. 517.

16. See G. J. Larson and R. S. Bhattacharya, eds. (1987), *Sāṃkhya: A Dualist Tradition in Indian Philosophy,* p. 15.

17. Feuerstein states (1979a: 3) that the *YS* is a product of the third century CE, although in a later work (1989, p. 169) he suggests the second century CE as a probable date.

18. Cf. Christopher K. Chapple (1994), "Reading Patañjali without Vyāsa: A Critique of Four *Yoga Sūtra* Passages," *JAAR* 62.1: 85. Chapple suggests in the above article that the *YS* was composed in the first or second century CE.

19. See Feuerstein (1989: 169).

20. Feuerstein (1979a: 3).

21. H. Āraṇya (1869–1947), author of a Sanskrit commentary (see n. 3 above) on the *YS,* claimed that his teacher, Svāmī Trilokī Āraṇya, was one of the distinguished teachers in the line of Yoga *guru*s established by Patañjali.

22. Feuerstein (1989: 170–171). Some of the arguments against Buddhist doctrine put forward by the classical Yoga school will be mentioned from time to time in this study.

23. See R. K. Mookerjie (1951: 258–325) for an analysis of education as conceived in the philosophical *sūtra* literature in Hinduism.

24. See n. 3 above.

25. Some earlier scholars who have questioned the unity of the *YS* are Paul Deussen (1920), S. Dasgupta (1922), and Otto Strauss (1925). More recently, Feuerstein (1979b, see n. 26 below) concedes to this problem also raised by Hauer (1958).

26. P. Deussen (1920: 1:510) tentatively suggested the following divisions: Text A: I.1–I.16; Text B: I.17–I.51; Text C: II.1–II.27; Text D: II.28–III.55; Text E: IV.1–IV.33. (According to most editions there are 34 *sūtra*s in chapter 4.) J. W. Hauer (1958: 221–230) investigated and restated Deussen's conclusions, discerning five texts, four of which he thinks reflect distinct schools of yogic practice, with the fifth as a late polemical accretion. The five texts according to Hauer are: (1) the *nirodha*-text (*YS* I.1–I.22) stressing dispassion/detachment *(vairāgya)* and practice *(abhyāsa)* necessary for "cessation" *(nirodha),* with the obstacles to these methods termed *'vṛttis'* (mental modifications); (2) the *īśvarapraṇidhāna*-text ("devotion to the Lord"), its method (I.23–I.51) and its corresponding obstacles *(antarāyas);* (3) the *kriyāyoga*-text (II.1–II.27) proposed to overcome the *kleśa*s (afflictions); (4) the *yogāṅga*s-text (II.28–III.55) which begins with the unwholesome "discursive thoughts" (*vitarka*s) and the cultivation of their opposites; and (5) *nirmāṇa-citta*-text (IV.1–IV.34) or "individualized/fabricated mind." The texts, he says, were edited into one piece, though he provides no clear motive for the editor's eclecticism. Frauwallner (1973: 344–345) differentiates between the *nirodha* form of Yoga described in the *Samādhi-Pāda* and the eight-limbed Yoga *(aṣṭāṅga-yoga)* of the *Sādhana-Pāda,* i.e., the former is perceived as taking a more negative approach calling for the suppression of "every mental activity" while the latter "seeks to raise the capac-

ity for knowledge to the highest." S. Dasgupta, while concluding that the first three *pādas* of the text were written early (the last chapter being a later addition), nevertheless asserts that the *YS* is "a masterly and systematic compilation" (1922: 229). Feuerstein (1979b: 37–104) argues that the *YS* could well be a composite of two distinct Yoga traditions. On the one hand there is the Yoga of action *(kriyā-yoga)* text running from *YS* I.1 to II.27 and again from III.3 or 4 to IV.34; and on the other hand, interrupting the above text, there is the eight-limbed Yoga text *(aṣṭāṅga-yoga)* extending from *YS* II.28 to III.2 or 3 and including *sūtra* III.55 (see n. 31 below).

27. G. Feuerstein (1989: 172).

28. C. Pensa, foreword to, *The Philosophy of Classical Yoga,* by G. Feuerstein (1980: vii).

29. Tola and Dragonetti (1987: xii) take a similar approach and consider Patañjali to be the author of the entire text of the *YS.*

30. See C. Chapple (1994) who is, as well, sensitive to these issues.

31. M. Eliade (1969) finds the unity of the *YS* to derive from mystical foundations, reading the work as the record of an extraordinary experience presumed to result from yogic experience. In a later work (1975: 14) he concedes that the text "may have been revised by many hands, to adapt it to new 'philosophical situations'." But despite the concession of possible recasting, Eliade's reading is highly unitary. He believes that the *YS* reflects a long tradition of reconfirmed yogic experience, whether or not a single person is its author. Adolf Janácek provides good reasons to question each of Hauer's arguments for dissecting the text. He claims (1959: 474) that the unity of the work lies in the fact that all the various practices advocated have a common purpose, which is "[to break] the links fettering together the subject and the object." Janácek (1951, 1954, 1957, 1958, and 1959) took pains to arrive at the recognition that the practices advocated in the *YS* all belong to a "voluntarist type of yoga," despite the many differences among them (1954, p. 82). Following from his suggestion that the *YS* could well be a composite of two distinct Yoga traditions (see note 26 above), Feuerstein then advances that the section dealing with *aṣṭāṅga-yoga* is quoted in the main body of the *YS* and is not a later interpolation as some scholars have submitted. If this were the case, "the widespread equation of Classical Yoga with the eightfold path would be a historical curiosity, since the bulk of the *Yoga-Sūtra* deals with kriyā-yoga" (Feuerstein, 1989: 329 n. 2). Yet Feuerstein cautions against his own (above) approach adding that "textual reconstructions of this kind are always tentative, and we must keep an open mind about this as about so many other aspects of Yoga and Yoga history" (ibid.). In an earlier work focusing on methodological issues, Feuerstein (1979b: 36–89) rightly draws attention to terminological repetitions along with uniformities of conception in all four chapters of the *YS* and makes a convincing case for a single author. As Feuerstein points out (1989: 329 n. 2), "[t]he advantage of this kind of methodological approach to the study of the *Yoga-Sūtra,* which presumes the text's homogeneity . . . is that it does not violate the work substantially, as is the case with those textual analyses that set out to prove that it is in fact corrupt or composed of fragments and interpolations." Based on their reading of the *YS* as outlined in the discussion of Patañjali's central theme being that of "subtilization," Chapple and Kelly (1990: 4–9) argue for a continuity throughout the text later noting that (p. 13) "it is clear from purely internal evidence that the text involves the overlay and interweaving of various yogic traditions

which became harmonized not by consistency but through their joint appearance through Patañjali."

32. For example, *YS* I.12-16 discuss practice *(abhyāsa)* and dispassion *(vairāgya); YS* I.20 deals with the application of faith *(śraddhā),* energy *(vīrya),* mindfulness *(smṛti),* ecstasy *(samādhi),* and insight (prajñā); YS I.23-32 and II.1, 32, and 45 make explicit the practice of devotion to *īśvara; YS* I.33 states appropriate attitudes and behavior in interpersonal relationships; *YS* I.34 and II.49-53 explain techniques of control over the breath *(prāṇāyāma); YS* I.35 speaks about steadying the mind in activity and I.36 instructs one to cultivate thoughts that are sorrowless and illuminating. There are many other forms of practice including the eight limbs of *Yoga (aṣṭāṅga-yoga)* in the second *pāda,* which will be discussed later on in this study.

33. See Chapple and Kelly (1990: 10-11).

34. Erich Frauwallner (1973: 335).

35. Chapple and Kelly (1990: 14).

36. *YS* I.1-4 (pp. 1, 4, and 7): *atha yogānuśāsanam; yogaś cittavṛttinirodhaḥ; tadā draṣṭuḥ svarūpe'vasthānam; vṛttisārūpyamitaratra.* The translation of *nirodha* as "cessation" is ambiguous and needs clarification. As I argue in chapter 4, it would be erroneous or misleading to understand "cessation" as being the definitive cessation of the existence of *vṛtti*s, i.e., the ontological cessation of *vṛtti*s. In *YS* I.2 *nirodha* refers to the cessation of the empirical effects of *vṛtti*s in the form of spiritual ignorance *(avidyā),* i.e., is an epistemological cessation of *vṛtti*s.

37. S. N. Dasgupta (1922: 229).

38. Ibid.

39. Eliade states (1969: 9), "they are not his discoveries, nor those of his time; they had been tested many centuries before him." He goes on to say that Patañjali's "sole aim is to compile a practical manual of very ancient techniques."

40. A number of scholars including Senart, Lindquist, la Vallée Poussin, Keith, and Eliade have pointed out parallels between Buddhist Yoga and Patañjali's Yoga. The presence of a wide-ranging network of Buddhist terminology in the *YS* shows, as Chapple argues (1990: 12), that Patañjali no doubt included yogic practices from Buddhist manuals—without acknowledging the Buddhist parallels—by incorporating, for example: the five practices given in *YS* I.20 of *śraddhā, vīrya, smṛti, samādhi* and *prajñā;* and the *brahmavihāra*s, outlined in *YS* I.33 *(maitrī, karuṇā, muditā, upekṣa),* and widely applied within Buddhism. There are also similarities between the *samādhi*s listed by Patañjali and the four *dhyāna*s in Buddhism as well as Patañjali's reference to seven *prajñā*s in *YS* II.27. The term *pariśuddha* ("complete purification"), used in *YS* I.43 (see notes 127 and 128 in chapter 5), corresponds to the fourth state of meditation listed in the *Dīgha Nikāya,* an important Buddhist text. The *Laṅkāvatāra Sūtra,* more or less contemporaneous with the *YS,* uses the metaphor of a clear jewel (cf. *YS* I.41) to describe the elevated state of the *bodhisattva* (II.8). See D. T. Suzuki (1932), *Laṅkāvatāra Sūtra.* (London: George Routledge and Sons). Buddhism tends to avoid positive statements such as the recognized notions within Hinduism of seer *(draṣṭṛ),* grasper *(grahītṛ),* or Self *(ātman, puruṣa).* Turning to epistemology, in the analysis of perception there is an interesting similarity between Yogācāra Buddhism and Patañjali's Yoga. In both, the separation between "grasper" and "grasping" must be overcome resulting in a transcendence or dissolution of the bifurcation between subject and object

(cf. *YS* I.41 and *Laṅkāvatāra Sūtra* IV.80, 213, and 215). For more on the parallels between Buddhism and Patañjali's Yoga, see Émile Senart (1900: 345–364), and L. de la Vallée Poussin (1936–37: 223–242). The relationship between Jainism and the *YS*, which is less explored by scholars, is certainly worthy of much more consideration. On this, C. Chapple (1990: 12) writes, "Three teachings closely associated with Jainism appear in Yoga: the doctrine of *karma,* the *telos* of isolation (*kevala* in Jainism, *kaivalyam* in Yoga), and the practice of nonviolence *(ahiṃsā).* In fact, the entire list of the five *yama*s (II.30) is identical with the ethical precepts taught by Mahāvira, the contemporary of the Buddha who established the foundations of modern Jainism."

41. Chapple and Kelly (1990: 15).

42. In Hindu tradition *Hiraṇyagarbha* is acknowledged as the founder of Yoga and is generally regarded by scholars as being mythic. Later Yoga commentators believed that there was an actual person named Hiraṇyagarbha who had written a work on Yoga, but this does not really tell us anything about the person, Hiraṇyagarbha.

43. See Woods (1914: xiv).

44. See *YB* (I.1) p. 1.

45. Cf. Woods (1914: 3), and Feuerstein (1979a: 25), who both translate *anuśāsana* as "exposition."

46. Monier-Williams (1899: 31).

47. Ibid., p. 1068.

48. Ibid., p. 1069.

49. *YB* (I.1) p. 1: *athetyayam adhikārārthaḥ*; see Monier-Williams (1899) p. 17 on *atha* and p. 20 on *adhikāra.*

50. See Mookerjie (1951: 262).

51. For example, as is the case in H. Āraṇya's works; see G. Larson (1987: 581).

52. See *YB* (I.51) p. 56.

53. J. W. Hauer, quoted by G. Feuerstein (1979b: 25).

54. G. Feuerstein (1980: ix). Feuerstein, in agreement with Hauer, writes in a later work (1989: 174) that Vyāsa "does not appear to have been in the direct lineage of Patañjali."

55. See, for example, C. Chapple (1994: 85–105), who criticizes Vyāsa's interpretation of several *sūtra*s (i.e., I.19–22; I.41; II.17–27; III.53) and proposes "that the standard interpretation given by Vyāsa needs to be reconsidered."

56. As Feuerstein himself admits; see (1979b: 23).

57. That is, developments prior to the *SK*. See E. H. Johnson (1937), A. B. Keith (1949), F. Edgerton (1924), and G. Larson (1969, 1987) for discussions on earlier Sāṃkhya.

58. The most comprehensive study of the Sāṃkhya tradition is by Gerald Larson and Ram Shankar Bhattacharya, eds. (1987). *Sāṃkhya: A Dualist Tradition in Indian Philosophy*. See also the older work (1969) by G. Larson entitled, *Classical Sāṃkhya: An Interpretation of its History and Meaning*. The term *"sāṃkhya"* means "enumeration," "relating to number," or "calculation" (see Monier-Williams, 1899: 1128). It also refers "to a specific Hindu school of dualist philosophizing that proceeds by a method of enumerating the contents of experience and the world for the purpose of attaining radical liberation *(mokṣa, kaivalya)* from frustration and rebirth" (G. Larson, 1987: 3).

59. See, for example, *Kaṭha Up* I.3.3–4 and I.3.10–11; see also *Śvet Up* II.8–10.

60. Radhakrishnan, *Upaniṣads,* pp. 720–721.

61. Larson (1987: 6).

62. Radhakrishnan, *Upaniṣads,* p. 746.

63. However, the precise number of enumerated principles varies widely. In *MBh* XII.239 and XII.267 (28), seventeen basic principles are enumerated; in *MBh* XII.298, the standard list of twenty-five are given.

64. Cf. Chakravarti (1951: 38-39).

65. See Radhakrishnan (1948: 176): "That state which is obtained by the Sāṃkhyas is also reached by the yogins. He who sees Sāṃkhya and Yoga as one, sees indeed."

66. Cf. Edgerton, trans. (1965: 325): "But both of these have the same practical result, and both are declared (to lead to) freedom from death. Men who are devoted to weak intelligence regard them as separate; but we regard them as certainly only one. The same thing which *Yoga*-followers perceive, is perceived also by *Sāṃkhya*-followers. Who looks upon *Sāṃkhya* and *Yoga* as one, knows the truth." Other passages which stress the oneness of Sāṃkhya and Yoga are *MBh* XII.295.42-43 and XII.293.29-30. Virtually identical are XII.304.4 and *BG* V.5.

67. Sanskrit text from Belvalkar *et al.,* eds. (1951-53), *The Mahābhārata,* pp. 1583-1584; *MBh* XII.289.7 and XII.289.9 state: *pratyakṣahetavo yogaḥ sāṃkhyāḥ śāstraviniś cayāḥ, ubhe caite mate tattve mama tāta yudhiṣṭhira. tulyaṃ śaicam tayor yuktaṃ dayā bhūteṣu cānagha, vratānāṃ dhāraṇaṃ tulyaṃ darśanaṃ na samaṃ tayoḥ.* In XII.289 (1) an indication is made whereby the two are clearly differentiated and XII.289 (2) tells us there are adherents within both schools which claim superiority for their interpretations. See Edgerton (1965: 291).

68. See Belvalkar (1951-53: 1061).

69. *MBh* XII.189.4-5.

70. *MBh* XII.189.17-18, 28; see also XII.294.7, where it is said that the superior strength of yogins is in their practice of meditation.

71. Radhakrishnan (1948: 176).

72. Ibid.; cf. *BG* XIII.29, which implies that Sāṃkhya by itself was a path to the liberation of the spirit and not just in conjunction with Yoga.

73. The sage Kapila is traditionally celebrated as the founder of Sāṃkhya, though in later texts, such as some of the Purāṇas, he is acknowledged as a great yogin. Kapila handed over this lore to his pupil Āsuri. Later *ācārya*s such as Pañcaśikha, Vārṣagaṇya, Vindyavāsin, Jaigīśavya, and Īśvara Kṛṣṇa belong to this tradition. We need briefly mention only some of the major influences on the Sāṃkhyan tradition stemming from the first century BCE. The *Ṣaṣṭitantra,* a tradition of "sixty topics," was either a format for the treatment of philosophical Sāṃkhya or the actual name of a text, an old form of which was attributed to Kapila or Pañcaśikha—ca. 100 BCE-200 CE. Vārṣagaṇya composed a revision of the *Ṣaṣṭitantra*—ca. 100-300 CE. In the first essay of his book entitled *Strukturen Yogischer Meditation* (Vienna: Verlag der Osterreichischen Akademie der Wissenschaften, 1977), G. Oberhammer examines "Sāṃkhyan meditation," by which he means those meditative structural approaches that have been handed down in the Sämkhya tradition, particularly that of Vārṣagaṇya. Oberhammer's analysis of this "yogic" orientation is based on relevant quotations found in the *Yuktidīpikā* and intends to show that the soteriology of the old Sāṃkhya tradition was not a purely rationalistic affair and that many of the Sāṃkhyan metaphysical categories can only be understood against a background of meditative praxis. Followers of Vārṣagaṇya include: (a) Vindyavāsin ca. 300-400 CE, who further revises

the Sāṃkhya system and participates in an intense polemic with the Buddhists. There is some speculation among scholars (e.g., P. Chakravarti, E. Frauwallner, and G. Larson) that the revision of Sāṃkhya given by Vindyavāsin eventually became the classical Yoga philosophy of Patañjali and Vyāsa (see also Aklujkar [1995] in n. 3 above); (b) Īśvara Kṛṣṇa ca. 350-450 CE, whose *SK* is based on Vārṣagaṇya's *Ṣaṣṭitantra* but corrected as a result of the Buddhist debates and the work of Vindyavāsin. See Larson (1987: 13, 131-146) for a discussion of dates and a philosophical analysis of these and other Sāṃkhyan thinkers. For more on Sāṃkhyan teachers see also: Keith (1949), *The Sāṃkhyan System,* p. 47; and H. D. Sharma (1933), "The Sāṃkhya-teachers," *Festschrift Moriz Winternitz,* pp. 225-231. A listing of Sāṃkhyan teachers may be found in *MBh* XII.306.58-62. See also V. M. Bedekar (1958), "The Teachings of Pañcaśikha in the Mahābhārata," *ABORI,* vol. 38, pp. 233-234. Īśvara Kṛṣṇa's *SK* apparently constitutes a definitive summary of the technical philosophical tradition of Sāṃkhya. Prior to the *SK,* Sāṃkhya, as a technical system, did exist, i.e., the *SK* comes at the end of the normative period of formulation rather than at the beginning; on this see Larson (1987: 9).

74. Dasgupta (1930: 15).

75. According to H. T. Colebrooke (1873: 1: 265), the only significant difference between Yoga and Sāṃkhya is the affirmation of the doctrine of *īśvara* by the former and its denial by the later. A host of other scholars do not fully acknowledge Yoga and Sāṃkhya as being distinct philosophical schools. See, for example, M. N. Dvivedī (1934: xviii), R. Garbe (1917: 148), S. Radhakrishnan (1951, 2: 342), M. Eliade (1969: 7), and N. Smart (1968: 26). S. Dasgupta (1930: 2) observes, however, that although the two schools are fundamentally the same in their general metaphysical positions, they hold quite different views on many points of philosophical, ethical and practical interest. Recent scholarship has tended to support Dasgupta's claim. See, for example, F. Catalina (1968: 19), K. B. R. Rao (1966: 9), and G. Koelman (1970: 57-66, 104, 237). See also notes 76, 77, and 78 below and accompanying text.

76. Feuerstein (1980: 109-118).

77. Ibid., p 111.

78. Larson (1987: 13) would obviously disagree with this dating. He suggests that the *SK* predates the *YS*. He lists Īśvara Kṛṣṇa's *SK* as (ca.) 350-450 CE and Patañjali's *YS* as (ca) 400-500 CE. Moreover, Larson feels that the *YS* philosophy is a school of Sāṃkhya. He writes (ibid., p. 19): "there is a basic and normative Sāṃkhya philosophy, concisely yet completely set forth in Īśvara Kṛṣṇa's *Sāṃkhyakārikā* and appropriated with a somewhat different inflection in Patañjali's *Yoga-Sūtra* for the sake of yogic praxis. The former can be called simply the tradition of Kārikā-Sāṃkhya and the latter, Pātañjala-Sāṃkhya." While admitting (ibid., p. 22) that the *YS* is "obviously a compilation of older *sūtra* collections" he further advances (ibid.) that, "Keith may well have been correct in suggesting that the appearance of the *Sāṃkhyakārikā* may have been the occasion for an attempt by the followers of Yoga to systematize their own older traditions." See Keith (1949: 70).

79. *SK* 19.

80. *YS* II.17-20. See discussion later in this chapter on *prakṛti* and *puruṣa*. One could, however, look upon the *vṛtti*s (*YS* I.6-11) as providing something of a proto-ontology equivalent in the first chapter.

81. *YS* II.16 (p. 78): *heyaṃ duḥkhamanāgatam.* "The suffering yet to come is to be overcome." It must be emphasized as well that the question of "how" also pre-

supposes the question of "why," why one would desire liberation from the saṃsāric realm. This question of "why" is answered, as we will see, in *YS* II.15, where we are told that from the perspective of the discerning yogin, all identity contained within the saṃsāric world is inherently dissatisfying.

82. *YB* IV.30 (p. 203). We will be saying more on this later.

83. See, for example, Śaṅkara's (ca. eighth century CE) use of *vyāvahārika* (the conventional empirical perspective) in contrast to *paramārthika* (the ultimate or absolute standpoint).

84. See in particular: Feuerstein (1980: 14, 56, 108); Eliade (1969: 94-95, 99-100); Koelman (1970: 224, 251); and G. Larson (1987: 13), who classifies Patañjali's Yoga as a form of Sāṃkhya.

85. F. Edgerton (1924), "The Meaning of Sāṃkhya and Yoga," *AJP* 45: 1-46.

86. I am adopting the term "maps" from G. Feuerstein; refer to n. 89 below and also Feuerstein (1989) pp. 176-178.

87. One might query, for example, whether the central expedient of *vijñāna* (*SK* 2), recommended by Īśvara Kṛṣṇa, to terminate suffering *(duḥkha)* is, in the last analysis, adequate for realizing the postulated goal of identity as Self. *Tattva-abhyāsa* or applied *vijñāna* is, however, equated by R. Parrot [see (1985), "The Experience called Reason in Sāṃkhya," *JIP* 13: 235-264] with wisdom as opposed to rational knowledge. Larson (1987: 27) states that the ethical goal of Sāṃkhya is to discriminate the presence of a transcendent consciousness *(puruṣa)* distinct from *prakṛti* and its tripartite process, and thereby to attain radical isolation *(kaivalya)* or liberation from ordinary human experience. But can *vijñāna* be synonomous with *prajñā* or yogic insight acquired in *samādhi* as described in the *YS* (I.17-18)? How, in Sāṃkhya, is the *bhāva* of (*SK* 23) *jñāna* actually brought about? K. B. R. Rao (1966: 432) speculated that it is the accentuated rationalism of classical Sāṃkhya that must be held responsible for the fact that this school of thought never actually acquired the same recognition and prestige as the other Hindu *darśana*s. Feuerstein (1980: 115-116) seriously doubts the efficacy of the classical Sāṃkhyan approach for arriving at genuine liberation, rendering *vijñāna* as "an intellectual act." He argues that *vijñāna,* as a sufficient means for attaining liberation, "is tacitly denied, by the adherents of Yoga." Koelman (1970: 237) also supports the claim that the method of *vijñāna* in the *SK* (2) is inferior to yogic praxis. He writes: "It is not by dint of thinking that one can empty the intellect; only another faculty, the will, can inhibit the working of the intellect. In this, Yoga has seen more clearly than *Sāṃkhya,* which considers liberation as a purely intellectual process."

88. Cf. *Kaṭha Up* VI.7-8.

89. Feuerstein (1980: 117).

90. Foreword to Feuerstein (1980: viii).

91. *TV* II.23 (p. 93): *pradhīyate janyate vikārajātamaneneti pradhānaṃ.* Translators have struggled to express the meaning of *mūlaprakṛti* with words such as "nature," "primordial nature," "primordial materiality," and "prime matter"; though these translations have generally been accepted, they are not precisely accurate and may even be misleading. The Sāṃkhyan dualism is quite distinct from the Cartesian dualism that bifurcates reality into mental and material aspects. The dualistic perspective of Sāṃkhya is made up of *puruṣa* as pure consciousness, and *prakṛti* as everything else, including the mental and the material. Psyche and the external world are not ultimately different. Both are forms of insentient (nonconscious, *acetana*) *prakṛti.* With the above explanation held in mind we shall adopt the simple term "matter" for *prakṛti.*

92. See S. Dasgupta (1922: 246–247), and Vācaspati Miśra on *SK* 3; see also *Sāṃkhya-Sūtra* I.61: *sattvarajastamasāṃ sāmyāvasthā prakṛti,* in R. Garbe, ed. (1943), *The Sāṃkhya-pravacana-bhāṣya* (Harvard Oriental Series, vol. 2, p. 29) of Vijñāna Bhikṣu as well as Vijñāna Bhikṣu's commentary *(SPB)* on *Sāṃkhya-Sūtra* I.61; see also *SPB* VI.39 and *passim.*

93. See Anima Sen Gupta (1969), *Classical Sāṃkhya: A Critical Study,* pp. 5–72.

94. See K. B. R. Rao (1966: 55–56).

95. In Advaita Vedānta, the effect—that which is observed in our world—is often understood to be an unreal appearance or manifestation of *brahman,* which alone is the ultimate reality. Therefore *brahman* is the real cause of all appearances, which only possess limited, empirical levels of reality. This approach to causality is termed *brahma-vivarta-vāda;* though the principle of *satkāryavāda* is accepted, each effect is understood as an unreal appearance of *brahman.* This is in marked contrast to Sāṃkhya and Yoga, which maintain that both the effect and the cause are on equal planes of reality. The above example is true of post-Śaṅkara Advaitins only. Śaṅkara did not hold *vivarta* but ascribed a lower level of reality, *vyāvahārikam sātyam,* to the phenomenal world. In the school of Viśiṣṭādvaita Vedānta, Rāmānuja conceived of souls and the material world as attributes or the body of the Absolute Cause, though real like the Cause; and in Dvaita Vedānta, Madhva considered souls as finite, dependent beings while the Supreme Cause is independent being.

96. *YB* IV.11 (p. 185): *na hy apūrvopajanaḥ.*

97. *YB* IV.12 (p. 186): *nāsty asataḥ saṃbhavaḥ, na cāsti sato vināśa.*

98. *TV* I.18 (p. 22): *kāryasarūpaṃ kāraṇaṃ yujyate na virūpam.*

99. *YS* IV.2 (p. 177): *jātyantarapariṇāmaḥ prakṛtyāpūrāt.* "The transformation into another life (i.e., birth) is implemented by [the] *prakṛti*[s]."

100. *YB* IV.2 (p. 177): *pūrvapariṇāmāpāya uttarapariṇāmopajanas teṣāṃ pūrvāvayavānupraveśād bhavati.*

101. See Radhakrishnan (1948: 105–106): *nā'sato vidyate bhāvo nā'bhāvo vidyate sataḥ, ubhayor api dṛṣṭo'ntas tv anayos tattvadaśibhiḥ. avināśi tu tad viddhi yena sarvam idaṃ tatam, vināśaṃ avyayasyā'sya na kaścit kartum arhati.* Cf. *Chānd Up* VI.1–4.

102. *YS* II.19 (p. 84).

103. *YS* III.13 (p. 124): *etena bhūtendriyeṣu dharmalakṣaṇāvasthāpariṇāmā vyākhyātāḥ.*

104. *YB* III.15 (p. 136): *cittasya dvaye dharmāḥ paridṛṣṭāś cāparidṛṣṭāś ca.* In *YB* III.52 (pp. 170–171) Vyāsa rejects the notion that "time" as normally conceived ("day," "night," "hour," etc.) is a real entity. The ultimate unit of time is the "moment" *(kṣaṇa).* Vyāsa tells us that a "moment" is the time taken to pass from one point of change in a substance to the next. A succession or sequence *(krama)* consists of a continuity of the unbroken flow of the moments in it. Yet there is no aggregation of "moments" and their "succession," i.e., hours, days, and nights are basically mental constructs empty of reality yet appear real to those people who have a conceptual or reified view of the world. It is only the *kṣaṇa* or "moment" that has reality and is the support or foundation of any succession of change over time. "Succession" is a continuity of "moments." At each moment in time a subtle change takes place (perceptible to the yogin) and it is the accumulated effect of these subtle changes of which we become aware. See also *YS* III.9, 15, 52 and IV.33 and Vyāsa's commentary on these *sūtras.* In classical Yoga the

idea of the "moment" attains significance in spite of the general rejection of Buddhist "impermanence" by "orthodox" Hindu schools in general.

105. *YS* III.14 (p. 132): *śāntoditāvyapadeśyadharmānupātī dharmī.* "The *dharma*-holder corresponds to the subsided, arisen or undetermined form."

106. *YS* III.14; see n. 105 above.

107. See *YB* III.14 (p. 134).

108. Wilhelm Halbfass (1992), *On Being and What There Is,* p. 61.

109. *YB* III.13 (p. 131): *tatredam udāharaṇaṃ mṛddharmī piṇḍākārād dharmād dharmāntaram upasaṃpadyamāno dharmataḥ pariṇāmate ghaṭākāra iti. ghaṭākāro'nāgataṃ lakṣaṇaṃ hitvā vartamānalakṣaṇaṃ pratipadyata iti lakṣaṇataḥ pariṇāmate. ghaṭo navapurāṇataṃ pratikṣaṇaṃ anubhavannavasthāpariṇāmaṃ pratipadyata iti.*

110. *YB* IV.13 (p. 187): *vartamānā vyaktātmano'tītānāgataḥ sūkṣmātmānaḥ.*

111. *YS* IV.12 (p. 186): *atītānāgataṃ svarūpato'sty adhvabhedād dharmāṇāṃ.* "Past and future exist in their own form due to differences between paths of the forms (*dharmas*) [generated by *prakṛti*]."

112. *YS* IV.18 (p. 193).

113. More discussion on the nature of *guṇas* including their manifestation as characteristics of personhood and human identity appears in chapter 3.

114. See van Buitenen (1956, 1957), "Studies in Sāṃkhya (I-III)," in *JAOS* 76, 77.

115. *YS* II.18 (p. 81): *prakāśakriyāsthitiśīlaṃ bhūtendriyātmakaṃ bhogāpavargārthaṃ dṛśyam.* "The seeable *[prakṛti]* whose qualities are of luminosity, activity, and inertia, has the nature of the elements and the senses and is for the purpose of experience and emancipation."

116. See n. 115 above.

117. *YB* II.18 (pp. 81-82): *prakāśaśīlaṃ sattvam. kriyāśīlaṃ rajaḥ. sthitiśīlaṃ tama iti. ete guṇāḥ parasparoparaktapravibhāgāḥ pariṇāminaḥ saṃyogaviyogadharmāṇa itaretaropāśrayeṇopārjitamūrtayaḥ parasparāṅgitve'py asaṃbinnaśaktipravibhāgās tulyajātīyātulyajātīyaśaktibhedānupātinaḥ pradhānavelāyām upadarśitasaṃnidhānā, guṇatve'pi ca vyāpāramātreṇa pradhānāntarṇītānumitāstitāḥ. puruṣārthakartavyatayā prayuktasāmarthyāḥ.*

118. G. Koelman (1970: 77).

119. Ibid.

120. G. Koelman's (ibid., p. 78) coinage. Cf. G. Feuerstein (1980: 36).

121. *YS* II.15 (p. 74): *pariṇāmatāpasaṃskāraduḥkhair guṇavṛttivirodhāc ca duḥkham eva sarvaṃ vivekinaḥ.*

122. See *YS* II.19. In other words, the predominant interpretation among scholars is that phenomenal existence is an inherently problematic, even constantly turbulent state of affairs. The danger in the above interpretation is that *prakṛti* all too easily becomes equated with or reduced to affliction *(kleśa)* itself.

123. See n. 121 above and text.

124. Patañjali uses the term *pratiprasava* twice, in *YS* II.10 and IV.34.

125. See Chapple and Kelly (1990: 60).

126. Feuerstein (1979a: 65).

127. Cf. T. Leggett (1990: 195) and U. Arya (1986: 146, 471).

128. *YS* II.19 (p. 84): *viśeṣāviśeṣaliṅgamātrāliṅgāni guṇaparvāṇi.* "The levels of the *guṇas* are the particularized, the unparticularized, the designator and the unmanifest."

129. *YB* II.19 (pp. 84–85): *tatrā''kāśavāyvagnyudakabhūmayo bhūtāni śabdasparśarūparasagandhatanmātrāṇāmaviśeṣāṇāṃ viśeṣāḥ. tathā śrotratvakcakṣujihvāghrāṇāni buddhīndriyāṇi, vākpāṇipādapāyūpasthāḥ karmendriyāṇi, ekādaśaṃ manaḥ sarvārtham, ity etāny asmitālakṣaṇasyāviśeṣasya viśeṣāḥ. guṇānām eṣa ṣoḍaśako viśeṣapariṇāmaḥ. ṣaḍaviśeṣāḥ. tadyathā śabdatanmātraṃ sparśatanmātraṃ rūpatanmātraṃ rasatanmātraṃ gandhatanmātraṃ ceti ekadvitricatuḥ pañcalakṣaṇāḥ śabdādayaḥ pañcāviśeṣāḥ, ṣaṣṭhaś cāviśeṣo'smitāmātra iti. ete sattāmātrasyā''tmano mahataḥ ṣaḍaviśeṣapariṇāmāḥ. yattatparamaviśeṣebhyo liṅgamātraṃ mahattattvaṃ tasminnete sattāmātre mahatyātmanyavasthāya vivṛddhikāṣṭhāmanubhavanti. pratisaṃsṛjyamānāśca tasminneva sattāmātre mahatyātmanyavasthāya yattanniḥsattāsattaṃ niḥsadasannirasadavyaktamaliṅgaṃ pradhānaṃ tatprātiyanti.*

130. *TV* II.19 (p. 85): *sattva rajastamasām sāmyāvasthā*. See also *TV* II.17 (p. 79): *pradhānasāmyam upagato'pi*. The state of equilibrium, balance, or equipoise is known as *sāmyāvasthā* or *pralaya* and is where the unmanifest *guṇa*s "neutralize" or balance one another's energy prior to all their manifestations.

131. See n. 129 above.

132. *TV* I.45 (p. 50).

133. *TV* II.19 (p. 85): *yāvatī kācit puruṣārthakriyā śabdādibhogalakṣaṇā, sattvapuruṣānyatākhyātilakṣaṇā vāsti sa sarvā mahati buddhau samāpyata ityarthaḥ.*

134. See n. 129 above and text.

135. See ibid.

136. G. Koelman (1970: 107).

137. Ibid.

138. On this see P. Chakravarti (1951: 134), who has made a strong case against the identification of the Patañjali referred to in the *Yuktidīpikā* with the author of the *YS*.

139. *SK* 24. Often in Hindu literature the term *ahaṃkāra* denotes the illusory sense of self confined to the nature of *prakṛti* as a body-mind and having various properties such as "my thoughts," "my feelings," "my actions," etc.

140. S. Radhakrishnan (1951), *Indian Philosophy,* vol 2, p. 434.

141. *YB* I.45 (p. 50): *teṣāhaṃkāraḥ. asyāpi liṅgamātraṃ sūkṣmo viṣayaḥ; teṣa* ("these") refers to the subtle elements (*tan-mātra*s).

142. *YS* II.6 (p. 64): *dṛgdarśanaśaktyor ekātmatevāsmitā [=eka-ātmatā-iva-asmitā].*

143. Vyāsa often uses the terms *buddhi* and *citta* synonomously, although we understand the former to be included in the later, as is explained in chapter 3.

144. *YB* II.6 (p. 64): *puruṣo dṛkśaktir buddhir darśanaśaktir ity etayor ekasvarūpāpattir ivāsmitā kleśa ucyate. bhoktṛbhogyaśaktyor atyantavibhaktayor atyantāsaṃkīrṇayor avibhagaprāptāv iva satyāṃ bhogaḥ kalpate. svarūpapratilambhe tu tayoḥ kaivalyam eva bhavati kuto bhoga iti. tathā coktam—"buddhitaḥ paraṃ puruṣam ākaraśīlavidyādibhir vibhaktam apaśyan kuryāt tatrā''tmabuddhiṃ mohena."* Vācaspati Miśra (*TV* II.6, p. 64) tells us that the above quotation used by Vyāsa is by the Sāṃkhya teacher, Pañcaśikha.

145. *YS* III.35 (p. 154): *sattvapuruṣayor atyantāsaṃkīrṇayoḥ pratyayāviśeṣo bhogaḥ . . .*

146. Āraṇya (1963), *Yoga Philosophy of Patañjali,* trans. by P. N. Mukerji, p. 195. When quoting Āraṇya, I will be using the translations by Mukerji.

147. *YS* IV.4 (p. 178): *nirmāṇacittānyasmitāmātrāt.*

148. *YS* IV.4 will be explained further in chapter 3.

149. S. Dasgupta (1920), *A Study of Patañjali,* p. 51.

150. Koelman (1970: 108).

151. Feuerstein (1980: 46).

152. For example, Koelman (1970: 108) writes: "Only when plurified or suppositated by the Ego-function *[ahaṃkāra]* can the Great Substance *(mahattattvam)* . . . be strictly called *buddhi.*" Koelman sees *buddhi* in an individuated sense only. Feuerstein (1980: 44) understands *buddhi,* in Patañjali's philosophy, as standing "for 'cognition' only and not for any ontological entity."

153. This "cosmic being," it could be argued, has been mythologized as Hiraṇyagarbha, who came to designate the "first-born" entity in the evolutionary series, as taught in Vedānta. According to the *MBh* (XII.291.17), Hiraṇyagarbha is none other than the higher mind or *buddhi.*

154. S. Chennakesavan (1980), *Concept of Mind in Indian Philosophy,* p. 134.

155. This experience is referred to in *YS* I.17 as *asmitā-samādhi.*

156. G. Feuerstein (1980: 41).

157. S. Dasgupta (1922).

158. See n. 141 above.

159. G. Koelman (1970: 115).

160. *TV* II.19 (p. 84): *pañca tanmātrāṇi buddhikāraṇakānyaviśeṣatvād asmitāvad iti.* "The five subtle elements have *buddhi* as their cause because they are unparticularized, like I-am-ness."

161. As outlined in the *SK* (24).

162. Āraṇya (1963: 196–197).

163. *YB* IV.2 (p. 177): *tatra kāyendriyāṇāṃ anyajatīyapariṇatānām . . . pūrvapariṇāmāpāya uttarapariṇāmopajanas teṣām apūrvāvayavānupraveśād bhavati.*

164. *YB* IV.2 (p. 177): *kāyendriyaprakṛtayaś ca svaṃ svaṃ vikāram anugṛhṇantyāpūrena dharmādi nimittam apekṣamāṇā iti.*

165. *YB* III.14 (p. 134): *deśakālā kāranimittāpabandhān na khalu samānakālam ātmanām abhivyaktir iti.* "Under the constraints of place, time, form, and cause, the essences do not manifest simultaneously."

166. As Vācaspati clarifies (*TV* III.14) p. 134.

167. Vijñāna Bhikṣu (*YV* IV.2) mentions such powers as the yogin's ability to multiply his body, implying a change of shape without intervening death and birth. See T. S. Rukmani (1989: 3–4).

168. See Johnston (1937: 26), and Larson (1969: 174).

169. *TV* IV.2 (p. 177): *manuṣyajātipariṇatānāṃ kāyendriyāṇāṃ yo devatiryagjātipariṇāmaḥ sa khalu prakṛtyāpūrāt. kāyasya hi prakṛtiḥ pṛthivyādīni bhūtāni. indriyāṇāṃ ca prakṛtir. asmitā. tadavayavānupraveśa āpūras tasmād bhavati.*

170. See n. 169 above.

171. See *TV* IV.2 (p. 177).

172. *YS* IV.3 (p. 177): *nimittam aprayojakaṃ prakṛtīnāṃ varaṇabhedas tu tataḥ kṣetrikavat.* It is understood here that the farmer does not initiate the flow of water but directs the flow by way of barriers. See n. 174 below.

173. Some aphorisms of Kaṇāda (*Vaiśeṣika-Sūtra*s IX.1.1 to 10) are specifically directed to refute the Sāṃkhya and Yoga doctrine of *satkāryavāda.* In Vaiśeṣika, the product does not preexist in its material cause. It is actually brought into existence in the process of causation.

174. *YB* IV.3 (pp. 177–178): *yathā kṣetrikaḥ kedārāntaraṃ piplāvayiṣuḥ samaṃ nimnaṃ nimnataraṃ vā nāpaḥ pāṇināpakarṣati āvaraṇaṃ tv āsāṃ bhinatti tasmin bhinne svayam evāpaḥ kedārāntaram āplāvayanti, tathā dharmaḥ prakṛtīnām āvaraṇam adharmaṃ bhinatti, tasmin bhinne svayam eva prakṛtayaḥ svaṃ svaṃ vikāram āplāvayanti.*

175. See *YB* IV.3 (p. 178).

176. *YB* IV.12 (p. 186): *sataś ca phalasya nimittaṃ vartamānīkaraṇe samarthaṃ nāpūrvopajanane. siddhaṃ nimittaṃ naimittikasya viśeṣānugrahaṇaṃ kurute nāpūrvam utpādayatīti.* "An efficient cause can bring to actuality a result already existent, but not produce what had not previously existed. A recognizable cause gives a particular aid towards what is effected; it produces something not indeed nonexistent before."

177. *YB* I.45 (p. 50): *nanvasti puruṣaḥ sūkṣma iti. satyam. yathā liṅgāt paramaliṅgasya saukṣmyaṃ na caivaṃ puruṣasya. kiṃ tu, liṅgasyānvayikāraṇaṃ puruṣo na bhavati hetus tu bhavati.*

178. *YB* II.19 (p. 86): *aliṅgāvasthāyāṃ na puruṣārthā heturnāliṅgāvasthāyāmādau puruṣārthatā kāraṇaṃ bhavatīti. na tasyāḥ puruṣārthatā kāraṇaṃ bhavatīti. nāsau puruṣārthakṛteti nityā''khyāyate. trayāṇāṃ tvavasthāviśeṣāṇāmādau puruṣārthatā kāraṇaṃ bhavati. sa cārthā heturnimittaṃ kāraṇaṃ bhavatītyanityā''khyāyate.*

179. Koelman (1970: 76).

180. *TV* IV.3 (p. 178): *na ca puruṣārtho'pi pravartakaḥ. kiṃ tu taduddeśeneśvaraḥ. uddeśyatāmātreṇa puruṣārthaḥ pravartaka ity ucyate. utpitsos tv asya puruṣārthasyāvyaktasya sthitikāraṇatvam yuktam . . . īśvarasyāpi dharmādhiṣṭhānārthaṃ pratibandhāpanaya eva vyāpāro veditavyaḥ.*

181. *YB* III.14; see n. 165 above.

182. *YB* IV.11 (p. 185): *heturdharmātsukhamadharmādduḥkhaṃ, sukhādrāgo duḥkhāddveṣas tataśca prayatnastena manasā vācā kāyena vā parispandamānaḥ paramanugṛhṇātyupahanti vā tataḥ punardharmādharmau sukhaduḥkhe rāgadveṣāviti pravṛttamidaṃ ṣaḍaraṃ saṃsāracakram. asya ca pratikṣaṇamāvartamānasyāvidyā netrī mūlaṃ sarvakleśānamityeṣa hetuḥ.*

183. See chapter 3 for a detailed explanation of the term *karman.*

184. As quoted in Feuerstein (1980: 118).

185. See Monier-Williams (1899), *A Sanskrit-English Dictionary,* p. 487.

186. Ibid., p. 334.

187. See Larson (1969).

188. *YS* II.25 (p. 96): *tadabhāvāt saṃyogābhāvo hānaṃ taddṛśeḥ kaivalyam.* "Without it (ignorance), there is no conjunction, and that abandonment (of ignorance) is the aloneness *(kaivalya)* of seeing."

189. *YS* II.20 (p. 87): *draṣṭā dṛśimātraḥ śuddho'pi pratyayānupaśyaḥ.* "The seer is seeing alone; although pure, it appears in the form of a cognition (idea, apprehension)." After stating in *YS* I.3 that our true nature and identity is the seer, *YS* I.4 informs us that unless we are aware as the seer, we yet conform in our identity to the changing nature of *vṛtti* or the modifications of the mind. See n. 36 above.

190. *YS* IV.18 (p. 193): *sadā jñātāś cittavṛttayas tatprabhoḥ puruṣasyāpariṇāmitvāt.* "The modifications of the mind are always known due to the immutability of their master, *puruṣa.*" In Yoga as portrayed in the epic literature of the *MBh,* the term *puruṣa* is widely referred to as the "knower" *(jña)* or the "field-knower" *(kṣetra-jña),* the "field" being *prakṛti.* See, for example, *BG* XIII.34. In *YB* II.17 Vyāsa uses the term

kṣetrajña for *puruṣa.* See *SK* 17 for the various proofs establishing the existence of *puruṣa* in the system of classical Sāṃkhya.

191. *YS* II.23.

192. *YS* IV.22.

193. *YS* IV.34.

194. *YS* II.20.

195. *YS* II.6.

196. *YS* III.35 (p. 154): *sattvapuruṣayor atyantāsaṃkīrṇayoḥ . . .*

197. *YS* III.49 (p. 167): *sattvapuruṣānyatā . . .*

198. *YS* IV.19 (p. 194): *na tat svābhāsaṃ dṛśyatvāt.* "That [*cittavṛtti,* i.e., mind, extrinsic identity] has no self-luminosity, because of the nature of the seeable [i.e., it is itself something known, perceived]." Cf. *SK* 20.

199. *YS* II.17 (p. 79): *draṣṭṛdṛśyayoḥ saṃyogo heyahetuḥ.* "The conjunction between the seer and the seeable is the cause of what is to be overcome [i.e., suffering, dissatisfaction *(duḥkha)*]."

200. *SK* 11; see Larson (1969: 263-264).

201. *SK* 19: *sākṣitvam . . . kaivalyam mādhyasthyam draṣṭṛtvam akartṛbhāva;* see Larson (1969) p. 265.

202. S. Dasgupta (1924), *Yoga as Philosophy and Religion,* p. 19.

203. See Edgerton (1965: 332).

204. *YB* I.24 (p. 26): *kaivalyaṃ prāptās tarhi santi ca bahavaḥ kevalinaḥ.* "There are many *kevalin*s who have attained liberation." Cf. *YB* II.22 (p. 90) and IV.33 (p. 205). It is of interest to note that *kevalin* is a Jaina term. Those who attain *kaivalya* according to Yoga are called *kaivalin* and not *kevalin.* On this matter U. Arya (1986: 289) writes: "It appears that Vyāsa is challenging the view of the Jains, who do not believe in a . . . God but do believe that those who reach the highest perfection through yoga and are called *kevalin*s become īśhvaras after death. In Vyāsa's view, Patañjali's definition of īśhvara does not apply to them."

205. See *TV* I.41 (p. 44).

206. S. Dasgupta (1930), *Yoga Philosophy in Relation to Other Systems of Indian Thought,* p. 167.

207. *YS* II.22 (p. 90).

208. See G. Feuerstein (1980: 23).

209. See, for example, *Muṇḍaka Up* I.2.9 and *Śvet Up* II.14.

210. See *SK* 18.

211. Larson (1987: 80).

212. Text from the *YV* (II.22) taken from T. S. Rukmani, trans. (1983), *Yogavārttika of Vijñāna Bhikṣu,* vol. 2: *Sādhanapāda,* p. 149: *buddhyā kṛtaḥ samāpito' rtho yasyeti.*

213. See *SPB* in R. Garbe, ed. (1943), *Harvard Oriental Series,* vol. 2, pp. 69-70.

214. Ibid., pp. 70-71.

215. *YB* II.18 (pp. 83-84): *tāvetau bhogāpavargau buddhikṛtau buddhāv eva vartamānau . . . buddher eva puruṣārthāparisamāptir bandhas tadarthāvasāyo mokṣa iti.*

216. *YS* II.18, 21.

217. See Radhakrishnan (1953: 167).

218. See Radhakrishnan (1948: 374).

219. See K. B. R. Rao (1966: 278); see P. M. Modi (1932: 81ff.) and G. Feuerstein (1980: 5–7) for studies on the twenty-six principles outlined in *MBh* XII.296.

220. *MBh* XII.296.7; see Edgerton (1965: 317).

221. *MBh* XII.296.20; see Edgerton (1965: 319) and Feuerstein (1980: 6).

222. *MBh* XII.296.11 and 13; see Edgerton, (1965: 318).

223. Feuerstein (1980: 6); see *MBh* XII.296.27.

224. See, for example, XII.296.11 and XII.306.53–54.

225. P. M. Modi (1932), *Akṣara: A Forgotten Chapter in the History of Indian Philosophy,* p. 81.

226. For instance, Feuerstein (1980: 116) conjectures that Īśvara Kṛṣṇa assumed a typical agnostic stance. What distinguishes epic Sāṃkhya and Yoga from their classical formulations is, above all, their theistic (panentheistic) orientation. It does not appear to be the case that *īśvara* is a necessary principle for all yogins, i.e., devotion to *īśvara* can be an optional approach to liberation in the first chapter of the *YS* (implied by the word *vā*, meaning "or" in *YS* I.23). Thus, the "nontheism" of classical Sāṃkhya, and "optional" theism of classical Yoga can be understood as deviations from a firmly established theistic base, reflected in the Upaniṣads. Feuerstein suggests (1989: 164), "The reason for this shift away from the original panentheism of [Sāṃkhya] and Yoga was a felt need to respond to the challenge of such vigorously analytical traditions as Buddhism by systematizing both [Sāṃkhya] and Yoga along more rationalistic philosophical lines." However, we must keep an open mind regarding this, especially in relation to Yoga where rational knowledge is clearly subservient to direct perception.

227. See *YS* I.23–29 below and *YS* II.45. Eliade and Feuerstein clearly endorse the theistic orientation of these *sūtra*s. Chapple and Kelly (1990: 3) do not impute that Patañjali's descriptions of *īśvara* constitute a theistic stance. However, they do not in turn underestimate the potential importance of the concept of *īśvara* in Patañjali's Yoga.

228. *YS* I.24 (p. 25): *kleśakarmavipākāśayair aparāmṛṣṭaḥ puruṣaviśeṣa īśvaraḥ.*

229. *YB* I.24 (p. 26): *sa tu sadaiva muktaḥ sadaiveśvara iti.*

230. *YS* I.25 (p. 29): *tatra niratiśayaṃ sarvajñabījam.*

231. *YS* I.26 (p. 31): *pūrveṣām api guruḥ kalenānavacchedāt.*

232. *YS* I.27 (p. 32): *tasya vācakaḥ praṇavaḥ.*

233. *YS* I.28 (p. 33): *tajjapas tadārthabhāvanam.*

234. *YS* I.29 (p. 33): *tataḥ pratyakcetanādhigamo'py antarāyābhāvaś ca.*

235. *YS* I.23 (p. 25): *īśvarapraṇidhānād vā.* "Or [*samādhi* is attained] by devotion to the Lord."

236. *YB* I.24 (p. 27): *yo'sau prakṛṣṭasattvopādānād īśvarasya śaśvatika utkarṣaḥ.*

237. This suggests one reason why such a being is called *īśvara*. *TV* I.24 (p. 27): *neśvarasya pṛthagjanasyevāvidyānibandhanaś cittasattvena svasvāmibhāvaḥ . . . tāpatrayaparītān pretyabhāvamahārṇavāj . . . jñānadharmopadeśena.*

238. *TV* I.24 (p. 27): *na punar avidyām avidyātvena sevamānaḥ . . .*

239. *TV* I.24 (p. 27): *na ceyam apahatarajastamomalaviśuddhasattvopādānaṃ vinetyālocya sattvaprakarṣam upādat te.*

240. *TV* I.24 (p. 26): *jñānakriyāśakti saṃpadaiśvaryam.*

241. *YB* I.25 (p. 30): *bhūtānugrahaḥ prayojanam*. For more on the meaning of "devotion to *īśvara*" see the section on *aṣṭāṅga-yoga* in chapter 4 of this study.

242. *YB* I.24 (p. 27): *tasya śāstraṃ nimittam. śāstraṃ punaḥ kiṃ nimittaṃ, prakṛṣṭasattva nimittam.* "This perfection—does it have a cause or is it without a cause?

The cause is sacred scripture. Then what is the cause of scripture? The cause is the perfection (of the divine mind)."

243. See *YB* I.23 (p. 25); *prasāda* can also mean "clarity," "serenity," "tranquility"—all qualities through which spiritual transformation is enhanced and freedom *(mokṣa)* is allowed to take place.

244. See G. Oberhammer (1964: 197–207).

245. M. Eliade (1969: 74).

246. Feuerstein (1980: 12).

247. Here we can mention a few scholars who at times underestimate the importance of *īśvara* in Patañjali's system. See, for example: R. Garbe (1917: 149); S. Radhakrishnan (1951, 2: 371); N. Smart (1968: 30); and G. Koelman (1970: 57).

248. *YS* II.17 ; see n. 199 above.

249. See *YS* II.15 and n. 121 above.

250. *YS* IV.22 (p. 197): *citer apratisaṃkramāyās tadākārāpattau svabuddhisaṃvedanam.* "When the unmoving higher consciousness assumes the form of that [mind] then there is perception of one's own intellect."

CHAPTER 3. THE MIND *(CITTA)*

1. On this see the *Sāṃkhya-Kārikā* of Īśvara Kṛṣṇa and G. Larson's (1987, 1969) explanation of these terms as used in classical Sāṃkhya.

2. A general schematic of perceptual processes is summarized in the *BG* (III.42) and *Kaṭha Up* (III.10 and VI.7).

3. In *YS* IV.31 Patañjali uses the words *āvaraṇa-mala* meaning "impure coverings" or "veils" of ignorance that obstruct the eternality of knowledge.

4. As G. Feuerstein (1980: 24) mistakenly asserts.

5. For a fruitful study of the creative potential of consciousness and activity in South Asian Indian thought, see C. Chapple (1986), *Karma and Creativity*. The following examples gathered from Chapple's study (ibid.: 34–35) illustrate the more creative dimension given to the mind in Upaniṣadic literature. The translations of the Upaniṣads are taken from S. Radhakrishnan (1953). The *Chānd Up* III.18.1 (p. 397) asserts that " one should meditate on the mind *(manas)* as *Brahman*." "For truly, beings here are born from mind *(manas)*, when born, they live by mind and into mind, when departing, they enter," states *Tait Up* III.4.1 (p. 555). In *Aitareya Up* III.1.3 (p. 523) we are told that the "world" is guided by and established in intelligence *(prajñāna)*. The *Kauṣītaki Up* (III.6) (pp. 779–780) states that when intelligence is applied to any faculty, a unity is experienced; all elements *(bhūta*s*)* depend on the mind. Yet the mind is not an autonomous power that creates out of nothing; as the *Kauṣītaki Up* (III.8) (p. 782) makes clear, a naive idealism is not implied.

6. See C. Chapple (1986: 35).

7. See, for example, the *Mait Up,* which sheds some light on the relationship between the mind and spiritual emancipation. Under the condition of ignorance, the mind is burdened with various propensities that conceal its potential power. In this deluded state a person is karmically predisposed to repeat patterns of affliction remaining entrapped in the saṃsāric world. One can, however, become freed from the enslavement to action caused by ignorance by tapping into the inherent powers of the mind.

Mait Up VI.34 (pp. 845–846) asserts that worldly existence and identity are generated by thought *(citta):* "One's own thought, indeed, is *saṃsāra;* let a man cleanse it by effort. What a man thinks, that he becomes, this is the eternal mystery." This purification process involves both thought and action and necessitates a restructuring of the intentions that lead to human action. Freedom *(mokṣa)* involves a radical transfomation of perspective so that the mind (and person) is no longer obsessed by the objects of sense due to the affects of past experience. The impure mind is purified, made tranquil, and the binding effects of *saṃsāra* are overcome. In the Sāṃkhya system the highest predisposition *(bhāva)* of the intellect *(buddhi)* is knowledge *(jñāna)* (*SK* 23), which alone can liberate the Sāṃkhyan from attachment and bondage.

8. See Monier-Williams, *A Sanskrit-English Dictionary,* p. 395.

9. Ibid.

10. See (e.g.) *ṚV* I.163.11 as well as *ṚV* V.79 and X.103.12; see also *Atharva Veda* I.34.2 (in the sense of "intent"—a love spell).

11. See (e.g.) *Mait Up* VI.34. See also *Chānd Up* VII.5.2 (where the term appears in the following compounds: *cittavant, citta-ātman,* and *citta-ekāyana*), and *Chānd Up* VII.5.3. Cf. Radhakrishnan (1953) and R. E. Hume (1921), who both often translate *citta* as "thought."

12. G. Feuerstein (1980: 58).

13. Cf. *BG* VI.18, where Radhakrishnan (1948: 199) translates *citta* as "mind," referring to the disciplined mind established in the Self *(ātman).* See also *BG* VI.19–20, and XIII.9, where *sama-cittatva* ("equal-mindedness") is regarded as a manifestation of knowledge *(jñāna).*

14. *YS* IV.19 (see n. 198 in chapter 2).

15. *TV* II.20 (p. 87): *buddhidarpaṇe puruṣapratibimbasaṃskrāntir eva buddhipratisaṃveditvaṃ puṃsaḥ.* I will be saying more on "reflection theory" in Yoga later in this chapter.

16. *YS* IV.22; see n. 250 in chapter 2.

17. *YS* IV.23 (p. 197): *draṣṭṛdṛśyoparaktam cittam sarvārtham.* "[Due to] the mind being colored by the seer and the seeable, [it can, therefore, know] all purposes."

18. Koelman (1970: 22) argues that the English word "consciousness" (cognate with the Latin *con-scire*) implies duality and should, therefore, be used when referring to the "mind." He adds (ibid), "The term 'awareness,' however . . . excludes by its very morphological structure that connotation of duality" and should be used when referring to *puruṣa.* However, by qualifying the term "consciousness" as being either: (1) empirical (phenomenal), i.e., mind, or (2) pure or immortal, the distinction between *citta* and *puruṣa* is clarified.

19. *YS* I.2 and I.6–11. The *vṛtti*s are discussed later in this chapter.

20. Vyāsa (*YB* II.6) and Vācaspati (see, for example, *TV* II.20) often use the terms interchangeably. G. Koelman suggests (1970: 103) that since Yoga purports to be a "technique" for the transcendence of all experiential states, it "is entitled to equate the mind with that where the resulting elaboration is impressed, it takes the *terminus a quo* in lieu of the *terminus ad quem.* This is the reason why . . . *(buddhi)* and mind *(manas)* are often used indiscriminately. This is also the reason why a more general, a more extensive term, comprising the whole complex organism of experience, occurs by far most frequently, viz. *citta.*"

21. See R. Prasāda (1912: 5), S. Dasgupta (1920, 1922), I. K. Taimni (1961: 6), S. Purohit Swami (1973: 25), H. Āraṇya (1963 :7), Bangali Baba (1976: 106), Tola and Dragonetti (1987: 3), C. Chapple and E. Kelly (1990: 33).

22. See Swami Vivekānanda (1966), J. H. Woods (1914), and H. Zimmer (1951).

23. See G. Koelman (1970: 99).

24. See M. Eliade (1969: 36) and G. Feuerstein (1979a: 26).

25. See G. Larson (1987: 27).

26. See J. W. Hauer (1958: 239).

27. See H. Jacobi (1929).

28. See C. H. Johnston (1912).

29. See M. N. Dvivedī (1930) and J. R. Ballantyne (1852–53).

30. See G. Jha (1907).

31. S. Dasgupta (1920: 92).

32. G. Koelman (1970: 100).

33. G. Feuerstein (1980: 58).

34. *YV* I.2 (p. 33): *cittaṃ antaḥkaraṇa sāmānyam ekasya ivāntaḥkaraṇasya vṛttibhedamātreṇa cātudhār vibhāgāt.*

35. *YS* I.2, 30, 33, 37; II.54; III.1, 9, 11, 12, 19, 34, 38; IV.4, 5, 15, 16, 17, 18, 21, 22, 23, 26.

36. *YS* I.35 (p. 39): *viṣayavatī vā pravṛttir utpannā manasaḥ sthitinibandhanī; YS* II.53 (p. 115): *dhāraṇāsu ca yogyatā manasaḥ.*

37. *YS* III.48 (p. 167): *tato manojavitvaṃ vikaraṇabhāvaḥ pradhānajayaś ca.*

38. See Koelman (1970: 104).

39. *YB* I.10 connects *manas* with sleep and *YB* I.34 with breath or life energy *(prāṇa); YB* I.36 links *manas* with sense-activity. See also *YB* II.15, 30; IV.3, 7, 11.

40. *YS* IV.21 (p. 196): *cittāntaradṛśye buddhibuddher atiprasaṅgaḥ smṛtisaṃkaraś ca.* "In trying to see the mind with another [mind] there is an overextending of the intellect from the intellect resulting in a confusion of memory." Refer to n. 16 above and text on *YS* IV.22.

41. As Vyāsa asserts in *YB* I.2 and which will be examined later.

42. See n. 17 above.

43. *YS* IV.4 (p. 178): *nirmāṇacittānyasmitāmātrāt.*

44. *YB* IV.3 (p. 178): *yadā tu yogī bahūnkāyān nirmimīte tadā kim eka manaskās te bhavanty athān eka manaskā iti.*

45. *YS* IV.1 (p. 176): *janmauṣadhimantratapaḥsamādhijāḥ siddhayaḥ.* "Powers arise due to birth, drugs, *mantra,* ascesis or from *samādhi.*"

46. *YB* IV.4 (p. 178): *asmitāmātraṃ cittakāraṇam upādāya nirmāṇacittāni karoti, tataḥ sacittāni bhavantīti.*

47. See *YB* IV.5 (p. 179).

48. *YS* IV.5 (p. 179): *pravṛttibhede prayojakaṃ cittamekamanekeṣām.*

49. See Feuerstein (1979a: 129).

50. See (1980: 46) and (1979a: 128).

51. See Feuerstein (1980: 58–59).

52. See *YS* III.55 (p. 175): *sattvapuruṣayoḥ śuddhisāmye kaivalyam iti.* "In the sameness (i.e., likeness) of purity between the *sattva* [of the mind] and the *puruṣa,* the aloneness (i.e., liberation) [is established]." See also Chapple and Kelly (1990: 108–109).

53. *YS* IV.14 (p. 188). *pariṇāmaikatvād vastutattvam.*

54. *YS* IV.15 (p. 190): *vastusāmye cittabhedāt tayor vibhaktaḥ panthāḥ. YS* IV.16 (p. 192): *na caikacittatantraṃ vastu tadapramāṇakaṃ tadā kiṃ syāt;* this *sūtra* is missing in some of the manuscripts (e.g., in Bhoja Rāja's *RM*) and it is possible that it is an original part of Vyāsa's commentary.

55. See n. 53 above and translation of *YS* IV.14 in the main text.

56. See *YB* IV.14 (pp. 188–189). Vyāsa no doubt was aware of the Buddhist school founded by Asaṅga (which probably postdates Patañjali). *YS* IV.14–16 may well refer to an earlier Vijñānavāda school. Chapple and Kelly (1990: 7) argue that Patañjali need not be seen as explicitly polemicizing against this "idealist" view, but as "merely advancing the Sāṃkhya perspective that all things stem from *prakṛti* through *pariṇāma.*"

57. *BG* XVIII.23–25; see Radhakrishnan (1948: 359–360).

58. See Monier-Williams (1899: 258).

59. This formula of three kinds of *karma* has been taught, for example, in the later Advaita Vedānta tradition; cf. H. Zimmer (1951), *Philosophies of India,* pp. 441–442.

60. *YS* III.22 (p. 147): *sopakramaṃ nirupakramaṃ . . . karma . . . vā.*

61. *YB* III.22 (p. 147): *āyurvipākaṃ karma dvividhaṃ sopakramaṃ nirupakramaṃ ca. tatra yathā''rdraṃ vastraṃ vitanitaṃ laghīyasā kālena śuṣyet tathā sopakramaṃ. yathā ca tad eva saṃpiṇḍitaṃ cireṇa saṃśuṣyed evaṃ nirupakramam.*

62. *YS* II.3 (p. 59): *avidyāsmitārāgadveṣābhiniveśāḥ kleśāḥ.*

63. *YS* II.12 (p. 67): *kleśamūlaḥ karmāśayo dṛṣṭādṛṣṭajanmavedanīyaḥ.*

64. *YS* II.13 (p. 68): *sati mūle tadvipāko jātyāyurbhogāḥ.*

65. *YS* II.14 (p. 73): *te hlādaparitāpaphalāḥ puṇyāpuṇyahetutvāt.*

66. *YB* II.15 (p. 74): *rāgajaḥ karmāśaya.*

67. *YB* II.15 (p. 76): *dveṣajaḥ karmāśaya.*

68. *YB* II.15 (p. 76): *karmāśayo lobhān mohāc ca.*

69. Monier-Williams (1899: 1120).

70. Ibid.

71. Ibid. See also J. Lipner (1994), *Hindus: Their Religious Beliefs and Practices,* p. 264.

72. Monier-Williams (1899: 1120).

73. See J. H. Wood (1914), G. Jha (1907), and S. Dasgupta (1920, 1924, 1930).

74. See P. Corrada (1969: 204).

75. See G. Koelman (1970: 278).

76. See Bangali Baba (1976: 9).

77. See G. Feuerstein (1979a: 57; 1980: 68).

78. *YS* IV.9 (p. 181): *jātideśākālavyavahitānām apy ānantaryaṃ smṛtisaṃskārayor ekarūpatvāt.*

79. *YB* IV.9 (p. 182): *jātideśākālavyavahitebhyaḥ saṃskārebhyaḥ smṛtiḥ. smṛteś ca punaḥ saṃskārā ity evam ete smṛtisaṃskārāḥ karmāśayavṛttilābhavaśādvyajyante.*

80. *YS* II.12–14; see notes 63 - 65 above.

81. *YS* IV.10 (p. 182): *tāsāmanāditvaṃ cā''śiṣo nityatvāt.* "They (the *saṃskāras*) are beginningless, due to the perpetuity of desire."

82. *YB* IV.9 (pp. 181–182): *yathā'nubhavās tathā saṃskārāḥ. te ca karma vāsanānurūpāḥ.* "As were the experiences, so are the *saṃskāras*. And they are in the form of the karmically derived habit patterns or *vāsanās*."

83. G. Larson (1993),"The *Trimūrti* of *Smṛti,*" *PEW* 43.3: 380. See also *YB* II.13 and *YS* IV.8-9.

84. See the section on *vṛtti* later in this chapter.

85. *YB* I.5 (p. 10): *tathā jātīyakāḥ saṃskārā vṛttibhir eva kriyante. saṃskāraiś ca vṛttaya iti. evaṃ vṛttisaṃskāracakram aniśam āvartate.*

86. See n. 182, chapter 2, on *YB* IV.11.

87. G. Feuerstein (1990), *Encyclopedic Dictionary of Yoga,* p. 309.

88. *YS* III.9 (p. 122): *vyutthānanirodhasaṃskārayor abhibhavaprādurbhāvau nirodhakṣaṇacittānvayo nirodhapariṇāmaḥ.*

89. *YS* III.10 (p. 123): *tasya praśāntavāhitā saṃskārāt.*

90. *YS* III.18 (p. 144): *saṃskārasākṣātkaraṇāt pūrvajātijñānam.*

91. G. Feuerstein (1980: 68).

92. *YS* III.50 (p. 168).

93. *YB* III.50 (p. 168): *dagdhaśālibījakalpāni.*

94. *YS* II.7 (p. 64): *sukhānuśayī rāgaḥ.*

95. *YS* II.8 (p. 65): *duḥkhānuśayī dveṣaḥ.*

96. *YB* II.15 (p. 76): *kā punaḥ saṃskāraduḥkhatā. sukhānubhavāt sukhasaṃskārāśayo duḥkhānubhavād api duḥkhsaṃskārāśaya iti. evaṃ karmabhyo vipake 'nubhūyamāne sukhe duḥkhe vā punaḥ karmāśayapracaya.*

97. *TV* II.13 (p. 68): *sukhaduḥkhaphalo hi karmāśayas tādarthyena tannāntarīyakatayā janmāyuṣī api prasūte. sukhaduḥkhe ca rāgadveṣānuṣakte tadavinirbhāgavartinī tadabhāve na bhavataḥ . . . tadiyam ātmabhūmiḥ kleśasalilāvasiktā karmaphalaprasavakṣetram . . .*

98. The term *vāsanā*, which will hitherto be translated as "habit pattern," is a derivative of the root *vas* meaning "to dwell, abide, remain." It is not by accident nor a mere coincidence that the term *vāsanā* basically represents selfhood under the influence of ignorance, i.e., as a mistaken identity that being extrinsic to *puruṣa,* is defined by or rather "dwells in" and is dependent on the "objects" of experience. It has been translated as "subconscious impression" (G. Jha, 1907), "residual potency" (R. Prasāda, 1912), "psychical subliminal impression" (Koelman, 1970: 50), "subliminal-trait" (G. Feuerstein, 1979a: 130) and "habit pattern" (C. Chapple and E. Kelly, 1990: 110).

99. *YS* IV.8 (p. 180): *tatas tadvipākanuguṇānām evābhivyaktir vāsanānām.* "Therefore [follows] the manifestation of those habit patterns which correspond to the fruition of that *[karma].*"

100. G. Feuerstein (1979a: 131).

101. *YB* I.24 (p. 26): *tadanuguṇā vāsanā āśayāḥ.*

102. Cf. *YS* IV.9 in n. 78 above.

103. *YB* II.13 (p. 71): *kleśakarmavipākānubhavanirvārtitābhistu vāsanābhiranādikālasaṃmūrchitamidaṃ cittaṃ vicitrīkṛtamiva sarvato matsyajālaṃ granthibhirivā'-'tatamityetā anekabhavapūrvikā vāsanāḥ.*

104. See n. 63 above.

105. See nn. 65 and 97 above.

106. See n. 89 above on *YS* III.10; Vyāsa's commentary—*YS* III.10—(p. 123) runs as follows: *nirodhasaṃskārābhyāsa pāṭavāpekṣā praśāntavāhitā cittasya bhavati.* "From practice [generating] *saṃskāra*s of cessation, there comes about a calm flow of the mind."

107. *YS* IV.7 (p. 180). *karmāśuklākṛṣṇaṃ yoginastrividhamitareṣām.*

108. See also *YS* II.14 and the terms *apuṇya* and *puṇya* in n. 65 above.

109. *YB* IV.7 (p. 180): *catuṣpadī khalviyaṃ karmajātiḥ. kṛṣṇā śuklakṛṣṇā śuklāśuklākṛṣṇā ceti. tatra kṛṣṇā durātmanām. śuklakṛṣṇā bahiḥsādhanasādhyā. tatra parapīḍānugrahadvāreṇaiva karmāśayapracayaḥ. śuklā tapaḥ svādhyāyadhyānavatām. sā hi kevale manasyāthattatvādabahiḥsādhanādhīnā na parānpīḍayitvā bhavati. aśuklākṛṣṇā saṃnyāsināṃ kṣīṇakleśānāṃ caramadehānām iti. tatrāśuklaṃ yogina eva phalasaṃnyāsādakṛṣṇam cānupādānāt. itareṣāṃ tu bhūtānāṃ pūrvam eva trividham iti.*

110. Including of course the higher form of *samādhi* called *asaṃprajñāta,* through which the mind is completely cleansed of ignorance; see *YS* I.18 and *YB* I.18.

111. The term *niṣ-kāma* (see discussion in chapter 1) is often translated as "desireless" and is used by Vijñāna Bhikṣu in *YV* IV.7; see *YV* (1989: 19).

112. See *YV* IV.7 (ibid.), where Vijñāna Bhikṣu distinguishes between true and false *saṃnyāsins*, i.e., of those who have transcended egoic identity and those who have merely put on the *saṃnyāsin*'s robes and act as if they have truly renounced. The true mark of renunciation, as Bhikṣu goes on to explain, is the purification of affliction. If affliction is sufficiently dissolved, then even one engaged in the duties of a householder can be freed from egoic attachment to the results of actions. See *YV* (1989: 20).

113. *YS* IV.24 (p. 199): *tadasaṃkhyeyavāsanābhiścitramapi parārthaṃ saṃhatyakāritvāt.*

114. *YS* II.21 (p. 89): *tadartha eva dṛśyasyā'tmā.* "The nature of the seeable is only for the purpose of this [seer]." Cf. *SK* 36–37 and *YS* II.18 as well as *YS* III.35 and IV.34.

115. *YB* IV.11 (p. 185): *manas tu sādhikāram āśrayo vāsanānām. na hy avasitādhikāre manasi nirāśrayā vāsanāḥ sthātum utsahante.*

116. *YB* IV.24 (pp. 199–200): *saṃhatyakāriṇā cittena na svārthana bhavitavyam, na sukhacittaṃ sukhārthaṃ na jñānaṃ jñānārtham ubhayam apy etat parārtham. yaś ca bhogenāpavargeṇa cārthanārthavan puruṣaḥ sa eva paro . . .*

117. *YS* II.23 (p. 91): *svasvāmiśaktyoḥ svarūpopalabdhihetuḥ saṃyogaḥ.* "The conjunction [between the seer and the seeable] is the cause of the apprehension of the own-form of the powers of owner and owned."

118. *YS* II.21: see n. 114 above.

119. *YB* IV.10 (pp. 183–184): *ghaṭaprāsādapradīpakalpaṃ saṃkocavikāsi cittaṃ śarīraparimāṇākāramātram ity apare pratipannāḥ. tathā cāntarābhāvaḥ saṃsāraś ca yukta iti. vṛttir evāsya vibhunaś cittasya saṃkocavikāsinīty ācāryaḥ.*

120. *YB* IV.10 (p. 184): *dharmādi nimittāpekṣam.*

121. *TV* IV.10 (p. 184): *tasmādāhaṃkārikatvāc cetaso'haṃkārasya ca gaganamaṇḍalavat trailokyavyāpitvād vibhutvaṃ manasaḥ. evaṃ cedasya vṛttir api vibhvīti sarvajñatāpattir ity ata uktam.* Cf. also *TV* IV.17 (p. 193).

122. G. Koelman (1970: 104).

123. Ibid.

124. H. Āraṇya (1963: 395).

125. *YS* III.49 (p. 167): *sattvapuruṣānyatākhyātimātrasya sarvabhāvādhiṣṭhātṛtvaṃ sarvajñātṛtvaṃ ca.* "Only from the discernment of the difference between *puruṣa* and the *sattva* is there sovereignty over all states of existence and omniscience."

126. *TV* IV.10; cf. Feuerstein (1980: 61), who argues that Vācaspati's notion of an omniscient *kāraṇa-citta* "makes the concept of *puruṣa* (Self) superfluous." It makes

more sense, however, to understand the *citta* in the above way as serving a cosmic purpose for the sake of the *puruṣa,* the "omniscient one" or "knower," without which the *kāraṇa-citta* would be incapable of registering any knowledge whatsoever. The *kārya-citta* could be conceived of as the individual mind(s) arising from the cosmic or root *citta.*

127. See notes 14 and 16 above on *YS* IV.19 and IV.22 respectively.

128. See n. 117 above.

129. See Monier-Williams (1899: 1009).

130. Ibid, p. 1010.

131. See Woods (1914: 8), Koelman (1970: 86), Feuerstein (1979a: 26), Chapple and Kelly (1990: 33); see also Halbfass (1991), *Tradition and Reflection: Explorations in Indian Thought,* p. 227.

132. See Taimni (1961: 6), Āraṇya (1963: 7), and Prasāda (1912: 5).

133. See Müller (1899: 337).

134. See Hauer (1958: 240).

135. See Purohit Swami (1973: 25).

136. See Tola and Dragonetti (1987: 3).

137. See Larson (1993: 377), who as well suggests "functions" as an appropriate translation for *vṛtti.*

138. See Hiriyanna (1949).

139. *YS* I.6 (p. 10): *pramāṇaviparyayavikalpanidrāsmṛtayaḥ.*

140. *YS* I.7–11 (pp. 10–16).

141. *YS* I.7 (p. 10): *pratyakṣānumānāgamāḥ pramāṇāni.*

142. *YS* I.8 (p. 12): *viparyayo mithyājñānam atadrūpapratiṣṭham.* "Error is incorrect knowledge not based on the [actual] form [of an object]."

143. See n. 62 above.

144. *YB* I.8 (p. 13): *sa kasmānna pramāṇam. yataḥ pramāṇena bādhyate. bhūtārtha viṣayatvāt pramāṇasya. tatra pramāṇena bādhanam apramāṇasya dṛṣṭam. tad yathā dvicandra darśanaṃ sadviṣayeṇaikacandradarśanena bādhyata iti. seyaṃ pañcaparvā bhavaty avidyā, avidyāsmitārāgadveṣābhiniveśāḥ kleśā iti. eta eva svasaṃjñābhis tamo moho mahāmohas tāmisro'ndhatāmisra.*

145. *YS* II.17; see n. 199 in chapter 2.

146. *YS* II.24 (p. 94): *tasya hetur avidyā.* "The cause of this [conjunction] is ignorance."

147. *YS* II.4 (p. 59) states: *avidyā kṣetraṃ uttareṣāṃ prasuptatanuvicchinnodārāṇām.* "Ignorance is the origin of the others (i.e., afflictions), which may be dormant, attenuated, intercepted, or fully active."

148. See n. 62 above.

149. See n. 168 below.

150. See n. 169 below.

151. I. K. Taimni (1961: 130).

152. *YS* II.5 (p. 61): *anityāśuciduḥkhānātmasu nityaśucisukhātmakhyātiravidyā.*

153. Text taken from Larson (1969); *SK* 47 (p. 275): *pañca viparyayabhedā bhavanty . . . ; SK* 48 (p. 275): *bhedas tamaso'ṣṭavidho mohasya ca daśavidho mahāmohaḥ. tāmisro'ṣṭādaśadhā tathā bhavaty andhatāmisraḥ.*

154. *TV* I.8.

155. *YV* I.8 and II.5.

156. *TV* I.8 (p. 13). *avidyā sāmānyam avidyāsmitādiṣu pañcasu parvasv ity arthaḥ.*

157. *YV* I.8 (p. 73): *pañcaparvā yāvidyā saṃsārānarthabījaṃ sā, iyam eva = mithyājñānarūpa vṛttir eva, etad viśeṣa eveti yāvat.* *YV* I.8 (p. 71): *bhramas thale jñānākārasyaiva viṣaye samāropa iti bhāvaḥ. saṃśayasyāpy atraivāntarbhāvaḥ.*

158. *YB* II.3 (p. 59): *kleśā iti pañca viparyayā ity arthaḥ. te spandamānā guṇādhikāraṃ draḍhayanti, pariṇāmam avasthā payanti, kāryakāraṇa srota unnamayanti, parasparānugrahatantrī bhūtvā karmavipākaṃ cābhinirharantīti.* The term *spanda* ("quiver," "vibration"), used by Vyāsa in the above description, refers not to activity or movement as ordinarily understood but rather to the first "movement" of (mis)identification with *guṇas*.

159. I am following the explanations provided by Vijñāna Bhikṣu (*YV* I.8) and/or Vācaspati Miśra (*TV* I.8) after having consulted U. Arya (1986: 168–170). For explanations of the *viparyayas* in Sāṃkhya, see Larson (1987: 57–58).

160. See *YV* I.8 (p. 74).

161. Ibid.: *aṣṭasvaṇimādyaiśvaryeṣvan ātmasvātmīyabuddhir asmitā.*

162. *YS* III.45 (p. 164): *tato'ṇimādiprādurbhāvaḥ kāyasaṃpattaddharmānabighātaś ca.* "Hence [from the conquest of the elements] arise the manifestation [of eight powers], such as becoming minute and so forth, perfection of the body, and unassailability of its [bodily] attributes." See Vyāsa's description of these powers in *YB* III.45 (pp. 164–165).

163. *YV* I.8 (p. 74): *svatvāsmitayoḥ paryāya tvāt,* i.e., *asmitā* is derived from *asmi* (I am). The beingness of "I" in this context means the same as belonging to "I" or ego-possession/attachment. To misperceive the *siddhis* as being an intrinsic aspect of self-identity and therefore to possess them as such is to feed into the delusion termed *moha.*

164. *YV* I.8 (pp. 74–75): *tathā dṛṣṭānuśravika bhedena daśasu śabdādi viṣayeṣu rāgo daśavidho mahāmohaḥ.* *TV* I.8 (p. 13): *tathā yogenāṣṭastavidham aiśvaryamupādāya siddho bhūtva dṛṣṭānuśravikāñśabdādīndaśa viṣayān bhokṣya ity evam ātmikā pratipattir mahāmoho rāgaḥ.*

165. *YV* I.8 (p. 75): *tathāṣṭaiśvaryasya viṣayadaśakasya ca paripanthinidveṣo'ṣṭādaśadhā tāmisraḥ.*

166. *TV* I.8 (p. 13): *evam aṇimādi guṇa saṃpattau dṛṣṭānuśravikaviṣayapratyupasthāne ca kalpānte sarvam etannaṅkṣyatīti yastrāsaḥ so'bhiniveśo'ndhatāmisraḥ.*

167. See Arya (1986: 170).

168. *YB* II.7 (p. 65): *sukhābhijñasya sukhānusmṛti pūrvaḥ sukhe tatsādhane vā yo gardhas tṛṣṇā lobhaḥ sa rāga iti.* "When one familiar with a pleasure now has a memory of it, one's eagerness for the pleasure or for the means to it, that thirst or greed, is [called] attachment." See also n. 94 above on *YS* II.7.

169. *YB* II.8 (p. 65): *duḥkhābhijñasya duḥkhānusmṛti pūrvā duḥkhe tatsādhane vā yaḥ pratigho manyurjighāṃsā krodhoḥ sa dveṣaḥ.* "When one familiar with a pain now has a memory of it, that aversion toward the pain or what causes it, the desire for retaliation, malice, revenge and anger, is [called] aversion." See n. 95 above on *YS* II.8.

170. *YS* II.9 (p. 65): *svarasavāhī viduṣo'pi tathā rūḍho'bhiniveśaḥ.* "Desire for continuity, arising even in the wise (sage), is sustained by its own inclination." Vyāsa seems to take the primary meaning of *abhiniveśa* to be fear of death (annihilation). Unlike *rāga* and *dveṣa,* and their resultant pleasure-pain impressions of which examples are easily found in this life itself, the *saṃskāra* of fear and anxiety involving death cannot be so easily accounted for, there being no such definitive experiences in this life.

Thus, for Vyāsa, the idea of a previous death and the experience of former lives is confirmed. *Abhiniveśa* arises naturally and spontaneously from the habit patterns *(vāsanā*s*)* of the past experiences of death pangs (*YB* II.9; pp. 65–66).

171. *YS* III.54 (p. 174).

172. Cf. for example, Koelman (1970: 183–184), and Feuerstein (1979a: 32); both appear to overlook this key insight into Yoga epistemology and its implications for understanding the meaning of Patañjali's whole system. See also our discussion on *nirodha* in chapter 4.

173. See *YV* I.8 (p. 71): *atra ca śāstre'nyathākhyātiḥ siddhānto na tu sāṃkhyavad avivekamātram.*

174. See n. 152 above.

175. *YB* II.5 (p. 63): *yathā nāmitro mitrābhāvo na mitramātraṃ kiṃ tu tadviruddhaḥ sapatanaḥ . . ., evaṃ aviḍyā na pramāṇaṃ na pramāṇābhāvaḥ kim tu vidyāviparītaṃ jñānāntaram avidyeti.*

176. *YS* I.9 (p. 13): *śabdajñānānupātī vastuśūnyo vikalpaḥ.*

177. See I. K. Taimni's (1961) usage.

178. See R. S. Mishra's (1972) usage.

179. *YB* I.7 (p. 12): *āptena dṛṣṭo'numito vārthaḥ paratra svabodhasaṃkrāntaye śabdenopadiśyate, śabdāt tadartha viṣayā vṛttiḥ śrotur āgamaḥ.*

180. *YB* I.9 (pp. 13–14): *sa na pramāṇopārohī na viparyayopārohī ca. vastuśūnyatve'pi śabdajñāna māhātmya nibandhano vyavahāro dṛśyate. tadyathā caitanyaṃ puruṣasya svarūpam iti. yadā citir eva puruṣas tadā kim atra kena vyapadiśyate. bhavati ca vyapadeśe vṛttiḥ. yathā caitrasya gaur iti. tathā pratiṣid-dhavastudharmo niṣkriyaḥ puruṣaḥ.*

181. Feuerstein (1979a: 32).

182. *YS* I.10 (p. 15): *abhāvapratyayālambanā vṛttir nidrā.*

183. *YB* I.10 (p. 15): *sā ca saṃprabodhe pratyavamarśāt pratyayaviśeṣaḥ. kathaṃ, sukham ahamasvāpsam.*

184. *YS* I.38 (p. 41): *svapnanidrājñānālambanaṃ vā.* "Or resting on the knowledge [derived] from dreams or sleep [the mind is made clear]."

185. *YS* I.11 (p. 16): *anubhūtaviṣayāsaṃpramoṣaḥ smṛtiḥ.*

186. *YB* I.11 (p. 16): *kiṃ pratyayasya cittaṃ smarati āhosvid viṣayasyeti.*

187. Ibid.: *grāhyoparaktaḥ pratyayo grāhyagrahaṇobhayākāranirbhāsas taj-jātīyakaṃ saṃskāram ārabhate.*

188. See n. 187 above.

189. *YB* I.11 (p. 16): *sa saṃskāraḥ svavyañjakāñjanas tadākārām eva grāhyag-rahaṇobhayātmikāṃ smṛtiṃ janayati.*

190. See *YV* I.11 (p. 88).

191. *YB* I.11 (p. 16): *tatra grahaṇākārapūrvā buddhiḥ.*

192. See *YV* I.11 (p. 88): *vyākhyāyānuvyavasāya . . .*

193. *YB* I.11 (p. 16): *grāhyākārapūrvā smṛtiḥ.*

194. *YB* I.11 (p. 17): *sarvāḥ smṛtayaḥ pramāṇaviparyayavikalpanidrāsmṛtīnām anubhavāt prabhavanti.*

195. See *TV* I.11 (p. 16).

196. Without explaining himself further, Bhoja Rāja asserts that of the five types of *vṛtti*s, the means of knowledge or valid cognition, error, and conceptualization occur in the wakeful state *(jāgrat)*. The experience of these three combined, masquerading as

direct perception (*pratyakṣa*), becomes the dream state (*svapna*). Sleep is a unique state in that it is marked by the absence of other *vṛtti*s even though it is in itself a *vṛtti*. Memory is the effect of any or all of these *vṛtti*s. *RM* I.11 (p. 4) states: *tatra pramāṇaviparyayavikalpā jāgrad avasthā. ta eva tadanubhava balāt prakṣīyamāṇāḥ svapnaḥ. nidrā tu asaṃvedyamānaviṣayā. smṛtiś ca pramānaviparyayavikalpanidrānimittā.*

197. *YV* I.11 (p. 90): *etāḥ sarvāḥ pramāṇādi vṛttayo buddhi dravyasya suvarṇasy eva pratimā''divad viṣayākārā dravyarūpāḥ pariṇāmaḥ . . .*

198. *YB* I.11 (p. 17): *sarvāś caitā vṛttayaḥ sukhaduḥkhamohātmikāḥ. sukhaduḥkhamohāś ca kleśeṣu vyākhyeyāḥ.*

199. *YB* I.11 (p. 17): *sukhānuśayī rāgaḥ, duḥkhānuśayī dveṣaḥ, mohaḥ punar avidyeti.*

200. *YS* I.5 (p. 9): *vṛttayaḥ pañcatayyaḥ kliṣṭākliṣṭāḥ.* "The modifications are fivefold; afflicted or nonafflicted."

201. *YSS* in G. Jha (1894: 3): *buddhivṛttiś ca pradīpasya śikhāvad buddher agrabhāgo yena cittasyaikāgratāvyavahāro bhavati. sa eva ca bhāga indriyadvāra bāhyārthe saṃyujya arthākareṇa pariṇāmate.*

202. *Sāṃkhya-Pravacana-Sūtra* V.107 (p. 488): *bhāgaguṇābhyāṃ tattvāntaraṃ vṛttiḥ sambandhārthaṃ sarpati iti.* Sanskrit text from N. Sinha, trans. (1915), *The Sāṃkhya Philosophy,* in *The Sacred Books of the Hindus,* Vol. 11.

203. In R. Garbe, ed. (1943), *Sāṃkhya-Pravacana-Bhāṣya or Commentary on the Exposition of the Sāṃkhya Philosophy by Vijñānabhikṣu,* vol. II; see *SPB* V.107 (p. 140).

204. *TV* III.47 (p. 166): *vṛttir ālocanaṃ viṣayākāra pariṇatir iti yāvat.*

205. *RM* I.2 (p. 2): *vṛttayo'ṅgāṅgibhāvapariṇāmarūpās tāsāṃ . . .*

206. *RM* I.5 (p. 3): *vṛttayaś cittasya pariṇāmaviśeṣāḥ.*

207. *TV* I.2 (p. 6): *yadā ca vivekakhyātir api heyā tadā kaiva kathā vṛttyantarāṇāṃ doṣabahulānām iti bhāvaḥ.*

208. *YB* I.5, 8, 11 and II.11.

209. See, for example, *YS* II.15: *guṇa-vṛtti;* see also *YS* II.50 and III.43.

210. Cf. Koelman (1970: 86), who appears to equate the term *vṛtti* with *pariṇāma*.

211. See n. 182 in chapter 2.

212. See n. 200 above.

213. *YB* I.5 (p. 9): *kleśahetukāḥ karmāśayapracaye kṣetrībhūtāḥ kliṣṭāḥ. khyātiviṣayā guṇādhikāra virodhinyo'kliṣṭāḥ.*

214. *TV* I.5 (p. 9): *kleśā asmitādayo hetavaḥ pravṛttikāraṇāṃ yāsāṃ vṛttīnāṃ tās tathoktāḥ. yad vā puruṣārthapradhānasya rajastamomayīnāṃ hi vṛttīnāṃ kleśakāraṇatvena kleśāyaiva pravṛttiḥ.*

215. *YV* I.5 (p. 57): *atra ca hetuḥ prayojanam. kleśaś cātra mukhya eva grāhyo duḥkhākhyaḥ. tathā ca kleśahetukāḥ duḥkhaphalikāviṣayākāravṛttaya ity arthaḥ.*

216. G. Feuerstein (1980: 66).

217. *YV* I.5 (p. 57): *akliṣṭa akleśaphalikāḥ.*

218. Cf. Āraṇya (1963: 18).

219. *TV* I.5 (p. 9): *vidhūtarajastamaso buddhisattvasya praśāntavāhinaḥ prajñāprasādaḥ khyātis tayā viṣayiṇyā.*

220. *YV* I.5 (p. 57): *khyātisādhanasyāpi saṃgrahāya viṣaya padam iti.*

221. *YV* I.5 (p. 57): *tāś ca guṇādhikāravirodhinyaḥ, guṇānāṃ sattvādīnām adhikāraḥ kāryārambhanaṃ tadvirodhinyo'vidyākāmakarmādirūpakāraṇanaśakatvāt. khyātiviṣayā vivekakhyāti sambaddhā ity arthaḥ.*

222. Rāmānanda Yati (1903), *Pātañjaladarśanam with a gloss called Maṇiprabhā*, p. 4.

223. See *YS* I.18 and *YB* I.18; *YS* III.50 states that the yogin must develop dispassion/detachment even toward discriminative discernment and its effects, i.e., omniscience and sovereignty over *prakṛti*.

224. *RM* I.5 (p. 3): *kleśair vakṣyamāṇalakṣaṇair ākrāntāḥ kliṣṭāḥ. tadviparītā akliṣṭāḥ.*

225. See Hauer (1958: 243).

226. See, for example, the writings of Taimni, Vivekānanda, Bangali Baba, Rāma Prasāda, Ballentyne, and Max Müller (1899: 337). Purohit (1973) uses "painful" and "pleasurable."

227. See *SPB* II.33 (p. 266) in N. Sinha, trans. (1915), *The Sāṃkhya Philosophy*.

228. See Aniruddha's commentary on the *Sāṃkhya-Sūtras* (p. 1104) in R. Garbe, ed. (1987), *Sāṃkhya Sūtra and Sāṃkhya System*.

229. *YB* II.19; see n. 178 in chapter 2.

230. See, for example, *YS* II.18, 21 and IV.24.

231. *YS* III.9; see n. 88 above.

232. *YB* I.2 (pp. 4–5): *cittaṃ hi prakhyāpravṛttisthitiśīlatvāt triguṇam prakhyārūpaṃ hi cittasattvaṃ rajastamobhyāṃ saṃsṛṣṭam aiśvaryaviṣayapriyaṃ bhavati. tad eva tamasānuviddham adharmājñānāvairāgyānaiśvaryopagaṃ bhavati. tad eva prakṣīṇamohāvaraṇaṃ sarvataḥ pradyotamānam anuviddhaṃ rajoleśamalāpetaṃ svarūpapratiṣṭhaṃ sattvapuruṣānyatākhyātimātraṃ . . .*

233. See *YS* I.15–16 and discussion on *vairāgya* in chapter 4.

234. See Monier-Williams (1899: 234).

235. See Larson (1969: 266).

236. Monier-Williams (1899: 170).

237. On the physical side, *sattva* gives rise to lightness, brightness, and other related material properties and is associated with the color white; *rajas* is responsible for mobility of various kinds and is associated with the color red; *tamas* produces darkness, inertia, decay, and related phenomena and is associated with the color black.

238. See chapters XVII and XVIII in the *BG*.

239. See Feuerstein (1979a: 81). More will be said on yogic liberation and its embodied, ethical implications in chapter 6.

240. *YV* I.5 (p. 58).

241. As, for example, in its role of bringing forth the two processes of the *sāttvika* and *tāmasa ahaṃkāra*, i.e., the manifestation of the subjective sensory world and the objective sensed world respectively.

242. See *TV* I.5 (p. 10).

243. *YB* I.5 (p. 10): *kliṣṭapravāhapatitā apy akliṣṭāḥ. kliṣṭacchidreṣv apy akliṣṭā bhavanti.*

244. See *TV* I.5 (p. 10).

245. See Āraṇya (1963: 18).

246. See *TV* I.5 (p. 10). The process of dispassion (detachment) will be explained in greater detail in chapters 4 through 6.

247. Some of the above examples are taken from Nārāyaṇa Tīrtha's *Yogasiddhāntacandrikā* as cited in Arya (1986: 143).

248. *YS* I.33 (p. 38): *maitrīkaruṇāmuditopekṣāṇāṃ sukhaduḥkhapuṇyāpuṇya-viṣayāṇāṃ bhāvanātaścittaprasādanam.*

249. *YB* I.33 (p. 39): *evamasya bhāvayataḥ śuklo dharma upajāyate. tataś ca cittaṃ prasīdati. prasannam ekāgraṃ sthitipadaṃ labhate.*

250. *YB* I.1 (p. 3). The states of mind according to Yoga will be discussed in chapter 4.

251. See n. 85 above.

252. See n. 36, chapter 2.

253. See n. 36, chapter 2.

254. *YS* II.17; see n. 199 in chapter 2.

255. See n. 121 in chapter 2.

256. See n. 117 above.

257. See *YS* III.35 (n. 196, chapter 2) and III.49 (n. 125 above).

258. See n. 277 below.

259. See n. 261 below.

260. See, for example, n. 265 below.

261. *YB* IV.23 (p. 198): *mano hi mantavyenārthenoparaktaṃ, tatsvayaṃ ca viṣayatvād viṣayiṇā puruṣeṇā''tmīyayā vṛttyā'bhisaṃbaddhaṃ, tadetaccittameva draṣṭṛdṛśyoparaktaṃ viṣayaviṣayinirbhāsaṃ cetanācetanasvarūpāpannaṃ viṣayātmakam apy aviṣayātmakam ivācetanaṃ cetanam iva sphaṭikamaṇikalpaṃ sarvārtham ity ucyate.*

262. *YB* I.4 (pp. 8–9); see n. 277 below.

263. Ibid.; see n. 277 below.

264. See F. Catalina (1968: 136).

265. *TV* I.4 (p. 8): *saṃnidhiś ca . . . yogyatā lakṣaṇaḥ. asti ca puruṣasya bhoktṛśaktiś cittasya bhogyaśaktiḥ.*

266. *YB* II.18 (p. 84): *etena grahaṇadhāraṇohāpoha tattva jñānābhiniveśā buddhau vartamānāḥ puruṣe'dhyāropitasad bhāvāḥ.*

267. *YB* I.4 (p. 8): *vyutthāne yāś cittavṛttayas tadaviśiṣṭavṛttiḥ puruṣaḥ.*

268. See n. 117 above.

269. *YB* II.23 (p. 91): *puruṣaḥ svāmī dṛśyena svena darśanārthaṃ saṃyuktaḥ. tasmāt saṃyogādṛśyasyopalabdhir yā sa bhogaḥ. yā tu draṣṭuḥ svarūpopalabdhiḥ so'pavargaḥ.*

270. *YB* II.23 (pp. 91–92): *darśanakāryāvasānaḥ saṃyoga iti darśanaṃ viyogasya kāraṇam uktam. darśanam adarśanasya pratidvaṃ dvītyadarśanaṃ saṃyoga nimittam uktam. . . . darśanasya bhave bandhakāraṇasyādarśanasya nāśa ity ato darśanaṃ jñānaṃ kaivalyakāraṇam uktam. kiṃ cedam adarśanaṃ nāma.*

271. See *YB* II.23 (pp. 92–93). The eight alternative explanations for *avidyā* listed by Vyāsa, which were probably prevalent during his time, are summarized as follows: (1) the prevailing of the *guṇa*s over the *puruṣa;* (2) the failure of *prakṛti* to bring the *puruṣa* to liberating sight; (3) the fact that the *guṇa*s are purposeful; (4) *avidyā* producing a mentality of its own kind; (5) the manifestation of the latent impressions of activity, the potency for stasis having ceased; (6) the need of *pradhāna* to make itself known; (7) the requirement of the presence of *puruṣa* for things knowable to be known, with an attendant apparent reflection of things knowable back upon the *puruṣa;* and (8) the identity of the failure-to-see with knowledge. Later in *YB* II.23 (p. 94), Vyāsa says that the above explanations are the alternatives contained in the [yogic] *śāstra* and that this multiplicity of opinion concerns a common object, namely the conjunction of the constituents *(guṇas)* [of *prakṛti*] with *puruṣa*. For more on the term *avidyā* see T. S.

Rukmani (1986), "Avidyā in the System of Yoga and an Analysis of the Negation in It," *The Adyar Library Bulletin,* pp. 526–534.

272. *YB* II.23 (p. 92): *avidyā svacittena saha niruddhā svacittasyotpattibījam.*

273. *YS* II.24 (p. 94): *tasya hetur avidyā.*

274. *YB* II.24 (p. 95): *viparyayajñānavāsanetyarthaḥ.*

275. *YB* II.23 (p. 94): *tatra vikalpabahutvametat sarvapuruṣāṇāṃ guṇāṇāṃ saṃyoge sādhāraṇaviṣayam. yastu pratyakcetanasya svabuddhi saṃyogaḥ.*

276. G. Larson (1969: 191).

277. *YB* I.4 (pp. 8–9): *cittaṃ ayaskāntamaṇikalpaṃ saṃnidhimātropakāri dṛśyatvena svaṃ bhavati puruṣasya svāminaḥ. tasmāc cittavṛttibodhe puruṣasyānādiḥ saṃbandho hetuḥ.*

278. *YB* II.18 (pp. 83–84): *yathā vijayaḥ parājayo vā yoddhṛṣu vartamānaḥ svāmini vyapadiśyate, sa hi tatphalasya bhokteti, evaṃ bandhamokṣau buddhāv eva vartamānau puruṣe vyapadiśyate, sa hi tatphalasya bhokteti.*

279. G. Koelman (1970: 143).

280. *TV* II.17 (p. 80): *prāgbhāvitayā saṃyogasyāvidyā kāraṇam sthitihetutayā puruṣārthaḥ kāraṇam tad (= bhogāpavargau puruṣārthatā) vaśena tasya (saṃyogasya) sthiteḥ.* We note here that the purpose "of" the Self *(puruṣa)* is an objective genetive and not a subjective genetive, i.e., *puruṣārtha* means "for the sake of *puruṣa.*" It is not that *puruṣa* actively has purposes.

281. Cf. *BG* XVIII.30–32, which discusses three types of understanding *(buddhi):* (1) a discerning *buddhi* that knows what is to be done, etc., and is sattvic; (2) a *buddhi* that understands incorrectly and whose nature is rajasic; and (3) a *buddhi,* whose nature being tamasic, is completely deluded.

282. *YB* II.6 (p. 64): *ātmabuddhiṃ mohena.*

283. *YB* IV.22 (p. 197): *apariṇāminī hi bhoktṛśaktir apratisaṃkramā ca pariṇāminy arthe pratisaṃkrānt eva tadvṛttimanupatati. tasyaś ca prāpta caitanyopagraha svarūpāyā buddhivṛtter anukārimātratayā, buddhivṛttyaviśiṣṭā hi jñānavṛttir ākhyāyate.*

284. Cf. *YB* IV.23 (p. 198), where Vyāsa uses the term *pratibimba* for "reflection."

285. *YB* II.17 (p. 79): *tadetad dṛśyam ayaskāntamaṇikalpaṃ saṃnidhimātropakāri dṛśyatvena svaṃ bhavati puruṣasya dṛśirūpasya svāminaḥ.*

286. See *YB* IV.22 (p. 197); Vyāsa is quoting some authority here. The verse quoted tells us that the secret cave in which *brahman* is hidden is neither the underworld, nor the mountain cave, nor darkness, nor the hidden caverns of the sea. The last stanza ends thus: *guhā yasyāṃ nihitaṃ brahma śāśvataṃ buddhivṛttimaviśiṣṭāṃ kavayo vedayante.*

287. *TV* I.7 (p. 11): *caitanyam eva buddhidarpaṇa . . .*

288. G. Koelman (1970: 137).

289. *TV* II.17 (p. 79): *citicchāyāpattir eva buddher buddhipratisaṃveditvam udāsīnasyāpi puṃsaḥ.* See also *TV* IV.23 (p. 198): *tacchāyāpattiḥ puruṣasya vṛttiḥ.* See also for *chāyā: TV* II.20, 21, 23; III.35 and IV.22. For a critique of the *cicchāyāpattivāda* adopted by Vācaspati Miśra see Vijñāna Bhiksu's comments in *YV* I.7 (p. 66).

290. See n. 283 above on *YB* IV.22; see also *YB* II.6 and Vācaspati's *STK* 5.

291. *YS* II.20 (p. 87): *draṣṭā dṛśimātraḥ śuddho'pi pratyayānupaśyaḥ.*

292. *YB* II.20 (pp. 87–88): *dṛśimātra iti dṛkśaktir eva viśeṣaṇāparāmṛṣṭety arthaḥ. sa puruṣo buddheḥ pratisaṃvedī. sa buddher na sarūpo nātyantaṃ virūpa iti. na tāvat sarūpaḥ. kasmat. jñātājñāta viṣaya tvāt pariṇāminī hi buddhiḥ. tasyaś ca viṣayo*

gavādirghaṭādirvā jñātaś cājñātaś ceti pariṇāmitvaṃ darśayati. sadājñāta viṣayatvaṃ tu puruṣasyāpariṇāmitvaṃ paridīpayati. kasmat. nahi buddhiś ca nāma puruṣaviṣayaś ca syādagṛhītā gṛhītā ceti siddhaṃ puruṣasya sadājñātaviṣayatvaṃ tataś cāpariṇāmitvam iti. See also *SK* I7 for the proofs establishing *puruṣa*.

293. *YB* II.20 (p. 88–89): *śuddho'py asau pratyayānupaśyo yataḥ. pratyayaṃ bauddham anupaśyati, tamanupaśyannatadātmā'pi tadātmaka iva pratyavabhāsate.*

294. *YB* II.15 (p. 77): *śāntaṃ ghoraṃ mūḍhaṃ vā pratyayaṃ triguṇam evā''rabhante.*

295. *YB* II.18 and II.15.

296. *YB* II.15 (p. 77): *evam ete guṇā itaretarāśrayeṇoparjita sukhaduḥkhamoha pratyayāḥ sarve sarvarūpā bhavantīti, guṇapradhānabhāvakṛtas tveṣāṃ viśeṣa iti . . . tadasya mahato duḥkha samudāyasya prabhavabījam avidyā.*

297. *TV* I.3 (p. 7). It is interesting to note that the terms *upādhi* and *aupādhika* are not strictly from the early Yoga philosophical system. They have been borrowed by Vācaspati Miśra without reserve from the Vedānta doctrinal system, thus creating a syncretic terminology. This by no means changes the Yoga doctrine itself, but only emphasizes grounds that are, according to Vācaspati, shared by both Vedānta and Yoga.

298. *TV* I.4 (pp. 7–8): *itaratra vyutthāne yāś cittavṛttayaḥ śāntaghoramūḍhās tā evāviśiṣṭā abhinnā vṛttayo yasya puruṣasya sa tathoktaḥ. . . . japākusumasphaṭikayor iva buddhipuruṣayoḥ saṃnidhānād abhedagrahe buddhivṛttīḥ puruṣe samāropya . . .*

299. Ibid. (p. 8): *yathā maline darpaṇatale pratibimbitaṃ mukhaṃ malinamāropya śocatyātmānaṃ malino'smīti.*

300. *TV* IV.22 (p. 198); see also *TV* III.35.

301. *TV* III.35 (p. 155): *buddheś caitanyabimbodgrāheṇa caitanyasya śāntādyākārādhyāropaḥ. TV* IV.23 (p. 198): *tasmāccittapratibimbatayā caitanyagocarā'pi cittavṛttirna caitanyāgocareti.*

302. *SPB* I.199.

303. See T. S. Rukmani (1988), "Vijñānabhikṣu's Double Reflection Theory of Knowledge in the Yoga System," *JIP* 16: 370.

304. *YV* I.4 (p. 48): *sā cārthākāratā buddhau pariṇāmarūpā . . . puruṣe ca pratibimbarūpā.*

305. *YV* I.4 (p. 50): *yathā ca citi buddheḥ pratibimbam evaṃ buddhāv api citpratibimbaṃ svīkāryamanyathā caitanyasya bhānānupapatteḥ; svayaṃ sākṣātsvadarśane karmakarttṛ virodhena buddhyāruḍhatayaivātmano ghaṭādivajjñeyatvābhyupāgamāt.*

306. *YV* I.4 (p. 45): *yady api puruṣaś cinmātro'vikārī tathā'pi buddher viṣayākāravṛttīnāṃ puruṣe yāni pratibimbāni tāny eva puruṣasya vṛttayaḥ, na ca tabhir avastubhūtābhiḥ pariṇāmitvam sphaṭikasy evātattvato'nyathābhāvād.*

307. The two divergent views of Vācaspati and Vijñāna Bhikṣu regarding the nature of experience by *puruṣa* are discussed further in *TV* IV.22 and *YV* IV.22 respectively. See also Rukmani (1988), "Vijñānabhiksu's Double Reflection Theory of Knowledge in the Yoga System," *JIP* 16: 367–375.

308. See n. 202 above.

309. See n. 334 below.

310. *YS* I.7; see n. 141 above.

311. *YS* IV.22–23.

312. See Monier-Williams (1899: 685).

313. *YB* I.7; see n. 315 below for text.

314. *YS* IV.17 (p. 193): *taduparāgāpekṣitvāccittasya vastu jñātājñātam.*

315. *YB* I.7 (p. 11): *indriyapraṇālikayā cittasya bāhyavastūparāgāt tadviṣayā sāmānyaviśeṣātmano'rthasya viśeṣāvadhāraṇa pradhānā vṛttiḥ pratyakṣaṃ pramāṇam. phalam aviśiṣṭaḥ pauruṣeyaś cittavṛttibodhaḥ.*

316. See Arya (1986: 150).

317. *YB* I.7 (p. 11): *pratisaṃvedī puruṣa . . .*

318. This is the explanation offered by Vācaspati Miśra and H. Āraṇya on *YB* I.7.

319. See, for example, *YS* III.17–19, 25–29, 33–36, 43, 49, 52, and 54. An example of *yogi-pratyakṣa* is the yogin's effecting the perception of *saṃskāra*s whereby knowledge of previous births is attained (*YS* III.18). Another example of yogic perception is the discriminative discernment *(vivekakhyāti)* that mind-*sattva* and *puruṣa* are different, as we are told in *YS* III.49 (see n. 125 above).

320. See *TV* I.7 and *YV* I.7.

321. See *YV* I.7 (p. 61).

322. Ibid.

323. In *TV* I.7 Vācaspati sees the definition of *pratyakṣa* in *YB* I.7 as a "pointer" to the implicit and more complete idea of direct perception or realization *(sākṣātkāra)*. Rāmānanda Yati understands *yogi-pratyakṣa* as taking place in *samādhi*. When the mind is clear and no longer dependent on external objects, there appears a clear reflection of pure consciousness.

324. See *YS* IV.22–23 and *YB* IV.22–23.

325. *YS* I.49 (p. 52): *śrutānumānaprajñābhyām anyaviṣayā viśeṣārthatvāt.*

326. *YS* I.48 (p. 51): *ṛtaṃbharā tatra prajñā*; see chapter 5 for further discussion on this topic.

327. *YB* I.49 (pp. 52–53): *śrutamāgamavijñānaṃ tatsāmānyaviṣayam. na hy āgamena śakyo viśeṣo'bhidhātuṃ, kasmāt, na hi viśeṣeṇa kṛtasaṃketaḥ śabda iti. tathā'numānaṃ sāmānyaviṣayam eva. . . . anumānena ca sāmānyenopasaṃhāraḥ. tasmāc chrutānumānaviṣayo na viśeṣaḥ kaścid astīti. na cāsya sūkṣmavyavahitaviprakṛṣṭasya vastuno lokapratyakṣeṇa grahaṇam asti. na cāsya viśeṣasyāpramāṇakasyābhāvo'stīti samādhiprajñā nirgrāhya eva sa viśeṣo bhavati bhūtasūkṣmagato vā puruṣagato vā.*

328. *YS* III.35; see n. 333 below.

329. As, for example, in the processes leading up to *savitarka-samāpatti* (*YS* I.42) and culminating in *nirvitarka-samāpatti* (*YS* I.43); on this see our discussion in chapter 5.

330. On the topic of levels of commitment to practice in Yoga refer to our discussion in chapter 1 on *YS* I.21–22 and Vyāsa's commentary.

331. *YS* IV.20 (p. 195): *ekasamaye cobhayānavadhāraṇam.*

332. *YS* IV.21; see n. 40 above.

333. *YS* III.35 (p. 154): *sattvapuruṣayor atyantāsaṃkīrṇayoḥ pratyayāviśeṣo bhogaḥ parārthatvāt svārthasaṃyamāt puruṣajñānam.*

334. *YB* III.35 (p. 155): *na ca puruṣapratyayena buddhisattvātmanā puruṣo dṛśyate. puruṣa eva taṃ pratyayaṃ svātmāvalambanaṃ paśyati, tathā hy uktam— "vijñātāram are kena vijānīyāt" iti.*

335. Chapple and Kelly (1990: 116); see also *BĀ Up* III.7.23.

336. C. Pensa in G. Feuerstein (1980: vi).

CHAPTER 4. *NIRODHA*

1. See n. 152 in chapter 3.
2. *YS* II.11 (p. 67): *dhyānaheyās tadvṛttayaḥ.*
3. By overcoming dissatisfaction (*YS* II.16) and its cause (*YS* II.17), classical Yoga can be seen to have the same purpose as classical Sāṃkhya and Buddhism.
4. *YS* I.2 (p. 4): *yogaś cittavṛttinirodhaḥ.*
5. As mentioned in chapter 2, in his open-ended approach Patañjali offers a diversity of practices that more or less complement each other. The openness of the *YS* is expressed, for example, in *YS* I.39 (p. 42): *yathābhimatadhyānādvā*, "Or [clarity of mind results] from meditation as desired."
6. See also Chapple (1986: 36–37) and Larson (1987: 26–29) on the classical systems of Sāṃkhya and Yoga; other comparisons or contrasts between these two *darśana*s are raised throughout our study.
7. Eliade (1969: 4).
8. *YB* II.15 (p. 76): *itaraṃ tu svakarmopahṛtaṃ duḥkham upāttam upāttaṃ tyajantaṃ tyaktaṃ tyaktaṃ upādadānam anādivāsanāvicitrayā cittavṛttyā samantato'nuviddham ivāvidyayā hātavya evāhaṃkāramamakārānupātinaṃ jātaṃ jātaṃ bāhyādhyātmikobhayanimittāstriparvāṇastāpā ānuplavante. tad evam anādinā duḥkhasrotasā vyuhyamānam ātmānaṃ bhūtagrāmaṃ ca dṛṣṭvā yogī sarvaduḥkhakṣayakāraṇaṃ samyagdarśanaṃ śaraṇaṃ prapadyata iti.*
9. Monier-Williams (1899: 884).
10. See, for example, G. Jha (1907: 3), H. Āraṇya (1963: 1), M. N. Dvivedī (1930: 2), M. Eliade (1969: 36).
11. See, for example, I. K. Taimni (1961: 6), T. Leggett (1990: 60).
12. See, for example, J. H. Woods (1914: 8), G. Koelman (1970: 237), G. Feuerstein (1979a: 26), T. S. Rukmani (1981: 31).
13. See, for example, J. Varenne (1976: 87), G. Larson (1987: 28); in a more recent work (1993: 377), Larson translates *nirodha* as "cessation" or "restraint."
14. See, for example, Tola and Dragonetti (1987: 5), Chapple and Kelly (1990: 33).
15. U. Arya (1986: 93). See also Purohit (1973), who translates *nirodha* as "controlling."
16. Other translations of *nirodha* include: "hindering" (Ballantyne, 1852), "Unterdrückung" (Jacobi, 1929: 587), and "Zur-Ruhe-bringen" or "Bewaltigung" (Hauer, 1958: 239).
17. See J. B. Sykes, ed. (1976), *The Concise Oxford Dictionary,* p. 299, where "dissolution" can mean the "undoing or relaxing of bond."
18. *YB* II.18 (p. 84); see n. 266 in chapter 3.
19. *YB* II.6 (p. 96); see n. 144 in chapter 2.
20. *YS* IV.34 (p. 207).
21. *YS* II.10 (p. 66): *te pratiprasavaheyāḥ sūkṣmāḥ.*
22. Cf. Feuerstein (1979a: 65) and Koelman (1970: 249).
23. Cf. Feuerstein (1979a: 65) and (1980: 36).
24. Koelman (1970: 249).
25. Ibid.
26. Ibid.

27. See *YB* III.50 (p. 168): *tadeteṣāṃ guṇānāṃ manasi karmakleśavipāka-svarūpeṇābhivyaktānāṃ caritārthānāṃ pratiprasave puruṣasyā''tyantiko guṇaviyogaḥ kaivalyaṃ.*

28. Cf. *YB* II.2 and II.27 as well as n. 27 above.

29. *YS* IV.32 (p. 204): *tataḥ kṛtārthānāṃ pariṇāmakramasamāptir guṇānāṃ.* "Then [with that eternality of knowledge] the *guṇa*s have fulfilled their purpose, and the succession of their changes is terminated."

30. Following from *dharmamegha samādhi* (*YS* IV.29: 202) there is the cessation of afflicted action; *YS* IV.30 (p. 202): *tataḥ kleśakarmanivṛttiḥ.* See further explanation on *YS* IV.29-30 in chapter 6.

31. *YS* IV.31 and *YB* IV.31 (p. 203).

32. *YV* I.2 (p. 33): *cittam antaḥkaraṇasāmānyam ekasyaivāntaḥkaraṇasya vṛttibhedamātreṇa caturdhā atra darśane vibhāgāt, tasya yāvallakṣyamāṇā vṛttayas tāsāṃ nirodhas tāsāṃ layākhyo'dhikāraṇasyaivāvasthāviśeṣo'bhāvasyāsman mate'dhi-kāraṇāvasthāviśeṣarūpatvāt, sa yoga ity arthaḥ.*

33. In Yoga, for example, the "absence" of a clay pot on the "ground" simply points to the nature of the clay or "ground" itself *(bhūtalasvarūpam);* cf. Rukmani (1981: 27 n. 2).

34. *RM* I.2 (p. 2): *nirodho vahirmukhapariṇātivicchedādantarmukhatayā pratilo-mapariṇāmena svakāraṇe layo yoga ity ākhyāyate.* While it may not be Bhoja's intention to support the notion of the nonexistence of *vṛtti*s in *nirodha,* his commentary (the *RM*) appears to lack the philosophical sophistication required for interpreting the meaning of *nirodha* along epistemological lines.

35. *YB* IV.12; see n. 97 in chapter 2.

36. *YS* II.26 (p. 96): *vivekakhyātir aviplavā hānopāyaḥ.* "The means of aban-donment [of *saṃyoga*] is the unfaultering discriminative discernment."

37. *YS* II.27 (p. 97): *tasya saptadhā prāntabhūmiḥ prajñā.*

38. *YB* II.27 (pp. 97-98).

39. *YB* II.27 (p. 98): *guṇā giriśikharataṭacyutā iva grāvāṇo niravasthānāḥ svakāraṇe pralayābhimukhāḥ saha tenāstaṃ gacchanti. na caiṣāṃ pravilīnānāṃ punar asty utpādaḥ prayojanābhāvād iti.*

40. See *YS* II.22.

41. See *YB* I.2.

42. *YS* II.25 (p. 96): *tadabhāvāt saṃyogābhāvo hānaṃ taddṛśeḥ kaivalyam.*

43. *YB* II.24 (p. 95): *viparyayajñānavāsanetyarthaḥ. viparyayajñānavāsanā vāsitā ca na kāryaniṣṭhāṃ puruṣakhyātiṃ buddhiḥ prāpnoti sādhikārā punar āvartate. sā tu puruṣakhyāti paryavasānāṃ kāryaniṣṭhāṃ prāpnoti, caritādhikārā nivṛttādarśanā ban-dhakāraṇābhāvānna punar āvartate.*

44. *YB* II.25 (p. 96): *tasyādarśanasyābhāvād buddhipuruṣasaṃyogābhāva ātyantiko bandhanoparama ity arthaḥ. etaddhānaṃ. taddṛśeḥ kaivalyaṃ puruṣasyāmiśrī-bhāvaḥ punar asaṃyogo guṇair ity arthaḥ. duḥkhakāraṇa nivṛttau duḥkhoparamo hānaṃ, tadā svarūpapratiṣṭhaḥ puruṣa ity uktam.*

45. Cf. *YB* II.2, 27 and IV.34.

46. G. Koelman (1970: 249).

47. As outlined in (1977) *The Complete Works of Swami Vivekānanda* (hereafter abbreviated *CWSV*) 8 vols. (Calcutta: Advaita Ashram).

48. For an examination of Swami Vivekānanda's understanding of *samādhi* as it relates to Patañjali's Yoga system, see A. Rambachan (1994), *The Limits of Scripture: Vivekananda's Reinterpretation of the Vedas,* pp. 98–112.

49. Vivekānanda also describes *samādhi* as a source of knowledge, giving the impression that he identifies the state with a particular level of mental activity (see, for example, *CWSV* 1: 185, where he describes *samādhi* as a state of mind; see also *CWSV* 2: 390 and *CWSV* 4: 59). This description is contradicted by several passages in which he repeatedly affirms that *samādhi* is consequent upon the death of the mind and characterized by a total absence of mental functions. There is an obvious tension in his writings in that this portrayal of *samādhi* is seen both as a state in which the mind still obtains and as a state where the mind ceases to exist.

50. Swami Vivekānanda, *CWVS* 1: 200.

51. *CWVS* 8: 40; see also *CWVS* 1: 234 and CWVS 7: 195.

52. *CWVS* 1: 188, 212–213.

53. *CWVS* 8: 36; see also *CWVS* 7: 140, 196.

54. *CWVS* 8: 48.

55. *CWVS* 7: 71.

56. *CWVS* 7: 195; see also *CWVS* 2: 255.

57. *CWVS* 8: 31.

58. *CWVS* 2: 256.

59. I do not think the issue being raised here is merely one of semantics but rather reflects a basic misunderstanding of Yoga philosophy itself and the actual process of thought- or mind-transcendence that takes place in Yoga. It is of interest to note that the practice of Yoga as usually understood in modern Western contexts is often confined to physical exercises or postures *(āsana),* perhaps accompanied by breathing exercises *(prāṇāyāma)* and techniques for concentration *(dhāraṇā)* of the mind. The deeper more subtle practice of meditation leading to *samādhi* is often ignored albeit for good reasons as it is often the case that the Yoga instructors are not qualified themselves nor are they experienced in higher meditative disciplines. Alternatively, for an inexperienced instructor to teach meditation to students of Yoga would be, from the perspective of the tradition of Yoga itself, pedagogically unsound and irresponsible. Moreover, if Yoga practice is presented as resulting ultimately in the annihilation or negation of the mind, it would not be unreasonable to presume that aspirants would resist the serious study and practice of Yoga, believing that Yoga would make them incapable of functioning effectively in the world. In an about-face in his perspective, Vivekānanda contradicts his more negative approach to the mind when (see *CWSV* 8: 47–48) he appears to instruct his listeners to make no effort to control their thoughts, but simply to watch them. In his authoritative book (1976) entitled *Yoga and the Hindu Tradition* (Chicago: University of Chicago Press), J. Varenne (pp. 6–7) questions the meaning of "cessation" *(nirodha)* in Yoga and rightly concludes that "Yoga is indeed the cessation of agitation of the consciousness." But he later goes on to support a more suppressive approach to the mind in Yoga. See, for example, where he writes (p. 114): "the chitta, whose activity yoga makes it an aim to destroy."

60. See the above listed interpretations of *nirodha* (notes 10–16). The exceptional interpretation here is Chapple and Kelly (1990: 8, 122), who, without "Vedānticizing" the Yoga system of Patañjali, imply that Yoga culminates in an embodied state or "experience" of liberation involving nonafflicted action.

61. P. Y. Deshpande (1978), *The Authentic Yoga,* pp. 22-23.
62. See *YB* II.15 in n. 294, chapter 3.
63. Dasgupta (1922: 268).
64. See *YB* I.2 and *YS* II.18.
65. See *YS* II.18 and *YB* I.2.
66. See *YB* II.15 in n. 294, chapter 3.
67. See Dasgupta (1922: 247); the term *prati-sañcara* is used in the *Tattvasamāsa-Sūtra* (6); see Larson (1987: 319).
68. *YS* II.18; see n. 115 in chapter 2.
69. As is often the case in the classical Sāṃkhya tradition and its interpretations.
70. See notes 115 and 128 in chapter 2.
71. *YS* II.21; see n. 114 in chapter 3.
72. *YB* I.1 (p. 2).
73. *YB* I.2 (p. 4). I will be presenting a detailed explanation of the various stages of *samādhi* in chapters 5 and 6.
74. *YB* I.2 (p. 4): *sarvaśabdāgrahaṇāt saṃprajñāto'pi yoga ityākhyāyate.*
75. This is easily inferred from *YB* I.2 (see chapter 3, n. 232); see also *TV* I.1 (p. 4): *rajastamomayī kila pramāṇādivṛttiḥ sāttvikīṃ vṛttimupādāya saṃprajñāte niruddhā.*
76. See *YB* IV.30 (pp. 202-203): *kleśakarmanivṛttau jīvanneva vidvānvimukto bhavati. kasmāt, yasmād viparyayo bhavasya kāraṇam. na hi kṣīṇaviparyayaḥ kaścit kenacit kvacijjāto dṛśyata iti.* "On cessation of afflicted action, the knower is liberated while yet living. Why? Because erroneous cognition *(viparyaya)* is the cause of rebirth [of egoity]. When error has vanished, no one is ever seen to be born anywhere." Here (again) there is room for an epistemological understanding—of "reborn," that is, one who is said to be reborn is misidentified as a body-self that takes birth and will eventually perish. The liberated yogin may have a body that is subject to birth and death yet the yogin is no longer misidentified as the body or as any other aspect of prakṛtic existence.
77. See *YS* IV.31; see also *YS* II.52 and III.43, where the expression *prakāśa-āvaraṇa* "covering of light" is used. Both *sūtra*s allude to the removal or dwindling of the "coverings" of *rajas* and *tamas* that conceal *prakāśa*—the inner light or illuminating quality of *sattva*-knowledge (the *guṇa* of *sattva*).
78. "Subtilization" is a term used by Chapple and Kelly (1990: 4).
79. See *YB* I.5 (p. 10).
80. *YS* II.15; *YS* IV. 9-10.
81. *YS* IV.8, 24.
82. *YB* II.24 (p. 95).
83. *YS* I.8 (p. 12).
84. See n. 76 above.
85. See *YB* II.23 (p. 92) and n. 272 in chapter 3.
86. See *YB* I.8 (p. 13) and n. 144 in chapter 3.
87. This correlates well with the term *sabīja* (*YS* I.46) used by Patañjali as will be seen in chapter 5 of this study.
88. Vyāsa (*YB* I.1, p. 4) refers to the supracognitive *samādhi*—wherein all *vṛtti*s and their effects are transcended—as *sarvavṛttinirodha.* There is no reason why *sarvavṛttinirodha* cannot be read as the complete cessation of the one seed-*vṛtti* of error *(viparyaya)* that, according to Vyāsa (*YB* I.8), contains all afflicted identity. The

cognitive *samādhi* is included as Yoga proper because it serves to dissolve misidentification with *vṛtti*s and is propaedeutic to the higher *samādhi*. The term *sarva* can refer to all the *vṛtti*s of identification that support misidentification or mistaken identity.

89. *YS* III.55 (p. 174): *sattvapuruṣayoḥ śuddhisāmye kaivalyam iti.* "In the sameness of purity between the *sattva* (of the mind) and *puruṣa,* there is aloneness."

90. *YS* I.12 (p. 17): *abhyāsavairāgyābhyāṃ tannirodhaḥ.*

91. *YB* I.11; see n. 198 in chapter 3.

92. See C. Pensa in Feuerstein (1980: viii) and also Feuerstein (1980: 78). K. S. Joshi (1965: 60) argues that *abhyāsa* and *vairāgya* can be seen as two poles of any form of Yoga.

93. *YB* I.12 (p. 17): *cittanadī nāmobhayatovāhinī vahati kalyāṇāya vahati pāpāya ca. yā tu kaivalyaprāgbhārā vivekaviṣayanimnā sā kalyāṇavahā. saṃsāraprāgbhārā'vivekaviṣayanimnā pāpavahā. tatra vairāgyeṇa viṣayasrotaḥ khilī kriyate. vivekadarśanābhyāsena vivekasrota udghāṭyata ity ubhayādhīnaś cittavṛttinirodhaḥ.*

94. See *YB* I.5 on *kliṣṭa* and *akliṣṭa.*

95. The interrelatedness of knowledge, ignorance, and moral aspiration is illustrated, for example, in the *Kaṭha Up* (I.2. 1-9), where two paths are outlined: (1) the path of ignorance that leads to self-indulgence and that falls into the power of the Lord of Death (Yama), and (2) the path of wisdom *(vidyā)* that leads to immortality and that is beyond Yama's grasp.

96. Feuerstein (1990: 381).

97. *BG* VI.35 (p. 206): *asaṃśayaṃ mahābāho mano durnigrahaṃ calam, abhyāsena tu kaunteya vairāgyeṇa ca gṛhyate.*

98. *YS* I.13 (p. 17): *tatra sthitau yatno'bhyāsaḥ.*

99. *YS* I.14 (p. 18): *sa tu dīrghakālanairantaryasatkārāsevito dṛḍhabhūmiḥ.*

100. It can probably be assumed here that knowledge *(vidyā)* presupposes a necessary preparation and includes a proficiency in the tradition, in the texts, and in the systematic method of practice.

101. *YB* I.14 (p. 18): *dīrghakālāsevito nirantarāsevitaḥ satkārāsevitaḥ, tapasā brahmacaryaṇa vidyayā śraddhayā ca saṃpāditaḥ satkāravāndṛḍhabhūmir bhavati.*

102. *YB* I.13 (pp. 17-18): *tadarthaḥ prayatno vīryamutsāhaḥ. tat saṃpipādayiṣayā tatsādhanānuṣṭhānamabhyāsaḥ.* Koelman notes (1970: 257) that while extraordinary will power is implied in all prescriptions and exercises in Yoga, nowhere is the word "will" *(icchā)* explicitly mentioned in the *YS* or the *YB*. It is one of the five activities of the intellect mentioned in the *Tattva-Samāsa-Sūtra*s (9).

103. *YB* I.13 (p. 17): *cittasyāvṛttikasya praśāntavāhitā sthitiḥ.*

104. *YV* I.13 (p. 94).

105. *TV* I.13 (p. 17): *rājasatāmasavṛttir ahitasya praśāntavāhitā vimalatā sāttvikavṛtti vāhitaikāgratā sthitiḥ.*

106. *RM* I.13 (p. 5): *vṛttir ahitasya cittasya svarūpaniṣṭhaḥ pariṇāmaḥ sthitistasyāṃ . . .*

107. *YB* I.14 (p. 18): *vyutthānasaṃskāreṇa drāgityevānabhe bhūtaviṣaya ityarthaḥ.*

108. S. Dasgupta (1930: 61).

109. *YS* I.15 (p. 18): *dṛṣṭānuśravikaviṣayavitṛṣṇasya vaśīkārasaṃjñā vairāgyam.*

110. *YV* I.15 (p. 96): *rāgābhāvamātraṃ doṣadarśanajanyo rāgābhāvo vā na nirodhahetur vairāgyaṃ rogādinimittakārūcitto yogānudayād, doṣadarśanajavairāgyādanantaramapi viṣayasāṃnidhyena citta kṣobhataḥ saubharyāderyogāniṣpatteś ca.*

"'*Vairāgya*' which is [understood as] the absence of attachment or which is the absence of attachment arising from seeing defects [in objects] is not a cause for cessation. [This is] because Yoga does not come into being based on a dislike of causes such as illnesses; [also] even after [achieving a certain] detachment arising from seeing the defects [in the objects] *ṛṣi*s like Saubhari failed to attain Yoga because of the agitation of [his] mind in the presence of the objects [of the senses]."

111. *YS* I.33 clearly shows the fallacy of developing such pseudo-notions of "detachment" in Yoga; see n. 248 in chapter 3.

112. *YV* I.15 (p. 98): *rāgadveṣaśūnyasya viṣayasākṣātkārasya yogyatā vaśīkāra-saṃjñā''khyaṃ vairāgyam . . .*

113. See notes 125 and 333 in chapter 3 on *YS* III.49 and III.35 respectively.

114. *YS* I.16 (p. 19): *tatparaṃ puruṣakhyāter guṇavaitṛṣṇyam.*

115. *YB* I.16 (pp. 19–20): *dṛṣṭānuśravikaviṣaya doṣadarśī viraktaḥ puruṣadarśanābhyāsāttacchuddhi pravivekāpyāyita buddhir guṇebhyo vyaktāvyaktadharmakebhyo virakta iti.*

116. See n. 117 below.

117. *YB* I.15 (pp. 18–19): *striyo'nnapānam aiśvaryam iti dṛṣṭaviṣaye vitṛṣṇasya svarga vaidehyaprakṛtilayatvaprāptāvānuśravikaviṣaye vitṛṣṇasya divyādivyaviṣayasaṃprayoge'pi cittasya . . . vaśīkārasaṃjñā vairāgyam.* U. Arya (1986: 206) paraphrases the word "women" *(striya)* as "the opposite sex" and "out of consideration for contemporary concerns." He goes on to write (pp. 206–207): "These texts were taught in monastic settings by yoga masters for whose male disciples the attraction of women must have been a common problem. Although there have been many great women yogīs (yoginīs) known to the tradition, it is somehow thought that men are not as strong an attraction to aspiring women as women are to men." Arya's point, I think, is well taken and discloses an unfortunate and already well-known bias—certainly present within Hinduism and other religious traditions of the world—which, focusing on religious literature written from a male perspective, tends to overlook the intrinsically spiritual nature and identity of women and does not address the issue of life as understood and experienced from a woman's perspective. If Vyāsa were a woman he undoubtedly would have addressed the issue of sexuality from a somewhat different perspective!

118. *SK* 45: *vairāgyāt prakṛtilayaḥ. . .*

119. *YB* I.16 (p. 20): *tatra yaduttaraṃ tajjñānaprasādamātram.*

120. *TV* I.16 (p. 20): *tadeva hi tādṛśaṃ cittasattvaṃ rajoleśamalenāpyaparāmṛṣṭamasyā''śrayo'ta eva jñānaprasāda . . . khyātiviśeṣe sati vartamānakhyātimānityarthaḥ.*

121. *YB* I.16 (p. 20): *yasyodaye sati yogī pratyudita khyātir evaṃ manyateprāptaṃ prāpaṇīyaṃ, kṣīṇāḥ kṣetavyāḥ kleśāḥ, chinnaḥ śliṣṭaparvā bhavasaṃkramaḥ, yasyāvicchedājjanitvā mriyate mṛtvā ca jāyata iti. jñānasyaiva parā kāṣṭhā vairāgyam. etasyaiva hi nāntarīyakaṃ kaivalyam iti.*

122. *YS* III.50 (p. 168): *tadvairāgyād api doṣabījakṣaye kaivalyam.*

123. *YS* III.49; see n. 125 in chapter 3.

124. *YV* I.16 (p. 101).

125. *YS* IV.29 (p. 202): *prasaṃkhyānye'pyakusīdasya sarvathā vivekakhyāter dharmameghaḥ samādhiḥ.* This *sūtra* will be discussed in chapter 6.

126. *YB* II.15 (p. 78): *tatra hātuḥ svarūpamupādeyaṃ vā heyaṃ vā na bhavitumarhati.* "Here, the true nature/identity of the one who is liberated cannot be something to be acquired or discarded."

127. *YB* II.27 (p. 97): *saptadheti aśuddhyāvaraṇamalāpagamaccittasya pratyayāntarānutpāde sati saptaprakāraiva prajñā vivekino bhavati.*

128. *YB* I.2 (p. 6): . . . *viraktaṃ cittaṃ tāmapi khyātiṃ niruṇaddhi.*

129. W. Halbfass (1991), *Tradition and Reflection: Explorations in Indian Thought,* p. 227.

130. *YS* II.27.

131. *YB* II.27 (p. 98): *svarūpamātrajyotir amalaḥ kevalī puruṣa . . .*

132. Ibid.: *etāṃ saptavidhāṃ prāntabhūmi prajñāmanupaśyanpuruṣaḥ. . .*

133. Ibid.: *pratiprasave'pi cittasya muktaḥ kuśala ityeva bhavati guṇātītatvāditi.*

134. *YS* II.29.

135. Monier-Williams (1899: 1159).

136. Ibid.

137. See M. N. Dvivedī (1930: 52), R. Prasāda (1912: 31).

138. See M. Müller (1899: 448), G. Jha (1907: 19).

139. See S. Dasgupta (1922: 271), Tola and Dragonetti (1987: 74), J. H. Woods (1914: 40).

140. See H. Zimmer (1951: 435), G. Koelman (1970: 188).

141. See M. Eliade (1969: 77), G. Feuerstein (1979a: 37).

142. See G. Feuerstein (1989: 195–196).

143. See n. 141 above.

144. R. C. Zaehner (1969), *The Bhagavad Gītā*, p. 143.

145. However, in a later work (1989: 183, 195) Feuerstein adopts the term "ecstasy" for *samādhi* (see n. 142 above and n. 5 in chapter 5 of our study).

146. *YB* II.1 (p. 57): . . . *samāhitacittasya yogaḥ. kathaṃ vyutthitacitto'pi yogayuktaḥ syādityetadārabhyate.*

147. *TV* II.1 (p. 57): *abhyāsavairāgye hi yogopāyau prathame pāda uktau. na ca tau vyutthitacittasya drāgityeva, saṃbhavat iti dvitīyapādopadeśyāmupāyāmapekṣate sattvaśuddhyarthaṃ.*

148. Monier-Williams (1899: 1040).

149. As can be inferred from *YB* I.5 and *YS* III.9.

150. There is an obvious tension between *vyutthāna* and *nirodha* in the *Yoga-Sūtra,* a tension that is not fully resolved until the highest stage of practice, namely *asaṃprajñāta-samādhi.* On this see chapter 5 and especially chapter 6.

151. See *YS* IV.18–22.

152. *YS* II.2 (p. 58): *samādhibhāvanārthaḥ kleśatanūkaraṇārthaś ca.*

153. *YS* II.1 (p. 57): *tapaḥsvādhyāyeśvarapraṇidhānāni kriyāyogaḥ.*

154. *YB* II.1 (p. 58): *svādhyāyaḥ praṇavādipavitrāṇāṃ japo mokṣaśāstrādhyayanaṃ vā.*

155. See references to G. Feuerstein in notes 26 and 31 in chapter 2; see also Feuerstein (1979a: 59).

156. For a comparative study of *kriyā-yoga* and *aṣṭāṅga-yoga* see Feuerstein (1979b: 37–104).

157. *YS* I.34 (p. 39): *pracchardanavidhāraṇābhyāṃ vā prāṇasya.*

158. *YS* I.37 (p. 41): *vītarāgaviṣayaṃ vā cittam.*

159. *YB* I.35 (p. 39).

160. *YS* 1.35 (p. 39): *viṣayavatī vā pravṛttir utpannā manasaḥ sthitinibandhanī.*

161. See n. 248 in chapter 3.

162. *YS* I.36 (p. 40): *viśokā vā jyotiṣmatī.* Vyāsa mentions (*YB* I.36: 40) that by concentrating on the heart-lotus *(hṛdaya-puṇḍarīka)* there is direct awareness of the *buddhi.* The percepton of luminous forms such as the sun may also take place through this form of concentration.

163. *YB* I.1 (p. 3): *kṣiptaṃ mūḍhaṃ vikṣiptam ekāgraṃ niruddham iti citta-bhūmayaḥ.*

164. See *TV* I.1 (p. 3): *mūḍham tu tamaḥsamudrekānnidrāvṛttimat.*

165. *YV* I.1 (p. 24): *kṣiptaṃ rajasā viṣayeṣveva vṛttimat. mūḍhaṃ tamasā nidrādivṛttimat.*

166. Cf. *TV* I.1 (p. 3) and *YV* I.1 (p. 24).

167. *YS* I.30 (p. 34): *vyādhistyānasaṃśayapramādālasyāviratibhrāntidarśanālab-dhabhūmikatvānavasthitatvāni cittavikṣepās te'ntarāyāḥ.* I have briefly elaborated on some of the meanings of the above terms as given by Vyāsa.

168. *TV* I.30; *YV* I.30.

169. *YB* I.30 (p. 34): *sahaite cittavṛttibhir bhavanti. eteṣāmabhāve na bhavanti pūrvāktāś cittavṛttayaḥ. . . . samādhipratilambhe hi sati tadavasthitaṃ syāditi.*

170. *YB* I.31 (p. 35): *duḥkhamādhyātmikamādhibautikamādhidaivikaṃ ca.*

171. *YS* I.31 (p. 35): *duḥkhadaurmanasyāṅgamejayatvaśvāsapraśvāsā vikṣepasa-habhuvaḥ.* See also *YB* I.31.

172. *YB* I.31 (p. 35): *ete vikṣepasahabhuvo vikṣiptacittasyaite bhavanti. samāhita-cittasyaite na bhavanti.* "Put or held together, joined, assembled, combined, united . . . composed, collected, concentrated . . . put in order, set right, adjusted" are some of the meanings Monier-Williams gives (1899: 1160) for *samāhita. Samāhita* implies a harmonizing of the mind or resolving of the conditions of agitation and conflict in the mind; on this see Arya (1986: 332).

173. *YB* I.1 (p. 3): *tatra vikṣipte cetasi vikṣepopasarjanībhūtaḥ samādhirna yoga-pakṣe vartate.*

174. G. Koelman (1970: 161).

175. *YB* I.1 (pp. 3–4): *yastvekāgre cetasi sadbhūtamarthaṃ pradyotayati kṣiṇoti ca kleśānkarmabandhanāni ślathayati nirodhamabhimukhaṃ karoti sa saṃprajñāto yoga ityākhyāyate.*

176. *YS* II.29 (p. 101): *yamaniyamāsanaprāṇāyāmapratyāhāradhāraṇādhyā-nasamādhayo'ṣṭāvaṅgāni.*

177. *YS* II.28 (p. 98): *yogāṅgānuṣṭhānād aśuddhikṣaye jñānadīptirāvivekakhyāteḥ.*

178. *YS* II.30 (p. 102): *ahiṃsāsatyāsteyabrahmacaryāparigrahā yamāḥ.*

179. *YS* II.35 (p. 107): *ahiṃsāpratiṣṭhāyāṃ tat saṃnidhau vairatyāgaḥ.* "When in the presence of one established in nonviolence, there is the abandonment of enmity."

180. *YS* II.36 (p. 107): *satyapratiṣṭhāyāṃ kriyāphalāśrayatvam.* "When established in truthfulness, [there is] correspondence between action [and its] fruition."

181. *YS* II.37 (p. 108): *asteyapratiṣṭhāyāṃ sarvaratnopasthānam.* "When established in non-stealing, all precious things appear for [the yogin]."

182. *YS* II.38 (p. 108): *brahmacaryapratiṣṭhāyāṃ vīryalābhaḥ.* "When established in sexual restraint, vitality is obtained."

183. *YS* II.39 (p. 108): *aparigrahasthairye janmakathaṃtāsaṃbodhaḥ.* "When steadied in nonpossessiveness [the yogin obtains] knowledge of the conditions of birth."

184. *YS* II.31 (p. 104): *jātideśakālasamayānavacchinnāḥ sarvabhaumā mahāvratam.*

185. *YS* II.32 (p. 104): *śaucasaṃtoṣatapaḥsvādhyāyeśvarapraṇidhānāni niyamāḥ.*

186. *YS* II.40 (p. 109): *śaucāt svāṅgajugupsā parairasaṃsargaḥ.* "Through purity [the yogin attains] distance toward his own body, and non-contamination by others." This *sūtra* is not meant to imply an aversion or dislike toward the body but rather a discerning and detached attitude based on a healthy respect for the body as a vehicle for the purification of consciousness; the yogin is no longer enslaved or consumed by a mere body-identification of self and does not pollute the body through unhealthy contact with others. *YS* II.41 (p. 109): *sattvaśuddhisaumanasyaikāgryendriyajayātma-darśanayogyatvāni ca.* "[Also:] purity of mind-*sattva,* cheerfulness, one-pointedness, mastery of the senses, and fitness for the vision of the self [are achieved]."

187. *YS* II.42 (p. 109): *saṃtoṣād anuttamaḥ sukhalābhaḥ.* "From contentment, unsurpassed happiness is gained."

188. *YS* II.43 (p. 110): *kāyendriyasiddhir aśuddhikṣayāt tapasaḥ.* "From austerity arises the dwindling of impurity and the perfection of the body and senses."

189. *YS* II.44 (p. 110): *svādhyāyād iṣṭadevatāsaṃprayogaḥ.* "Through personal, scriptural (i.e., self-) study [the yogin establishes] contact with the desired deity." See also n. 154 above.

190. *YS* II.45 (p. 110): *samādhisiddhir īśvarapraṇidhānāt.* "Through devotion to *īśvara* arises perfection in *samādhi.*"

191. This is, however, a matter for interpretation. See, for example, references to Feuerstein in notes 26 and 31 of chapter 2.

192. *YS* II.33 (p. 105): *vitarkabādhane pratipakṣabhāvanam.*

193. *YS* II.34 (p. 106): *vitarkā hiṃsādayaḥ kṛtakāritānumoditā lobhakrodhamoha-pūrvakā mṛdumadhyādhimātrā duḥkhājñānānantaphalā iti pratipakṣabhāvanam.*

194. See, for example, n. 248 in chapter 3 and text for n. 161 above.

195. See *YB* II.33 (p. 105).

196. B.-A. Scharfstein (1974), *Mystical Experience,* pp. 131–132.

197. *YS* II.46 (p. 110): *sthirasukhamāsanam.* "The posture should be firm and comfortable." Vyāsa (*YB* II.46) mentions postures such as the lotus position.

198. *YS* II.47 (p. 111): *prayatnaśaithilyānantasamāpattibhyām.* "[It is accompanied] by the relaxation of effort and by unification with the infinite." It appears that the posture can be perfected when the mind is in *samādhi,* that is, at a later stage; or the posture can be perfected at an earlier stage by the relaxation of effort. See *YB* II.47 (p. 111).

199. *YS* II.48 (p. 111): *tato dvandvānabhighātaḥ.* "From that [the yogin] becomes immune to the pairs of opposites."

200. *YS* II.49 (p. 112): *tasminsati śvāsapraśvāsayor gativicchedaḥ prāṇāyāmaḥ.* "*Prāṇāyāma* is to be in this [posture] and 'cut-off' the flow of inhalation and exhalation." The breath is only an external aspect or form of manifestation of *prāṇa* which is the "life-force" or "vital energy" that interpenetrates and sustains the body and its functions. For more on the term *prāṇa* see Feuerstein (1989: 258–259).

201. The first three as outlined in *YS* II.50 (p. 112) are: "external" *(bāhya),* "internal" *(abhyantara),* and "stopped" *(stambha).*

202. The fourth form (*YS* II.51: 113) is a withdrawal from the external and internal conditions of the breath: *bāhyābhyantaraviṣayākṣepī caturthaḥ.*

203. *YS* II.52 (p. 114): *tataḥ kṣīyate prakāśāvaraṇam; YB* II.52 (p. 114): . . . *kṣīyate vivekajñānāvaraṇīyaṃ karma.*

204. *YS* II.53 (p. 115): *dhāraṇāsu ca yogyatā manasaḥ.* This *sūtra* invites comparison with *YS* I.34, where it is said the mind is made steady through controlled expulsion and retention of the breath. See n. 157 above.

205. *YS* II.54 (p. 115): *svaviṣayāsaṃprayoge cittasvarūpānukāra ivendriyāṇāṃ pratyāhāraḥ.*

206. *YS* II.55 (p. 116): *tataḥ paramā vaśyatendriyāṇām.* "From that, the supreme obedience of the senses [arises]."

207. *YB* II.54 (pp. 115-116): *yathā madhukararājaṃ makṣikā utpatantamanūtpatanti niviśamānamanu niviśante tathendriyāṇi cittanirodhe niruddhānīty eṣa pratyāhāraḥ.*

208. *YS* III.1 (p. 118): *deśabandhaś cittasya dhāraṇā.* "Concentration is the binding of the mind to a [single] place."

209. *YB* III.1 (p. 118).

210. It appears that *ekāgratā* (*YS* III.11-12) is initiated in the practice of *dhāraṇā*, deepens in meditation *(dhyāna)* and matures in the stages of cognitive *samādhi.* Thus, Vyāsa refers to the fourth state of mind, which matures in *saṃprajñāta,* as *ekāgra,* "one-pointed." See also n. 52 in chapter 5.

211. *YS* III.2 (p. 119): *tatra pratyayaikatānatā dhyānam.* "The unbroken continuity or extension of one idea with regard to that [object of concentration] is meditation." Feuerstein (1990: 96) translates "one-directional flow" for *eka-tānatā.*

212. T. R. Kulkarni (1972), *Upanishads and Yoga,* p, 119.

213. Quoted by G. Feuerstein (1980: 84-85).

214. J. H. Clark (1983), *A Map of Mental States,* (London: Routledge and Kegan Paul) p. 29.

215. See n. 216 below.

216. *YS* III.3 (p. 119): *tad evārthamātranirbhāsaṃ svarūpaśūnyam iva samādhiḥ.*

217. *YS* III.11 (p. 123): *sarvārthataikāgratayoḥ kṣayodayau cittasya samādhipariṇāmaḥ.* "When there is the dwindling of all objectivity, and the arising of one-pointedness, there takes place in the mind the transformation of *samādhi.*" For more on *ekāgratā,* refer to notes 51 and 52 in chapter 5.

218. Undistorted insight *(prajñā)* initially occurs in the *nirvitarka* and *nirvicāra* forms of cognitive *samādhi.* The processes leading to insight will be explained in chapter 5.

219. *YS* III.4 (p. 120): *trayamekatra saṃyamaḥ.*

220. *YS* III.5 (p. 120): *tajjayāt prajñālokaḥ.* "From mastery of that *[saṃyama],* the light (illumination) of insight."

221. *YS* III.6 (p. 120): *tasya bhūmiṣu viniyogaḥ.* "Its application is by stages."

222. See *YS* I.41. An analysis of *YS* I.41 will be given in chapter 5.

223. See *YS* I.41 and *YS* I.42-44 where the stages of *samāpatti* are outlined. An analysis of the stages of "unification" *(samāpatti)* is given in chapter 5.

224. *YS* I.45. The yogin can merge with unmanifest *prakṛti* as in the case of the *prakṛti-laya*s (*YS* I.19).

225. *YS* III.7 (p. 121): *trayamantaraṅgaṃ pūrvebhyaḥ.* "[Distinct] from the prior [five] ones are the three inner limbs."

226. We can infer from *YS* III.7 that the first five limbs of the *aṣṭāṅga-yoga* are "external" aids compared to the last three.

227. *YS* III.8 (p. 122): *tad api bahiraṅgaṃ nirbījasya.* "Yet these are outer means in relation to the seedless [enstasy]." The notion of "seedless" will be discussed in chapters 5 and 6.

228. *YS* II.28; see n. 177 above.

229. G. Feuerstein (1979a: 80).

230. *YB* II.32 (p. 104): *tatra śaucaṃ mṛjjalādijanitaṃ medhyābhyavaharaṇādi ca bāhyam. ābhyantaraṃ cittamalānāmākṣālanam.*

231. See n. 186 above on *YS* II.41 and purity of the mind-*sattva.*

232. See n. 190 above on *YS* II.45.

233. *YB* II.45 (p. 110): *īśvarārpitasarvabhāvasya samādhisiddhiryayā sarvamīpsitamavitathaṃ jānāti deśāntare dehāntare kālāntare ca. tato'sya prajñā yathābhūtaṃ prajānātīti.*

234. *YB* I.23 (p. 25): *praṇidhānād bhaktiviśeṣādāvarjita īśvarastamanugṛhṇātyabhidhyānamātreṇa. tad abhidhyānamātrād api yogina āsannatamaḥ samādhilābhaḥ samādhiphalaṃ ca bhavatīti.*

235. *YB* II.1 (p. 58): *īśvarapraṇidhānaṃ sarvakriyāṇāṃ paramagurāvarpaṇaṃ tatphalasaṃnyāso vā.*

236. See the last section of chapter 2.

237. *YS* I.23 (p. 25): *īśvarapraṇidhānād vā.* The *sūtra* appears to present a choice between (1) the five methods *(upāyas)* of *YS* I.20: faith, energy, mindfulness, cognitive *samādhi,* and insight, and (2) *YS* I.23: devotion to *īśvara.*

238. See n. 2 above. Here I take issue with Feuerstein (1979a: 66), who deduces that all *vṛttis* are "overcome" or restricted in *dhyāna* (the stage of practice prior to *samādhi*), thereby refuting the assertions found in the major Sanskrit commentaries or subcommentaries that the *vṛttis* are ultimately mastered only through *samādhi.* *YS* II.11 actually states that the mental processes arising from the *kleśas* are overcome through *dhyāna.* The *vṛttis* caused by the *kleśas* must be taken here to be of the *kliṣṭa* or afflicted type and dominated by *rajas* and *tamas.* All *vṛttis* including the sattvic or nonafflicted *(akliṣṭa)* type are mastered only in *samādhi.* It is the grosser tendencies and affects of the afflictions that are removed through meditation until having been made subtle they (the *kleśas*) are dissolved in the process of *pratiprasava* (*YS* II.10), i.e., through *samādhi.* Vyāsa (*YB* II.11) includes the practice of *prasaṃkhyāna,* which refers to a high-level state in *samādhi* needed to bring about the final elimination of the misidentification with *vṛtti* in its more subtle afflicted seed-form. Feuerstein rigidly separates *dhyāna* from *samādhi,* which Vyāsa does not. Feuerstein also wrongly holds (1980: 74) that *pratyayas,* since they exist in *samādhi,* are more subtle than *vṛttis* (for more here see notes 82, and 84–85 in chapter 5). Feuerstein understands *YS* I.2 as "a preliminary definition of *Yoga*" (1980: 73) "intended to kick off the discussion" (1979a: 26), and that *YS* I.3 ("Then there is abiding in the seer's own form") does not in fact follow from *YS* I.2; in otherwords, there is, according to Feuerstein, an "unexpected hiatus" (ibid.: 28) between these two *sūtras.*

239. See *YS* II.15–17.

240. For more on the embodied implications of freedom in Patañjali's Yoga, see chapter 6.

241. See notes 197–204 above.

242. Feuerstein (1974: 72) rightly argues for a circular arrangement among the eight members where the center of the circle is the goal of Yoga: *kaivalya.* G. Koelman

(1970: 162–163) takes up "Yoga Technique," discussing *kriyā-yoga, yogāṅga,* and the levels of *samādhi* in terms of a typology of levels: (i) the somatic level (p. 162), which has as its goal the "pacification of the body"; (ii) the ethical level (p. 167), intended for the purification and stabilization of the mind; (iii) the psychological level (p. 182), for ensuring "the liberating disjunction of the Self from its conditioning prakṛtic organism"; (iv) the metaphysical level (p. 247), which is identical with emancipation, the realization of *puruṣa.* Koelman's model is useful and in a way complements Patañjali's distinction between the "external members" *(bahir-aṅga)* and "internal members" *(antar-aṅga)* of the eight-limbed path. However, in his analysis it appears that the final stages become incompatible with the earlier ones resulting in a disengagement from or disintegration of human existence rather than an integration and engagement of the liberated identity of the yogin with empirical reality.

243. This is, unfortunately, what has often been done.

244. See Chapple and Kelly (1990: 15).

CHAPTER 5. COGNITIVE *SAMĀDHI*

1. See *YS* I.46. As can be easily inferred from *YS* III.8, *saṃprajñāta* is, compared to the "seedless" *(nirbīja) samādhi,* an outer limb of Yoga; see n. 227 in chapter 4.

2. Vyāsa (*YB* I.1–2 and I.17) and the main commentators after him understand *YS* I.17 to refer to *samādhi* that is linked with objects or mental content; or, as Feuerstein puts it (1979a: 37), *saṃprajñāta* is "object-oriented." *YS* I.18 is interpreted by Vyāsa as providing information on another kind of *samādhi* that he calls *asaṃprajñāta* and is devoid of all objective supports. See also the section on a preliminary look at the meaning and practice of *samādhi* in chapter 4 of our study.

3. The term *asaṃprajñāta* does not appear in the *YS*. But the term *saṃprajñāta* appears in *YS* I.17 with the term *anya* ("other") in the following *sūtra* glossed by the major commentators as *"asaṃprajñāta-samādhi."* Clearly, *asaṃprajñāta-samādhi* is the best candidate there.

4. As translated by Arya (1986: 248). The translation of *asaṃprajñāta* as "acognitive" is, however, highly problematic as it can all too easily lead one to conclude that this *samādhi* is an unconscious or mindless state that makes one incapable of functioning effectively in the world.

5. Obviously both kinds of *samādhi* can be called ecstatic in that they occur outside of or expand beyond the ordinary sense or limits of self or ego. However, in Yoga, *puruṣa* alone is true identity; there is no second principle of authentic selfhood. In line with this fundamental philosophical premise I have designated the two kinds of *samādhi* as ecstasy and enstasy. Lumping together both kinds or categories of *samādhi* as "enstasis" (see Eliade, 1969: 79, 84) or "enstasy" (Feuerstein, 1979a: 37–38) blurs the important distinction made in Yoga between *saṃprajñāta* and *asaṃprajñāta.* More recently, Feuerstein (1989: 11) translates *samādhi* as "ecstasy," which he readily admits does not have exactly the same connotations as "enstasy." He is, however, more emphatic about the distinction in an even more recent work (1990: 106). See our discussion in chapter 4 on a preliminary look at the meaning and practice of *samādhi.*

6. Eliade (1969: 84).

7. Monier Williams (1899: 1152). *Sam* is sometimes prefixed to nouns in the sense of *sama* and can mean (ibid.): "same," "equal," "full," "complete," "whole," "entire."

8. Ibid., p. 652.

9. Ibid., p. 425; note also the abstract noun *prajñā*, which means (ibid.: 659): "wisdom, intelligence, knowledge, discrimination."

10. Ibid., p. 1174.

11. *YB* I.16 (p. 20): *athopāyadvayena niruddhacittavṛtteḥ kathamucyate saṃprajñātaḥ samādhir iti.*

12. *YV* I.17 (p. 104): *upāyadvayenābhyāsavairāgyābhyāṃ niruddharājasatamasavṛtteḥ.*

13. As Vyāsa makes clear in *YB* I.1. See also Vācaspati's (*TV* I.1) comments as well as n. 12 above and n. 238 in chapter 4.

14. *YS* I.17 (p. 20): *vitarkavicārānandāsmitārūpānugamāt saṃprajñātaḥ.*

15. *YB* I.17 (p. 21): *vitarkaścittasyā"lambane sthūla ābhogaḥ. sūkṣmo vicāraḥ. ānando hlādaḥ. ekātmikā saṃvidasmitā. tatra prathamaś catuṣṭayānugataḥ samādhiḥ savitarkaḥ. dvitīyo vitarkavikalaḥ savicāraḥ. tṛtīyo vicāravikalaḥ sānandaḥ. cāturthastadvikalo'smitāmātra. . . . sarva ete sālambanāḥ samādhayaḥ.*

16. G. Feuerstein (1980: 89). See the discussion in chapter 2 on *satkāryavāda* and refer to *SK* 9; cf. *SK* 22 on the causal succession of the categories of existence that appears to give an ontological emphasis to the Sāṃkhyan system.

17. Both Vācaspati Miśra (*TV* I.17) p. 21 and Vijñāna Bhikṣu (*YV* I.17) p. 105 often use the term *sākṣātkāra* for yogic perception.

18. *TV* I.17 (p. 21): *yathā hi prāthamiko dhānuṣkaḥ sthūlameva lakṣyaṃ vidhyatyatha sūkṣmamevaṃ prāthamiko yogī sthūlameva pāñcabhautikaṃ caturbhujādi dhyeyaṃ sākṣātkārotyatha sūkṣmam iti. evaṃ cittasyā"lambane sūkṣma ābhogaḥ sthūlakaraṇabhūtasūkṣmapañcatanmātraliṅgāliṅga viṣayo vicāraḥ.*

19. *YSS* (pp. 44–45): *ayaṃ tūtsarga eveti prāgevoktam. yatho yadīśvaraprasādāt sadguruprasādād vā ādāv eva sūkṣmabhūmikāyām avasthiti yogyatā svacittasya dṛśyate tadā na sthūlādi pūrvapūrvabhūmikāyā mumukṣubhiḥ kālakṣepaḥ kartayaḥ.*

20. See *YB* II.15 (p. 76): *akṣipātrakalpo hi vidvān iti;* see also *YB* II.16 (p. 79).

21. *YS* II.4 (p. 59): *avidyā kṣetramuttareṣāṃ prasuptatanuvicchinnodārāṇām.*

22. *YB* IV.29 (p. 202): *saṃskārabīja.*

23. See *YB* II.4 (p. 59).

24. *YB* II.4 (p. 60).

25. Ibid.: *rāgakāle krodhasyādarśanāt.*

26. Ibid. (p. 61): *viṣaye yo labdhavṛttiḥ sa udāraḥ.*

27. See note 152 in chapter 4.

28. *YB* II.4 (p. 61): *yadavidyayā vastvākāryate tadevānuśerate kleśā viparyāsapratyayakāla upalabhyante kṣīyamāṇāṃ cāvidyāmanu kṣīyanta . . .*

29. *YB* II.26 (p. 97): *sattvapuruṣānyatāpratyayo vivekakhyātiḥ.*

30. See *YS* IV.27 (p. 201): *tacchidreṣu pratyayāntarāṇi saṃskārebhyaḥ.*

31. *YB* IV.27 (p. 201): *pratyayāntarāṇyasmīti vā mameti vā jānāmīti . . . kṣīyamāṇabījebhyaḥ pūrvasaṃskārebhya iti.*

32. *YS* IV.28 (p. 201): *hānameṣāṃ kleśavad uktam.*

33. Cf. *YS* II.26.

34. VB IV.28 (p. 202): *yathā kleśā dagdhabījabhāvā na prarohasanarthā bhavanti tathā jñānāgni nā dagdhabījabhāvaḥ pūrvasaṃskāro na pratyayaprasūr bhavati.*

35. The term "de-identification" does not imply here that the power or capacity of the mind to identify with the objects of experience has been taken away from the yogin or permanently discarded.

36. As *YS* I.21-22 make clear. See the section on "pedagogy" in chapter 1.

37. Here I have consulted Arya's (1986: 224-225) formulation of Patañjali's model. See chapter 2 (n. 129) of our study for a more detailed explanation of the ontological schematic outlined in *YS* II.19 and *YB* II.19.

38. G. Feuerstein (1979a: 14).

39. Ibid.

40. See, for example, *Kaṭha Up* VI.7-8.

41. *YS* IV.3; see n. 172 in chapter 2.

42. See *YS* II.28 and *YB* II.28.

43. This refers to the *samāpatti*s of *YS* I.42-44.

44. *YS* III.4-5; see notes 219 and 220 in chapter 4.

45. *YS* I.47-50; see the discussion on *nirvicāra-samādhi* later in this chapter.

46. The analogy of the "red-hot ball of iron" is given by Vijñāna Bhikṣu; see *YV* I.17 (p. 110): *taptāyaḥ piṇḍavad ekībhāvena sthūlasākṣātkāre puruṣaparyantānāṃ sarveṣāmeva bhānāt.* "In the direct perception of the gross object there is perception of everything up to *puruṣa* because of an identity, as in [the case of] a red-hot ball of iron."

47. *YS* I.15; see n. 109 in chapter 4.

48. Patañjali does state in *YS* IV.1 that the *siddhi*s (supranormal powers) can be the result of birth, herbs, *mantra* recitation, ascesis, or *samādhi*. But nowhere in the *YS* does Patañjali claim that drugs can replace the self-discipline and commitment required for the attainment of *samādhi*. Furthermore, the *siddhi*s are not the true goal of Yoga.

49. See C. G. Jung (1936), "Yoga and the West," in *Collected Works,* vol. 11, and (1973), *Letters,* vol. 1, pp. 262-263; see also C. G. Jung (1963), *The Integration of the Personality,* (London: Kegan Paul), p. 26, and (1978), *Psychology and the East*. For a critique of Jung's views, especially on his equating *samādhi* with the psychologist's "unconscious," see Swami Akhilananda (1947), *Hindu Psychology: Its Meaning for the West,* p. 167; see also H. Jacobs (1961), *Western Therapy and Hindu Sadhana: A Contribution to Comparative Studies on Psychology and Metaphysics,* p. 164. Paralleling Kant, Jung argued from the perspective of the epistemological limitations of human nature (i.e., one cannot know "the thing-in-itself") and the more theological claim within, for example, Christianity, that human nature is inescapably flawed. For a general discussion of Jung's views on Eastern thought and practice, see Coward (1985), *Jung and Eastern Thought*. While Jung's position is obviously prejudiced, he was right to warn against Westerners merely imitating the East and carelessly or impulsively abandoning their historical roots; see, for example, Jung (1953), "Psychological Commentary on the *Tibetan Book of the Dead,*" in *Collected Works,* vol. 11, 2nd ed. (Princeton, N.J.: Princeton University Press, 1969).

50. See n. 217, chapter 4 on *YS* III.11; Vyāsa writes (*YB* III.11: 123): *sarvārthatā cittadharmaḥ. ekāgratā'pi cittadharmaḥ.* J. H. Woods translates the compound *sarva-arthatā* as "dispersiveness."

51. *YS* III.12 (p. 124): *tataḥ punaḥ śāntoditau tulyapratyayau citta-syaikāgratāpariṇāmaḥ.*

52. *YB* III.12 (p. 124): *samādhicittamubhayoranugataṃ . . . sa khalvayaṃ dharmiṇaś cittasyaikāgratāpariṇāmaḥ.* The transformation *(pariṇāma)* termed

"*samādhi*" (*YS* III.11) may be used by Patañjali to include the early stages of cognitive *samādhi* when the state of one-pointedness initially arises in the mind. Through continued practice, cognitive *samādhi* is more matured, and the mind attains to prolonged periods of one-pointedness, as *YS* III.12 seems to imply.

53. As can be inferred from Patañjali's analysis in *YS* I.41. See n. 65 below.

54. Ian Kesarcodi-Watson (1982), "*Samādhi* in Patañjali's Yoga-Sūtras," *PEW* 32.1: 79–80.

55. Ibid., p. 80.

56. Janácek (1951) quoted by Pensa (1969: 200). Elsewhere Pensa (1973: 39) emphasizes that the powers cannot be "separated from the essentially organic and unitary structure of *Yoga*."

57. Feuerstein (1979a: 104).

58. *YS* III.36 (p. 156): *tataḥ prātibhaśrāvaṇavedanādarśāsvādavārtā jāyante.*

59. *YS* III.37 (p. 156): *te samādhāvupasargā vyutthāne siddhayaḥ.* Cf. *Mahābhārata* XII.232.22 and XII.266.7, which advise that these "intuitive illuminations" arising from one's spiritual practice should be ignored or conquered.

60. See Chapple and Kelly (1990: 95).

61. Cf. *BG* III.42, where the senses are described as being great, the mind as being above the senses, the intellect as being superior to the mind, and even greater than the intellect is said to be the Self.

62. *YB* III.45 (p. 165): *na ca śakto'pi padārthaviparyāsaṃ karoti.* The ethical implications of Vyāsa's statement should not go unnoticed and suggest that those who abuse power while claiming to be yogins are not true yogins.

63. *YB* III.55 (p. 175): *tadā puruṣasyopacaritabhogābhāvaḥ śuddhiḥ. etasyāmavasthāyāṃ kaivalyaṃ bhavatīśvarasyānīśvarasya vā. . . . nahi dagdhakleśabījasya jñāne punarapekṣā kācidasti.*

64. The practice referred to here is the meditative practice on one principle (*ekatattvābhyāsa, YS* I.32), dealt with in *YS* I.32–39, and meant for stabilizing the mind and preventing the obstacles or distractions (*YS* I.30–31) from arising. Vyāsa includes *vairāgya* here (*YB* I.31) even though it is not mentioned in *YS* I.32 itself. It appears that from the point of their introduction in *YS* I.12 and onward both *abhyāsa* and *vairāgya* can be seen to include the necessary expedients and preconditions for all yogic attainments and insights.

65. *YS* I.41 (p. 43): *kṣīṇavṛtter abhijātasyeva maṇer grahītṛgrahaṇagrāhyeṣu tatsthatadañjanatā samāpattiḥ.*

66. Woods (1914); Rukmani (1981: 206).

67. Āraṇya (1963: 99).

68. Bangali Baba (1976: 21).

69. R. Prasāda (1912: 64).

70. Sri Purohit Swami (1973).

71. Dvivedī (1934).

72. Taimni (1961).

73. Hauer (1958: 243).

74. Feuerstein (1979a: 51).

75. Koelman (1970: 197).

76. Leggett (1990: 152).

77. Chapple and Kelly (1990: 52).

78. Monier-Williams (1899: 1161).

79. *YB* I.41 (p. 43): *abhijātasyeva maṇer iti dṛṣṭāntopādānam. tathā sphaṭika upāśrayabhedāttattadrūpoparakta upāśrayarūpākāreṇa nirbhāsate tathā grāhyālambanoparaktaṃ cittam grāhyasamāpannaṃ grāhyasvarūpākāreṇa nirbhāsate.*

80. *YS* III.14; see notes 105 and 106 in chapter 2.

81. *YS* III.13; see n. 103 in chapter 2.

82. *YB* I.41 (p. 43): *kṣīṇavṛtter iti pratyastamitapratyayasyetyarthaḥ.*

83. *YV* I.41 (p. 208): *kṣīṇavṛtter apagatavṛttyantarasya cittasyetyarthaḥ.*

84. *TV* I.41 (p. 43): *abhyāsavairāgyābhyāṃ kṣīṇarājasatāmasapramāṇādivṛtteś cittasya. . . . tadanena cittasattvasya svabhāvasvacchasya rajastamobhyāmanabhibhava uktaḥ.* "[From which the modifications have subsided] describes the mind as existing in the state in which that class of modifications (*pramāṇa,* valid cognition) that are of a rajasic or a tamasic nature have subsided as a result of practice and dispassion. In this manner it is stated that the *sattva* of the mind, which is by nature pure, is not overpowered by *rajas* (disturbing activity) and *tamas* (inertia, dullness)."

85. This explanation for the relationship between *vṛtti* and *pratyaya* contrasts with Feuerstein's hierarchical summarization of the process of *nirodha* in that Feuerstein (1979a: 28) sees *"pratyaya-nirodha"* ("restriction of the presented-ideas") as a level of "restriction" that takes place after *"vṛtti-nirodha"* ("restriction of the fluctuations").

86. See n. 82 above; see also *YV* I.41 (p. 209): *pratyayasya pratyayāntarasyetyarthaḥ, samāpatter api pratyayatvāt.*

87. *YB* I.41 (p. 43): *bhūtasūkṣmoparaktaṃ bhūtasūkṣmasamāpannaṃ bhūtasūkṣmasvarūpābhāsaṃ bhavati. tathā sthūlālambanoparaktaṃ sthūlarūpāsamāpannaṃ sthūlarūpābhāsaṃ bhavati. tathā viśvabhedoparaktaṃ viśvabhedasamāpannaṃ viśvarūpābhāsaṃ bhavati.*

88. See *YV* I.41 (p. 210); cf. *YS* I.40 (p. 42): *paramāṇuparamamahattvānto'sya vaśīkāraḥ.* "The yogin's mastery [extends] from the most minute to the greatest."

89. Vācaspati Miśra also holds this opinion; see *TV* I.41 (p. 43).

90. *YB* I.41 (p. 43): *tathā grahaṇeṣvapīndriyeṣvapi draṣṭavyam. grahaṇālambanoparaktaṃ grahaṇasamāpannaṃ grahaṇasvarūpākāreṇa nirbhāsate.*

91. As Vijñāna Bhikṣu notes in *YV* I.41 (p. 210): *indriyāṇāṃ sūkṣmaṃ buddhyahaṃkārāv iti bhāṣyakāro vakṣyati.*

92. *YB* I.41 (pp. 43–44): *tathā grahītṛpuruṣālambanoparaktaṃ grahītṛpuruṣasamāpannaṃ grahītṛpuruṣasvarūpākāreṇa nirbhāsate. tathā muktapuruṣālambanoparaktaṃ muktapuruṣasamāpannaṃ muktapuruṣasvarūpākāreṇa nirbhāsata iti.*

93. *YV* I.41 (p. 211): *grahītṛtvaṃ buddher api vyapadiśyata iti tadvyāvarttanāya puruṣapadam.*

94. See n. 129 in chapter 2 on *YB* II.19 and Āraṇya (1963: 102, 197).

95. Vācaspati's reflection theory, however, tends to shift the locus of knowledge to the *buddhi* or intellect.

96. See Arya (1986: 376–377).

97. Chapple and Kelly (1990: 52) give a translation of *YS* I.41 that is at variance with Vyāsa's interpretation, translating *YS* I.41 as follows: "[The accomplished mind] of diminished fluctuations, like a precious (or clear) jewel assuming the color of any near object, has unity among grasper, grasping, and grasped." Stating that Vyāsa posits three types of "unity" *(samāpatti),* they argue (ibid.) for only "one form of unity where . . . all three aspects of grasping, etc., collapse, regardless of what is grasped, gross or

subtle." *YS* I.41 can be interpreted as positing one unity among grasper, grasping, and grasped, but this can be the case only after sufficient purification of the mind has taken place. As a study of *vitarka* and *vicāra* (which follows this section) makes clear, the earlier stages of *samāpatti* (in the *"sa"* forms) do not entail the necessary purity of mind to enable a full-fledged unity of the three components of the above triad to take place. Much of what goes on at the lower-level *samāpattis* is a removal of misidentification (ignorance) so that unification among the grasper, grasping, and the grasped can arise. Vyāsa understands *samāpatti* as a multileveled practice that progressively purifies and illuminates consciousness, thereby allowing insight and pure "seeing" to arise. In fact, the stages of *samāpatti* are considered by Patañjali to fall under the category of *samādhi* with seed (*sabīja, YS* I.46), the potential still remaining for the "seeds" of ignorance to "sprout." When sufficient purification of consciousness in relation to the grasped, grasping, and grasper has transpired, only then can there be an authentic unification among grasper, grasping, and grasped. *Samāpatti* does not *begin* with this unification. Vyāsa is pointing out where ignorance can arise in forms of cognitive *samādhi* and how that ignorance can be eradicated. His emphasis here is pedagogical as well as epistemological. *Samāpatti* involves a process of the increasing sattvification of consciousness where the yogin's attention is led from the grosser to the most subtle aspects of the "seeable" (including the ego and intellect) through which insight *(prajñā)* dawns and the discriminative discernment between *sattva* and *puruṣa* comes about. Vyāsa's perspective, however, can be seen to incorporate the above view held by Chapple and Kelly: When sufficient purification and illumination of consciousness have taken place, on whatever level, be it that of the grasped, grasping, or grasped, there is a unification of all three implying no epistemological distortion. But the stages of purification in *samādhi* are important and must not be overlooked in Yoga. For a critique of Vyāsa's reading of *YS* I.41 (and other passages of the *YS*) see C. Chapple (1994), "Reading Patañjali Without Vyāsa: A Critique of Four *Yoga Sūtra* Passages." *JAAR* 62.1: 85–105.

98. See n. 18 above.

99. Here I will elaborate upon what Vijñāna Bhikṣu has said (see n. 19 above). The question arises as to whether the methodical and analytical approach of *YS* I.17 is essential in order to prepare the yogin for *asaṃprajñāta-samādhi*. Patañjali allows for dedication to *īśvara,* a devotional practice that can result in purification and, according to the commentators, "favor" from *īśvara*. On the topic of "godhead," the commentators have for the most part expressed their own religious perspectives and have attempted to find a place for it within the scheme of Patañjali and Vyāsa. The realization of the various aspects or descent *(avatāra)* of the deity may be categorized in two ways: In one approach the yogin is engaged in meditational practice and *samādhi* to such a degree that the purified consciousness may ascend and project itself to the subtle worlds that are the domains of particular aspects of the deities. In the other, the deity is so pleased by the devotee's *japa* (repetition of the name *Om [praṇava]* or simply mental concentration on a *mantra*) and meditation/contemplation (as in *YS* I.27–28) that it projects an appearance of itself in order to bestow the grace of its descent and presence to the devotee. As an experiential fact in Yoga the two, however, cannot be separated. The ascent of the yogin's consciousness through self-effort and the descent of "divine grace" both are aids in the cultivation of *samādhi.* If a yogin's practice *(sādhana)* or "cultivation" *(bhāvana)* is focused on a particular deity, it is required that the yogin

take this same supportive factor *(ālambana)* through all the four stages of *saṃprajñāta* in the order in which they occur (see *YV* I.17: 105). The order in which the four stages are practiced and mastered is important. However, according to Vijñāna Bhikṣu, Patañjali seems to imply that if the yogin's awareness spontaneously ascends to a "higher ground" through dedication to *īśvara,* then it need not be necessary to climb methodically and laboriously over the lower steps (see n. 19 above). Thus, the "favor" obtained through devotion to *īśvara* may be understood as an efficacious expedient and "shortcut" that can bypass the more formal method as presented in *YS* I.17. Although the possibility of such an instantaneous realization of a higher state is conceded to by Vyāsa (*YB* I.23), for the purposes of this study it is assumed that an ongoing method is normally requisite for attaining mental purification and insight in order that the yogin may become fit for the realization of *puruṣa.* In the tradition of Patañjali, all objects of *samādhi* are either parts or composites of *grāhya, grahaṇa,* or *grahītṛ.* For example, a candle flame for concentration is part of the fire element. An icon may be considered a composite product of all five gross elements. The so-called "theism" of Yoga encouraged the later commentators such as Vijñāna Bhikṣu to state more clearly that the mental image of *virāṭ*, the universal form of *īśvara,* or the figure of a deity or descent *(avatāra)* is often used as the object of concentration. Although at first glance these mental images may not appear to be included in the scheme of Patañjali, the theology of the Purāṇa texts explains that *īśvara* may take forms that appear material-like to the devotees, even though the spiritual power and energy utilized for such appearances is actually "nonmaterial," i.e., more subtle. As seen from the point of view of the devotee seeking experiences leading to illuminations in *saṃprajñāta-samādhi,* the form of such a "divine manifestation" is a visible one subject to experiences involving the senses; therefore, concentration on such an image is concentration on the *viśeṣa*s. Vijñāna Bhikṣu (*YV* I.17: 110), citing the *Garuḍa-Purāṇa* (I.229.25) as one of the authoritative traditional texts that regards the general order of the *samādhi*s, tells us that in the early stages of Yoga one should concentrate on Lord Viṣṇu "with form." Then, once the mind has mastered the gross form of the object, it should slowly be turned toward the subtle. One of the main tasks of the spiritual preceptor or *guru* is to guide the disciple *(śiṣya)* in selecting an appropriate object of meditation—the one that will be most helpful to that particular disciple. One not attracted to such mental images of a deity may begin one's concentration on other parts or composites of the *viśeṣa*s by adopting a form of meditation as desired (*YS* I.39). For more on the status and role of *īśvara* in the *YS* see our discussion in chapter 2.

100. J. H. Woods (1914).
101. Vivekānanda (1966); Taimni (1961).
102. Bangali Baba (1976: 9).
103. Hauer (1958: 24).
104. R. Prasāda (1912: 31).
105. Sri Purohit Swami (1973).
106. Feuerstein (1979a: 37); Koelman (1970: 198).
107. Tola and Dragonetti (1987: 52).
108. Chapple and Kelly (1990: 40).
109. Āraṇya (1963: 48).
110. R. Śarmā (1967).
111. *TV* I.17 (p. 21): *svarūpasākṣātkāravatī prajñā''bhogaḥ.*

112. See, for example, *YV* I.17 (p. 106): *viśeṣeṇa tarkaṇamavadhāraṇaṃ* . . . ; see also n. 115 below.

113. See n. 15 above and related text.

114. See Monier-Williams (1899: 145).

115. *YV* I.17 (p. 106): *sthūlayorbhūtendriyayoradṛṣṭāśrutāmatāśeṣaviśeṣasākṣātkāraḥ sa vitarka ityarthaḥ.*

116. See n. 112 above.

117. *YS* I.42 (p. 44): *tatra śabdhārthajñānavikalpaiḥ saṃkīrṇā savitarkā samāpattiḥ.*

118. *YB* I.42 (pp. 44–45): *tadyathā gauriti śabdo gaurityartho gauriti jñānamityavibhāgena vibhaktānāmapi grahaṇaṃ dṛṣṭam. vibhajyamānāś cānye śabdadharmā anye'rthadharmā anye vijñānadharmā ityeteṣām vibhaktaḥ panthāḥ.*

119. *TV* I.42 (p. 44): *tadevamavinirbhāgena vibhaktānāmapi śabdārthajñānānāṃ grahaṇaṃ loke dṛṣṭaṃ draṣṭavyam.*

120. *YB* I.42 (p. 45): *tatra samāpannasya yogino yo gavādyarthaḥ samādhiprajñāyāṃ samārūḍhaḥ sa cecchabdārthajñānavikalpānuviddha upāvartate sā saṃkīrṇā samāpattiḥ savitarketyucyate.*

121. See *RM* I.42 (p. 14). See also *YS* III.17, which points out the confusion arising from the overlapping or superimposition of words, objects, and ideas on one another; from *saṃyama* ("constraint") on the distinctions of them, there is knowledge of the sound (i.e., utterance) of all beings.

122. See *YV* I.42 (pp. 212–215).

123. Koelman (1970: 199).

124. Feuerstein (1979a: 53).

125. As suggested by Tola and Dragonetti (1987: 160).

126. Vyāsa (*YB* I.42: 45) refers to *nirvitarka* as *"paraṃ pratyakṣam"*—the higher perception of the yogin.

127. *YS* I.43 (p. 46): *smṛtipariśuddhau svarūpaśūnyevārthamātranirbhāsā nirvitarkā.* See *YS* III.3 cited in n. 216 of chapter 4.

128. *YB* I.42 (p. 45): *yadā punaḥ śabdasaṃketasmṛtipariśuddhau śrutānumānajñānavikalpaśūnyāyāṃ samādhiprajñāyāṃ svarūpamātreṇāvasthito'rtha* . . .

129. Vācaspati (*TV* I.42: 45) uses the word *tyakta,* "abandoned." Vijñāna Bhikṣu, however, uses the expression (*YV* I.43: 218): *saṃketasmṛtistyajyate,* meaning "gives up the memory of convention."

130. In *RM* I.43 (p. 14) Bhoja uses the term *pravilaya.*

131. *YB* I.42 (p. 45): *tatsvarūpākāramātratayaivāvacchidyate. sā ca nirvitarkā samāpattiḥ. tat paraṃ pratyakṣam. tacca śrutānumānayorbījam. tataḥ śrutānumāne prabhavataḥ. na ca śrutānumānajñānasahabhūtaṃ. taddarśanaṃ. tasmād asaṃkīrṇaṃ pramāṇāntareṇa yogino nirvitarkasamādhijaṃ darśanam.*

132. Koelman (1970: 210).

133. See *TV* I.42 (p. 45).

134. Ibid.

135. See *YV* I.43 (p. 219); see also Vyāsa's commentary on *YS* I.49 in n. 327 of chapter 3.

136. *YB* I.43. In fact, Patañjali declares that all the forms of *prakṛti,* whether manifest or not, whether present or latent, have the three *guṇa*s for their essence. He states in *YS* IV.13 (p. 187): *te vyaktasūkṣmā guṇātmānaḥ.* "These [forms], manifest and subtle, are of the nature of the *guṇas.*" *YS* IV.14 (p. 188, see n. 53 in chapter 3) goes

on to assert: "From the homogeneity in the transformation [of the *guṇas*] there is the 'thatness' of an object." Vyāsa (*YB* I.43 and IV.13-16) refutes views (see below) held by certain opponents and reasserts the Sāṃkhyan view (i.e., *satkāryavāda*) that seeks to retain an ontological continuity between an effect and its material cause. The Nyāya-Vaiśeṣika schools adhere to *ārambhavāda* (the doctrine of a "new beginning"), which is based on the perspective that qualities begin afresh in the effects that are produced when atoms of various elements combine, and that their prior absence in the anterior (the cause) is evident; that is, that it is known that those qualities were not there previous to their appearances in newly created objects. While both the above doctrines agree that the effect is new formally, in the later it is regarded as also new *qua* being. See Potter, ed. (1977), *Encyclopedia of Indian Philosophies,* 2: 58-59. The Buddhists of the Sautrāntika and Vaibhāṣika schools hold that an object (e.g., a jar) is simply a combination of uncountable numbers of atoms, not their transmuted product, and that there are not cause and effect relationships between the atoms and the jar. This is known as the "aggregation doctrine" *(saṅghāta-vāda).* Vyāsa sees Patañjali as taking a stand against the Buddhist Yogācāra school, which has been viewed by some as a form of pure idealism in that it is argued that this school, sometimes referred to as Vijñānavāda, holds that all perceived objects exist merely as ideas within a universal mind *(ālaya-vijñāna),* thereby negating the reality of the manifest objective world. *YS* IV.14 and 16 can be interpreted as a tacit refutation of the above idealism. For more here see notes 54-56 and related text in chapter 3.

137. As suggested by Tola and Dragonetti (1987: 164).

138. See n. 15 above for the text of *YB* I.17.

139. See Woods (1914), Taimni (1961), Koelman (1970: 202), Feuerstein (1979a: 37), Chapple and Kelly (1990: 40).

140. See Vivekānanda (1966).

141. See Bangali Baba (1976: 9).

142. See Hauer (1958: 241).

143. See S. Purohit Swami (1973).

144. See R. Prasāda (1912: 32).

145. See Tola and Dragonetti (1987: 51).

146. See Monier-Williams (1899: 389).

147. See n. 15 above for the text of *YB* I.17.

148. Āraṇya (1963: 49) writes: "As the fundamental principles and subtle yogic ideals are realized through such thinking, the concentration on subtle objects is called *vicārānugata samādhi.*"

149. *YS* I.44 (p. 48): *etayaiva savicārā nirvicārā ca sūkṣmaviṣayā vyākhyātā.*

150. *YB* I.44 (pp. 48-49): *tatra bhūtasūkṣmakeṣvabhivyaktadharmakeṣu deśakālanimittānubhavāvacchinneṣu yā samāpattiḥ sā savicāretyucyate.*

151. For an examination of the concept of time in Indian systems of thought, see A. N. Balshev (1983), *A Study of Time in Indian Philosophy.*

152. *TV* I.44 (p. 48): *nimittaṃ pārthivasya paramāṇorgandhatanmātrapradhānebhyaḥ pañcatanmātrebhya utpattiḥ*, i.e., cause—for instance, the atom of earth is produced by the five subtle elements among which the subtle element of smell is predominant. Even though the word *nimitta* normally refers to an efficient cause, here it can be understood to be taken in the broader sense of any causative factor including the process of the subtle elements producing respective effects.

153. *YB* I.44 (p. 49): *tatrāpyekabuddhinirgrāhyamevoditadharmaviśiṣṭaṃ bhūtasūkṣmamālambanībhūtaṃ samādhiprajñāyamupatiṣṭhate.*

154. Ibid.: *yā punaḥ sarvathā sarvataḥ śantoditāvyapadeśyadharmānavacchinneṣu sarvadharmānupātiṣu sarvadharmātmakeṣu samāpattiḥ sā nirvicāretyucyate.*

155. See n. 153 above.

156. *YB* I.44 (p. 49): *evaṃ svarūpaṃ hi tadbhūtasūkṣmametenaiva svarūpeṇā''lambanībhūtameva samādhiprajñāsvarūpamuparañjayati. prajñā ca svarūpaśūnyevārthamātrā yadā bhavati tadā nirvicāretyucyate.*

157. *TV* I.44 (p. 49): *atra saṃketasmṛtyāgamānumānavikalpānuvedhaḥ sūcitaḥ.*

158. *YV* I.44 (p. 233): *pūrvabhūmikāyāṃ tyaktavikalpasyottarabhūmikāyāmasaṃbhavād.*

159. *YB* I.44 (p. 49): *evamubhayoretayaiva nirvitarkayā vikalpahānirvyākhyāteti.*

160. *YB* III.50: see n. 93 in chapter 3; see also notes 30–34 of this chapter.

161. Cf. the Mahāyāna Madhyamaka Buddhist doctrine of "emptiness" *(śūnyatā),* which disallows essentiality to both subject and object.

162. See Feuerstein (1980: 89).

163. *YS* I.47 (p. 51): *nirvicāravaiśāradye'dhyātmaprasādaḥ.*

164. *YS* I.48 (p. 51): *ṛtaṃbharā tatra prajñā.*

165. *YB* I.48 (p. 51): *na ca tatra viparyāsajñānagandho'pyastīti.*

166. See *YSS* (p. 2), where Bhikṣu asserts that *nirodha* not only involves the *vṛttis* of *YS* I.6 but also includes *vṛttis* which have to do with desire or will *(icchā);* cessation *(nirodha)* implies both a moral and affective as well as a cognitive purification.

167. *YB* I.47 (p. 51): *aśuddhyāvaraṇamalāpetasya prakāśātmano buddhisattvasya rajastamobhyāmanabhibhūtaḥ svacchaḥ sthitipravāho vaiśāradyam. yadā nirvicārasya samādhervaiśāradyamidaṃ jāyate tadā yogino bhavatyadhyātmaprasādo bhūtārthaviṣayaḥ kramānanurodhī sphuṭaḥ prajñālokaḥ.*

168. See Monier-Williams (1899: 223).

169. See n. 175 in chapter 4.

170. *YV* I.1 (p. 26): *savitarkādikrameṇaiva sākṣātkāravṛddhyā caramabhūmikāyāmṛtambharaprajñodayena bhūmikācatuṣṭaya eva sākṣātkārasaṃbandhād iti.*

171. Swami Nikhilananda (1951: 95).

172. *YS* I.45 (p. 50): *sūkṣmaviṣayatvaṃ cāliṅgaparyavasānam.*

173. *YB* I.45 (p. 50): *pārthivasyāṇorgandhatanmātraṃ sūkṣmo viṣayaḥ. . . . teṣāmahaṃkāraḥ. asyāpi liṅgamātraṃ sūkṣmo viṣayaḥ. liṅgamātrasyāpyaliṅgaṃ sūkṣmo viṣayaḥ. na cāliṅgātparaṃ sūkṣmamasti.* "In the case of an atom of earth, the subtle element of odor is a subtler object [for the *vicāra* meditation]. . . . Subtler than these [subtle elements] is the ego-sense *(ahaṃkāra).* Subtler than that is the designator (the great principle—*liṅga-mātra* or *mahat*). More subtle than that is the unmanifest *(aliṅga, pradhāna).* There is nothing more subtle [i.e., prakṛtic] beyond the unmanifest."

174. See *YS* I.19 (p. 22): *bhavapratyayo videhaprakṛtilayānām;* see n. 117 on *YB* I.15 in chapter 4 and the discussion later in this chapter on the status of the *prakṛtilayas*, especially the text referring to notes 216–220.

175. See n. 172 above.

176. *YB* I.45 (p. 50): *nanvasti puruṣaḥ sūkṣma iti. satyam. yathā liṅgātparamaliṅgasya saukṣmyaṃ na caivaṃ puruṣasya. kiṃ tu, liṅgasyānvayikāraṇaṃ puruṣo na bhavati, hetus tu bhavatīti. ataḥ pradhāne saukṣmyaṃ niratiśayaṃ vyākhyātam.*

177. See Arya (1986: 408).

178. *ānando hlādaḥ*; see n. 15 above on *YB* I.17 and related text.

179. Koelman (1970: 207).

180. Cf *SK* 25.

181. See n. 15 above for Vyāsa's text.

182. *YV* I.17 (p. 107): *tadānīm cānandagocara evāha sukhīti cittavṛttirbhavati na sūksṃavastusvapīti vicārānugatād viśesaḥ.* "At that time there is only *ānanda* as the object; the modification of the mind of the form 'I am happy' is there; and there is no modification with regard to even subtle objects. Thus it is different from the Yoga connected with *vicāra*."

183. See *YB* I.19 (p. 22) where Vyāsa seems to imply that at this level of *samādhi* the *videha* has attained a degree of mastery of the "subtle worlds" made up of the six *aviśeṣas*.

184. *TV* I.17 (p. 21): *prakāśaśīlatayā khala sattvapradhānādahaṃkārādindriyāṇyutpannāni. sattvaṃ sukhamiti tānyapi sukhānīti tasminnābhogo hlāda iti.*

185. *YV* I.17 (pp. 108–109). Feuerstein (1989: 196) appears to follow Vācaspati Miśra's interpretation of *ānanda-* and *asmitā-samādhi* by dividing these stages of *samādhi* into two categories, namely: *sānanda-samāpatti* ("ecstatic coincidence with bliss") and *nirānanda-samāpatti* ("ecstatic coincidence beyond bliss") as well as *sāsmitā-samāpatti* ("ecstatic coincidence with 'I-am-ness'") and *nirasmitā-samāpatti* ("ecstatic coincidence beyond 'I-am-ness'").

186. *TV* I.17 (p. 21): *asmitāprabhavānīndriyāṇi. tenaiṣāmasmitā sūkṣmaṃ rūpam. sā cā"tmanā grahītrā saha buddhirekātmikā saṃvit.* See main text referring to n. 193 below.

187. See *YV* I.17 (p. 107).

188. *YV* I.17 (p. 106): *prakṛtimahadahaṃkārapañcatanmātrarūpā bhūtendriyayoḥ sūkṣmā . . . sa vicāra.*

189. Āraṇya writes (1963: 49): "The object or basis of this concentration [on bliss] is a particular feeling of [sattvic] happiness felt all over the mind and the senses due to a particular state of calmness."

190. Ibid, p. 50.

191. *RM* I.17 (p. 6): *yadā tu rajastamoleśānuviddhamantaḥkaraṇasattvaṃ bhāvyate tadā guṇabhāvāccitiśakteḥ sukhaprakāśamayasya sattvasya bhāvyamānasyodrekāt sānandaḥ samādhir bhavati.*

192. Ibid: *na cāhaṃkārāsmitāyor abhedaḥ śaṅkanīyaḥ. yato yatrāntaḥkaraṇamahamityullekhena viṣayānvedayate so'haṃkāraḥ. yatrāntar mukhatayā pratilomapariṇāme prakṛtilīne cetasi sattāmātramavabhāti sā'smitā.*

193. See n. 186 above for text.

194. *YB* I.17 (p. 21): *ekātmikā saṃvidasmitā.*

195. See the section on *saṃyoga* in chapter 3 of our study and also *YS* II.17 cited in n. 199 of chapter 2.

196. See n. 191 above.

197. *YB* I.36 (p. 41): *tāthā' smitāyāṃ samāpannaṃ cittaṃ nistaraṅgamahodadhikalpaṃ śāntamanantam . . .*

198. Ibid: *yatredamuktam—"tamaṇumātramātmānamanuvidyāsmītyevaṃ tāvatsaṃprajānīte" iti.*

199. See, for example, *Kaṭha Up* II.8; *Mait Up* VI.20, 38 and VII.7; *Muṇḍaka Up* II.2, 2 and III.1.9; see also *BG* VIII.9.

200. See, for example, *BĀ Up* IV.4.20 and 22; *Kaṭha Up* II.22.

201. See, for example, *Kaṭha Up* II.20 and *Śvet Up* III.9.

202. See our discussion in chapter 2 on *YB* II.19 (cited in n. 129).

203. On this see Āraṇya (1963: 365), who states: "When the powers of omnipotence and omniscience are acquired the yogin becomes like Almighty Īśvara. That is the highest state of the Intellect. Puruṣa with such adjuncts, i.e., such adjuncts and their seer combined, is called Mahān Ātmā or the Great Self. The adjuncts by themselves are also called Mahat-tattva."

204. See notes 164, 165, and 170 above.

205. See Monier-Williams (1899: 856). From another perspective, one can say that by *adding* or including the consciousness of *puruṣa* or authentic identity in Yoga, one's life becomes complete, full, whole.

206. See reference to *YB* II.18 in n. 215 of chapter 2.

207. *YS* I.47; see n. 163 above.

208. *YB* I.41; see n. 92 above.

209. *TV* I.41 (pp. 43–44): *asmitāspadaṃ hi grahītā puruṣa iti bhāvaḥ.*

210. Koelman (1970: 215).

211. See n. 15 above.

212. *YV* I.17 (p. 109): *eka evātmā'syāṃ viṣayatvenāstītyekātmikā. [tathā coktam-] ekālambane yā cittasya kevalapuruṣākārā saṃvit sākṣātkāro'smītyetāvanmātrākāratvādasmitetyarthaḥ.* Bhikṣu later qualifies *asmitā* as being of two kinds: pertaining to *jīvātman* (qualified being) or pertaining to *param-ātman* (unqualified being).

213. See, for example, *YS* III.35 (p. 154): *parārthatvāt svārthasaṃyamāt puruṣajñānam;* refer to n. 333 in chapter 3.

214. Cf. n. 197 above.

215. *YS* II.26.

216. *YB* I.19 (p. 23): *tathā prakṛtilayāḥ sādhikāre cetasi prakṛtilīne kaivalyapadamivānubhavanti.*

217. See the discussion on *viparyaya* in chapter 3.

218. *YB* II.19 (p. 86): *aliṅgāvasthāyāṃ na puruṣārtho heturnāliṅgāvasthāyāmādau puruṣārthatā kāraṇaṃ bhavatīti. na tasyāḥ puruṣārthatā kāraṇaṃ bhavatīti. nāsau puruṣārtha kṛteti . . .*

219. *YS* I.21–22. Chapple and Kelly (1990: 41–42) argue that the *prakṛti-laya*s are to be deemed "mild" *(mṛdu)* or weak in their practice compared to the "moderate" *(madhya)* intensity or type of practice as outlined in *YS* I.20 and the "ardent" (*adhimātratva, YS* I.22) or "strongly intense" type of yogin (*tīvra-saṃvega, YS* I.21).

220. *YS* I.19 (p. 22): *bhavapratyayo videhaprakṛtilayānām.* "Of the ones who are absorbed in *prakṛti* and of those who are bodiless, [there is] an idea/intention of becoming." See also n. 117 and text in chapter 4 of this study which mentions the "bodiless" *(videha)* yogins along with the *prakṛti-laya*s.

221. Feuerstein (1979a: 38).

222. In doing so I have responded to Feuerstein's query on this matter. He writes (1980: 90): "It is unclear how he [Vyāsa] envisages the correlation between these postulated types [of ecstasy in *YS* I.17] and the four varieties of *samāpatti* as cited in *YS* I. 42–44. Does he [Vyāsa] take *ānanda* and *asmitā-samādhi* to be instances of *nirvicāra-samāpatti*?"

223. *TV* I.46 (pp. 50–51): *tena grāhye catasraḥ samāpattayo grahītṛgrahaṇayośca tasra ityaṣṭau siddhā bhavantīti.* Feuerstein (1989: 196; see n. 185 above) appears to endorse Vācaspati Miśra's reading of eight stages.

224. *YV* I.17 (p. 107): *yaścittasya vicārānugatabhūmyārohātsattvaprakarṣeṇa jāyamāne hlādākhyasukhaviśeṣa ābhogaḥ sākṣātkāro bhavati sa ānandaviṣayakatvādānanda ityarthaḥ;* see also n. 182 above.

225. *YV* I.17 (pp. 108–109).

226. *YV* I.17 (p. 109): *asyā asmitāyā api sāsmitanirasmitarūpo vibhāgo nāsti.*

227. See Koelman (1970: 198ff).

228. Ibid., p. 223.

229. Feuerstein (1980: 91).

230. *YS* I.46 (p. 50).

231. *YB* I.46 (p. 50): *tāścatasraḥ samāpattayo bahirvastubījā iti samādhirapi sabījaḥ.*

232. *RM* I.46 (p. 15): *tā evoktalakṣaṇāḥ samāpattayaḥ saha bījenā''lambanena vartata iti sabījaḥ saṃprajñātaḥ samādhirityucyate, sarvāsāṃ sālambanatvāt.*

233. This is also the interpretation of Ballantyne, Taimni, and Āraṇya, although they do not affirm, as explicitly as Bhoja Rāja does, the equivalence: *bīja = ālambana.*

234. Cf. Dvivedī, Vivekānanda, and those explicitly mentioned below.

235. Hauer (1958: 243, 466 n. 11).

236. *MP* I.46 (p. 23): *bandhabīja.*

237. *YV* I.46 (p. 240): *bahirvastunyanātmadharmāḥ. saṃskāradharmādayo duḥkhabījāni jāyante ābhya iti bahirvastubījāḥ.*

238. *YSS* (p. 26): *dhyeyarūpālambanayogāt tadāpi vṛttibījasaṃskārotpatteś ceti.*

239. Parts of Vyāsa's remaining commentary appear to support Vijñāna Bhikṣu's understanding of the term *bīja;* see, for example, *YB* III.50 and IV.28.

240. This has been discussed in some detail in chapter 3 (refer, for example, to n. 274) and chapter 4.

241. *YB* I.46 (p. 50): *tāścatasraḥ samāpattayo bahirvastubījā iti samādhirapi sabījaḥ. tatra sthūle'rthe savitarkā nirvitarkaḥ, sūkṣme'rthe savicāro nirvicāra iti caturdhopasaṃkhyātaḥ samādhir iti.*

242. See Arya (1986: 409). Though it appears that the *samāpatti*s are referred to as *"samādhi,"* Vijñāna Bhikṣu (*YV* I.46) makes it clear that *samāpatti* and *samādhi* are not to be confused as synonyms. While *samāpatti* only occurs at the time (at least provisionally during the process of purification) in which *saṃprajñāta-samādhi* takes place, it can be understood as the effect or the quality of the mind during *saṃprajñāta-samādhi.* As such, *samādhi* is the cessation of distraction and misidentification, a one-pointedness of mind, whereas *samāpatti* refers to the unification or identity of the mind with the object of contemplation resulting from this one-pointedness. In other words, *samāpatti* is both contained in, and arises from *samādhi.* The two represent and are experienced as a continuum of awareness and identity.

243. The term *nirbīja* is used in *YS* I.51 and III.8.

CHAPTER 6. THE "ALONENESS" OF THE KNOWER

1. *YB* II.28 (p. 99): *teṣāmanuṣṭhānātpañcaparvaṇo viparyayasyāśuddhirūpasya kṣayo nāśaḥ.* See discussion on the *kleśa*s in chapter 3.

2. *YS* II.28.

3. *YB* I.12–13.

4. *YB* I.5; see n. 85 in chapter 3 and the discussion in the main text on *kliṣṭa-* and *akliṣṭa-vṛtti*.

5. See *YS* II.41, where the expression *sattvaśuddhi* is used.

6. *YS* III.50 and IV.34.

7. C. Pensa (1969: 207).

8. Ibid., p. 205.

9. As Vijñāna Bhikṣu maintains, the *śāstra*s mention many expiations (*prāyaścitta*s) for the eradication of demerit or evil *(pāpa)* that has begun to fructify; see *YV* I.1 and I.50 on pp. 29 and 256 respectively.

10. See, for example, *Chānd Up* III.16.1.

11. On this see *YB* IV.10 (pp. 184–185) where Vyāsa points to various internal means in Yoga (such as meditations on friendliness, faith, and so on, culminating in knowledge and detachment) as being independent of and superior to external means (such as various performed deeds leading to praise or salutations, and so on). The "mental" means adopted in Yoga are said to be productive of the highest *dharma.* See also the *BG* (IV.33), which declares the superiority of the "knowledge-sacrifice" over sacrifice of material things.

12. *YS* I.48; see n. 164 in chapter 5.

13. *YS* I.47; see n. 163 in chapter 5.

14. *YV* I.48 (p. 245): *tasminsamāhitacittasyeti purvoktasabījayoga* . . .

15. This is also implied in the practice of *saṃyama* ("constraint"), involving concentration, meditation, and *samādhi* (*YS* III.4).

16. *YS* III.49; see n. 125 in chapter 3.

17. *YS* I.50 (p. 53): *tajjaḥ saṃskāro'nyasaṃskārapratibandhī.*

18. *YB* I.50 (pp. 53–54): *samādhiprajñāpratilambhe yoginaḥ prajñākṛtaḥ saṃskāro navo navo jāyate. . . . samādhiprajñāprabhavaḥ saṃskāro vyutthāna-saṃskārāśayaṃ bādhate. vyutthānasaṃskārābhibhavāttatprabhavāḥ pratyayā na bhavanti. pratyayanirodhe samādhirūpatiṣṭhate. tataḥ samādhijā prajñā, tataḥ prajñākṛtāḥ saṃskārā iti navo navaḥ saṃskārāśayo jāyate. tataśca prajñā, tataśca saṃskārā iti. kathamasau saṃskārātiśayaścittaṃ sādhikāraṃ na kariṣyatīti. na te prajñākṛtāḥ saṃskārāḥ kleśakṣayahetutvāccittamadhikāraviśiṣṭaṃ kurvanti. cittaṃ hi te svakāryādavasādayanti. khyātiparyavasānaṃ hi cittaceṣṭitam iti.*

19. See *YB* I.5 as cited in n. 85 of chapter 3, and refer to n. 18 above.

20. *YB* I.12; refer to n. 93 in chapter 4.

21. *YB* IV.25 (p. 200): *tatrā"tmabhāvabhāvanā ko'hamāsaṃ kathamahaṃāsaṃ kiṃsvididaṃ kathaṃsvididaṃ ke bhaviṣyāmaḥ kathaṃ vā bhaviṣyāma iti.*

22. *YS* IV.25 (p. 200): *viśeṣadarśina ātmabhāvabhāvanānivṛttiḥ.*

23. *YS* IV.26 (p. 201): *tadā vivekanimnaṃ kaivalyaprāgbhāraṃ cittam.*

24. *RM* I.50 (p. 15): *tattvarūpatayā'nayā janitāḥ saṃskārā balavattvādatatt-varūpaprajñājanitānsaṃskārānbādhituṃ* . . .

25. *YV* I.50 (p. 254): *adṛdhaiśca prāthamikaiḥ saṃprajñātasaṃskāraistasya bādhārthāntanutāparaṃ paraiva kriyate.*

26. See n. 25 above. *YS* II.2 refers to the attenuation *(tanū-karaṇa)* of affliction brought about by *kriyā-yoga;* see notes 152 and 153 in chapter 4.

27. *YS* II.18.

28. *YS* IV.24.

29. *YS* II.18.

30. *YB* III.35; see n. 334 in chapter 3.

31. *YS* I.18 (p. 21): *virāmapratyayābhyāsapūrvaḥ saṃskāraśeṣo'nyaḥ.*

32. *YB* I.18; see n. 40 below.

33. *TV* I.18 (p. 21): *virāmo vṛttīnām abhāvas tasya pratyayaḥ kāraṇaṃ . . .*

34. *YV* I.18 (p. 112): *vṛttyā'pi viramyatāmiti pratyayo virāmapratyayaḥ, paraṃ vairāgyaṃ jñāne'pyalaṃbuddhirjñānamapi śamyatvity evaṃ rūpā . . .*

35. Āraṇya writes (1963: 52): "The meaning of attaining such cessation is the practice, i.e., constant repetition in the mind of the idea of supreme detachment."

36. *RM* I.18 (p. 6): *viramyate'neneti virāmo vitarkādicintātyāgaḥ.*

37. *YV* I.18 (p. 112): *tasyā abhyāsāt paunaḥ punyājjāyata ityādyaviśeṣaṇārthaḥ. TV* I.18 (p. 21): *tasyābhyāsastadanuṣṭhānaṃ paunaḥpunyaṃ tadeva pūrvaṃ yasya sa tathoktaḥ.*

38. *RM* I.18 (pp. 6-7): *virāmapratyayastasyābhyāsaḥ paunaḥpunyena cetasi niveśanam.*

39. Āraṇya (1963: 52).

40. *YB* I.18 (pp. 21-22): *sarvavṛttipratyastamaye saṃskāraśeṣo nirodhaścittasya samādhirasaṃprajñātaḥ. tasya paraṃ vairāgyamupāyaḥ. sālambano hyabhyāsastatsādhanāya na kalpata iti virāmapratyayo nirvastuka ālambanī kriyate.*

41. See, for example, J. H. Woods (1914: 12) and G. Jha (1907: 20) where "*asaṃprajñāta*" has been described as "unconscious." See also n. 49 and text in chapter 5, which offers a critique of Jung's position on *samādhi.*

42. Dasgupta (1924: 124).

43. Koelman (1970: 239).

44. Ibid., p. 131.

45. *YS* I.51 (p. 54): *tasyāpi nirodhe sarvanirodhānnirbījaḥ samādhiḥ.*

46. *YB* I.51 (pp. 55-56): *sa na kevalaṃ samādhiprajñāvirodhī prajñākṛtānāmapi saṃskārāṇāṃ pratibandhī bhavati. kasmāt, nirodhajaḥ saṃskāraḥ samādhijānsaṃskārān-bādhata iti. nirodhasthitikālakramānubhavena nirodhacittakṛtasaṃskārāstitvamanumeyam. vyutthānanirodhasamādhiprabhavaiḥ saha kaivalyabhāgīyaiḥ samskāraiścittaṃ svasyāṃ prakṛtāvavasthitāyāṃ pravilīyate. tasmātte saṃskārāścittasyādhikāravirodhino na sthitihetavo bhavantīti. yasmādavasitādhikāraṃ saha kaivalyabhāgīyaiḥ saṃskāraiś-cittaṃ nivartate, tasminnivṛtte puruṣaḥ svarūpamātrapratiṣṭho'taḥ śuddhaḥ kevalo mukta ityucyata iti.*

47. Refer to notes 225-227 in chapter 4 and the discussion in chapter 5.

48. *YB* I.51; see n. 46 above for text.

49. As stated in *YS* I.14.

50. *YS* III.10; see chapter 3, n. 89 and related text.

51. *YB* III.10 (p. 123): *[nirodha] . . . saṃskāramāndye vyutthānadharmiṇā saṃskāreṇa nirodhadharmasaṃskāro'bhibhūyata iti.* See also n. 106 in chapter 3.

52. As Vijñāna Bhikṣu suggests (*YV* I.51: 259).

53. Pensa states (1969: 208): "*asaṃprajñāta-samādhi* figures as an accelerator of the yogic way, not as an essential instrument."

54. See the section in chapter 4 on *aṣṭāṅga-yoga.*

55. See n. 40 above.

56. *YS* III.50; see n. 122 in chapter 4 and *YB* III.50 and I.2.

57. *YS* III.49; see n. 125 in chapter 3. Patañjali goes on to state in *YS* III.51 (p. 168): *sthānyupanimantraṇe saṅgasmayākaraṇaṃ punaraniṣṭaprasaṅgāt.* "Upon the

invitation of those well established, there is no cause for attachment and pride because of the renewed association with the undesired [realms]." The meaning of this *sūtra* takes us back to the meaning of dispassion (*YS* I.15; see n. 109 in chapter 4). The comments made by Chapple and Kelly (1990: 104) are worth noting. They write: "Even if one is tempted to re-enter the realm of attachment, the momentum to do so has ceased, because one is constantly aware of the undesirable outcome of such a return." Of course, the "undesirable outcome" refers to sorrow or dissatisfaction *(duḥkha)*.

58. *YB* I.16; see n. 121 in chapter 4.

59. See notes 37–39 in chapter 4.

60. *YB* III.35 (p. 155): *tasmācca sattvātpariṇāmino'tyantavidharmā viśuddho'nyaścitimātrarūpaḥ puruṣaḥ. . . . yastu tasmādviśiṣṭaścitimātrarūpo'nyaḥ pauruṣeyaḥ pratyayastatra saṃyamātpuruṣaviṣayā prajñā jāyate.*

61. *YSS* (p. 55): *tam imaṃ saṃyamaṃ vihāyātmāsākṣātkārasyanya upāyo nāsti.*

62. *YB* III.35 (see n. 334 in chapter 3); see also n. 127 in chapter 4 on *YB* II.27.

63. *YB* II.24 (see n. 43 in chapter 4); see also *YS* IV.24 (n. 113 in chapter 3) as well as notes 115 and 116 in chapter 3.

64. See n. 46 above and related text.

65. Āraṇya (1963: 123) writes: "It might be argued that as stoppage of cognition is not a form of knowledge, how can there be latent impressions thereof" and "*nirodha* is nothing but broken fluctuation, and the latent impression is of that break of fluctuation. Complete renunciation can give rise to latent impressions, which only bring stoppage of mutation and thus stop the mind from fluctuating. There is going on incessantly a break between the appearance and the disappearance of modifications of the mind, which break is only lengthened in concentration on *nirodha samādhi*."

66. *RM* I.51 (p. 16): *tasyāpi saṃprajñātasya nirodhe pravilaye sati sarvāsāṃ cittavṛttīnāṃ svakāraṇe pravilayādyā yā saṃskāramātrād vṛttirūdeti tasyāstasyā neti netīti kevalaṃ paryudasanānnirbījaḥ samādhirāvirbhavati.*

67. See, for example, *BĀ Up* II.3.6; III.9.26; IV.2.4; IV.4.22; IV.5.15.

68. See *YSS* (p. 4), where Vijñāna Bhikṣu states: *nirodho na nāśo'bhāvasāmānyaṃ vā.*

69. See especially the argument presented in the section on *nirodha* in chapter 4.

70. *YSS* (p. 4): *vṛttyeva nirodhenāpi saṃskāro janyate.*

71. *YS* IV.34.

72. *RM* I.18 (p. 7): *nirdahati evamekāgratājanitānsaṃskārānnirodhajāḥ svātmānaṃ ca nirdahanti.*

73. See n. 109 in chapter 4.

74. See Vyāsa's commentary on *YS* III.10 in n. 51 above.

75. *YB* I.18 (p. 22): *tadabhyāsapūrvakaṃ hi cittaṃ nirālambanamabhāvaprāptamiva bhavatītyeṣa nirbījaḥ samādhirasaṃprajñātaḥ.*

76. See especially the section on *vṛtti* in chapter 3.

77. *YS* II.18, 21, and 22.

78. See, for example, Koelman (1970: 249) and Feuerstein (1979a: 58, 142, and 144) who both imply that the psychophysical being of the yogin becomes incapacitated, disintegrates or is negated in the liberated state.

79. *Saṃskāras* are, in effect, the hidden *(adṛṣṭa)* impressions which activate and shape our human, prakṛtic existence and are canalized by efficient causes such as vir-

tuous or unvirtuous actions. As Vyāsa says (*YB* IV.2: 177), *nimitta* = *dharmādi*. See our discussion on *karma, saṃskāra,* and *vāsanā* in chapter 3.

80. The term *kaivalya* comes from *kevala,* meaning "alone." Feuerstein (1979a: 75) also translates *kaivalya* as "aloneness" but with a metaphysical or ontological emphasis that implies the absolute separation of *puruṣa* and *prakṛti.*

81. See R. Prasāda (1912: 142).

82. See C. Pensa (1969: 209).

83. See T. Leggett (1990: 252).

84. See S. Phillips (1985), *JIP* 13: 402.

85. See M. Eliade (1969: 93).

86. See Tola and Dragonetti (1987: xvii) and T. S. Rukmani (1989: 139). Koelman (1970: 251) adopts the term "isolation" as in a solipsistic state. Varenne (1976) uses the term "isolation," (p. 67) as well as the expression "absolute solitude" (p. 138). Chapple and Kelly (1990) also use the term "isolation," implying, however, "an embodied experience [as] given in [*YS*] I:3" (p. 122) wherein the seer abides in its own form or true identity. While noting (p. 8) that the purity resulting from Yoga "guarantees nonafflicted action," it does not appear to have been the intent of Chapple and Kelly in their analysis and translation of the *YS* to consider further the nature of *kaivalya* as an embodied state of liberation.

87. *YS* II.25 (p. 96): *tadabhāvāt saṃyogābhāvo hānaṃ taddṛśeḥ kaivalyam.*

88. *YS* II.20 and IV.18.

89. *YS* IV.34 (p. 207): *puruṣārthaśūnyānāṃ guṇānāṃ pratiprasavaḥ kaivalyaṃ svarūpapratiṣṭhā vā citiśaktir iti.*

90. See n. 89 above.

91. *YS* III.55 (p. 174): *sattvapuruṣayoḥ śuddhisāmye kaivalyamiti*. See also n. 52 in chapter 3 for translation. On a cautionary note, one must be careful not to characterize the state of *sattva* itself as liberation or *kaivalya,* for without the presence of *puruṣa* the mind (as reflected consciousness) could not function in its most transparent aspect as *sattva*. It is not accurate, according to Yoga philosophy, to say that the *guṇa* of *sattva* is equivalent to liberation itself. The question of the nature of the *guṇa*s from the enlightened perspective is an interesting one. In the *Bhagavadgītā* (II.45) Kṛṣṇa advises Arjuna to become free from the three *guṇa*s and then gives further instructions to be established in eternal *sattva* (beingness, light, goodness, clarity, knowledge), free of dualities, free of acquisition-and-possession, Self-possessed *(nirdvandvo nityasattvastho niryogakṣema ātmavān)*. It would appear from the above instructions that the nature of the *sattva* referred to here transcends the limitations of the nature of *sattva guṇa,* which can still have a binding effect in the form of attachment to joy and knowledge. It is, however, only by first overcoming *rajas* and *tamas* that liberation is possible.

92. See n. 48 in chapter 3.

93. See Chapple and Kelly (1990: 109).

94. *YS* IV.6 (p. 179): *tatra dhyānajamanāśayam.*

95. *YB* III.50.

96. *YB* III.55 (p. 175): *nahi dagdhakleśabījasya jñāne punarapekṣā kācidasti.* "When the seeds of afflictions have been scorched there is no longer any dependence at all on further knowledge."

97. H. Āraṇya writes (1963: 123) that in the state of *nirodha* the *guṇas* "do not die out but their unbalanced activity due to non-equilibrium that was taking place . . . only ceases on account of the cessation of the cause (*avidyā* or nescience) which brought about their contact."

98. *YB* IV.25 (p. 201): *puruṣastvasatyāmavidyāyāṃ śuddhaścittadharmaira-parāmṛṣṭa*.

99. *YB* I.41; see n. 92 in chapter 5.

100. See J. Gonda (1960: 312).

101. Vyāsa (*YB* II.13) likens the mind and its *vāsanās* to a fishing net with its knots; see n. 103 in chapter 3.

102. *YB* II.24; see n. 43 in chapter 4.

103. *YS* II.26.

104. *YS* III.49.

105. Vijñāna Bhikṣu insists (YV IV.34: 141) that *kaivalya* is a state of liberation for both *puruṣa* and *prakṛti,* each reaching its respective natural or intrinsic state. He then, however, cites the *Sāṃkhya-Kārikā* (62) where it is stated that no *puruṣa* is bound, liberated, or transmigrates. It is only *prakṛti* abiding in her various forms that transmigrates, is bound and becomes liberated. See also n. 106 below and main text.

106. *YB* II.18; see n. 215 in chapter 2 for text.

107. *YS* I.51 and III.8.

108. *RM* I.1 (p. 1).

109. Müller (1899: 309).

110. See, for example, Eliade (1969), Koelman (1970), Feuerstein (1979a), and Larson (1987).

111. *YS* II.9; see n. 170 in chapter 3.

112. I am here echoing some of the points made by Chapple in his paper entitled, "*Citta-vṛtti* and Reality in the *Yoga Sūtra,*" in *Sāṃkhya-Yoga: Proceedings of the IASWR Conference, 1981,* pp. 103–119. See also Chapple and Kelly (1990: 5) where the authors state: "*kaivalyam* . . . is not a catatonic state nor does it require death." *SK* 67 acknowledges that even the "potter's wheel" continues to turn because of the force of past impressions *(saṃskāras);* but in Yoga, higher dispassion and *asaṃprajñāta-samādhi* eventually exhaust all the impressions or karmic residue. Through a continued program of ongoing purification Yoga allows for the possibility of an embodied state of freedom utterly unburdened by the effects of past actions. As such Yoga constitutes an advance over the apparently fatalistic perspective in Sāṃkhya where the "wheel of *saṃsāra*" continues (after the initial experience of liberating knowledge) until, in the event of separation from the body, *prakṛti* permanently disappears from view and unending "isolation" *(kaivalya)* is attained (*SK* 68). In any case, the yogic state of supra-cognitive *samādhi* goes beyond the liberating knowledge of *viveka* in the Sāṃkhyan system in that the yogin must develop dispassion even toward discriminative discernment itself. For more on an analysis of the notion of liberation in Sāṃkhya and Yoga, see C. Chapple's chapter on "Living Liberation in Sāṃkhya and Yoga," in *Living Liberation in Hindu Thought,* ed. by Andrew O. Fort and Patricia Y. Mumme.

113. Cf. *SK* 64.

114. Thus, as Chapple (1983: 112) writes, although both *puruṣa* and *prakṛti* "are seen as fulfilling separate and discrete functions . . . both are necessary and present, even in the act of 'truly seeing'." Vyāsa (*YB* II.17) has also used the term "knower-of-the-field" *(kṣetrajña),* meaning the seer. Cf. *BG* XIII.34, where the one who sees the

field *(kṣetra, prakṛti)* as distinct from the knower of the field *(kṣetrajña, puruṣa)* is said to be wise. The author wishes to acknowledge the work of Chapple (1983) in helping to formulate some of the ideas mentioned in this part of the discussion.

115. Klaus Klostermaier (1994), *A Survey of Hinduism,* p. 402.

116. *YS* II.29; see the discussion in chapter 4 on *aṣṭāṅga-yoga.*

117. *YB* II.28 (pp. 99-101).

118. *YB* II.28 (p. 101): *dhṛtikāraṇaṃ śarīramindriyāṇam. tāni ca tasya. mahābhūtāni śarīrāṇāṃ, tāni ca parasparaṃ sarveṣāṃ tairyagyaunamānuṣadaivatāni ca parasparārthatvāt.*

119. *YS* I.48; see n. 164 in chapter 5.

120. Refer to n. 205 in chapter 5.

121. Cf. *BG* VI.23, where Yoga is defined as the "disengagement from the union with suffering" *(duḥkha-saṃyoga-viyoga).*

122. *YS* II.22; see n. 207 and related text in chapter 2.

123. Āraṇya (1963: 384).

124. *YS* III.54 (see n. 179 below) and *YS* III.55 (see n. 91 above).

125. *YB* I.18; see n. 40 above.

126. *YS* I.3; see n. 36 in chapter 2.

127. See n. 89 above.

128. Our position thus counters the often held notion that in *kaivalya* the yogin can no longer act and has become, in effect, disembodied.

129. See K. Klostermaier (1989), "Spirituality and Nature," in *Hindu Spirituality: Vedas Through Vedānta* ed. by Krishna Sivaraman, pp. 319-337.

130. See Feuerstein (1980: 98-101) and Klostermaier (1986), "Dharmamegha Samādhi: Comments on Yogasūtra IV. 29," in *PEW* 36.3: 253-262.

131. This has been clearly articulated by Feuerstein (1980: 99) and is evident from statements in Vyāsa's commentary; see *YB* I.2, 15 as well as II.2 and IV.29.

132. *YS* III.49-50.

133. *YS* I.15-16 and III.50.

134. See n. 57 above on *YS* III.51.

135. *YB* IV.29 (p. 202): *yadā'yaṃ brāhmaṇaḥ prasaṃkhyāne'pyakusīdastato'pi na kiṃcitprārthayate. tatrāpi viraktasya sarvathā vivekakhyātireva bhavati . . .*

136. *YS* IV.29 (p. 202): *prasaṃkhyāne'pyakusīdasya sarvathā vivekakhyāter dharmameghaḥ samādhiḥ.* It is noteworthy that Vyāsa (*YB* II.15) likens Yoga (p. 78) to medicine with its four parts: illness, the cause of illness, the state of good health, and the remedy. Thus Yoga is portrayed as a "fourfold division" whose four parts *(caturvyūha)* are: (1) *saṃsāra,* which (along with its sorrowful states) is to be discarded; (2) the conjunction *(saṃyoga)* between *puruṣa* and *prakṛti* / *pradhāna,* which is the cause of what is to be discarded; (3) liberation, which is the complete cessation of the conjunction; and (4) right knowledge, which is the means to liberation. But see also n. 126 in chapter 4 of our study, which draws on a quote from the same passage (*YB* II.15) declaring that the true nature/identity of the one (i.e., *puruṣa*) who is liberated is not something to be obtained or discarded. The inalienable identity of *puruṣa* puts it in a "category" that transcends the dualistic categories of means and ends, causes and effects, obtaining and discarding. In a stimulating and incisive essay on this topic, W. Halbfass (1991: 243-263) points out the limitations of the applicability to Yoga of the medical/therapeutic paradigm. In particular he writes (p. 253): "The denial of *hāna* ['discarding'] and *upādāna* ['obtaining'] with regard to the ultimate goal of Yoga is a

denial of the fundamental premises of the medical, therapeutic orientation; in a sense, it revokes the 'fourfold scheme' and the therapeutic paradigm itself. Indeed, it is not only through the adoption of this paradigm, but also through its transcendence, that Yoga and other schools of Indian thought articulate their self-understanding." Of course the fundamental "disease" that Yoga seeks to overcome is *avidyā* and its manifestation as *saṃyoga*.

137. *YB* IV.29 (p. 202): *saṃskārabījakṣayānnāsya pratyayāntarāṇyutpadyante*.

138. See n. 40 above.

139. See Feuerstein (1980: 98).

140. *YS* III.49 and III.54

141. *YS* IV.7; see notes 107–112 in chapter 3. See also *YS* IV.30 (n. 142 below).

142. *YS* IV.30 (p. 202): *tataḥ kleśakarmanivṛttiḥ*. Thus, it may be said that to dwell without defilement in a "cloud of *dharma*" is the culminating description by Patañjali of what tradition later referred to as living liberation *(jīvanmukti)*. To be sure, there is a "brevity of description" in the *YS* regarding the state of liberation. Only sparingly, with reservation (one might add, caution) and mostly in metaphorical terms does Patañjali speak about the qualities exhibited by the liberated yogin. Chapple (1996: 116, see below) provides three possible reasons for this "brevity of description" regarding living liberation in the context of the *YS* (and Sāṃkhya, i.e., the *SK* of Īśvara Kṛṣṇa): (1) He states: "(T)he genre in which both texts were written does not allow for the sort of narrative and poetic embellishment found in the epics and Purāṇas." (2) Perhaps, as Chapple suggests, "a deliberate attempt has been made to guarantee that the recognition of a liberated being remains in the hands of a spiritual preceptor." What is to be noted here is that the oral and highly personalized lineage tradition within Yoga stresses the authority of the *guru,* which guards against false claims to spiritual attainment on the part of others and thereby "helps to ensure the authenticity and integrity of the tradition." (3) A further reason for brevity "could hinge on the logical contradiction that arises due to the fact that the notion of self is so closely identified with *ahaṃkāra* [the ego or prakṛtic sense of self]. It would be an oxymoron for a person to say [']I am liberated.[']" The Self *(puruṣa)* is of course not an object that can be seen by itself thus laying emphasis, as Chapple points out, on the ineffable nature of the liberative state that transcends mind-content, all marks, and activity itself.

143. *YS* IV.31 (p. 203): *tadā sarvāvaraṇamalāpetasya jñānasyā''nantyājjñeyamalpam.*

144. See *YV* I.1; *YSS* (p. 2) states: *asaṃprajñātayogasya cākhilavṛttisaṃskāradāhadvārā prārabdhasyāpy atikrameṇeti.*

145. See n. 144 above and *YV* 1.1 (p. 31).

146. *YS* IV.7 and *YB* IV.7 (see notes 107 and 109 respectively in chapter 3).

147. *YB* IV.30 (see n. 76 in chapter 4).

148. *YV* IV.30 (pp. 123–124). Elsewhere in his *YSS* (p. 17) Vijñāna Bhikṣu tells us that the yogin who is "established in the state of *dharmamegha-samādhi* is called a *jīvanmukta*": *dharmameghaḥ samādhiḥ . . . asyāmavasthāyāṃ jīvanmukta ityucyate.* Vijñāna Bhikṣu is critical of Vedāntins (i.e., Śaṅkara's Advaita Vedānta school) who, he says, associate the *jīvanmukta* with ignorance *(avidyā-kleśa)*—probably because of the liberated being's continued link with the body—despite Yoga's insistence on the complete overcoming of the afflictions.

149. See Āraṇya (1963: 433; also p. 226).

150. This is the essence of Kṛṣṇa's teaching in the *BG* on *karma-yoga;* see, for example, *BG* IV.20 and our discussion on the *BG* in chapter 1.

151. *YB* I.16; see n. 119 in chapter 4.

152. See R. C. Zaehner (1974), *Our Savage God,* pp. 97–98.

153. See B.-A. Scharfstein (1974), *Mystical Experience,* pp. 131–132.

154. See Feuerstein (1979a: 81).

155. *YS* I.33.

156. *YS* II.35.

157. See *YS* II.5 (n. 152 in chapter 3), where Patañjali indirectly describes *puruṣa* as being a joyful state, i.e., a state of intrinsic happiness or satisfaction *(sukha)* that, like other inalienable aspects of *puruṣa* such as purity and permanency, is not to be confused with an emotional state. To be sure, *kaivalya* is not an emotional condition that, being of the nature of the mind, comes and goes, changes. It would be highly misleading to suggest that *kaivalya* implies either an alienation/isolation from the world or a state of loneliness, for these are states of mind and afflicted states at that. Such a misrepresentation of Yoga only buttresses the ill-founded notion that Yoga is an escape from the world.

158. See *YB* II.6 and IV.21, 22.

159. On this point see n. 4 and related text in chapter 3.

160. For example, *YS* I.33 (see n. 248 in chapter 3) can be seen as a preparatory discipline for an ethical embodiment of liberation in Yoga.

161. Thus the term "Yoga" (like the terms *"nirodha"* and *"samādhi"*) is ambiguous in that it means both the process of purification and illumination and the final "goal" of liberation or "aloneness." Due to Yoga's traditional praxis-orientation it becomes all too easy to reduce Yoga to a "means only" approach to well-being and spiritual enlightenment. In the light of its popularity in the Western world today, in which technique and practice have been emphasized often to the exclusion of philosophical/theoretical understanding and a proper pedagogical context, there is a great danger in simply reifying practice whereby practice becomes something the ego does for the sake of its own security. Seen here, practice—often then conceived as a superior activity in relation to all other activities—becomes all-important in that through the activity called "practice" the ego hopes and strives to become "enlightened." Practice thus becomes rooted in a future-oriented perspective largely motivated out of a fear of not becoming enlightened; it degenerates into a form of selfishly appropriated activity where "means" become ends-in-themselves. Moreover, human relationships become instruments for the greater "good" of Self-realization. Thus rationalized, relationships are seen as having only a tentative nature and value. The search for enlightenment under the sway of this kind of instrumental rationality/reasoning (i.e., the attempt to "gain" something from one's practice, namely, enlightenment) never really goes beyond the level of ego and its compulsive search for permanent security, which of course, according to Yoga thought, is an inherently afflicted state of affairs. To be sure, the concern in Yoga is to (re)discover *puruṣa,* to be restored to true identity thus overcoming dissatisfaction, fear, and misidentification by uprooting and eradicating the dis-ease of ignorance *(avidyā).* Yet (see n. 136 above), as W. Halbfass puts it, true identity "cannot be really lost, forgotten or newly acquired" (1991: 252) for liberation "is not to be produced or accomplished in a literal sense, but only in a figurative sense" (ibid.: 251). Sufficient means for the sattvification of the mind are, however, both desirable and

necessary in order to prepare the yogin for the identity shift from egoity to *puruṣa*. By acknowledging that "aloneness" cannot be an acquired state resulting from or caused by yogic methods and techniques, and that *puruṣa* cannot be known (*YB* III.35), acquired or discarded/lost (*YB* II.15), Yoga in effect transcends its own result-orientation as well as the dualistic categories of means and ends.

162. *YB* I.20 (pp. 23–24): *śraddhā cetasaḥ saṃprasādaḥ. sā hi jananīva kalyāṇī yoginaṃ pāti.*

163. See notes 163–169 in chapter 5. See also the discussion in chapter 1 on *ṛta*.

164. Often yogic knowledge or teachings are extended by the principles of analogy and isomorphism between the macrocosm (the universe at large) and the microcosm that is the human organism. A striking example of this isomorphism is to be found in the *Yoga-Darśana Upaniṣad* (IV.48–53), where the eternal *tīrtha* (sacred font, holy water, place of pilgrimage) is considered inferior to the *tīrtha* in the body, and mountains and other places of spiritual significance (e.g., Vārāṇasī) are identified with various parts of the human body.

165. *YS* IV.19, 22, 23.

166. See n. 198 in chapter 2 and also *SK* 20.

167. C. Chapple claims that Sāṃkhya has also been misinterpreted. See his chapters entitled "The Unseen Seer and the Field: Consciousness in Sāṃkhya and Yoga" in *The Problem of Pure Consciousness*, ed. by Robert K. C. Forman and "Living Liberation in Sāṃkhya and Yoga," in *Living Liberation in Hindu Thought*, ed. by Andrew O. Fort and Patricia Y. Mumme.

168. *YB* IV.30; see n. 76 in chapter 4 for text.

169. See, for example, Eliade (1969: 32–33) and Koelman (1970: 251), who both maintain this solipsistic view, i.e., of *puruṣa* understood as a monadic state.

170. See Vyāsa's description of *saṃsāra* as a "six-spoked wheel" (*YB* IV.11 in n. 182 of chapter 2), and the root meaning of *duḥkha* (see notes 185–186 and relevant text in chapter 2) as referring to a "wheel" with a "bad axle-hole."

171. *YB* III.49 (p. 168): *ityeṣā viśokā nāma siddhiryāṃ prāpya yogī sarvajñaḥ kṣīṇakleśabandhano vaśī viharati.*

172. *YS* III.55; see n. 91 above.

173. See Koelman (1970: 249–250).

174. See Feuerstein (1979a: 142, 144).

175. *YB* II.23.

176. *YS* IV.18.

177. *YB* IV.21, 22.

178. *YB* III.49 (pp. 167–168): *sarvātmāno guṇā vyavasāyavyavaseyātmakāḥ svāminaṃ kṣetrajñaṃ . . .*

179. *YS* III.54 (p. 174): *tārakaṃ sarvaviṣayaṃ sarvathāviṣayamakramaṃ ceti vivekajaṃ jñānam.*

180. Although the historical identity of Patañjali the Yoga master is not known, we are assuming that Patañjali was, as the tradition would have it, an enlightened Yoga adept; for more on Patañjali see the introductory section in chapter 2.

181. Koelman (1970: 258). Ethical conduct can be seen as a prerequisite to and/or as a natural concomitant of spiritual realization. This is the case in nondualistic Vedānta where according to the text entitled *Vivekacūḍāmaṇi* (v. 37), those who have achieved spiritual insight are inherently beneficial, "just as the spring season" *(vasantavad);* this of course echoes notions within Mahāyāna Buddhism.

182. See *BG* III.33, where the wise—those who have overcome ignorance—are said to function in a natural "conformity" or alignment with their prakṛtic constitution, following or "attuned to" *prakṛti* without suppression.

183. *BG* IV.20.

184. This is certainly one of the most praiseworthy aspects within Mahāyāna Buddhism. The four *brahmavihāra*s cited in *YS* I.33—obviously well known by Patañjali and authorities within Buddhism—as well as some of the ethical teachings (i.e., the *yama*s and *niyama*s) outlined in the *aṣṭāṅga-yoga* section of the *Sādhana-Pāda* support the notion of an altruistic approach within Yoga.

185. Refer to notes 121-122 and text in chapter 3.

186. Refer to chapter 3, p. 106.

187. As I have argued in chapter 2.

188. As I have suggested in chapter 2.

189. *YB* III.35 (pp. 154-155): *buddhisattvaṃ prakhyāśīlaṃ samānasattvopanibandhane rajastamasī vaśīkṛtya sattvapuruṣānyatāpratyayena pariṇatam;* see also *YB* II.26.

190. See n. 93 in chapter 4.

191. *YS* III.35 (p. 154): *sattvapuruṣayor atyantāsaṃkīrṇayoḥ pratyayāviśeṣo bhogaḥ . . .*

192. *YS* IV.16; see n. 54 in chapter 3.

193. See Koelman (1970: 260). While, historically, forms of Yoga practice as set out in the *YS* have found a legitimate place within different schools of Vedānta as well as later schools of Yoga, one must take caution not to evaluate Yoga on the basis of mere technique alone.

194. See, for example, *BĀ Up* III.4.2.

195. See also our discussion of Patañjali in chapter 2 and Chapple's noteworthy comment: refer to n. 41, chapter 2.

196. See W. Halbfass (1988), *India and Europe: An Essay in Understanding,* p. 393.

197. *YB* III.6 (p. 121): *yoga evopādhyāyaḥ. . . . "yogena yogo jñātavyo yogo yogātpravartate. yo'pramattastu yogena sa yoge ramate ciram."*

198. J. Tabor (1983), *Transformative Philosophy: A Study of Śaṅkara, Fichte and Heidegger,* p. 26.

199. W. Halbfass (1992: 38, also 232-234).

200. This is appropriate in that, from *prakṛti*'s perspective, *puruṣa* is a mysterious, ineffable silence. It appears that *īśvara* as symbolized by the *praṇava* (the syllable *Om, YS* I.27) is the closest approximation to that silence.

201. *YS* IV.18-19, 22-23.

202. *YB* III.55 (p. 175): *tatpuruṣasya kaivalyaṃ, tadā puruṣaḥ svarūpamātrajyotiramalaḥ kevalī bhavati.*

203. *YB* II.27 and III.35.

CONCLUSION

1. G. Feuerstein (1990: 82).

2. J. Varenne (1976: 145) suggests that specialized texts within the tradition of Yoga such as the *Bhagavadgītā, Yoga-Sūtra,* and *Yoga Upaniṣads* should be viewed as being complementary to one another in order to arrive at a synthetic understanding of

Yoga within Hinduism. He argues for an underlying unity as well as a diversity of possible approaches in Yoga. One area for potentially fruitful research in Yoga would be to explore closely the relationship between Patañjali's Yoga and later expressions of Yoga as outlined, for example, in the *Yoga Upaniṣads* and Kashmiri Śaiva Yoga. Further research also needs to be carried out concerning the nature of the relationship between Patañjali's Yoga, Buddhism, and Jainism.

BIBLIOGRAPHY

PRIMARY SOURCES

A. Editions, Commentaries, and Translations of the *Yoga-Sūtra* and Other Classical Yoga Texts

Āraṇya, Swāmi Hariharānanda (1963). *Yoga Philosophy of Patañjali.* Translated into English by P. N. Mukerji. Calcutta: Calcutta University Press.

Arya, U. (1986). *Yoga-Sūtras of Patañjali with the Exposition of Vyāsa: A Translation and Commentary.* Vol. 1: *Samādhi-Pāda.* Honesdale, Pa.: Himalayan International Institute.

Ballantyne, James Robert (1852–53). *The Aphorisms of the Yoga Philosophy of Patañjali with Illustrative Extracts from the Commentary by Bhoja Rāja.* Allahabad: Presbyterian Mission Press.

Baba, Bangali (1976). *Yogasūtra of Patañjali with the Commentary of Vyāsa.* Delhi: Motilal Banarsidass.

Chapple, Christopher K. and Yogi Ananda Viraj (Eugene P. Kelly Jr.) (1990). *The Yoga Sūtras of Patañjali: An Analysis of the Sanskrit with Accompanying English Translation.* Delhi: Sri Satguru Publications.

Deshpande, P. Y. (1978). *The Authentic Yoga: A Fresh Look at Patañjali's Yoga-Sūtras with a New Translation, Notes and Comments.* London: Rider.

Dvivedī, Manilal N., ed. and trans. (1930). *The Yoga-Sūtras of Patañjali.* Adyar, Madras: Theosophical Publishing House.

Feuerstein, Georg (1979a). *The Yoga-Sūtra of Patañjali: A New Translation and Commentary.* Folkstone, England: Wm. Dawson and Sons.

Gosh, Shyam (1980). *The Original Yoga as Expounded in Śiva-saṃhitā, Gheraṇḍa-saṃhitā and Pātañjala Yoga-sūtra.* New Delhi: Munshiram Manoharlal.

Hauer, Jakob W. (1958). *Der Yoga.* Stuttgart, Germany: W. Kohlhammer.

Isbert, Otto Albrecht (1955). *Raja Joga, der ködnigliche Weg der Selbstmeisterung in Westlicher Sicht und Praxis.* Gelnhausen, Germany: Verlags-Union Bündingen-Haingründau.

Iyengar, B. K. S. (1993). *Light on the Yoga-Sūtras of Patañjali.* London: Aquarian/Thorsons.

Jha, G., trans. (I894). *An English Translation with Sanskrit Text of the Yogasāra-Saṅgraha of Vijñāna Bhikṣu.* Bombay: Tattva-Vivechaka Press.

——— (1907). *The Yoga-Darśana.* Bombay: Rajaram Tukaram Tatya.

Johnston, Charles (1912). *The Yoga Sūtras of Patañjali*. New York: Quarterly Book Dept.

Judge, William Q. (1920). *The Yoga Aphorisms of Patañjali*. Los Angeles: United Lodge of Theosophists.

Jyotir Maya Nanda, Swāmi (1978). *Raja Yoga Sūtras*. Miami, Fla.: Yoga Research Foundation.

Leggett, Trevor (1990). *The Complete Commentary by Śaṅkara on the Yoga Sūtra-s: A Full Translation of the Newly Discovered Text*. London and New York: Kegan Paul International.

Mangoldt, Ursula von (1957). *So Spricht das Yoga-Sutra des Patanjali*. Munich: O. W. Barth.

Mitra, Rājendralāla (1881-83). *Yoga Aphorisms of Patañjali, with the Commentary of Bhoja Rāja*. Bibliotheca Indica Series, no. 93. Calcutta: Asiatic Society of Bengal.

Pātañjalayogadarśana, with Vyāsa's *Bhāṣya,* Vācaspati Miśra's *Tattva-Vaiśāradī* and Vijñāna Bhikṣu's *Yoga-Vārttika* (1971). Edited by Śrī Nārayaṇa Miśra. Varanasi: Chowkhambā.

Pātañjalayogadarśana, with the *Tattva-Vaiśāradī and the Commentary of Vyāsa* (1963). Edited by Ram Shankar Bhattacharya. Varanasi: Bhāratīya Vidyā Prakāśan.

Pātañjalayogadarśana, with the *Yoga-Pradīpikā* of Baladeva Miśra (1931). Edited by Dhundhiraja Shastri. Varanasi: Chowkhambā.

Pātañjalayogadarśana, with the *Vyāsa-Bhāṣya,* the *Tattva-Vaiśāradī,* the *Pātañjala Rahasya of Rāghavānanda Sarasvatī,* the *Yoga-Vārttika* of Vijñāna Bhikṣu, and the *Bhāsvatī* of H. Āraṇya (1935). Edited by Gosvāmī Dāmodara Shāstrī. Varanasi: Chowkhambā.

Pātañjalayogadarśana, with the *Rāja-Mārtaṇḍa* of Bhoja Rāja, *Pradīpikā* of Bhāvāgaṇeśa, *Vṛtti* of Nāgojī Baṭṭa, *Maṇi-Prabhā* of Rāmānanda Yati, *Pada-Candrikā* of Ananta-Deva Pandit, and *Yoga-Sudhākara* of Sadāśivendra Sarasvatī (1930). Edited by Dhundhiraja Shastri. Varanasi: Chowkhambā.

Pātañjalayogadarśana, with the *Yoga-Siddhānta-Candrikā and Sūtrārtha-Bodhinī* of Nārāyaṇa Tīrtha (1911). Edited by Ratna Gopāla Bhaṭṭa. Varanasi: Chowkhambā.

Pātañjalayogadarśana, with the *Tattva-Vaiśāradī* of Vācaspati Miśra, edited by Rajaram Bodas; and *Vṛtti (Bṛhati)* of Nāgojī Bhaṭṭa (1917), edited by Vasudeva Shastri Abhyankar. Bombay Sanskrit and Prakrit Series, no. 46. Bombay: Government Central Press.

Pātañjalayogadarśana, with the *Vyāsa-Bhāṣya* of Vyāsa, the *Tattva-Vaiśāradī* of Vācaspati Miśra and the *Rāja-Mārtaṇḍa* of Bhoja Rāja (1904). Edited by Kāśīnātha Śāstrī Āgāśe. Ānandāśrama Sanskrit Series, no. 47. Poona: Ānandāśrama.

Prabhavananda, Swami, and Christopher Isherwood (1953). *How to Know God: The Yoga Aphorisms of Patañjali*. London: Allen and Unwin.

Prasāda, Rāma, trans. (1912). *The Yoga-sūtras of Patañjali with the Commentary of Vyāsa and the Gloss of Vācaspati Miśra*. Vol. 4 of *The Sacred Books of the Hindus, Translated by Various Sanskrit Scholars*. Edited by Major B. D. Basu. Allahabad: Panini Office.

Rukmani, T. S., trans. (1981–89). *Yogavārttika of Vijñānabhikṣu: Text with English Translation and Critical Notes along with the Text and English Translation of the Pātañjala Yogasūtras and Vyāsabhāṣya*. Vol. 1: *Samādhipāda* (1981); Vol. 2: *Sādhanapāda* (1983); Vol. 3: *Vibhūtipāda* (1987); and Vol. 4: *Kaivalyapāda* (1989). New Delhi: Munshiram Manoharlal.

Śarma, Rām (1967). *Yoga-Darśana*. Barelī, Uttar Pradesh: Saṃskṛti Saṃsthān.

Shree Purohit, Swami (1973). *Aphorisms of Yoga*. London: Faber and Faber.

Shyam, Swami (1980). *Patanjali Yog Darshan*. Montreal, Canada: Be All Publications.

Taimni, I. K. (1961). *The Science of Yoga*. Adyar, Madras, India and Wheaton, Ill.: Theosophical Publishing House.

Tola, Fernando and Carmen Dragonetti (1987). *The Yogasūtras of Patañjali: On Concentration of Mind*. Translated by K. D. Prithipaul. Delhi: Motilal Banarsidass.

Venkatesananda, Swami (1978). *Enlightened Living: A New Interpretative Translation of the Yoga Sūtra of Maharṣi Patañjali*. Delhi: Motilal Banarsidass.

Vijñānāśrama, Svāmī (1961). *Pātañjala Yogadarśana*. Ajmer, Rajasthan: Madanlāl Lakṣmīnivās Caṃḍak.

Vivekānanda, Swami (1966). *Rāja-Yoga or Conquering the Internal Nature*. Calcutta: Advaita Ashrama.

Woods, James Haughton, trans. (1914). *The Yoga System of Patañjali*. Harvard Oriental Series, vol. 17. Cambridge, Mass.: Harvard University Press.

——— (1915). "The Yoga Sūtras of Patañjali as Illustrated by the Commentary entitled 'The Jewel's Lustre' or Maṇiprabhā." *Journal of the American Oriental Society* 34: 1–114.

Yardi, M. R. (1979). *The Yoga of Patañjali*. Bhandarkar Oriental Series no. 12. Poona, India: Bhandarkar Oriental Research Institute.

Yati, R. (1903). *Pātañjaladarśana, with a Gloss Called Maṇi-Prabhā*. Benares Sanskrit Series, no. 75. Benares: Vidya Vilas Press.

Yogasūtrabhāṣyavivaraṇa [Pātañjalayogaśāstravivaraṇa] of Śaṇkara-Bhagavat-Pāda (1952). Edited with an introduction by S. Rama Sastri and S. R. Krishnamurti Sastri. Madras Government Oriental Series, 94. Madras: Government Oriental Manuscripts Library.

B. Other Primary Source Material

Abhinavagupta (1918). *Tantrasāra*. Edited by M. S. Kaul, Kashmir Series of Texts and Studies, no. 17.

Avalon, Arthur, ed. (1929). *Tantric Texts*. Madras: Ganesh and Co.

Basu, B. D., ed. (1914). *The Yoga Śāstra: Śiva Saṃhitā*. Vol. 15 of *The Sacred Books of the Hindus*. Allahabad: Panini Office.

Belvalkar, S. K. *et al.*, eds. (1951–53). *The Mahābhārata*. Śāntiparvan fascicules 22, 23, 24. Poona: Bhandarkar Oriental Research Institute.

Bhattacharya, Ram S., ed. (1967). *Sāṃkhyakārikā*. Varanasi: Motilal Banarsidass.

——— (1964). *Sāṃkhyasūtram*. Vārāṇasī: Prācyabhāratīprakāśanam.

Bloomfield, Maurice, trans. (1897). *Hymns of the Atharva Veda. Sacred Books of the East*. Vol. 42. Oxford: Oxford University Press.

Buitenen, J. A. B. van, trans. (1981). *The Bhagavad Gītā in the Mahābhārata: Text and Commentary.* Chicago: University of Chicago Press.

Deutsche, Eliot (1968). *The Bhagavad Gītā: Translated with Introduction and Critical Essays*. New York: Holt, Rhinehart & Winston.

Edgerton, Franklin, trans. (1965). *The Beginnings of Indian Philosophy*. London: George Allen and Unwin.

Eggeling, Julius, trans. (1882–1900). *Śatapatha Brāhmaṇa. Sacred Books of the East.* Vols. 12, 26, 41, 43, 44. Oxford: Oxford University Press.

Gambhīrānanda, Swāmī, trans. (1965). *Brahma-Sūtra-Bhāṣya of Śaṅkarācārya*. Calcutta: Advaita Ashrama.

Garbe, R., ed. (1943). *Sāṃkhya-Pravacana-Bhāṣya or Commentary on the Exposition of the Sāṃkhya Philosophy by Vijñānabhikṣu*. Cambridge, Mass.: Harvard University Press.

———, ed. (1987). *Sāṃkhya Sūtra and Sāṃkhya System, Aniruddha's and Mahādeva's Commentaries*. 2nd ed. New Delhi: Trirup Prakashan [first publ. 1884].

Hume, Robert C., trans. (1921). *The Thirteen Principal Upaniṣads*. London: Oxford University Press.

Jha, G., ed. and trans. (1934). *The Tattva-Kaumudī*. Poona: Oriental Book Agency.

———, trans. (1984). *The Nyāya-Sūtras of Gautama*. Reprint of Vol. 4. Delhi: Motilal Banarsidass [first pub. in *Indian Thought,* 1912–1919].

Mādhavācārya (1882). *The Sarva-Darśana Saṃgraha; or, Review of the Different Systems of Hindu Philosophy*. Translated by Edward Byles Cowell and Archibald Edward Gough. London: Trübner and Co.

Mahadeva Sastri, A., ed. and trans. (1920). *The Yoga Upaniṣads with the Commentary of Srī Upaniṣad-Brahma-Yogin*. Adyar Library Series, 6. Madras: Adyar Library and Research Centre.

Mainkar, T. G., ed. and trans. (1964). *The Sāṃkhyakārikā of Īśvarakṛṣṇa with the Sāṃkhyakārikābhāṣya of Gauḍapāda*. Poona: Oriental Book Agency.

O'Flaherty, Wendy Doniger (1981). *The Rig Veda: An Anthology.* London: Penguin Books.

Radhakrishnan, Sarvepalli (1948). *The Bhagavadgītā*. London: George Allen and Unwin.

——— (1953). *The Principal Upaniṣads*. London: George Allen and Unwin.

Radhakrishnan, Sarvepalli and Charles A. Moore, eds. (1957). *A Source Book in Indian Philosophy*. Princeton, N. J.: Princeton University Press.

Roy, Pratap Chandra, ed. and trans. (1970). *The Mahābhārata*. New Delhi: Munshiram Manoharlal.

Sarma, V. P. and S. Vangiya, eds. (1970). *Sāṃkhyakārikā [with Mātharavṛtti and Jayamaṅgalā]*. Varanasi: Chowkhambā Sanskrit Series Office.

Śāstri, K. S., ed. (1938). *The Yogayājñavalkya*. Trivandrum Sanskrit Series, 134. Trivandrum: Government Press.

Satya Prakash Sarasvati, Swami and Satyakam Vidyalankar, trans. (1977, 1987). *Ṛg-Veda Saṃhitā*. Vols. 2, 5, 6, and 13. New Delhi: Veda Prathishthana.

Sinha, Nandalal, trans. (1911) *The Vaiśeṣika Sūtras of Kaṇāda.* In *The Sacred Books of the Hindus,* vol. 6. Allahabad: Panini Office.

———, trans. (1915). *The Sāṃkhya Philosophy.* In *The Sacred Books of the Hindus,* vol. 11. Allahabad: Panini Office.

Whitney, William Dwight, trans. (1905). *Atharva-Veda Saṃhitā: Translated with a Critical and Exegetical Commentary*. Revised and brought nearer to completion and edited by Charles Rockwell Lanman. Cambridge, Mass.: Harvard University Press.

SECONDARY SOURCES

Akhilananda, Swami (1947). *Hindu Psychology: Its Meaning for the West.* London: Routledge & Sons.

Allchin, B. and R. Allchin (1982). *The Rise of Civilisation in India and Pakistan.* Cambridge: Cambridge University Press.

Alper, Harvey P., ed. (1989). *Understanding Mantras*. Albany: State University of New York Press.

Apte, V. S. (1970). *Sanskrit-English Dictionary.* Delhi: Motilal Banarsidass.

Avalon, A. (1978). *Shakti and Shakta.* New York: Dover Publications.

Ayyanger, T. R. S., trans. (1952). *The Yoga Upaniṣads*. Adyar: Vasanta Press.

Bahm, Archie J. (1967). *Union with the Ultimate.* New York: Unger.

Balshev, A. N. (1983). *A Study of Time in Indian Philosophy*. Wiesbaden: Otto Harrassowitz.

Bastow, David (1978). "An Attempt to Understand Sāṃkhya-Yoga." *Journal of Indian Philosophy* 5: 191–207.

Bedekar, V. M. (1960–61). "The Dhyānayoga in the Mahābhārata (XII.188)." *Munshi Indological Felicitation Volume, Bhāratīya Vidyā* 20–21: 115–125.

Berry, Thomas (1971). *Religions of India.* New York: Bruce Publishing Company.

Bharati, Agehananda (1967). *The Tantric Tradition.* New York: Doubleday.

Bhattacharji, Sukumari (1970). *The Indian Theogony: A Comparative Study of Indian Mythology from the Vedas to the Purāṇas.* Cambridge: Cambridge University Press.

Bhattacharya, Krishnachandra (1956). *Studies in Philosophy.* Vol. 1. Calcutta: Progressive Publishers.

Bhattacharya, S. (1968). "The Concept of *Videha* and *Prakṛti-Laya* in the Sāṃkhya-Yoga System." *Annals of the Bhandarkar Oriental Research Institute* 48–49: 305–312.

Bronkhorst, Johannes (1981). "Yoga and Seśvara Sāṃkhya." *Journal of Indian Philosophy* 9: 309–320.

——— (1983). "God in Sāṃkhya." *Wiener Zeitschrift für die Kunde Südasiens und Archiv für indische Philosophie* 27: 149–164.

Buitenen, J. A. B. van (1956). "Studies in Sāṃkhya I." *Journal of the American Oriental Society* 76: 153–157.

——— (1957). "Studies in Sāṃkhya II." *Journal of the American Oriental Society* 77: 15–25.

——— (1957). "Studies in Sāṃkhya III." *Journal of the American Oriental Society* 77: 88–107.

——— (1964). "The Large Ātman." *Journal of the History of Religions* 4: 103ff.
Catalina, Francis V. (1968). *A Study of the Self Concept of Sāṃkhya-Yoga Philosophy.* Delhi: Munshiram Manoharlal.
Chakravarti, P. (1951). *Origin and Development of the Sāṃkhya System of Thought.* Calcutta: Metropolitan Printing and Publishing House.
Chapple, Christopher K. (1983). "*Citta-vṛtti* and Reality in the *Yoga Sūtra.*" In *Sāṃkhya-Yoga: Proceedings of the IASWR Conference, 1981.* Stony Brook, New York: Institute for Advanced Studies of World Religions, pp. 103–119.
——— (1986). *Karma and Creativity.* Albany: State University of New York Press.
——— (1993). *Nonviolence to Animals, Earth, and Self in Asian Traditions.* Albany: State University of New York Press.
——— (1994). "Reading Patañjali without Vyāsa: A Critique of Four *Yoga Sūtra* Passages." *Journal of the American Academy of Religion* 62.1: 85–105.
——— (1996). "Living Liberation in Sāṃkhya and Yoga." In *Living Liberation in Hindu Thought*, edited by Andrew O. Fort and Patricia Y. Mumme. Albany: State University of New York Press, pp. 115–134.
Chennakesavan, S. (1980). *Concept of Mind in Indian Philosophy.* New Delhi: Motilal Banarsidass.
Chettimattam, John B. (1967). *Consciousness and Reality: An Indian Approach to Metaphysics.* Bangalore: The Bangalore Press.
Clark, J. H. (1983). *A Map of Mental States.* London: Routledge and Kegan Paul.
Colebrooke, H. T. (1873). *Miscellaneous Essays.* Vol. 1. London: Trubner and Co.
Coster, G. (1957). *Yoga and Western Psychology: A Comparison.* London: Oxford University Press.
Coward, Harold (1985). *Jung and Eastern Thought.* Albany: State University of New York Press.
Daniélou, A. (1954). *Yoga: The Method of Re-Integration.* London: Christopher Johnson.
Dasgupta, Shashibhusan (1962). *Obscure Religious Cults.* Calcutta: Firma K.L. Mukhopadhyay.
Dasgupta, Surendranath (1920). *A Study of Patañjali.* Calcutta: Calcutta University Press.
——— (1922). *History of Indian Philosophy.* Vol. 1. Cambridge: Cambridge University Press.
——— (1924). *Yoga as Philosophy and Religion.* London: Trubner and Co.
——— (1930). *Yoga Philosophy in Relation to Other Systems of Indian Thought.* Calcutta: Calcutta University Press.
Datta, Dhirendra M. (1972). *The Six Ways of Knowing.* Calcutta: Calcutta University Press.
Deussen, Paul (1920). *Allgemeine Geschichte der Philosophie.* Vol. 1, pt. 3. Leipzig: F. A. Brockhaus.
Dharmarāja, Adhvarīndra (1963). *Vedānta-Paribhāṣā.* Trans. by S. Madhavānanda. Calcutta: Ramakrishna Mission.
Divanji, P. C. (1953, 1954). "The Yogayājñavalkya." *Journal of the Bombay Branch of the Royal Asiatic Society,* 28 (1953): 99–158, 215–268; 29 (1954): 96–128.
Edgerton, Franklin (1924). "The Meaning of Sāṅkhya and Yoga." *American Journal of Philology* 45: 1–46.

——— (1959). "Did the Buddha Have a System of Metaphysics?" *Journal of the American Oriental Society* 79: 81ff.

Eliade, Mircea (1969). *Yoga: Immortality and Freedom.* Trans. by Willard R. Trask. 2nd ed. Bollingen Series no. 56. Princeton, N.J.: Princeton University Press.

——— (1975). *Patañjali and Yoga.* Trans. by Charles Lam Markmann. New York: Schocken Books.

Falk, Maryla (1941). *The Unknown Early Yoga and the Birth of Indian Philosophy.* Madras: University of Madras Press.

Feuerstein, Georg (1974). *The Essence of Yoga: A Contribution to the Psycho-History of Indian Civilization.* London: Rider and Company.

——— (1975). *Textbook of Yoga.* London: Rider and Company.

——— (1979b). *The Yoga-Sūtra of Patañjali: An Exercise in the Methodology of Textual Analysis.* New Delhi: Arnold-Heinemann.

——— (1980). *The Philosophy of Classical Yoga.* Manchester, England: Manchester University Press.

——— (1984). "Worshipping the Guru's Feet." *The Laughing Man* 4.4: 7-11.

——— (1989). *Yoga: The Technology of Ecstasy.* Los Angeles, California: J. P. Tarcher.

——— (1990). *Encyclopedic Dictionary of Yoga.* New York: Paragon House.

Feuerstein, Georg and Jeanine Miller (1971). *A Reappraisal of Yoga: Essays in Indian Philosophy.* London: Rider and Company.

Frauwallner, Erich (1953). *Geschichte der indischen Philosophie.* Vol. 1. Salzburg, Austria: 0. Muller.

——— (1973). *History of Indian Philosophy*. Vol. 1. Trans. by V. M. Bedekar. Delhi: Motilal Banarsidass.

Gambhīrānanda, Swāmī, trans. (1986). *Śvetāśvatara Upaniṣad: With the Commentary of Śaṅkarācārya.* Calcutta: Advaita Ashrama.

Garbe, Richard (1894). *Sāṃkhya and Yoga.* Strassburg: K. J. Trubner.

——— (1917). *Die Sāṃkhya Philosophie.* 2nd ed. Leipzig: H Haessel.

——— (1922). "Yoga." *Encyclopedia of Religion and Ethics,* ed. James Hastings. Vol. 12: 831-833. New York: Charles Scribners and Sons.

Ghosh, J. (1930). *Sāṃkhya and Modern Thought.* Calcutta: The Book Company.

Glassenapp, H. von (1958). *Die Philosophie der Inder.* Stuttgart, Germany: Alfred Kröner.

Gonda, Jan (1960). *Die Religionen Indiens.* Vol. 1. Stuttgart, Germany: W. Kohlhammer Verlag.

——— (1963). *The Vision of the Vedic Poets.* The Hague: Mouton.

——— (1975). *Vedic Literature (Saṃhitās and Brāhmaṇas)*. Vol. 1, fasc. I in *History of Indian Literature*, ed. J. Gonda. Wiesbaden: Otto Harrassowitz.

Govinda, Lama Anagarika (1972). *The Way of the White Clouds.* New Delhi: B. I. Publications.

Hacker, Paul (1968). "Śaṅkara der Yogin und Śaṅkara der Advaitin: Einige Beobachtungen." *Beiträge zur Geistesgeschichte Indiens: Festschrift E. Frauwallner: Wiener Zeitschrift für die Kunde Süd—und Ostasiens und Archiv für indische Philosophie* 12/13: 119-148.

Halbfass, Wilhelm (1988). *India and Europe: An Essay in Understanding*. Albany: State University of New York Press.

——— (1991). *Tradition and Reflection: Explorations in Indian Thought*. Albany: State University of New York Press.

——— (1992). *On Being and What There Is: Classical Vaiśeṣika and the History of Indian Ontology*. Albany: State University of New York Press.

Hauer, Jakob W. (1931). "Das IV Buch des Yogasūtra." *Studia Indo-Iranica: Ehrengabe für Wilheim Geiger,* ed. W. Wüst. Leipzig: Otto Harrassowitz.

——— (1922). *Die Anfange der Yogapraxis im Alten Indien.* Stuttgart, Germany: W. Kohlhammer.

Hiriyana, M. (1932). *Outlines of Indian Philosophy*. London: George Allen and Unwin.

——— (1949). *The Essentials of Indian Philosophy.* London: George Allen and Unwin.

Hopkins, E. Washburn (1901). "Yoga Technique in the Great Epic." *Journal of the American Oriental Society* 22: 333–379.

Hopkins, Thomas J. (1971). *The Hindu Religious Tradition.* Belmont, Calif.: Dickenson.

Hulin, Michael (1978). *Sāṃkhya Literature.* Vol. 6, fasc. 3 in *History of Indian Literature*, ed. J. Gonda, Wiesbaden: Otto Harrossowitz.

Hultzsch, E. (1927). "Sāṃkhya und Yoga im Śiśupālavadha." *Aus Indiens Kultur: Festgabe für Richard von Garbe,* ed. J. von Negelein. Erlangen: Palm and Enke.

Humphries, Francis (1981). Review: Georg Feuerstein, *The Philosophy of Classical Yoga. Bulletin of the School of Oriental and African Studies,* 44.2: 393–394.

lyengar, B. K. S. (1976). *Light on Yoga.* New York: Schocken Books.

Jacob, George Adolphus (1981). A *Concordance to the Principal Upanishads and Bhagavadgītā.* Bombay: Government Central Book Depot.

Jacobi, Hermann (1911). "The Dates of the Philosophical Sūtras of the Brahmans." *Journal of the American Oriental Society* 31:1–29.

——— (1929). "Uber das ursprüngliche Yoga-System." *Sitzungsberichte der Preusischen Akademie der Wissenschaften.* Berlin: Akademie Verlag, pp. 581–624.

Jacobs, H. (1961). *Western Therapy and Hindu Sadhana: A Contribution to Comparative Studies on Psychology and Metaphysics.* London: George Allen and Unwin.

Jaini, Padmanabh S. (1979). *The Jaina Path of Purification.* Berkeley: University of California Press.

Janácek, Adolf (1951). "The Methodological Principle in Yoga According to Patañjali's Yoga-Sūtras." *Archiv Orientální* 19: 514–567.

——— (1954). "The 'Voluntaristic' Type of Yoga in Patañjali's Yoga-Sūtras." *Archiv Orientální* 22: 69–87.

——— (1957). "The Meaning of Pratyaya in Patañjali's Yoga-Sūtras." *Archiv Orientální* 25: 201–261.

——— (1958). "Two Texts of Patañjali and a Statistical Comparison of Their Vocabularies." *Archiv Orientální* 26: 88–101.

——— (1959). "To the Problems of Indian Philosophical Texts." *Archiv Orientální* 27: 463–475.

Jarrell, H. R. (1981). *International Yoga Bibliography 1950 to 1980.* Metuchen, N.J.: Scarecrow Press.

Johnston, E. H. (1930). "Some Sāṃkhya and Yoga Conceptions of the Śvetāśvatara Upaniṣad." *Journal of the Royal Asiatic Society* 84: 855–878.

——— (1937). *Early Sāṃkhya.* London: The Royal Asiatic Society.

Joshi, K. S. (1965). "On the Meaning of Yoga." *Philosophy East and West* 15.1: 53-64.

——— (1965). "The Concept of Saṃyama in Patañjali's Yogasūtra." *Yoga-Mīmāṃsā* 8.2: 1-18.

Jung, C. G. (1936). "Yoga and the West." In *Collected Works.* Vol. 11. Princeton, N.J.: Princeton University Press, 1969.

——— (1973). *Letters.* Vol. 1. Edited by G. Adler. London: Routledge and Kegan Paul.

——— (1978). *Psychology and the East.* Princeton, N.J.: Princeton University Press.

Kane, P. V. (1962). *History of the Dharmaśāstra.* Vol. 5, part 2. Poona: Bhandarkar Oriental Research Institute.

Kaviraj, Gopinath (1924). "The Doctrine of Pratibhā in Indian Philosophy." *Annals of the Bhandarkar Oriental Research Institute* 5: 1-18, 113-132.

Keith, A. B. (1925). *Religion and Philosophy of the Veda and Upaniṣads.* Harvard Oriental Series, vol. 31. Cambridge, Mass.: Harvard University Press.

——— (1949). *Sāṃkhya System: A History of the Sāṃkhya Philosophy.* Calcutta: Y.M.C.A. Publishing House.

Kenghe, C. T. (1958). "The Concept of Prakṛti in the Sāṃkhya Philosophy." *Poona Orientalist* 23: Iff.

——— (1968). "The Problem of Pratyayasarga in Sāṃkhya and Its Relation to Yoga." *Annals of the Bhandarkar Oriental Research Institute* 48-49: 365-373.

Kesarcodi-Watson, Ian (1982). "Samādhi in Patañjali's Yoga-Sūtras." *Philosophy East and West* 32.1: 77-90.

Klostermaier, Klaus K. (1984). "Time in Patañjali's Yogasūtra." *Philosophy East and West* 34.2: 205-210.

——— (1986). "Dharmamegha Samādhi: Comments on Yogasūtra IV.29." *Philosophy East and West* 36.3: 253-262.

——— (1989). "Spirituality and Nature." In *Hindu Spirituality: Vedas through Vedanta,* ed. Krishna Sivaraman. New York: Crossroad Publishing, pp. 319-337.

——— (1994). *A Survey of Hinduism.* 2nd ed. Albany: State University of New York Press.

Koelman, Gaspar M. (1970). *Pātañjala Yoga: From Related Ego to Absolute Self.* Poona, India: Papal Anthenaeum.

Kulkarni, T. R. (1972). *Upanishads and Yoga.* Bombay: Bharatiya Vidya Bhavan.

Kumar, Shiv (1981). "Knowledge and Its Genesis in Sāṃkhya-Yoga." *Annals of the Bhandarkar Oriental Research Institute* 62: 17ff.

Lad, Ashok (1967). *The Conception of Liberation in Indian Philosophy.* Gwalior, India: Shri Krishna Press.

Larson, Gerald J. (1969). *Classical Sāṃkhya: An Interpretation of Its History and Meaning.* Delhi: Motilal Banarsidass [contains text and trans. of the *Sāṃkhya-Kārikā*].

——— (1978). Review: Gaspar M. Koelman (1970), *Pātañjala Yoga: From Related Ego to Absolute Self. Philosophy East and West* 28.2: 236-239.

——— (1993). "The Trimūrti of Smṛti in Classical Indian Thought." *Philosophy East and West* 43.3: 373-388.

Larson, Gerald J. and Ram S. Bhattacharya, eds. (1987). *Sāṃkhya. A Dualist Tradition in Indian Philosophy.* Vol. 4 of *The Encyclopedia of Indian Philosophies.* Princeton, N.J.: Princeton University Press.
La Vallée Poussin, Louis de (1936–37). "Le Bouddhisme et le Yoga de Patañjali." *Mélanges chinois et bouddhiques* 5: 223–242.
Lester, R. C. (1976). *Rāmānuja on the Yoga.* Adyar Library Series, 106. Madras: Adyar Library and Research Centre.
Lipner, Julius J. (1986). *The Face of Truth: A Study of Meaning and Metaphysics in the Vedāntic Theology of Rāmānuja.* Albany: State University of New York Press.
——— (1994). *Hindus: Their Religious Beliefs and Practices.* London and New York: Routledge.
Majumdar, Abhay (1930). *The Sāṃkhyan Conception of Personality.* Calcutta: Calcutta University Press.
Mariau, Daniel (1979). "The Upaniṣad of the Dagger." *Bulletin of the Yoga Research Centre.* 1: 17–24.
Marshall, J. (1931). *Mohenjo Daro and the Indus Civilization.* 3 vols. London: Oxford University Press.
Matilal, Bimal K. (1986). *Perception: An Essay on Classical Indian Theories of Knowledge.* Oxford: Clarendon Press.
Mayeda, Sengaku (1988). Review of Trevor Leggett (1983), *Śaṅkara on the Yoga-Sūtras (Vol. 2: Means): The Vivaraṇa Sub-commentary to Vyāsa-bhāṣya on the Yoga-Sūtra-s of Patañjali: Sādhana-pāda. Philosophy East and West* 37: 440–443.
Miller, David (1976–77). "The Guru as the Centre of Sacredness." *Sciences Religeuses/Studies in Religion,* 6.5: 527–533.
Miller, Jeanine (1974). *The Vedas: Harmony, Meditation and Fulfilment.* London: Rider and Company.
Mishra, R. S. (1972). *The Textbook of Yoga Psychology.* London: Lyrebird Press.
Mlecko, Joel D. (1982). "The Guru in Hindu Tradition." *NUMEN: International Journal for the History of Religions* 29.1: 33–61.
Modi, P. M. (1932). *Akṣara: A Forgotten Chapter in the History of Indian Philosophy.* Baroda, India: Baroda State Press.
Monier-Williams, Sir M. (1899). A *Sanskrit-English Dictionary.* Oxford: Oxford University Press.
Mookerji, R. K., ed. (1951). *Ancient Indian Education.* London: Macmillan.
Mukerji, J. N. (1930). *Sāṃkhya: The Theory of Reality.* Calcutta: Jitendra Nath.
Müller, Max (1899). *The Six Systems of Indian Philosophy.* London: Longmans, Green and Co.
Nakamura, H. (1980–81). "Śaṅkara's Vivaraṇa on the Yogasūtra-Bhāṣya." *Adyar Library Bulletin* 44–45: 475–485.
Nicolás, Antonio T. de. (1976). *Avatāra: The Humanization of Philosophy through the Bhagavad Gītā.* New York: Nicolas Hays.
——— (1976). *Meditations Through the Ṛg Veda.* New York: Nicolas Hays.
———, trans. (1990). *The Bhagavad Gītā.* York Beach, Maine: Nicolas Hays.
Nikhilananda, Swami (1951). "Concentration and Meditation as Methods in Indian Philosophy." In *Essays in East-West Philosophy,* ed. C. A. Moore. Honolulu: University of Hawaii Press, pp. 89–102.

Oberhammer, Gerhard (1964). "Gott, Urbild der emanzipierten Existenz im Yoga des Patañjali." *Zeitschrift für Katholische Theologie* 86: 197–207.

——— (1965). "Meditation und Mystik im Yoga des Patañjali." *Wiener Zeitschrift für de Kunde Süd- und Ostasiens und Archiv für indische Philosophie* 9: 98–118.

——— (1977). *Strukturen Yogischer Meditation.* Vol. 13. Vienna: Verlag der Osterreichischen Academie der Wissenschaften.

O'Flaherty, Wendy Doniger, ed. (1980). *Karma and Rebirth in Classical Indian Traditions.* Berkeley: University of California Press.

Otto, Rudolf (1963). *The Idea of the Holy.* New York: Oxford University Press.

Pandeya, R. C. (1967). *Yuktidīpikā.* Delhi: Motilal Banarsidass.

Pandit, M. P. (1965). *The Kulārṇava Tantra.* Madras, India: Ganesh.

Panikkar, Raimundo (1977). *The Vedic Experience: Mantra-mañjarī.* Berkeley and Los Angeles: University of California Press.

Parrott, Rodney J. (1985). "The Experience Called 'Reason' in Classical Sāṃkhya." *Journal of Indian Philosophy* 13: 235–264.

Pensa, Corrado (1969). "On the Purification Concept in Indian Tradition, with Special Regard to Yoga." *East and West,* n.s., 19: 194–228.

——— (1973). "The Powers (Siddhis) in Yoga." *Yoga Quarterly Review* 5: 9–49.

——— (1980). Foreword to *The Philosophy of Classical Yoga,* by Georg Feuerstein. Manchester, England: Manchester University Press, pp. vi-viii.

Phillips, Stephen H. (1985). "The Conflict of Voluntarism and Dualism in the Yogasūtras." *Journal of Indian Philosophy* 13: 399–414.

Pines, S. and T. Gelblum (1966, 1977). "Al-Bīrūnīs Arabic Version of Patañjali's Yoga-Sūtra." *Bulletin of the School of Oriental and African Studies* 29: 302–325; 40: 522–549.

Potter, Karl H., ed. (1977). *Indian Metaphysics and Epistemology: The Tradition of Nyāya-Vaiśeṣika up to Gaṅgeśa.* Vol. 2 of *The Encyclopedia of Indian Philosophies.* Princeton, N.J.: Princeton University Press.

———, ed. (1983). *Bibliography of Indian Philosophies.* Rev. ed. Vol. 1 of *The Encyclopedia of Indian Philosophies.* Delhi: Motilal Banarsidass.

Prasad, Jwala (1930). "The Date of the Yoga-sūtras." *Journal of the Royal Asiatic Society* 84: 365–375.

——— (1956). *History of Indian Epistemology.* Delhi: Munshiram Manoharlal.

Prem, Sri Krishna (1948). *The Yoga of the Bhagavat Gita.* London: John M. Watkins.

Radhakrishnan, Sarvepalli (1951). *Indian Philosophy.* 2 vols. London: George Allen and Unwin.

Raju, P. T. (1985). *Structural Depths of Indian Thought.* Albany: State University of New York Press.

Rambachan, A. (1994). *The Limits of Scripture: Vivekananda's Reinterpretation of the Vedas.* Honolulu: University of Hawaii Press.

Rao, K. B. Ramakrishna (1966). *Theism of Pre-Classical Sāṃkhya.* Mysore, India: University of Mysore Press.

Ravindra, R. (1978). "Is Religion Psychotherapy?—An Indian View." *Religious Studies* 14: 389–397.

Ranganathananda, Swami (1982). "The Science of Consciousness in the Light of Vedānta and Yoga." *Prabuddha Bhārata,* June: 257–263.

Renou, Louis, ed. (1963). *Hinduism.* New York: Washington Square Press.

Rukmani, T. S. (1980). "Vikalpa as Defined by Vijñānabhikṣu in the Yogavarttika." *Journal of Indian Philosophy* 8.4: 385–392.
——— (1988). "Vijñānabhikṣu's Double Reflection Theory of Knowledge in the Yoga System." *Journal of Indian Philosophy* 16: 367–375.
——— (1992). "The Problem of the Authorship of the *Yogasūtrabhāṣyavivaraṇam.*" *Journal of Indian Philosophy* 20.4: 419–423.
Sahay, Mahajot (1964). "Pātañjala-Yogasūtras and the Vyāsa-Bhāṣya: An Examination." *Vishveshvaranand Indological Journal* 2: 254–260.
Saksena, S. K. (1944). *Nature of Consciousness in Hindu Philosophy.* Benares: Nand Kishore and Bros.
——— (1970). *Essays on Indian Philosophy.* Honolulu: University of Hawaii Press.
Sangharakshita, B. (1980). A *Survey of Buddhism.* Boulder, Colo: Shambhala.
Sanyal, J. M., trans. (1973). *The Srimad-Bhagavatam of Krishna-Dwaipayana Vyasa.* New Delhi: Munshiram Manoharlal.
Scharfstein, B.-A. (1974). *Mystical Experience.* Baltimore, Md.: Penguin Books.
Schubring, Walther (1962). *The Doctrine of the Jainas.* Trans. Wolfgang Beurlen. Delhi: Motilal Banarsidass.
Schumann, H. W. (1973). *Buddhism: An Outline of Its Teachings and Schools.* London: Rider and Co.
Sen, Sanat Kumar (1968). "Time in Sāṃkhya-Yoga." *International Philosophical Quarterly* 8: 406–426.
Senart, Émile (1900). "Bouddhisme et Yoga." *Revue de l'Histoire des Religions* 62 (November): 345–364.
——— (1915) "*Rajas* et la theorie indienne des trois *guṇa.*" *Journal asiatique* 11: 151ff.
Sen Gupta, Anima (1959). *Evolution of the Sāṃkhya School of Thought.* Lucknow, India: Pioneer Press.
——— (1969). *Classical Sāṃkhya: A Critical Study.* Patna, India: The University Press.
Sharma, Chandrahar (1960). *A Critical Survey of Indian Philosophy.* Varanasi: Motilal Banarsidass.
Sinari, R. A. (1965). "The Method of Phenomenological Reduction and Yoga." *Philosophy East and West* 15.3–4: 217–228.
——— (1984). *The Structure of Indian Thought.* First Indian edition. Delhi: Oxford University Press [first edition 1970].
Singh, Mohan (1959). "Yoga and Yoga Symbolism." *Symbolon: Jahrbuch für Symbolforschung* 2: 121–143.
Sinha, Jadunath (1952, 1956). *A History of Indian Philosophy.* 2 vols. Calcutta: Central Book Agency.
Smart, Ninian (1964). *Doctrine and Argument in Indian Philosophy.* London: George Allen and Unwin.
——— (1968). *The Yogi and the Devotee.* London: George Allen and Unwin.
Sovani, V. V. (1935). A *Critical Study of the Sāṃkhya System.* Poona Oriental Series no. 11. Poona: Oriental Book Agency.
Stace, W. T. (1961). *Mysticism and Philosophy.* London: Macmillan.
Stcherbatsky, Theodore (1923). *The Central Conception of Buddhism and the Meaning of the Word "Dharma."* London: Royal Asiatic Society.

——— (1965). *The Conception of Buddhist Nirvāṇa.* The Hague: Mouton and Co.

Sutherland, S., L. Houlden, P. Clarke and F. Hardy, eds. (1988). *The World's Religions.* London: Routledge.

Sykes, J. B., ed. (1976). *The Concise Oxford Dictionary of Current English.* 6th ed. Oxford: Clarendon Press.

Taber, John (1983). *Transformative Philosophy: A Study of Śaṅkara, Fichte and Heidegger.* Honolulu: University of Hawaii Press.

Takagi, S. Shingen (1966). "On 'Kriya-Yoga' in the Yoga-Sūtra." *Journal of Indian and Buddhist Studies* 15.1: 441-451.

Underhill, E. (1960). *Mysticism: A Study in the Nature and Development of Man's Spiritual Consciousness.* London: Methuen.

Varenne, Jean (1976). *Yoga and the Hindu Tradition.* Chicago: University of Chicago Press.

Vesci, Uma (1985). *Heat and Sacrifice in the Vedas.* Delhi: Motilal Banarsidass.

Vetter, T. (1989). "Zum ersten Kapital der Yogasūtras." *Weiner Zeitschrift für die Kunde Süd- und Ostasiens (Südasiens) und Archiv für indische Philosophie* 33: 159-176.

Vivekānanda, Swami (1977). *The Complete Works of Swami Vivekānanda.* 8 vols. Calcutta: Advaita Ashrama.

Welden, Ellwood Austin (1910). "The Sāṃkhya Term Liṅga." *American Journal of Philology* 31: 445-459.

——— (1914). "The Sāṃkhya Teachings in the Maitrī Upaniṣad." *American Journal of Philology* 35: 32-51.

Werner, K. (1977). *Yoga and Indian Philosophy.* Delhi: Motilal Banarsidass.

Wezler, A. (1974). "Some Observations on the Yuktidīpikā." *Deutscher Orientalistenag* 18: 434-455.

——— (1983). "Philological Observations on the So-Called Pātañjalayogasūtrabhāṣyavivaraṇa." *Indo-Iranian Journal* 25: 17-40.

——— (1984). "On the Quadruple Division of the Yogaśāstra, the Caturvyūhatva of the Cikitsāśāstra and the 'Four Noble Truths' of the Buddha." *Indologica Taurinensia* 12: 289-337.

Wheeler, M. (1968). *The Indus Civilisation.* 3rd ed. Cambridge: Cambridge University Press.

Whicher, Ian (1995). "Cessation and Integration in Classical Yoga." *Asian Philosophy* 5.1: 47-58; also in (1996) *Morals and Society in Asian Philosophy*, ed. Brian Carr (Richmond, U. K.: Curzon Press, pp. 92-108).

——— (1997). "Nirodha, Yoga Praxis and the Transformation of the Mind." *Journal of Indian Philosophy* 25.1: 1-67.

——— (1997). "The Mind *(Citta):* Its Nature, Structure and Functioning in Classical Yoga (1)." *Saṃbhāṣā (Nagoya Studies in Indian Culture and Buddhism)* 18: 35-62.

——— (1998). "The Mind *(Citta):* Its Nature, Structure and Functioning in Classical Yoga (2)" *Saṃbhāṣā (Nagoya Studies in Indian Culture and Buddhism)* 19: 1-50.

——— (1998). "Yoga and Freedom: A Reconsideration of Patañjali's Classical Yoga." *Philosophy East and West* 48.2: 272-322.

Williams, Paul (1989). *Mahāyāna Buddhism: The Doctrinal Foundations.* London: Routledge.

Wilson, H. H., trans. (1870). *The Vishnu Purana.* Vol. 5. London: Trubner and Co.
Winternitz, M. (1967). *History of Indian Literature.* Vol. 3. Delhi: Motilal Banarsidass.
Wood, E. (1962). *Yoga.* Harmondsworth, England: Penguin Books.
Zaehner, R. C. (1969). *The Bhagavad-Gītā.* Oxford: Oxford University Press.
——— (1974). *Our Savage God.* London: Collins.
Zigmund-Cerbu, A. (1963). "The Ṣaḍaṅgayoga." *Journal of the History of Religions* 3: 128–134.
Zimmer, Heinrich R. (1951). *Philosophies of India.* Edited by Joseph Campbell. Bolingen Series, 26. Princeton, N.J.: Princeton University Press.

INDEX

Abhimāna (pride/false identity), 67, 85, 142
Abhinavagupta, 27
Abhiniveśa. See Death, fear of; Desire, for continuity
Abhiṣeka (ritual empowerment), 35
See also Dīkṣā (initiation)
Abhyāsa (practice), 3, 17, 172-181, 186, 266, 272, 306
See also Practice, of Yoga
Abstinences, 190
Action(s) *(karma),* 97-105, 284
and bondage, 22-23, 97-98, 104
and *citta* (mind), 98-99, 100-103, 121
and classes of *karma* in classical Yoga, 103-104
Yoga *darśana* and, 4
fruits *(phala)* of one's, 97, 102, 285
*guṇa*s and, 97, 104
as improper *(vikarman),* 23, 24
and inaction *(akarman),* 23, 24
and *karmāśaya* (latent karmic residue), 98-100, 101, 102
mental, 22, 29-30, 97, 99-103
as meritorious *(puṇya)*/demeritorious *(apuṇya),* 98, 104
and morality, 23-24, 37, 75-76, 97, 99-100, 124-125, 312-313
naiṣkarmya-karma (ego-transcending action), 22, 24
nonafflicted, 3, 22, 32, 84, 121-130, 187-188, 284
rājasa-karman, 97
and renunciation, 22, 32, 103-104
ritual, 10, 15, 17, 28, 97
and *saṃskāra*s (impressions), 99-103, 110-111, 260-262
sāttvika-karman, 97, 124-125
Self and, 15
selfless/nonegoistic *(niṣkāma karma),* 23, 98, 104, 284
skill in, 29-30, 280
tāmasa-karman, 97
of worship, 10
of yogin, 103-104
See also Kriyā; Rajas; Saṃsāra
Adhikārin. See Disciple, qualified
Adhiṣṭhātṛtva (sovereignty), 106, 180, 262
Adhyāropa (superimposition), 132, 142, 171, 288
Adhyātma (inner self), 235-236, 249
Adhyātma-prasāda (clarity of the inner self), 235, 288
Adhyātma-yoga (Yoga of the inner self), 18
Advaita Vedānta, 55, 133, 297-298, 321, 330
See also Vedānta
Affliction(s) *(kleśa*s*),* 65
and *asmitā* (I-am-ness), 68-69, 70-71, 111, 112-115
and *citta* (mind), 98-99, 111-112, 121, 124-129, 167-170, 187-188
five types of, 111-115
importance of theory of, 111
and *karma* / *saṃskāra*s, 99-103, 110-111
and *nirodha,* 155-160, 166-172, 172-174
and practice/dispassion, 172-181
and *saṃsāra,* 111-115, 121
various states of, 205-206
and *vṛtti* (modification/functioning of mind), 110, 111-115, 172-181, 187-188, 198
yogic understanding of, 112-115, 195-199, 209-210, 259-260
See also Aversion *(dveṣa); Abhiniveśa; Asmitā;* Attachment; Ignorance; Nonaffliction *(akleśa)*
Āgama. See Testimony, valid
Agehananda Bharati, 6
Agni, 10
Ahaṃkāra (sense of self), 67, 77, 104, 332
ānanda-samādhi and, 238-243
asmitā (I-am-ness) and, 71, 241-242, 243
asmitā-mātra (mere I-am-ness) and, 66-72, 95-96
and *citta* (mind), 95-96
and Descartes' *cogito,* 91
and *rājasa-karman* (action), 97
sattvic, 239
senses and, 219
tamasic, 239
vicāra-samādhi and, 229-230